Sponsors

EPILEPSY ADVISORY COMMITTEE

Chairman
Richard D. Walter

Executive Secretary
J. Kiffin Penry

Milton Alter

Lillian R. Elveback

James R. Fouts

Brian B. Gallagher

Richard L. Masland

Dominick P. Purpura

Theodore Rasmussen

Ewart A. Swinyard

Donald B. Tower

Glenn E. Ullyot

NATIONAL INSTITUTE OF NEUROLOGICAL DISEASES AND STROKE

Director
Edward F. MacNichol, Jr.

AMERICAN EPILEPSY SOCIETY

President
Gian E. Chatrian

Secretary-Treasurer
B. J. Wilder

Experimental Models of Epilepsy —

A Manual for the

Laboratory Worker

Editors:

Dominick P. Purpura, M.D.
*Professor and Chairman of the
Department of Anatomy, and
Director of the
Rose F. Kennedy Center for Research in
Mental Retardation and Human Development,
Albert Einstein College of Medicine, New York City*

J. Kiffin Penry, M.D.
*Chief, Applied Neurologic Research Branch, and
Head, Section on Epilepsy,
Collaborative and Field Research,
National Institute of Neurological Diseases and
    Stroke,
National Institutes of Health
Bethesda, Maryland*

Donald B. Tower, M.D.
*Chief, Laboratory of Neurochemistry,
National Institute of Neurological Diseases and
    Stroke,
National Institutes of Health,
Bethesda, Maryland*

Dixon M. Woodbury, Ph.D.
*Professor and Head of Pharmacology,
University of Utah College of Medicine,
Salt Lake City, Utah*

Richard D. Walter, M.D.
*Professor, Department of Neurology,
University of California Medical Center,
Los Angeles, California*

Raven Press, Publishers • New York

Standard Book Number 0–911216–26–X
Library of Congress Catalog Card Number 72–181308

Dedicated to the memory of

Don W. Esplin
(1927–1971)

Don W. Esplin will best be remembered for his signal contributions to our understanding of the basic physiological mechanisms underlying the action of drugs in the central nervous system. His early work concerning the interaction of diphenylhydantoin and post-tetanic potentiation became a classic within his own lifetime and was among the considerations which led him to receive the John J. Abel Award of the American Society for Pharmacology and Experimental Therapeutics. It may be recalled that post-tetanic potentiation is a transient facilitation of synaptic efficacy occurring after strong repetitive stimuli. Don demonstrated that diphenylhydantoin had a specific action and reduced post-tetanic potentiation at doses which were without effect on other parameters of synaptic transmission or axonal conduction.

His fascination with the physiology of the nervous system led him to study the action of a variety of convulsant drugs on excitatory and inhibitory mechanisms, especially within the spinal cord. These experiments progressed and led logically to the development of his most recent contributions.

The summer before his untimely death in December 1971 saw the publication of a series of experiments in which he and Barbara Zablocka-Esplin, his wife and collaborator, were involved for a period of almost five years. These fundamental studies dealt with the kinetics of neurohumoral transmission associated with synaptic mechanisms in the spinal cord and were published in a single issue of the *Journal of Neurophysiology*.

Don left a rich legacy for generations of neuropharmacologists to come, which can easily be found in his publications. Despite his sophistication of thought and the clarity of his writing, his published works will serve to remind us that we have been deprived of the opportunity to know Don, a unique experience that at the same time challenged and provoked.

The breadth and sensitivity of his viewpoint and perspective was best expressed by Don himself in a passage from the fourth edition of *The*

Pharmacological Basis of Therapeutics, the classic textbook edited by
Louis S. Goodman and Alfred Gilman:

"The complexity of the CNS, as compared to other organs and systems
of the body, humbles all who study it. Despite remarkable advances in
neuropharmacology, the dearth of definitive information on the mechanisms
by which specific drugs affect neuronal functions necessitates a considerable
degree of empiricism in the therapeutic approach to both organic and functional diseases of the nervous system. Schemes purporting to show precisely how a drug acts to restore neuronal dysfunction, whether in scientific
or promotional literature, must be regarded with considerable skepticism.

"The problem of understanding the anatomical and functional complexities of the human nervous system poses the ultimate challenge for the
mind of man. Progress in discovering and creating chemicals to ameliorate
the undesirable consequences of functional and organic disturbances of the
nervous system is steady but also marked by frequent reverses. While no
limit should be placed upon our ultimate expectations, the problems of inadequate drug efficacy, drug toxicity, multiple actions of drugs, and side
effects of drugs will plague therapeutics for a considerable time to come."

Perhaps longer, lacking his illumination . . .

lawrence m. halpern

Preface

No disorder of brain function has revealed more about the organization of the human brain and behavior than that subsumed under the term epilepsy. And none has been the subject of more intense experimental inquiry. Epileptic manifestations are unique among the various disturbances of brain function in providing the neurobiologist with a wealth of opportunities to examine the intimate neuronal mechanisms underlying a major health problem. At the same time, studies of convulsant activities provide fruitful approaches to the analyses of neuronal structure and function and of biochemical, genetic, and environmental factors contributing to normal and abnormal neuronal synchronization processes. It is little wonder then that the search for knowledge concerning the basic mechanisms of the epilepsies has been so closely related to the historical development of neurobiological research in general. From the most fundamental investigations concerning the elementary properties of neurons and glia have come new clues to the mechanisms of epilepsy, and vice versa.

Recognition of the foregoing relationship between experimental epilepsy and neurobiological research might be considered sufficient justification in itself for the attempt made in this volume to call attention to the various experimental models of epilepsy that have contributed to our understanding of normal and abnormal neuronal functions at different levels of organizational complexity. To be sure, this was an overriding motivation. But the purpose here goes somewhat beyond this in the intent of the editors and contributors to make available to the laboratory worker a manual of experimental models that is as critical in approach as detailed in methodology. Too often the description of methods and materials employed in producing a particular experimental model of epilepsy has been lost or poorly detailed in the original account of the model. Subsequent reports of the series generated from individual laboratories generally contribute little further information on methodologies. How often the inquiring reader has been frustrated by the statement—"methods similar to those used previously were employed in the present investigation" . . . only to find the previously mentioned investigation similarly described! Nor has it been customary for proponents of a particular experimental model of epilepsy to indicate the limitations and disadvantages of their model. And how many times does the reader learn about the failures to produce a particular model in the hands of its proponent? From these brief introductory remarks it will be appreciated that each of the contributors to the manual was requested to develop a chapter that would provide the young investigator interested in experimental epilepsy with sufficient information to reproduce the model or to become better aware of its complexities. To the extent that the laboratory worker is made aware of the problem of reproducing and perfecting the various models described here, so will the success of this volume be judged. Beyond this is the expectation that the young investigator attracted to the field of experimental epilepsy will discover additional approaches sufficiently valuable to warrant major new departures in the quest for experimental models of epilepsy. Hopefully, such approaches will emerge from the wide variety of experimental models described in this volume, many of which have a direct bearing on the problems of human epilepsy.

The limitations of space and the publication schedule imposed practical requirements in the scope of the material, and any deficiencies thereof may be credited to the editors. The material included, however, represents the conceptions and judgments of the individual authors and does not necessarily reflect the views and opinions of the editors and the sponsors.

The Editors

Contents

Contributors

Robert L. Collins
The Jackson Laboratory
Bar Harbor, Maine 04609

Stanley M. Crain
Department of Physiology
Albert Einstein College of Medicine
Yeshiva University
Bronx, New York 10461

David R. Curtis
John Curtin School of Medical Research
Australian National University
P.O. Box 334
Canberra City, A.C.T. 2601, Australia

Don W. Esplin
Department of Pharmacology and
*   Therapeutics*
McGill University
Montreal, Quebec, Canada

Carl F. Essig
National Institute of Mental Health
* Clinical Research Center*
Lexington, Kentucky 40507

Gilbert H. Glaser
Department of Neurology
Yale University School of Medicine
New Haven, Connecticut 06510

Lawrence M. Halpern
Department of Pharmacology
University of Washington School of
*   Medicine*
Seattle, Washington 98105

Herbert H. Jasper
Université de Montreal
Case Postale 6128
Montreal 101, Quebec, Canada

Aristides A. P. Leão
Institute of Biophysics
Federal University of Rio de Janeiro
Rio de Janeiro, Brazil

Edward Lewin
Division of Neurology
University of Colorado Medical Center
Denver, Colorado 80220

Elliott M. Marcus
Department of Neurology
Tufts University School of Medicine
Boston, Mass. 02111

C. Ajmone Marsan
Branch of Electroencephalography
* and Clinical Neurophysiology*
National Institute of Neurological
* Diseases and Stroke*
National Institutes of Health
Bethesda, Maryland 20014

Henry McIlwain
Department of Biochemistry
Institute of Psychiatry
De Crespigny Park
London, SE5 8AF, England

B. S. Meldrum
Départment de Neurophysiologie
  Appliquée
Institut de Neurophysiologie et de
  Psychophysiologie
C.N.R.S.
31, Chemin J. Aiguier
13 — Marseilles, 9 éme, France

R. Naquet
Départment de Neurophysiologie
  Appliquée
Institut de Neurophysiologie et de
  Psychophysiologie
C.N.R.S.
31, Chemin J. Aiguier
13 — Marseilles, 9 éme, France

David A. Prince
Department of Neurology
Stanford University Medical Center
Stanford, California 94305

Dominick P. Purpura
Department of Anatomy
Albert Einstein College of Medicine
Yeshiva University
Bronx, New York 10461

Z. Servít
Institute of Physiology
Czechoslovak Academy of Sciences
Prague, Czechoslovakia

William E. Stone
Department of Physiology

University of Wisconsin Medical
  School
Madison, Wisconsin 53706

Ewart A. Swinyard
Departments of Pharmacology
College of Pharmacology, and
  College of Medicine
University of Utah
Salt Lake City, Utah 84112

Arthur A. Ward, Jr.
Department of Neurological Surgery
University of Washington School of
  Medicine
Seattle, Washington 98105

B. J. Wilder
Department of Medicine
Veterans Administration Hospital and
  University of Florida College of
  Medicine
Gainesville, Florida 32601

C. D. Withrow
Department of Pharmacology
University of Utah College of
  Medicine
Salt Lake City, Utah 84112

J. D. Wood
Department of Biochemistry
University of Saskatchewan
Saskatoon, Saskatchewan, Canada
  57N OWO

Dixon M. Woodbury
Department of Pharmacology
University of Utah College of
  Medicine
Salt Lake City, Utah 84112

1

Topical Convulsant Metals

Arthur A. Ward, Jr.

OUTLINE

I. INTRODUCTION

Because of narrative clinical reports that allergic hypersensitivity might play a role in certain convulsive disorders in man coupled with experimental reports that the production of an Arthus reaction in the cortex would induce seizures, Kopeloff et al. (1942) undertook a systematic study of this problem. By immunologic means, they showed that seizures could be induced but that an enduring state of convulsive reactivity was not produced. Since it was well known that alum-precipitated proteins are particularly effective in the production of antibodies, they then undertook experiments utilizing alum-precipitated egg white applied to the cortex of monkeys. In the initial four rhesus monkeys, Jacksonian seizures were observed some 4 to 9 weeks after the operation, and such epileptiform attacks could be elicited intermittently over a period of many months. In analyzing the variables involved, it became clear that alumina cream alone applied to one hemisphere was responsible for the recurrent, generalized, convulsive seizures in these animals.

In the intervening 30 years, Lenore and Nicholas Kopeloff have extensively exploited their initial serendipitous observations and, more recently in collaboration with Joseph Chusid, have provided us with a large body of knowledge regarding this unique model of the epileptic process. Up to the present time, no other technique has been developed by which chronic, recurrent, spontaneous convulsive seizures can be induced in experimental animals. Since the history of science clearly indicates that insight into natural phenomena is so often dependent on the availability of suitable experimental models which can be analytically studied, it is appropriate that those of us working on the neurobiology of epilepsy recognize our debt to the Kopeloffs.

In addition to the alumina cream technique, the action of other metallic compounds has been studied. In 1960, Kopeloff reported that the implantation of cobalt into the cortex of the mouse would induce seizures for a period of time and these studies have been extended to other species by other investigators. Also in 1960, Blum and Liban reported that the intracerebral injection of tungstic acid gel would induce recurrent seizures which again were of limited duration. The potential epileptogenicity of pure metals implanted in the motor cortex of the monkey has been investigated by Chusid and Kopeloff (1962) in some detail. Although they were unable to induce clinical seizures in the monkey by the intracortical implantation of pellets of cobalt, they did observe occasional spontaneous clinical seizures, which recurred for 1 to 6 months, following the intracortical implantation of the pure metals, antimony and nickel, both of which produced a severe, necrotizing lesion. Subclinical EEG foci were induced by implantation of aluminum, bismuth, cadmium, iron, mercury, molybdenum, tantalum, titanium, tin, tungsten, vanadium, and zirconium. In these instances, seizures could often be precipitated by activation with pentylenetetrazol or picrotoxin for periods of 6 to 18 months after implantation. Neither spontaneous nor induced seizures were produced by beryllium, chromium, cobalt, copper, gold, lead, magnesium, manganese, silicon, silver, or zinc. Thus it is possible that further studies utilizing various forms of the first group of metallic compounds listed above might be rewarding.

This discussion will deal at some length with the alumina cream technique since this is the only experimental preparation which exhibits spontaneous seizures of focal onset occurring recurrently over a period of months and years. The discussion will then deal with the cobalt and the tungstic acid gel techniques which induce seizures for relatively short periods of time.

II. ALUMINA CREAM METHOD

A. Technique

The original preparation utilized by the Kopeloffs consists of a precipitate of alumina cream produced by treating ammonium alum at room temperature with dilute ammonium hydroxide. Commercial aluminum oxide powder washed with saline, autoclaved, and used as a moist sediment has also proved to be effective. However, we and others have found it most convenient to utilize commercially available aluminum hydroxide gel, one form of which (Amphojel) is equivalent to 4% aluminum oxide and consists of a mixture of two forms of gel, one of which is said to be antacid and the other a demulcent gel. It should be noted that some commercial preparations contain other therapeutically active compounds in addition to the aluminum hydroxide.

It appears that the essential condition is that the alumina cream come in contact with a volume of neurons in the CNS containing cell bodies and dendrites. Thus, in the cerebral cortex, it may be placed in the subarachnoid space or injected intracortically. There is no evidence to indicate that seizures can be induced if the alumina is restricted to white matter.

In the original report of Kopeloff et al. (1942), the alumina cream was applied to the precentral cortex in a hollow, circular disc of laminated linen of fiber. These discs were tooled on a lathe to an outside diameter of 16 mm, inside diameter of 13 mm, height 2.5 mm, inside depth 1.5 mm, and a capacity of approximately 0.2 ml. The discs were autoclaved and filled aseptically with the alumina. Sterile operations were performed exposing the dura overlying the desired cortical region, the dura incised, and the disc filled with alumina slipped beneath the dura against the brain. The overlying dura was then sutured and the wound closed.

We subsequently modified the technique by introducing the compound into the cortical grey matter by injection and this modification was reported at about the same time by Kopeloff et al. (1955). In our laboratories, the monkey is anesthetized (see Halpern, Chapter 8), and under aseptic conditions the sensorimotor cortex is exposed by trephining the bone and incising the dura in a partial circle. At four points in the pre- and postcentral gyri, autoclaved aluminum hydroxide gel is injected into the cortex with a small syringe and 27-gauge hypodermic needle to produce a minimally detectable bolus at each puncture site. Great care is taken to prevent spillage of the alumina onto the pial surface, and a layer of absorbable gelatin film is placed between the cortex and overlying dura as well as between the dura and overlying bone disc to minimize scarring and to thereby facilitate atraumatic subsequent exposure at the time of acute experiment or at autopsy. In such monkeys, spontaneous clinical seizures appear after a variable delay, usually 35 to 60 days. The frequency of the seizures is roughly proportional to the degree of cortical pathology induced. If a larger number of focal, punctate injections of alumina are performed, the seizures, once they occur, may increase in frequency to status epilepticus. Aggressive treatment with anticonvulsants is then necessary to maintain a viable preparation.

Differential epileptogenicity within the CNS

There is a large body of evidence obtained from studies of acute seizure phenomena in animals induced by topical convulsant drugs or electrical stimulation (French et al., 1956) as well as from clinical experience in human epilepsy that indicates that seizure activity is more easily induced in certain specific parts of the nervous system. This also appears to be true of the chronic epileptic process induced in animals by alumina cream.

The sensorimotor cortex is one of these susceptible regions and most of the studies of alumina foci have involved this cortical region, particularly in the monkey (Kopeloff et al., 1942, 1954, 1955; Ward et al., 1948; Ward, 1969). Although the differential susceptibility of precentral versus postcentral gyrus has not been systematically examined, it is our feeling that injections into postcentral gyrus produce a higher yield of monkeys with spontaneous seizures as compared to those with foci restricted to precentral gyrus alone. Foci involving both pre- and postcentral gyri may be more epileptogenic than either alone. This cortical region is also somewhat epileptogenic in the cat in which spontaneous clinical seizures can be induced (Mayman et al., 1965; Schmalbach, 1970), although less easily than in the monkey. Intracortical injections in this region in the dog induce a focus where seizures have been reported during barbiturate withdrawal (Essig, 1962), whereas similar foci in rats nonsusceptible to audiogenic seizures result in the occurrence of audiogenic seizures in one-third of the animals (Servit and Sterc, 1958).

Epileptogenic foci in the temporal lobe can also be induced with alumina cream. Injections in the anterior portion of the temporal lobe in the monkey and cat are said to induce either motor seizures or "psychomotor fits" (Youmans, 1956); injections into the amygdala can induce clinical seizures characterized by automatisms (Sloan et al., 1953). Stereotactic implantation of alumina cream in the amygdaloid complex of the cat has been reported to induce behavioral seizures in more than one-half of the animals while "grand mal" fits were observed in one-half of the animals (Gastaut et al., 1959; Naquet et al., 1960). Seizures resembling psychomotor seizures have also been reported from similar foci in the dog (Aida, 1956).

Other regions of cerebral cortex appear to be less susceptible. Only in the monkey have chronic recurring clinical seizures been reported from foci elsewhere than in sensorimotor cortex. Although epileptogenic foci have been induced in parietal (Chusid et al., 1955) and in preoccipital cortex (Chow and Obrist, 1955), it is of interest that in both instances the clinical seizures were motor seizures. Although negative data are infrequently reported, it appears that it is difficult to induce spontaneous seizures with alumina applied to cortical regions other than sensorimotor cortex, even in the monkey.

Kopeloff et al. (1950) have observed that in the monkey, injection of alumina cream (0.1 to 0.2 ml) into thalamus, putamen (bilateral), subcallosal fasciculus, and white matter adjacent to the cingulate gyrus induced recurrent convulsive seizures similar to those induced from the motor cortex. No seizures were observed after injection into the lateral nuclear groups of thalamus, hypothalamus, tegmentum of pons and decussation of the brachium conjunctivum, caudate, or putamen (unilateral). Faeth and Walker (1957) also observed no spontaneous clinical seizures after injection of alumina into the basal ganglia in the monkey.

A few random reports have dealt with other types of clinical seizures. Shirao (1969) injected alumina into the substantia nigra in cats and observed myoclonic seizures in two animals of the series studied. Guerrero-Figueroa et al. (1963*b*) implanted alumina into the intralaminar nuclei and reticular formation in kittens and adult cats. In kittens, they observed bursts of 3/sec spike-and-wave discharges and "absence" behavior; older cats did not develop these patterns. No statement is made as to how long the "absence" attacks persisted. This seems to be the only report of the production of an experimental model of "petit mal" seizures in the experimental animal by alumina cream.

Finally, Kennard (1950*a*, *b*, 1953) has shown that neuronal hyperactivity can be induced in the spinal cord by the intramedullary injection of alumina cream into the cord or instillation of this compound into the subarachnoid space over the cord. Since such neuronal hyperactivity involves sensory systems, the clinical expression of the process includes hyperalgesia, hyperesthesia, and spontaneous episodes of pain (Kennard, 1953; Dyken, 1964). The hyperactive neurons in such spinal foci exhibit many of the physiological properties of epileptic neurons in cortical foci induced with alumina (Loeser, 1971).

There have been no reports of the consequences of alumina applied to cerebellum. However, it is assumed that it is not possible to induce an epileptogenic focus in the cerebellum and that, in fact, activation of Purkinje neurons may well inhibit generalized seizures or seizures of cortical origin.

C. Role of age

The factor of age does not appear to have been systematically investigated in any of the models of epilepsy induced by alumina in the monkey. It is our impression that foci in the sensorimotor cortex of the monkey are induced with greater ease in younger adolescents than in the older or mature animals. The induction of "absence" seizures in kittens is heavily dependent on the age of the animal (Guerrero-Figueroa et al., 1963*b*). After alumina implantation into intralaminar nuclei and reticular formation, young kittens developed the 3/sec pattern as early as 18 hr, whereas the latency was as long as 12 days in animals at the upper limit of the age group (near 30 days). The spike-and-wave pattern did not develop in animals older than 30 days.

D. Species differences

The occurrence of spontaneous seizures arising from a focus in the cerebral cortex appears to be unusual in any species below the primate. This generalization appears also to be true of cortical foci induced by alumina. Although at one time it was felt that the intracortical injection of alumina into any portion of cortex might induce electrographic abnormalities but would not result in spontaneous clinical seizures in subprimates, seizures arising from alumina-induced cortical foci have been reported in the cat by Mayman et al. (1965) and Schmalbach (1970). However, it would appear that such clinically effective foci are induced with some difficulty, even in the sensorimotor cortex, and the yield is low for preparations exhibiting long-lasting, spontaneous seizures. There are no reports of spontaneous seizures induced by intracortical alumina in lower forms. Servit and Sterc (1958) did succeed in converting some rats nonsusceptible to audiogenic seizures into animals now susceptible to audiogenic seizures by local application of alumina to cortex. The induction of cortical epileptogenic foci generating spontaneous seizures appears to be unrewarding in animals other than primates although such seizures can be induced with some difficulty in the cat. In the monkey, however, cortical epileptogenic foci can be induced with relative ease and a large body of knowledge has been generated dealing with various features of the epileptic process utilizing the alumina focus in the cortex of the monkey as the experimental preparation (see Kopeloff et al., 1954; Ward, 1969).

The induction of epileptic foci in subcortical nuclei, however, has been reported not only in monkeys but in a variety of subprimate species. There appears to have been no systematic study of species susceptibility but the majority of reports have utilized the cat, possibly more for reasons of economy and convenience than because of greater seizure susceptibility of subcortical structures in this species.

E. Natural history and clinical phenomenology

After the operation for the intracerebral injection of the alumina cream into the sensorimotor cortex of the rhesus monkey, no clinical changes are noted in the immediate postoperative period. Spontaneous clinical seizures appear after a variable delay, usually 35 to 60 days. If a more intense epileptogenic focus has been induced by many intracortical injections of alumina, the clinical manifestations may appear in 2 to 3 weeks; conversely, if a limited alumina focus has been induced, the first clinical seizure may not be observed for as long as 6 to 8 months. EEG examination reveals abnormalities in the form of spikes or sharp wave activity prior to overt epilepsy.

The clinical pattern of seizures is characteristic of the location of the scar as in human epilepsy of focal onset. Since the most accessible portion of the sensorimotor cortex contains the cortical representation for contralateral face and arm, the seizures in such animals usually begin with focal twitching in contralateral face or hand. These commonly progress by Jacksonian spread to involve the musculature of the entire contralateral side and become generalized. When a relatively intense epileptogenic focus has been induced, the clinical manifestations may include what appears to be the simian counterpart of human epilepsia partialis continua in which the contralateral hand and forearm is almost continuously engaged in short, myoclonic-like jerks recurring at frequencies ranging from greater than 1/sec to 1/10 sec. Such preparations can often be precipitated into major seizures with relatively minor stress or excitement with the development of the usual propagating pattern of seizure activity. As in human seizures of focal cortical onset, the initial onset of a clinical seizure in the monkey consists of synchronous movements of the contralateral face or hand which increase in intensity and frequency in those muscles as well as spreading to adjacent muscle groups. As the frequency increases, the muscular contractions almost fuse into a "tonic" contraction during the height of the seizure. This "tonic" phase of the clinical fit may last for 30 sec to several minutes. During this phase, strong generalized jerks are superimposed and some cyanosis and excess salivation may be evident. The muscular contractions then abruptly cease throughout the entire body. In some animals there is a linear relationship between the severity of the seizure and the duration as noted in Fig. 1 (right side; monkey #803) whereas in others this is not the case (Lockard and Barensten, 1967). Postictally, the monkey is relatively hypotonic, nonresponsive to external stimuli, and often hyperventilates. In some animals there is prompt recovery but in others there is a prolonged period of postictal stupor.

The seizures occur spontaneously, and the frequency is roughly proportional to the degree of cortical pathology induced. If a relatively large epileptic focus is induced, the seizures, once they occur, may gradually increase in frequency to status epilepticus; aggressive treatment with anticonvulsant drugs is then necessary to maintain a viable preparation. In the majority of animals, once the seizures are established, they recur spontaneously, presumably for the life-span of the animal since a relatively constant pattern of seizure frequency has been observed in such monkeys for at least 7 years (Kopeloff et al., 1954; Ward, 1969).

F. Precipitating factors

As observed by Kopeloff et al. (1964), it has been a common observation by all investigators working with this monkey model that seizures may be precipitated by such stress stimuli as severe noisy prodding for a minute or so, or attempting to catch the animal. This has been confirmed by objec-

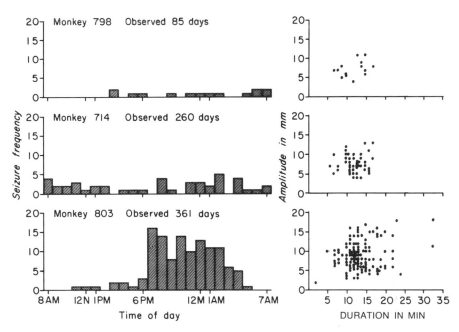

FIG. 1.   Clinical seizure frequency of epileptic monkeys as a function of time-of-day (*left*), and the severity vs. duration of clinical seizures (*right*).   From Lockard and Barensten (1967) with permission of the publisher.

tive behavioral studies undertaken by Lockard and Barensten (1967). Monkeys with chronic, alumina-induced epilepsy were housed in primate restraining chairs instrumented with displacement transducers.   The transducers were connected to a multichannel polygraph operating continuously at low speed.   The activity transducer output also triggered an electronic control gate which recognizes the signature of gross motor seizures (Barensten and Lockard, 1969).   This device activates a video-tape recorder which gives unattended, 24-hr clinical verification of the seizures.   In this fashion, every clinical seizure can be recorded and the clinical pattern visually validated.   During a year of such continuous recording, one monkey was given periods of avoidance conditioning for approximately 2 hr per day for 2 weeks at a time utilizing a schedule previously developed for another study of behavioral stress.   The seizure frequency of this monkey during the weeks of avoidance conditioning was as much as 2.25 times its seizure frequency during comparable control weeks.

Such behavioral studies (Lockard and Barensten, 1967) have also indicated that the seizures in some monkeys have a pronounced diurnal variation.   When all seizures are recorded, the examples in Fig. 1 (left side) indicate that the frequency graphs for monkeys 798 and 803 reveal two possibly related trends. First, for each subject, seizures repeatedly occurred during the quietest period of the day, i.e., what would normally be night for these animals. Although it is not obvious from the frequency graph, these trends may also hold for subject 714 as many of its morning seizures seemed to be precipitated by the maintenance activities of the animal technician which occurred only at this time.

In certain female monkeys, the seizures tend to cluster around the time of estrus. In some preparations, the monkey appears to be able to abort focal seizures in the hand by voluntary movement of that member; in other animals, spontaneous seizures are strikingly absent during the fixed daily feeding period (Halpern and Ward, 1969).

The occurrence of nocturnal seizures in some animals and the relation to estrus in certain female epileptic monkeys is variable and unpredictable. The factors involved are unknown as they are in the many human examples of the same phenomena. However, the role of stress in precipitating seizures appears to apply in varying degree in all animals. In those having frequent seizures, the susceptibility to stress appears to be high; in those with relatively infrequent attacks, the role of stress in precipitating seizures may be less apparent.

The convulsive threshold to rapid intravenous injection of pentylenetetrazol (Metrazol ®) is significantly lower (2.8 to 6.3 mg/kg) in epileptic monkeys than in a control group of normal monkeys (8.5 to 29 mg/kg) as reported by Kopeloff et al. (1954); this is also true for other drugs (Kopeloff et al., 1957). Furthermore, many observers have noted that intramuscular injections of pentylenetetrazol (9 to 25 mg/kg) will induce clinical seizures in monkeys with foci which may be electrographically active but which do not spontaneously generate clinical seizures. Such drug precipitation will often induce seizures in monkeys with foci in relatively nonepileptogenic cortex not exhibiting spontaneous attacks, and may precipitate attacks in cats and lower species in which alumina foci have been induced which also do not generate spontaneous fits. However, since this drug will induce seizures in all mammals in appropriate doses, ambiguity inevitably arises when seizures are so induced in animals with alumina foci who are otherwise seizure-free.

Although the precipitation of seizures by sensory stimuli has not been reported for cortical alumina foci in any species, Guerrero-Figueroa et al. (1963a) have reported the inhibitory effect of certain types of sensory stimuli on the 3/sec spike-and-wave induced in kitten by alumina injection into nonspecific thalamic nuclei and also point out that the paroxysmal discharges in these animals can be evoked by photic and acoustic stimuli.

G. Properties of alumina focus in cortex

In monkeys exhibiting spontaneous clinical seizures some months after the intracortical injection of alumina, the epileptogenic focus is characterized by the occurrence of epileptic spikes when recording the gross electrical activity from either the exposed brain or scalp. When recording from the pial surface, the focal interictal spiking is often localized at one edge of the area of alumina injection. The activity of single neurons in this focus is characterized by a variety of patterns of neuronal hyperactivity. In the unanesthetized monkey, the most common pattern consists of recurrent bursts of high-frequency discharge such as seen in Fig. 2. Here the bursts

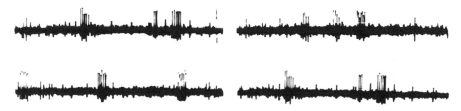

FIG. 2. Extraneuronal microelectrode recording of spontaneous discharges of neurons in focus of awake, epileptic monkey. Bursts are not stereotyped and show no special features of timing.

are seen to be unstructured and are not stereotyped. Often at the center of the focus one can record regular, repetitive bursts which may be remarkably constant in number and temporal relationships and in which the firing pattern has an unusual structure (Calvin et al., 1968). The distinguishing feature is an unusually long interval between the first and second spikes of these epileptic bursts, with the later spikes of the burst time-locked to the second spike as seen in Fig. 3. Under other experimental conditions involving acute experiments, the use of paralyzing drugs, and direct cortical exposure, the patterns of firing may be characterized by tonic discharge, waxing and waning in frequency, or irregular bursts of high-frequency firing (Ward, 1969). These properties of epileptic cells in the alumina focus do not appear to be peculiar to cortical neurons. After alumina injection into the dorsal horn of the spinal cord, patterns of abnormal hyperactivity can also be recorded which may be indistinguishable from those recorded in cortex as seen in Fig. 4. Both high-frequency bursts and prolonged trains of tonic discharge may be recorded during acute experiments many months

cell 6

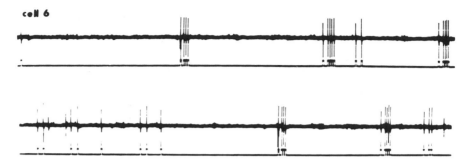

FIG. 3. Spontaneous burst firing of neuron in epileptic focus of awake monkey. Bursts are characterized by a long first interval between the first spike and the after-burst. (Bottom trace is a pulse triggered by each discharge for purposes of computer analysis.)

after the alumina implantation (J. D. Loeser, *unpublished observations*).

Histologically, the injection sites contain well-circumscribed deposits of alumina which are bordered by astrocytic gliosis and acellular areas (Sterova, 1966). In the adjacent electrographic focus, there is an overall decrease in neuronal elements and an increase in glial forms (Ward et al., 1948). The neurons remaining have distinct morphological alterations specifically related to the dendrites consisting of less dendritic branching, and the dendritic shafts are almost completely divested of their normal

139 DAYS L–5 ALUMINA INJECTION DORSAL HORN

A

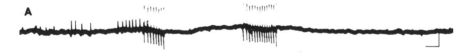

B

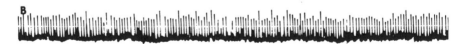

FIG. 4. Spontaneous discharges of neurons in cord near site of alumina injection. *A:* Burst firing just caudal to spinal focus. *B:* Tonic firing just rostral to focus. (Loeser, *unpublished observations.*)

dendritic spines (Westrum et al., 1965). These latter changes appear to be peculiar to the electrographic focus and not to other parts of the cortical scar.

There has been no systematic attempt to compare the properties of the alumina focus with other experimental models of the epileptic process. The obvious and cardinal distinguishing feature is that although the application of topical convulsant drugs or electrical stimulation can induce acute seizures, the alumina focus appears to be the only model of chronic, spontaneous clinical seizures. From an electrographic standpoint, many of the properties of the actual propagating seizure can be reproduced by other techniques. However, the interictal phenomena may be more unique. Although burst firing of cortical neurons can be induced by topical convulsants such as penicillin (Prince, 1968), this and other models do not reproduce the long-first-interval burst firing characteristic of cells in the primary alumina focus. In addition, a constant relationship between the slow wave or EEG spike and the unit burst firing is characteristic of seizure activity induced by certain convulsant drugs. At the alumina focus, such a relationship between surface EEG and unit firing is often lacking although the local field potential recorded by an extracellular microelectrode may show a variable correlation to the burst firing. Finally, topical cooling of normal cerebral cortex induces a sequence of changes in neuronal firing patterns. Similar cooling of tungstic acid and strychnine foci induce the same sequence of events as noted in normal cortex. In contrast, topical cooling of alumina foci precipitates seizure activity with small drops of intracortical temperature and the sequence of changes is both qualitatively and quantitatively different from those seen in normal cortex or in foci induced by other techniques (J. Moseley, G. Ojemann, and A. A. Ward, Jr., *in preparation*). This would be consistent with the reported changes in ATPase activity which are different in alumina foci as compared to other experimental models (Harmony et al., 1968).

H. Validation of the alumina model

A model is useful to the extent that it is an accurate surrogate for the natural phenomenon. It is therefore relevant to compare this model in the monkey to epilepsy in the human.

Morphologically, the neuronal depopulation and astrocytic gliosis at the focus is the same as that seen in human cortical scars. More importantly, the alterations in dendritic morphology seen in the Golgi impregnation of monkey foci can be seen at the maximal electrographic focus in man. Physiologically, the high-frequency burst firing, including the unusual structuring of the burst characterized by the long first interval, is common to the focus in both monkey and man.

In both the monkey model and man, the seizures appear some months after the cortical insult and, once established, may persist indefinitely. In both, the seizures may be more frequent at certain times of the day or night in some instances; in the female, the seizures may cluster around the time of menstruation. Although seizures may be more frequent during periods of stress in the human, the response to stress may be more obvious in the monkey.

Those anticonvulsant drugs which are effective in humans with seizures of cortical onset are also effective in monkeys with cortical foci.

It would thus appear that when it has been possible to test a specific property of the monkey model against the phenomenon in man, confirmation has been obtained.

I. Research potential of the model

The chronic epileptogenic focus in the cortex of the monkey provides an experimental preparation where the substrate of the epileptic process may be examined by any discipline in the neurosciences. The morphology of the focus can be studied and a variety of electrophysiological studies of neuronal membrane, the firing properties of epileptic neurons, local synaptic interactions, and neuron-glia interactions can be studied (Ward, 1969; Prince and Futamachi, 1970). The chronicity of the epileptic process permits studies of the poorly understood phenomenon of the mirror focus (Wada and Cornelius, 1960; Guerrero-Figueroa et al., 1964). The neurochemistry of the focus can be studied (Tower, 1969; Harmony et al., 1968); and a variety of behavioral studies of the effects of the local interictal epileptic process on brain function can also be studied (Chow and Obrist, 1954; Stamm and Pribram, 1960; Stamm and Warren, 1961; Driver et al., 1968). Finally, this chronic model of epilepsy, having a relatively stable frequency of seizures, provides an unusual test bed for testing anticonvulsant drugs (Berman et al., 1968); Lockard, *unpublished observations*). Such studies can also be extended to investigate the interaction between anticonvulsant drug therapy and the underlying epileptic process since Servit (1960) has reported the prophylactic effects of anticonvulsant drugs in reducing the incidence of seizures subsequent to the induction of epileptic foci. The use of this model to validate new forms of therapy is not limited to pharmacological studies since the model can also be used to investigate the therapeutic effectiveness of new types of surgical therapy including the stereotactic production of lesions in subcortical relays that may be essential for the precipitation or propagation of seizures.

J. Critique

The process which is broadly called epilepsy in the human (when it arises in cortex) can be roughly subdivided into the events which transpire at the focus responsible for the interictal activity, the processes by which such activity is precipitated into a propagating seizure, and the mechanisms of propagation into a clinically evident seizure. The clinical seizure is the dramatic event and often the word "epilepsy" becomes synonymous with the clinical fit. However, these occur at relatively rare intervals and are only a consequence of the sequence of processes which precede them. In cortical epilepsy, at least, the clinical seizure does not occur if there is no epileptogenic focus—and it is the interictal activity at the focus whose understanding is fundamental to a solution of the problem.

In this setting, it would appear that the alumina cream model presents the best opportunities for studying these processes underlying the epileptic focus. In contrast, it may present few unique opportunities for studying the processes involved in the actual propagating, clinical seizure where other models may be equally good surrogates for nature and have the additional advantages of economy, rapid induction, ease of manipulation and control of variables. Finally, since there is a long delay between the induction of the alumina focus and the appearance of clinical seizures, the model is poorly suited to experiments where the acute production of seizures is the goal.

The seizures induced in the alumina model are spontaneous and recurrent for indefinite periods and thus the model best lends itself to studies where these properties are essential to the experimental design. The best model of human epilepsy is obviously human epilepsy itself. The alumina epileptic monkey appears to share many of the characteristics of epilepsy with the human and also shares many of the inconveniences and limitations of human studies. However, the epileptogenic focus in the monkey can usually be localized discretely while the focus can rarely be defined as clearly in man. Thus the model may, in some circumstances, be superior. However, if the goal of a study can be analytically dissected down to specified processes which other models of epilepsy exhibit, then, clearly, acute experiments are best carried out utilizing such other models. Nevertheless, ultimately data must be confirmed in the phenomenon of nature and the alumina model of chronic epilepsy (particularly in the monkey) appears at present to represent a satisfactory surrogate for the phenomenon of seizures of cortical origin in the human.

III. COBALT METHOD

A. Technique

In 1960, Kopeloff reported that implantation of the pure metal cobalt into the cortex of the mouse would induce seizures and the technique was subsequently utilized extensively by Dow and his colleagues. In their first description (Dow et al., 1962), a small quantity (approximately 30 mg) of commercially available cobalt powder (200 mesh) was applied to an area of 10 to 15 mm² on frontal cortex of the rat in the motor area. The studies were subsequently extended to the cat (Henjyoji and Dow, 1965) where 50 to 100 mg of metallic cobalt powder (lab grade CX1775 — Matheson, Coleman and Bell) was applied topically to the anterior sigmoid gyrus over an area of 30 to 50 mm². Dawson and Holmes (1966) placed a small amount (50 to 100 μg) of finely divided cobalt powder on the motor cortex of the rat but they did not feel that particle size was important.

Fischer et al. (1967) felt that the reliability of the technique was improved if a cobalt-gelatin stick were inserted into the cortex. The sticks are prepared as follows. A suspension of metallic cobalt powder in warm 5% gelatine is allowed to sediment and is then decanted onto a horizontal slide to form a layer 0.75-mm thick. The solidified film is dehydrated in acetone, fixed in formaldehyde vapors, and kept in 80% alcohol. Sticks measuring 0.75 × 0.75 × 1.5 mm are then cut from the film using a razor blade. After trepanation and removal of dura under aseptic precautions, the stick is inserted into the cortex perpendicularly and the wound closed.

To induce subcortical foci with cobalt, Mancia and Lucioni (1966) utilized cobalt powder (200 mesh) sterilized at 150°C for 1½ hr. A dose of about 10 mg was put into the hub of a needle, and this bolus was implanted using the stylus as a plunger.

B. Phenomenology

Many of the reported studies using cobalt have been concerned with the electrophysiological events induced by this technique; data are more limited regarding the clinical seizures and their natural history. In the rat, Dow et al. (1962) mention that clonic movements of the contralateral body are seen by the second week after cobalt implantation. These lasted only 1 to 2 days, and generalized seizures were seen in only a few animals. EEG spiking occurred within 10 to 20 days, but the intensity decreased within 4 to 6 weeks with subsequent gradual disappearance of epileptic EEG activity. Dawson and Holmes (1966), using a relatively large amount of cobalt on cortex of rat, found that limb jerks started to appear after 24 hr and occurred with increasing frequency until the 10th day and thereafter declined.

In the cat, Henjyoji and Dow (1965) reported that seizure activity occurred spontaneously or could be provoked within 30 hr of the operation. The spontaneous fits were focal and clonic in nature; they occurred more frequently after various forms of provocation, and these authors found that shaking of the involved forelimb was the most effective technique. Clonic movements of the contralateral corner of mouth or half-face was seen at the peak of the epileptic response at first or second day. The maximum duration of focal motor seizures was 25 to 30 sec. After the fourth to fifth day, no clinically evident seizure activity could be observed. Generalized fits occurred in only a few cats.

The induction of seizures in limbic structures is possible with cobalt. Mutani (1967a,b) implanted cobalt into ventral amygdala and ventral hippocampus. The foci in amygdala were electrically active for about 1 month, those in hippocampus for about 2 months. The focus became active in about 48 hr and, when clinical seizures later appeared, they were characterized as feline psychomotor attacks. The animal would become motionless, staring, unresponsive with tachypnea; there was postictal confusion, automatic walking, digging, and pleasure reactions. Some of these clinical seizures apparently occurred spontaneously, others were induced with supplemental convulsant drugs.

There has been no systematic study of species susceptibility to epilepsy induced by cobalt. Implantation in or on motor cortex of the mouse, rat, and cat induced seizures. There is only one report of cobalt-induced epilepsy in primates, and that is in the squirrel monkey where EEG paroxysmal activity was recorded (Grimm et al., 1970). Clusid and Kopeloff (1962) were unable to induce clinical seizures by intracortical implantation of pellets of solid cobalt in the rhesus monkey. However, the major variable may be the surface area of the metal in contact with neuronal tissue, and it appears that, if the powder is used, seizure activity can be induced in primates at least as easily as in other forms.

There has also been no systematic study of differential epileptogenicity using cobalt. It is clearly effective in motor cortex, but Dawson and Holmes (1966) noted that no clinical jerks were observed if cobalt was applied to cortical sites far from the sensorimotor strip in the rat. It will induce both EEG abnormalities and clinical seizures when implanted into medial temporal lobe structures in the cat (Henjyoji and Dow, 1965; Mutani, 1967b). If cobalt is implanted into midline thalamic structures or brainstem reticular formation (Mancia and Lucioni, 1966) or onto visual cortex (Dimov, 1966), EEG changes are observed but no clinical seizures.

Histologically, cobalt induces a severe, necrotizing destructive process in brain (Dow et al., 1962; Henjyoji and Dow, 1965; Engel, 1968). This cellular destruction is progressive and involves all elements. Dow et al. (1962) have speculated that cobalt may be effective because of interference with cellular enzymatic processes rather than by any mechanical effect induced by its presence or the secondary scarring which follows. The slow progression of the destructive process may be a consequence of the relative insolubility of the metal.

C. Potential applications and critique

The implantation of pure cobalt powder clearly induces an active epileptic process. The EEG evidence of abnormal activity appears in hours, and clinical seizures, if they occur at all, are seen in at least several days. The natural history of the clinical seizure process is poorly documented, but it may last only several days although the EEG abnormalities may gradually disappear over a period of many weeks.

Thus this model is useful for those studies requiring an epileptic process that is semichronic; however, it has the drawback that it cannot be used for acute observations. Unfortunately, data are not available to indicate that there are any properties of this model not shared by other techniques that induce epileptic-like activities acutely. Thus, for certain types of specific observations on specific phenomena, there may be only the inconvenience of the somewhat delayed onset of the phenomena. However, if the experimental design requires an epileptic process lasting longer than a few hours, this model clearly has advantages over other models such as those utilizing topical applications of convulsant drugs. It can thus be used for neurochemical studies of enzyme changes (Fischer et al., 1968) as well as studies of the phenomenon of the mirror focus (Fischer et al., 1967; Engel, 1968) where continuous bombardment of the homotopic focus for more than a few hours is desirable.

Finally, some of the advantages of a preparation exhibiting seizures of acute onset can be combined with a chronic epileptic process by injecting a mixture of cobalt powder and alumina cream (Levin et al., 1968; Dimov and Lanoir, 1969).

IV. TUNGSTIC ACID

The paucity of literature dealing with the use of the tungstic acid gel technique as a model of the epileptic process is difficult to explain since it was first described as an epileptogenic agent in 1960 by Blum and Liban. This, in part, may be due to concern regarding the ease of preparation of the compound.

A. Technique

Tungstic acid is thought to be found in three forms, only one of which is biologically active. The monohydrate is biologically inactive. The hydrous forms can be prepared as a bulky precipitate or as a colloidal gel by virtue of its different particle size. Only the colloidal form is biologically active. Preparation of the latter form involves mixing cold, dilute aqueous solutions of sodium tungstate and hydrochloric acid. The resulting white flocculant precipitate is then washed free of excess acid with cold distilled water. A detailed description of two methods for preparation of the colloidal gel have been published by Black et al. (1967).

The material must be kept cold until immediately before injection into cortex, subcortical nuclear masses, or spinal cord. To accomplish this, the gel may be kept in a 0.5-ml or micrometer syringe in the refrigerator until immediately before use. It is then brought to the animal and the volume in the needle expressed and discarded. The needle is then inserted in the desired target, a quantity of 0.01 ml injected, and the needle left in place for about 1 min. The syringe may be capped and returned to the refrigerator where it may be stored for 6 weeks or more.

B. Phenomenology

No behavioral changes are observed attributable to the lesion for 2 to 3 hr after injection. Then, over a period of about an hour, motor or sensory signs appropriate to the site of injection begin and develop to their maximum. If carefully controlled volumes of gel are utilized, the seizures may continue up to 12 hr, but with larger doses the seizures progress to status epilepticus and the animal dies. Others have noted seizure activity lasting from 4 days to 9 weeks (Blum et al., 1961). If the dosage is controlled so that the seizures do not progress to status, the seizure abnormalities disappear, leaving no clinically detectable deficit (Black et al., 1967).

Prior to the onset of the clinical seizures, electrographic changes are noted. There is no observable change in the EEG or single-unit activity during the first 18 to 20 min after injection. Then a gradual increase in unit activity can be recorded with extraneuronal micro-electrodes, which progresses over the next hour or two to a rapid, tonic burst-firing pattern reminiscent of the epileptic units reported by Schmidt et al. (1959) in the chronic alumina focus in the monkey.

Tungstic acid gel has been injected into the cortex, brainstem, and spinal cord of the rat, cat, and monkey and has produced, in every instance, a predictable response. Even in the frog, periodic convulsions can be induced.

Histologically, a central area of acute necrosis is seen within 3 to 6 hr surrounded by a zone of abnormal, pyknotic neurons. The size of the lesion induced by an injection mass of 0.01 ml of tungstic acid is a sphere approximately 2.8 mm in diameter. Within 36 to 48 hr, a well-encapsulated cavity is seen at the site of injection surrounded by a zone of inflammatory cells, fibrin, and glial response.

C. Potential applications and critique

Tungstic acid injected into the CNS induces an intense epileptic process with dramatic electrophysiological hyperactivity. Neither the electrographic hyperactivity nor the clinical seizures are appreciably modified by anticonvulsant drugs, including the barbiturates. If the gel is suitably prepared, the epileptic activity is very consistently induced with a short and very predictable pattern of action. The relatively short latency of action of this agent is an obvious advantage in experiments of an acute nature (Mori, 1968). Unlike other topical epileptogenic agents, especially tetanus toxin and strychnine, no generalized systemic manifestations are seen and all of the effects can be neurologically attributed to activity at the site of injection. Furthermore, the presence of a permanent, discrete lesion for histological control and the complete recovery of the animal from this transient seizure state make correlations possible between pathological site and the clinical manifestations.

V. ACKNOWLEDGMENT

This work was supported by U.S. Public Health Service Research Grant NS04053 from the National Institute of Neurological Diseases and Stroke.

VI. REFERENCES

Aida, S. (1956): Experimental research on the function of the amygdaloid nuclei in psychomotor epilepsy. *Folia Psychiatrica et Neurologica Japonica,* 10:181–207.

Barensten, R. I., and Lockard, J. S. (1969): Behavioral experimental epilepsy in monkeys. II. Video-tape control gate for the detection and recording of motor seizures. *Electroencephalography and Clinical Neurophysiology,* 27:89–92.

Berman, A. J., Pomina, A. C., and Nepomuceno, N. R. (1968): Anticonvulsant properties of nitrazepam (Mogadon). *Electroencephalography and Clinical Neurophysiology,* 24:187.

Black, R. G., Abraham, J., and Ward, A. A., Jr. (1967): The preparation of tungstic acid gel and its use in the production of experimental epilepsy. *Epilepsia,* 8:58–63.

Blum, B., and Liban, E. (1960): Experimental baso-temporal epilepsy in the cat. Discrete epileptogenic lesions produced in the hippocampus or amygdaloid by tungstic acid. *Neurology,* 10:546–554.

Blum, B., Magnes, J., Bental, E., and Liban, E. (1961): Electroencephalographic studies in cats with experimentally produced hippocampal epilepsy. *Electroencephalography and Clinical Neurophysiology,* 13:340–353.

Calvin, W. H., Sypert, G. W., and Ward, A. A., Jr. (1968): Structured timing patterns within bursts from epileptic neurons in undrugged monkey cortex. *Experimental Neurology,* 21:535–549.

Chow, K. L., and Obrist, W. D. (1954): EEG and behavioral changes on application of AL(OH)$_3$ cream on preoccipital cortex of monkeys. *Archives of Neurology and Psychiatry,* 72:80–87.

Chusid, J. G., Kopeloff, L. M., and Kopeloff, N. (1955): Motor epilepsy of parietal lobe origin in the monkey. *Neurology,* 5:108–112.

Chusid, J. G., and Kopeloff, L. M. (1962): Epileptogenic effects of pure metals implanted in motor cortex of monkeys. *Journal of Applied Physiology,* 17:696–700.

Dawson, G. D., and Holmes, O. (1966): Cobalt applied to the sensory motor area of the cortex cerebri of the rat. *Journal of Physiology,* 185:455–470.

Dimov, S. D. (1966): Changes in the cerebral bioelectric activity of rabbits following application of cobalt to the brain cortex (formation and development of epileptogenic focus). In: *Comparative and Cellular Pathophysiology of Epilepsy,* edited by Z. Servit. Excerpta Medica, Amsterdam.

Dimov, S., and Lanoir, J. (1969): The effects of chronic occipital epileptogenic lesions (cobalt alumina) in *Papio papio. Revue Neurologique,* 120:480–481.

Dow, R. S., Fernandez-Guardiola, A., and Manni, E. (1962): The production of experimental cobalt epilepsy in the rat. *Electroencephalography and Clinical Neurophysiology,* 14: 399–407.

Driver, M., Ettlinger, G., Moffett, A. M., and St. John-Loe, P. (1968): Epileptogenic lesions in the monkey. *Journal of Physiology,* 196:93P–94P.

Dyken, P. R. (1964): Hyperpathic disorder from intrathecal alumina gel injections. *Archives of Neurology,* 11:521–528.

Engel, J., Jr. (1968): Secondary epileptogenesis in rats. *Electroencephalography and Clinical Neurophysiology,* 25:494–498.

Essig, C. F. (1962): Focal convulsions during barbiturate abstinence in dogs with cerebrocortical lesions. *Psychopharmacologia,* 3:432–437.

Faeth, W. H., and Walker, A. E. (1957): Studies on effect of the injection of alumina (alumina oxide) cream into the basal ganglia. *Archives of Neurology and Psychiatry,* 78:562–567.

Fischer, J., Holubar, J., and Malik, V. (1967): A new method of producing chronic epileptogenic cortical foci in rats. *Physiologia Bohemoslovaca,* 16:272–277.

Fischer, J., Holubar, J., and Malik, V. (1968): Dehydrogenase patterns of the experimental epileptogenic cortical focus in the rat. A correlation of histochemical and electrophysiological findings. *Acta Histochemica,* 31:296–304.

French, J. D., Gernandt, B. E., and Livingston, R. B. (1956): Regional differences in seizure susceptibility in monkey cortex. *Archives of Neurology and Psychiatry,* 75:260–274.

Gastaut, H., Naquet, R., Meyer, A., Cavanagh, J. B., and Beck, E. (1959): Experimental psychomotor epilepsy in the cat. Electroclinical and anatomopathological correlations. *Journal of Neuropathology and Experimental Neurology,* 18:270–293.

Grimm, R. J., Frazee, J. G., Kawasaki, T., and Savic, M. (1970): Cobalt epilepsy in the squirrel monkey. *Electroencephalography and Clinical Neurophysiology,* 29:525–528.

Guerrero-Figueroa, R., Barros, A., and De Balbian Verster, F. (1963a): Some inhibitory effects of attentive factors on experimental epilepsy. *Epilepsia,* 4:225–240.

Guerrero-Figueroa, R., Barros, A., De Balbian Verster, F., and Heath, R. G. (1963b): Experimental 'petit mal' in kittens. *Archives of Neurology,* 9:297–306.

Guerrero-Figueroa, R., Barros, A., Heath, R. G., and Gonzalez, G. (1964): Experimental subcortical epileptiform focus. *Epilepsia,* 5:112–139.

Halpern, L. M., and Ward, A. A., Jr. (1969): The hyperexcitable neuron as a model for the laboratory analysis of anticonvulsant drugs. *Epilepsia,* 10:281–314.

Harmony, T., Urba-Holmgren, R., Urbay, C. M., and Szava, S. (1968): (Na-K)-ATPase activity in experimental epileptogenic foci. *Brain Research,* 1:672–680.

Henjyoji, E. Y., and Dow, R. S. (1965): Cobalt-induced seizures in the cat. *Electroencephalography and Clinical Neurophysiology,* 19:152–161.

Kennard, M. A. (1950a): Chronic focal hyper-irritability of sensory nervous system in cats. *Journal of Neurophysiology,* 13:215–222.

Kennard, M. A. (1950b): Chronic experimental hyperalgesia in cats. *Folia Psychiatry Neurologica et Neurochirugica Neerlandica,* 53:320–327.

Kennard, M. A. (1953): Sensitization of the spinal cord of the cat to pain-inducing stimuli. *Journal of Neurosurgery,* 10:169–177.

Kopeloff, L. M. (1960): Experimental epilepsy in the mouse. *Proceedings of the Society for Experimental Biology and Medicine,* 104:500–504.

Kopeloff, L. M., Barrera, S. E., and Kopeloff, N. (1942): Recurrent convulsive seizures in animals produced by immunologic and chemical means. *American Journal of Psychiatry,* 98:881–902.

Kopeloff, L. M., Chusid, J. G., and Kopeloff, N. (1954): Chronic experimental epilepsy in *Macaca mulatta. Neurology,* 4:218–227.

Kopeloff, L. M., Chusid, J. G., and Kopeloff, N. (1955): Epilepsy in *Macaca mulatta* after cortical or intracerebral alumina. *Archives of Neurology and Psychiatry,* 74:523–526.

Kopeloff, L. M., Chusid, J. G., and Kopeloff, N. (1957): Convulsant threshold dosages of picrotoxin and strychnine sulfate in normal and epileptic monkeys. *Journal of Applied Physiology,* 11:465–476.

Kopeloff, N., Whittier, J. R., Pacella, B. L., and Kopeloff, L. M. (1950): The epileptogenic effect of subcortical alumina cream in the rhesus monkey. *Electroencephalography and Clinical Neurophysiology,* 2:163–168.

Levin, P., Wyss, F. E., Scollo-Lavizzari, G., and Hess, R. (1968): Evolution of seizure patterns in experimental epilepsy. *European Neurology,* 1:65–84.

Lockard, J. S., and Barensten, R. I. (1967): Behavioral experimental epilepsy in monkeys. I. Clinical seizure recording apparatus and initial data. *Electroencephalography and Clinical Neurophysiology,* 22:482–486.

Mancia, M., and Lucioni, R. (1966): Experimental epilepsy: EEG and behavioral changes induced by subcortical introduction of cobalt powder in chronic cats. *Epilepsia,* 7:308–317.

Mayman, C. I., Manlapaz, J. S., Ballantine, H. T., Jr., and Richardson, E. P., Jr. (1965): A neuropathological study of experimental epileptogenic lesions in the cat. *Journal of Neuropathology and Experimental Neurology,* 24:502–511.

Mori, K. (1968): Changes in slow bioelectric potentials of epileptogenic foci produced by tungstic acid gel. *Archiv Fur Japanische Chirurgie,* 37:583–591.

Mutani, R. (1967a): Cobalt experimental amygdaloid epilepsy in the cat. *Epilepsia,* 8:73–92.

Mutani, R. (1967b): Cobalt experimental hippocampal epilepsy. *Epilepsia,* 8:223–240.

Naquet, R., Alvim-Costa, C., and Toga, M. (1960): Etude clinique, électroencephalographique et anatomopathologique de l'épilepsie "psychomotrice" induite chez le chat par une injection de crème d'alumine. A propos d'une nouvelle série expérimentale. *Revue Neurologique,* 103:216–217.

Prince, D. A. (1968): The depolarization shift in "epileptic" neurons. *Experimental Neurology,* 21:467–485.

Prince, D. A., and Futamachi, K. J. (1970): Intracellular recordings from chronic epileptogenic foci in the monkey. *Electroencephalography and Clinical Neurophysiology,* 29:496–509.

Schmalbach, K. (1970): An animal model of the epileptic process. *Pharmakopsychiatrie Neuro-Psychopharmakologie,* 3:162–175.

Schmidt, R. P., Thomas, L. B., and Ward, A. A., Jr. (1959): The hyper-excitable neurone. Microelectrode studies of chronic epileptic foci in monkey. *Journal of Neurophysiology,* 22:285–296.

Servit, Z. (1960): Prophylactic treatment of post-traumatic audiogenic epilepsy. *Nature,* 188:669–670.

Servit, Z., and Sterc, J. (1958): Audiogenic epileptic seizures evoked in rats by artificial epileptogenic foci. *Nature,* 181:1475–1476.

Shirao, T. (1969): Effects of alumina cream lesions in the substantia nigra or on the cortex of cats. *Acta Medica Kagoshima,* 11:79–96.

Sloan, N., Ransohoff, J., and Pool, J. L. (1953): Clinical and EEG seizures following chronic –irritative lesions of the medial temporal region in monkeys. *Electroencephalography and Clinical Neurophysiology,* 5:320–321.

Stamm, J. S., and Pribram, K. H. (1960): Effects of epileptogenic lesions in frontal cortex on learning and retention in monkeys. *Journal of Neurophysiology,* 23:552–563.

Stamm, J. S., and Warren, A. (1961): Learning and retention by monkeys with epileptogenic implants in posterior parietal cortex. *Epilepsia,* 2:229–242.

Stercova, A. (1966): Dynamics of neurohistological changes in an epileptogenic focus produced by alumina cream in the rat. In: *Comparative and Cellular Patho-Physiology of Epilepsy,* edited by Z. Servit. Excerpta Medica, Amsterdam.

Tower, D. B. (1969): Neurochemical mechanisms. In: *Basic Mechanisms of the Epilepsies,* edited by H. H. Jasper, A. A. Ward, Jr., and A. Pope. Little, Brown and Co., Boston.

Wada, J. A., and Cornelius, L. R. (1960): Functional alteration of deep structures in cats with chronic focal cortical irritative lesions. *Archives of Neurology,* 3:425–447.

Ward, A. A., Jr. (1969): The epileptic neuron: Chronic foci in animals and man. In: *Basic Mechanisms of the Epilepsies,* edited by H. A. Jasper, A. A. Ward, Jr., and A. Pope. Little, Brown and Co., Boston.

Ward, A. A., Jr., McCulloch, W. S., and Kopeloff, N. (1948). Temporal and spatial distribution of changes during spontaneous seizures in monkey brain. *Journal of Neurophysiology,* 11:377–386.

Westrum, L. E., White, L. E., and Ward, A. A., Jr. (1964): Morphology of experimental epileptic focus. *Journal of Neurosurgery,* 21:1033–1046.

Youmans, J. R. (1956): Experimental production of seizures in the macaque by temporal lobe lesions. *Neurology,* 6.179–186.

2

The Production of Epileptogenic Cortical Foci in Experimental Animals by Freezing

Edward Lewin

OUTLINE

I. INTRODUCTION

It has long been recognized that spontaneous convulsive seizures may be induced in laboratory animals by briefly freezing a small area of cerebral cortex. Openchowski (1883) first reported producing seizures in this manner in both rabbits and dogs. Speransky (1943) developed a technique which utilized compressed carbon dioxide for cortical freezing, and described his observations on seizures produced in dogs in a number of publications, beginning in 1926, and later summarized in English. Both Schneider and Epstein (1931) and Nims et al. (1941) employed either dry ice or an ethyl chloride spray to create a freezing lesion, and the latter workers first reported the results of electroencephalographic (EEG) recordings following these procedures. Morrell (1960) described the emergence of secondary foci developing in homotopic cortex contralateral to freezing foci. Purpura and his co-workers utilized freezing cortical lesions for biochemical as well as for extensive electrophysiological investigations (Purpura et al., 1958a,b; Berl et al., 1959; Smith and Purpura, 1960). More recently, biochemical as well as morphological studies of epileptogenic foci induced by freezing have continued in attempts to find correlates with the resulting electrophysiological disturbances. The effects of the administration of anticonvulsant drugs to animals with cortical foci have also been investigated. Moreover, the fact that freezing of the cortical surface is an effective means of experimentally producing cerebral edema has resulted in additional morphological and biochemical studies which, although primarily concerned with edema, should relate to epileptogenesis as well. In the following sections, some of these investigations will be reviewed.

II. METHODS

Although a number of techniques have been employed to produce local cortical freezing, either a dry ice-cooled metal rod or an ethyl chloride spray has been most frequently used for this purpose.

Smith and Purpura (1960) described the use of a metal rod, 2 mm in diameter, attached to a chamber containing dry ice. The rod is placed on the pial surface and allowed to remain until ice crystals appear in the area immediately surrounding the rod. The rod and pia are then washed with warm Ringer's solution in order to remove the rod without tearing the pia or underlying cortex. Stalmaster and Hanna (in press) have fabricated a similar device in which the refrigerant chamber and rod were turned on a lathe from a single block of aluminum. The inner and outer diameters of the chamber are $1/2$ and $3/4$ inch, respectively, and the rod is 2 mm in diameter. The chamber is insulated by placing it within a block of cellulose sponge coated with Silastic adhesive sealant into which an opening corresponding to the size of the chamber has been cut. Four freezing contacts are fashioned from annealed silver wire and are soldered to a sleeve made from rolled sheet silver, which, in turn, is attached to the aluminum rod. These workers have found that the sleeve arrangement permits some thermal loss and allows longer freezing times and, thus, better-controlled lesions. When there is either a dry ice-acetone or a dry ice-alcohol mixture in the chamber, exposures of 100 sec have produced lesions confined to cortical layers I and II. Methods utilizing dry ice-cooled metal rods or wire have the great advantage of producing lesions of uniform size when applied for measured intervals of time.

The use of an ethyl chloride spray, as employed in rabbits and in cats, has been detailed by Morrell and Florenz (1958; Morrell, 1959). After a small burr hole is made, a fine spray of ethyl chloride is directed onto the pia until the cortex whitens. Alternatively, the ethyl chloride spray is applied to the intact dura for 1 to 2 min. In the rat, after light ether anesthesia is induced, the spray is directed onto the dura for only a 15-sec period and then repeated immediately following thawing (Lewin, 1967), while applying a stream of air adjacent to the skull opening with a laboratory vacuum. The spray bottle is held at least 30 cm from the dura in order to minimize the effect of the force of the spray. The animal should be protected as much as possible from inhalation of ethyl chloride, which is a rapidly acting general anesthetic agent. Respiratory arrest should be anticipated and can be easily treated using a rubber bulb as a respirator. This method is simple and requires no special equipment, since ethyl chloride is conveniently available in spray bottles used clinically for local anesthesia. However, this technique has been criticized because of its lack of temperature control and the consequent difficulty in producing lesions of uniform size and depth.

III. CLINICAL AND ELECTROPHYSIOLOGICAL MANIFESTATIONS

The epileptogenicity of cortical foci induced by freezing has been variously defined by the subsequent clinical convulsive activity which develops, or by the resulting "epileptic" electrophysiological phenomena, or by both.

As noted above, the early observations of Openchowski and of Speransky on the effects of cortical freezing were concerned only with the clinical seizures which followed this procedure. Speransky (1943) described generalized seizures beginning 1 to 5 hr after freezing in dogs, and the frequency and severity of the seizures were apparently enhanced by morphine administration. Other reports have confirmed the early onset of clinical convulsions (Keith and Bickford, 1954; Morrell, 1959), focal as well as generalized seizures being observed. However, only a minority of

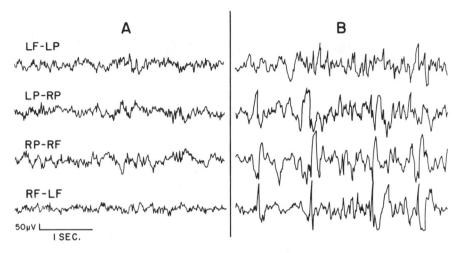

FIG. 1. *A:* Control EEG in albino rat. *B:* Forty min after right somatosensory freezing lesion in same animal (site of lesion between RF and RP). Note prominent spikes with phase reversal around RF. LF, left frontal; LP, left posterior; RP, right posterior; RF, right frontal.

the animals subjected to cortical freezing will develop spontaneous seizures (Lewin and McCrimmon, 1967).

Abnormal EEG discharges unaccompanied by clinical seizures more often result from local cortical freezing. Although the electrophysiological disturbances which follow this procedure are highly variable, focal "epileptic" discharges, when prominent, frequently have become established within a few minutes to several hours after freezing (Keith and Bickford, 1954; Morrell, 1959; Smith and Purpura, 1960; Lewin and McCrimmon, 1967), as shown in Figs. 1 and 2. In some animals, bilateral rather than focal discharges have developed. Spikes and sharp waves have often been more striking during drowsiness and sleep than in the awake EEG. Purpura et al. (1958a,b) have found that the epileptiform discharge always arises within the area of cortex in which an alteration of blood-brain barrier has occurred as defined by Evans blue staining. Maximal EEG abnormality has usually developed within the first 8 to 12 hr after freezing; spontaneous focal discharges become less frequent after this time. The subsequent course of the focus has been unpredictable, but, as the lesion has aged, the resting EEG has tended to approach normal. However, focal discharges have been activated for many weeks with pentylenetetrazol or with bemegride, as well as by photic stimulation in the case of occipital lesions.

The development of "secondary" discharges from the hemisphere contralateral to the induced focus has been carefully studied by Morrell (1960)

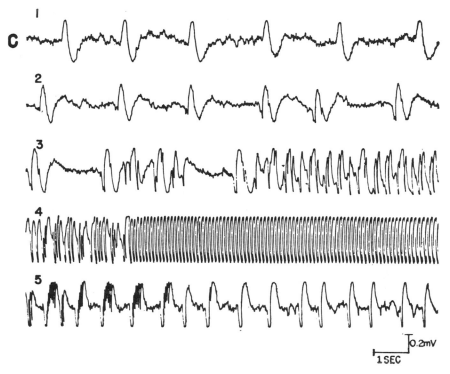

FIG. 2. Monopolar recording from a freezing lesion in a cat showing transition of diphasic potentials (1) to complex multiphasic potentials (2,3) terminating in a sustained "focal seizure" (4), followed by recovery with reversal of polarity of focal discharges. From Smith and Purpura (1960), with permission of the publisher.

in rabbits and in cats. Secondary foci appeared at about 24 hr in the rabbit and within 72 hr in the cat. Using EEG criteria, the contralateral focus became independent between 3 and 7 days in the rabbit and between 3 days and 8 weeks in the cat. Frequently, the secondary focus was ultimately more active electrically than the primary. Excision of the primary focus or section of the corpus callosum sometimes was effective in preventing the appearance of a contralateral focus if performed within 3 weeks of freezing. Secondary discharges similar to those observed in the rabbit and cat developed following cortical freezing in the rat, usually within the first 24 hr (Lewin and McCrimmon, 1967). The early appearance of apparently independent secondary foci has permitted the study of epileptogenic cortex other than at the site of cortical exposure and freezing.

Morrell (1961) and Goldensohn and Purpura (1963) have probed

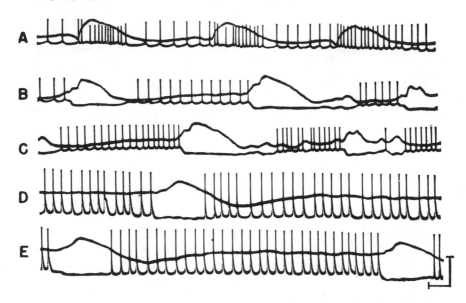

FIG. 3. Monopolar recordings of local EEG discharges from the surface of an epileptogenic lesion induced by freezing in a cat (upper traces) correlated with intracellular recordings from three neurons (lower traces). *A:* Neuron exhibiting minimal depolarization and acceleration of firing during surface negativity (negativity upward). *B* and *C:* A second neuron showing membrane hyperpolarization and inhibition of discharge during all phases of surface waves. *D* and *E:* A third neuron, superficial to those shown in *A, B,* and *C,* showing inhibition of discharge during surface negativity. Calibration: horizontal bar, 0.1 second; vertical bar, 0.5 mV for surface traces and 50 mV for intracellular records. From Goldensohn and Purpura (1963), copyright 1963 by the American Association for the Advancement of Science.

freezing cortical foci with micro-electrodes in attempts to correlate surface EEG events with the behavior of individual neurons. Morrell sampled single units extracellularly and found a variable relation to EEG discharges. Some neurons showed an increased rate of firing at the time of EEG paroxysms, whereas others with high resting rates were inhibited during the same discharges. Goldensohn and Purpura recorded intracellularly from individual neurons and similarly found units both with increased and decreased firing rates during surface discharges, accompanied by depolarization and hyperpolarization, respectively (Fig. 3). Their observations paralleled those made in penicillin-induced foci by Enomoto and Ajmone Marsan (1959).

Recently, Morrell and his colleagues (Morrell et al., 1965; Proctor et al., 1966) prepared rabbits and cats with freezing lesions made with a cryogenic probe in a number of subcortical structures, including caudate nucleus, lateral geniculate body, and several thalamic nuclei. Recordings were made with depth electrodes. Primary subcortical foci were produced, and, in addition, secondary discharges in other subcortical areas were prominent, some animals having as many as five such foci. The authors have pointed out the possible importance of their findings in patients undergoing stereotactic freezing procedures for the relief of movement disorders. However, the relation of these depth models to human convulsive disorder remains to be elucidated.

IV. PATHOLOGICAL ALTERATIONS

The histopathological alterations which result from cortical freezing are of considerable interest. Initially, the lesion is hyperemic and swollen. Supravital dyes such as Evans blue and trypan blue, when injected intravenously or subcutaneously, have been found to penetrate the edematous cortex (Purpura et al., 1958a,b; Torack et al., 1959). An increase in periodic acid Schiff (PAS) staining has been noted in the superficial layers of cortex as well as in underlying white matter (Klatzo et al., 1958). When the cortex has been subjected to more intense and prolonged freezing, hemorrhagic necrosis has been produced (Rosomoff et al., 1965). As the lesion has evolved, variable neuronal derangement has been seen, and glial proliferation has become evident and ultimately has resulted in a glial scar (Torack et al., 1959).

Electron microscopy has demonstrated that the edema developing within the first 24 to 48 hr in cortex was intracellular in contrast to the enlargement of the extracellular space present in white matter (Torack et al., 1959; Lee and Bakay, 1966). Within the cortex, large swollen astrocytic cells and processes have been seen adjacent to apparently unaffected neural elements. The marked astrocytic swelling has accounted almost entirely for the grossly apparent increase in cortical volume.

V. CHEMICAL CHANGES

Experimentally produced epileptogenic cortical foci provide models in which biochemical abnormalities can be correlated with the resulting physiological manifestations. Although a number of such studies have been done, current understanding of the biochemistry of epileptogenesis in freezing lesions remains fragmentary.

Among the first chemical studies of cortical freezing lesions were those of glutamic acid metabolism conducted by Berl et al. (1959). These investigators found a 30 to 75% decrease in glutamic acid, glutamine, and glutathione in lesions in which focal discharge developed; less pronounced changes were present in those without electrical abnormality. Of interest, γ-aminobutyric acid (GABA) was not decreased. However, GABA, when given intravenously, abolished paroxysmal discharges, particularly those of low frequency (Purpura et al., 1958*a,b*). The effectiveness of intravenous GABA has confirmed the alteration in blood-brain barrier demonstrated with vital dyes, as GABA does not enter normal cortex when administered in this manner.

Sodium, potassium, and water content have been measured in cortex at various intervals after freezing. Not unexpectedly, at 8 hr after an ethyl chloride lesion, sodium and water content were increased while potassium was decreased (Lewin et al., 1969), confirming the early edema demonstrated histologically and by electron microscopy. At 24 hr (Pappius and Gulati, 1963) and at 48 hr (Nakazawa, 1969) following more severe freezing, remarkably little abnormality in these parameters remained evident in cortex although edema was present in underlying white matter. It appears, therefore, that the transient cortical edema which follows freezing is present during the period in which the most marked electrophysiological abnormalities occur but is not a feature of the chronic lesion.

The activities of a number of enzymes have been determined in cortex following freezing. Bingham et al. (1969), in an investigation of cerebral edema, estimated several lysosomal and nonlysosomal enzymes at 6 and at 12 hr after extensive freezing through the intact skull. In samples which included underlying white matter as well as cortex, beta-glucuronidase activity was increased while the activities of acid phosphatase and acid cathepsin were decreased. Among the nonlysosomal enzymes, alkaline phosphatase activity was elevated, but a neutral protease was diminished. The significance of the disparity in the behavior of the three lysosomal enzymes studied was not clear.

It has been suggested that a defect in cation transport may be an important factor in epileptogenesis. Therefore, measurements of sodium-potassium-activated ATPase (Na,K-ATPase) in freezing cortical foci have been of interest, because of the probable association of this enzyme with the energy assisted movement of sodium and potassium. Somewhat unexpectedly, an increase in Na,K-ATPase activity was found within the first 8 hr after freezing (Lewin and McCrimmon, 1967). The greatest elevations were in cortical layers III, IV, and V (Lewin and McCrimmon, 1968). At 24 hr, this increase was no longer present. Moreover, when the intracortical distribution of Na,K-ATPase activity was studied in cortex contralateral to the lesion, a significant increase was demonstrated in layers III to VI at 8 hr after freezing, a finding which may be related to the development of secondary foci. It is not known whether the increase in Na,K-ATPase activity was in neural or glial elements or both, although glia normally possess low levels of Na,K-ATPase activity. (Hess et al., 1963). The increase in the activity of this enzyme found at the time of the most active EEG paroxysms may have been an adaptive response to either an elevation in intracellular sodium or to an increase in neuronal discharge.

Escueta and Reilly (1971) studied potassium transport in synaptosomes prepared from both primary and mirror foci. Freezing had been carried out at least 7 days before sacrifice. The ability of synaptosomes from primary freezing lesions to accumulate potassium was impaired, and net potassium influx into synaptosomes from secondary foci was also decreased. These results suggest that freezing produces a chronic alteration in the membrane properties of synaptic terminals.

VI. ANTICONVULSANT DRUGS

Freezing cortical foci has been utilized to study the effects of anticonvulsant drugs on both the electrophysiology and the chemistry of epileptogenic cortex.

Morrell et al. (1959) administered several commonly used drugs to rabbits with freezing lesions and looked for changes in the primary discharge, in the spread to basal nuclei, and in pentylenetetrazol activation. Trimethadione initially enhanced and later suppressed focal spike discharge whereas neither phenobarbital nor diphenylhydantoin altered the primary focus. Both trimethadione and phenobarbital inhibited spread to basal structures and counteracted activation by pentylenetetrazol, but diphenylhydantoin did not appear to have either effect.

Both diphenylhydantoin and phenobarbital, when given to rats prior to freezing, prevented the increase in Na,K-ATPase activity in the cortical focus discussed in Section IV above (Lewin et al., 1969). In contrast, sodium pentobarbital, a barbiturate which is thought not to possess anticonvulsant properties, did not reverse this elevation in enzyme activity (Lewin, *unpublished*). The effect of diphenylhydantoin in the freezing lesion seems inconsistent with the observed stimulation of Na,K-ATPase by this drug under certain ionic conditions (Festoff and Appel, 1968; Lewin and Bleck, 1971) and also with the demonstrated increase in potassium influx in synaptosomes from freezing cortical foci following diphenylhydantoin administration (Escueta and Reilly, 1971). Although the increase in cortical Na,K-ATPase following freezing and its prevention by certain anticonvulsant agents are as yet unexplained, it is possible that the behavior of this enzyme might prove to be useful in the evaluation of future anticonvulsant drugs.

VII. DISCUSSION AND CONCLUSIONS

Characteristics of epileptogenic foci produced by local cortical freezing may be compared to those of other epileptic models. Features which are shared with discharging lesions induced with either alumina gel (Kopeloff et al., 1954; Chow and Obrist, 1954) or with cobalt powder (Dow et al., 1962) include accentuation of paroxysmal activity during drowsiness, activation by analeptic drugs, and the appearance of secondary foci in cortex contralateral to the primary lesion. However, the development of maximal epileptic discharge within the first 8 to 12 hr after freezing contrasts with the days to weeks required following the application of these metals.

When placed on the surface of the brain, penicillin results in the onset within minutes of high-amplitude spike discharges, often accompanied by clinical seizures. However, the effect of penicillin probably disappears as the drug is removed, and unlike freezing, penicillin does not induce a chronic focus.

Recently, the epileptogenicity of ouabain, an inhibitor of cation transport and of Na,K-ATPase, has been recognized (Bignami and Palladini, 1966). When this cardiac glycoside is applied to the cortical surface, an active focal spike discharge, often accompanied by contralateral focal seizures, results (Lewin, 1970). The ouabain focus resembles the freezing lesion in that cortical edema and glial swelling are features of both (Cornog et al., 1967; Lewin, 1971). The glial response is of interest as it has been proposed that astrocytes are involved in the transport of water and electrolytes between the vascular system and the neural elements of the brain (Gerschenfeld et al., 1959). Furthermore, Pollen and Trachtenberg (1970) have suggested that in post-traumatic focal epilepsy, astrocytic dysfunction, by permitting excessive local accumulations of extracellular potassium, leads to neuronal depolarization and hyperexcitability. However, the role of glia in the epileptic process remains conjectural.

The freezing of mammalian tissues leads to the formation of ice crystals which, unless extremely low temperatures are used, may be primarily extracellular in location (Meryman, 1956). The growth of extracellular crystals results in intracellular dehydration, which, in turn, may produce cellular injury, particularly during rewarming. Cell membranes as well as other structures may share in this injury.

It seems likely that a major derangement resulting from cortical freezing occurs in cell membranes and results in disturbances of water and ion movement. The defects in synaptosome potassium transport in freezing foci, discussed in Section IV, support this view. The early increases in Na,K-ATPase activity also point to membrane changes, perhaps implying that the sodium-potassium pump is in some way uncoupled from the enzymatic breakdown of ATP. The striking astrocytic swelling which follows freezing indicates membrane alterations in these cells. A disorder of cation transport in convulsive states has been proposed by Tower (1960), based in part on his finding that surgically removed human epileptic cortex was unable to extrude sodium (Tower, 1955). The epileptogenicity of ouabain is additional evidence for this concept. Current evidence suggests that interference with cation membrane transport may be of great importance in the epileptogenicity of freezing cortical foci.

In summary, local cortical freezing is an effective means of producing an animal model of focal convulsive disorder. It is hoped that this model will continue to yield important insights into the epileptic process.

VIII. REFERENCES

Berl, S., Purpura, D. P., Girado, M., and Waelsch, H. (1959): Amino acid metabolism in epileptogenic and non-epileptogenic lesions of the neocortex (cat). *Journal of Neurochemistry*, 4:311–317.

Bignami, A., and Palladini, G. (1966): Experimentally produced cerebral status spongiosus and continuous pseudorhythmic electroencephalographic discharges with a membrane-ATPase inhibitor in the rat. *Nature*, 209:413–414.

Bingham, W. G., Jr., Paul, S. E., and Sastry, K. S. S. (1969): Effects of cold injury on six enzymes in rat brain. *Archives of Neurology*, 21:649–660.

Chow, K. L., and Obrist, W. D. (1954): EEG and behavioral changes on application of Al(OH)$_3$ cream on preoccipital cortex of monkeys. *Archives of Neurology and Psychiatry*, 72:80–87.

Cornog, J. L., Jr., Gonatas, N. K., and Feierman, J. R. (1967): Effects of intracerebral injection of ouabain on the fine structure of rat cerebral cortex. *American Journal of Pathology*, 51:573–590.

Dow, R. S., Fernández-Gaurdiola, A., and Manni, E. (1962): The production of cobalt experimental epilepsy in the rat. *Electroencephalography and Clinical Neurophysiology*, 14: 399–407.

Enomoto, T. F., and Ajmone Marsan, C. (1959): Epileptic activation of single cortical neurons and their relationship with electroencephalographic discharges. *Electroencephalography and Clinical Neurophysiology*, 11:119–218.

Escueta, A. V., and Reilly, E. L. (1971): The effects of diphenylhydantoin on potassium transport within synaptic terminals of the epileptogenic foci. *Neurology*, 21:418.

Festoff, B. W., and Appel, S. H. (1968): Effect of diphenylhydantoin on synaptosome sodium-potassium-ATPase. *Journal of Clinical Investigation*, 47:2752–2758.

Gerschenfeld, H. M., Wald, F., Zadunaisky, J. A., and DeRobertis, E. D. P. (1959): Function of astroglia in the water-ion metabolism of the central nervous system: An electron microscope study. *Neurology*, 9:412–425.

Goldensohn, E. S., and Purpura, D. P. (1963): Intracellular potentials of cortical neurons during focal epileptogenic discharges. *Science*, 139:840–842.

Hess, H. H., Schneider, G., Warnock, M., and Pope, A. (1963): Lack of effect of Na^+ plus K^+ on Mg^{2+}-stimulated ATP phosphohydrolase activity of human astrocytomas. *Federation Proceedings*, 22:333.

Keith, H. M., and Bickford, R. G. (1954): Observations on the properties of an electrical focus induced by freezing the animal cortex. *American Journal of Physiology*, 179:650–651.

Klatzo, I., Piraux, A., and Laskowski, E. J. (1958): The relationship between edema, blood-brain barrier and tissue elements in a local brain injury. *Journal of Neuropathology and Experimental Neurology*, 17:548–564.

Kopeloff, L. M., Chusid, J. G., and Kopeloff, N. (1954): Chronic experimental epilepsy in *Macaca mulatta. Neurology*, 4:218–227.

Lee, J. C., and Bakay, L. (1966): Ultrastructural changes in the edematous central nervous system: II. Cold-induced edema. *Archives of Neurology*, 14:36–49.

Lewin, E. (1970): Epileptogenic foci induced with ouabain. *Electroencephalography and Clinical Neurophysiology*, 29:402–403.

Lewin, E. (1971): Epileptogenic cortical foci induced with ouabain: Sodium, potassium, water content, and sodium-potassium-activated ATPase activity. *Experimental Neurology*, 30:172–177.

Lewin, E., and Bleck, V. (1971): The effect of diphenylhydantoin administration on sodium-potassium-activated ATPase in cortex. *Neurology*, 21:647–651.

Lewin, E., Charles, G., and McCrimmon, A. (1969): Discharging cortical lesions produced by freezing: The effect of anticonvulsants on sodium-potassium-activated ATPase, sodium, and potassium in cortex. *Neurology*, 19:565–569.

Lewin, E., and McCrimmon, A. (1967): ATPase activity in discharging cortical lesions induced by freezing. *Archives of Neurology*, 16:321–325.

Lewin, E., and McCrimmon, A. (1968): The intralaminar distribution of sodium-potassium-activated ATPase activity in discharging cortical lesions induced by freezing. *Brain Research*, 8:291–297.

Meryman, H. T. (1956): Mechanics of freezing in living cells and tissues. *Science*, 124:515–521.

Morrell, F. (1959): Experimental focal epilepsy in animals. *Archives of Neurology*, 1:141–147.

Morrell, F. (1960): Secondary epileptogenic lesions. *Epilepsia*, 1:538–560.

Morrell, F. (1961): Microelectrode studies in chronic epileptic foci. *Epilepsia*, 2:81–88.

Morrell, F., Bradley, W., and Ptashne, M. (1959): Effect of drugs on discharge characteristics of chronic epileptogenic lesions. *Neurology*, 9:492–498.

Morrell, F., and Florenz, A. (1958): Modification of the freezing technique for producing experimental epileptogenic lesions. *Electroencephalography and Clinical Neurophysiology*, 10:187–188.

Morrell, F., Proctor, F., and Prince, D. A. (1965): Epileptogenic properties of subcortical freezing. *Neurology*, 15:744–751.

Nakazawa, S. (1969): Biochemical studies of cerebral tissues in experimentally induced edema. *Neurology*, 19:269–276.

Nims, L. F., Marshall, C., and Nielsen, A. (1941): Effect of local freezing on the electrical activity of the cerebral cortex. *Yale Journal of Biology and Medicine*, 13:477–484.

Openchowski, P. (1883): Sur l'action localisée du froid, appliqué à la surface de la région corticale du cerveau. *Comptes Rendus des Séances et Mémoires de la Société de Biologie,* 35:38–43.

Pappius, H. M., and Gulati, D. R. (1963): Water and electrolyte content of cerebral tissues in experimentally induced edema. *Acta Neuropathologica,* 2:451–460.

Pollen, D. A., and Trachtenberg, M. C. (1970): Neuroglia: Gliosis and focal epilepsy. *Science,* 167:1252–1253.

Proctor, F., Prince, D., and Morrell, F. (1966): Primary and secondary spike foci following depth lesions. *Archives of Neurology,* 15:151–162.

Purpura, D. P., Girado, M., Smith, T. G., and Gomez, J. A. (1958a): Effects of systemically administered ω-amino and guanidino acids on spontaneous and evoked cortical activity in regions of blood-brain barrier destruction. *Electroencephalography and Clinical Neurophysiology,* 10:187–188.

Purpura, D. P., Girado, M., Smith, T. G., and Gomez, J. A. (1958b): Synaptic effects of systemic γ-amino butyric acid in cortical regions of increased vascular permeability. *Proceedings of the Society for Experimental Biology and Medicine,* 97:348–353.

Rosomoff, H. L., Clasen, R. A., Hartstock, R., and Bebin, J. (1965): Brain reaction to experimental injury after hypothermia. *Archives of Neurology,* 13:337–345.

Schneider, A., and Epstein, B. (1931): The effects of local freezing of the central nervous system of the cat. *Archives of Neurology and Psychiatry,* 25:1263–1270.

Smith, T. G., Jr., and Purpura, D. P. (1960): Electrophysiological studies on epileptogenic lesions of cat cortex. *Electroencephalography and Clinical Neurophysiology,* 12:59–82.

Speransky, A. D. (1943): *A Basis for the Theory of Medicine.* International Publishers, New York.

Stalmaster, R. M., and Hanna, G. R. (*in press*): Epileptic phenomena of cortical freezing in the cat. Persistent multifocal effects of discrete superficial lesions. *Epilepsia* (*in press*).

Torack, R. M., Terry, R. D., and Zimmerman, H. M. (1959): The fine structure of cerebral fluid accumulation: I. Swelling secondary to cold injury. *American Journal of Pathology,* 35:1135–1147.

Tower, D. B. (1955): Nature and extent of the biochemical lesion in human epileptogenic cerebral cortex: An approach to its control in vitro and in vivo. *Neurology,* 5:113–130.

Tower, D. B. (1960): *Neurochemistry of Epilepsy.* Charles C Thomas, Springfield.

3

Topical Convulsant Drugs and Metabolic Antagonists

David A. Prince

OUTLINE

I. INTRODUCTION

Local electrical and clinical epileptiform discharges may be produced experimentally by applying any of a large number of epileptogenic agents to a complex neuronal system such as mammalian cerebral cortex. The acute epileptogenic focus which results has many advantages for the investigator: the relatively uncomplicated technique required for its preparation; the speed with which it becomes established (minutes in most instances); the absence of gross damage and histological changes in the nervous tissue (with certain exceptions, e.g., Bignami and Pallidini, 1966); the regular spontaneous generation of interictal discharges which are "triggerable" by controlled natural or electrical stimulation of afferents to the focus (e.g., Matsumoto, 1964; Prince, 1966); the frequent transitions between interictal and ictal activity which occur spontaneously and may be easily evoked (Matsumoto and Ajmone Marsan, 1964a); and the reversibility of some acute foci over hours or under the influence of specific antagonists (Gutnick and Prince, 1971) which may allow the same preparation to be studied repeatedly during periods of "normal" and epileptogenic activity (Caveness, 1969). These factors facilitate the application of this technique to phylogenetic (Servit et al., 1968; Servit and Strejckova, 1970) and ontogenetic (Bishop, 1950; Caveness, 1969; Prince and Gutnick, 1971, 1972; Purpura, this volume) studies.

The fact that many substances produce electrographically similar epileptiform activity raises certain important issues for the investigator. For example, to what extent will the results obtained depend upon the epileptogenic agent employed? Do the various agents have different basic modes of action? Which most closely approximates the pathophysiology in human focal epilepsy? These questions are relevant if the model is to be applied to drug evaluation studies or used as the basis for parallel electrophysiological and neurochemical investigations of epileptogenesis. For the most part, the answers are unknown, even in the case of the most studied topical convulsants such as strychnine or penicillin (see Ajmone Marsan, 1969, for discussion). The questions themselves are overly simplified. For example, clinical epilepsy is a symptom complex rather than a disease; many varieties of pathology may give rise to convulsions. These may turn out to have a common underlying pathophysiology (e.g., a disturbance in a metabolic process within affected neurons); however, considering the multiple complex processes which regulate such things as membrane potential and permeability, impulse generation, and synaptic activities, there is no particular reason to expect that a single pathophysiology underlies all clinical epilepsy.

The gross differences in the responsiveness of the spectrum of clinical epilepsies to different classes of anticonvulsant medication also raise serious questions about a "single defect" hypothesis. In any case, this key issue is unresolved. Why then should we expect to find in a particular experimental model system a "best fit" for the human epileptogenic process? Each model rather provides an opportunity to study some aspect of the generation of synchronous discharge by groups of neurons and the effects of this activity on normal brain function. Each particular epileptogenic agent may also be regarded as a tool for elucidating a set of induced cellular abnormalities which result in epileptogenesis. The investigator should choose that system which is best suited to a particular experimental problem. For example, if one is studying the projection and spread of epileptiform activity from a focus to distant areas, the agent used may be of little consequence, providing that drug spread can be adequately controlled (see below). On the other hand, the investigator interested in cell behavior within a drug-induced epileptogenic focus must be aware that generalization of the results to other model systems or to other areas of the same nervous system may not be warranted since even the same agent may produce convulsant effects by different actions at different sites. The heterogeneity in the properties of nerve membranes and synaptic mechanisms in various cells of different species (Grundfest, 1966a,b) makes generalization of the effects of a convulsant agent from a so-called "simple" system to the mammalian central nervous system equally hazardous.

A number of the above considerations also apply to the models of generalized epileptiform activity produced by the large array of metabolic inhibitors (Table 2; section II below) available to the investigator. These agents induce convulsions by interfering with a variety of basic metabolic processes, and the epileptologist should be aware that the results of his study may be dependent to a large degree upon the model selected.

In spite of the limitations in experimental approach discussed above and in section II A, it should ultimately be possible to categorize groups of convulsant agents according to the specific varieties of induced abnormality by which they give rise to epileptogenesis, such as the capacity to produce repetitive firing in terminals, blockade of inhibitory synaptic mechanisms, and defects in ionic pumps. It may then be possible to use this basic catalog of disturbances as a test system against which systematic nonempirical evaluation of existing and potential therapeutic agents will be possible.

Although the main purpose of this volume is to provide information about various systems available for studying epileptogenesis *per se*, it should be emphasized that the study of epileptogenic discharge and the pathological neuronal organization which generates it provides a useful tool for understanding relationships between elements of normal neuronal networks.   Intracellular studies have emphasized the dynamic interactions which take place between the epileptic neuronal aggregate and synaptically related organizations.   In a sense, epileptogenic discharges are labeled, internally generated signals which use normal connectivity for their generation and spread, and thus may more closely imitate the normal temporal sequence and distribution of synaptic activities than a volley evoked by electrical stimulation.

II. TOPICAL CONVULSANT DRUGS AND METABOLIC ANTAGONISTS

A few of the more commonly used topical convulsant and metabolic antagonists are listed in Tables 1 and 2, respectively, together with selected references to electrophysiological, biochemical, and other studies.   The actions of these and other agents are considered in recent reviews (Grundfest, 1957, 1966a,b; Tower, 1960, 1969; Merlis, 1962; Esplin and Zablocka, 1965; Kreindler, 1965; Servit, 1966; Esplin and Zablocka-Esplin, 1969; Gastaut et al., 1969; Jasper et al., 1969; Stone, 1969; Ajmone Marsan, 1969; Prince, 1969b).   Topical convulsants not listed in Table 1 include estrogens (Marcus et al., 1966, 1968; Hardy, 1970); mescaline (Crighel and Stoica, 1961; Ochs et al., 1962; Crighel, 1968), and others (see Ajmone Marsan and Abraham, 1963, 1964, 1965, and Ajmone Marsan, 1966, for review).

Numerous other metabolic antagonists are available, including convulsant amino acids (DaVanzo et al, 1964a,b; McFarland and Wainer, 1965; Tews and Stone, 1965); convulsant barbiturates (Swanson, 1934; Swanson and Chen, 1939; Knoefel, 1945; Domino et al., 1955; Domino, 1957, Downes and Williams, 1969; Downes et al., 1970); convulsant ethers (Butler et al., 1964; Adler, 1965; Mori et al., 1971); fluorofatty acids (Kandel and Chemoweth, 1952; Benitez et al., 1954; Pscheidt et al., 1954; Lahiri and Quastel, 1963); hyperbaric oxygen (Granpierre et al., 1967; Giretti et al., 1969; Porta and Barbarani, 1969; Wada et al., 1970; Von Schnakenburg and Nolte, 1970; Thompson and Akers, 1970; Kowalski et al., 1971); pyridoxine antagonists (Killam and Bain, 1957; Killam, 1957; Bain and Williams, 1960; Gammon et al., 1960; Tews, 1969; Tower, 1969 — review); and convulsant phenols (Angel and Rogers, 1968; Banna and Jabbur, 1970).

A. Experimental methods

Various aspects of the use of topical epileptogenic agents will be discussed here, using penicillin as an example; most of the discussion is relevant to any one of the other drugs. Some aspects of the techniques for preparation and use of gross- and microelectrodes for recording from acute epileptogenic foci are discussed in the Appendices.

1. Drug application

The drug to be applied should be dissolved in physiological saline which has been modified so that the solution remains isotonic (Appendix I). pH should also be adjusted with appropriate buffers. These measures are necessary if results are to be comparable from experiment to experiment or laboratory to laboratory, and if one is to be certain that the effects produced are due to the drug itself. Depending on the nature of the investigation, additional control solutions may be required. For example, an isotonic solution of penicillin is most conveniently prepared by replacing a quantity of NaCl in the Ringer's solution with an equivalent amount of Na penicillin. The resulting solution has a pH of 5.5 to 7.0 and contains reduced Cl^- which is replaced by a large, presumably impermeant anion (penicillin). Such a solution could conceivably have effects on the preparation quite apart from those of penicillin (Hutter and Warner, 1967; Takeuchi and Takeuchi, 1971). With higher concentration of epileptogenic agent, these distortions in the ionic content of the applied solution may be very substantial (see Appendix I). The need for a control solution (for example, one with an equivalent amount of NaCl replaced by Na acetate) is obvious, particularly when the preparation consists of an isolated neuron (Ayala et al., 1970a) or simple synaptic system (Ayala et al., 1971; Futamachi and Prince, 1971) where the perfusion solution essentially becomes the extracellular fluid in direct contact with the cell membrane. For example, in a study of the effects of penicillin in neuromuscular transmission in the crayfish tonic abdominal flexor muscles (Futamachi and Prince, 1971), it was found that a penicillin-Van Harreveld's solution (about 30,000 U/cc) produced an increase in membrane resistance as well as an increase in the amplitude of summated excitatory junctional potentials as compared to normal Van Harreveld's solution. Without any other observations, one might conclude that the increase in membrane resistance was related to the increase in excitatory synaptic action. However, when the normal Van Harreveld's solution was replaced with a solution which contained acetate ion in an amount equivalent to the penicillin ion in order to control for the effect of

TABLE 1. *Topical convulsant agents*

Agent	Electrophysiology, cells	EEG	Biochemistry, pharmacology	Other
Acetylcholine	Krnjevic et al. (1970) Krnjevic (1969) Ferguson and Jasper (1971) Spehlmann and Chang (1969)	Spehlmann and Chang (1969) Ferguson and Jasper (1971) Echlin (1959) Bernard et al. (1969) Chatfield and Dempsey (1942) Forster (1945) Brenner and Merritt (1942) Grossman (1963) Spehlmann et al. (1971) Baker and Benedict (1968)	Tower (1969, review) Celesia and Jasper (1966) Stone (1957)	Permeability, blood flow: Barlow (1970) Papy and Naquet (1971) Shalit (1965)
Pentylenetetrazol, (Metrazol ®)	Borys and Esplin (1969) Machek and Fischer (1966) Negishi et al. (1963) Creutzfeldt et al. (1966) Sugaya et al. (1964) Johnson and O'Leary (1965)	Kopeloff and Chusid (1965) Papy and Naquet (1971) Bach-y-Rita et al. (1969) Barlow (1970) Creutzfeldt (1969) Speckman and Caspers (1969) Bures et al. (1968) Baker et al. (1965) Payan et al. (1966) Machek and Fischer (1966)	Barlow (1970) Bignami et al. (1966) Tews et al. (1963) Torda (1954) Carter and Stone (1961) Ferngren (1968)	
Penicillin	Walsh (1971) Ayala et al. (1971) Ayala et al. (1970a,b) Crowell (1970)	Udvarhelyi and Walker (1965) Gummit and Matsumoto (1968)	Louis et al. (1971) Pintillie et al. (1967) Epstein and O'Connor (1966)	

	Prince (1968a,b; 1969) Matsumoto and Ajmone Marsan (1964a,b) Matsumoto et al. (1969) Matsumoto (1964) Prince and Wilder (1967) Dichter and Spencer (1969a,b) Futamachi and Prince (1971) Gutnick and Prince (1972) Prince and Gutnick (1971, 1972) Davidoff (1972)	Holubar (1964) Vastola et al. (1969) Gumnit and Takahashi (1965) Rovit and Swiecicki (1965) Prince (1966) Ralston (1958)		
Picrotoxin	Negishi et al. (1963) Galindo (1969) Tebecis and Phillis (1969) Usunoff et al. (1969) Johnson and O'Leary (1965)	Ramwell and Shaw (1965) Baker and Kratky (1967) Usunoff et al. (1969) Negishi et al. (1963)	Hathway et al. (1965) Ferngren (1968)	Anatomy: Sikdar and Ghosh (1964)
Strychnine	Pollen and Lux (1966) Pollen and Ajmone Marsan (1965) Li (1959) Davidoff et al. (1969) Roper et al. (1969) Washizu et al. (1961) Johnson and O'Leary (1965)	Baker et al. (1965) Udvarhelyi and Walker (1965) Creutzfeldt (1969) Li (1959) Bishop (1950)		Anatomy: Sikdar and Ghosh (1964) Permeability, blood flow: Mchedlishvili et al. (1970) Barlow (1970) Review: Ajmone Marsan (1969)

TABLE 2. *Metabolic antagonists*

Agent	Electrophysiology, cells	EEG	Behavior	Biochemistry, Pharmacology	Anatomy
Ammonium (NH_4^+)	Lux et al. (1970) Lux (1971)	Gastaut et al. (1968b) Ishida (1967)		Pintillie et al. (1967) Tews et al. (1963) Hathway et al. (1965) Lahiri and Quastel (1963) Tews and Stone (1965) Omer (1971) McKhann and Tower (1961) Benitez et al. (1954)	
Hydrazides		Killam (1957) Baker and Kratky (1967) Sakai et al. (1964) Bonavita et al. (1964) Kopeloff and Chusid (1965)		Killam and Bain (1957) Killam (1957) Sakai et al. (1964) Uchida and O'Brien (1964a,b) Weir et al. (1964) Bonavita et al. (1964) Sze and Lovell (1970) Roa et al. (1964)	Knyihar et al. (1971)
Hypoglycemia	Creutzfeldt and Meisch (1963)	Waltregny (1969) Tokizane and Sawyer (1957) Berkowitz et al. (1960) Gastaut et al. (1968a) Van Meter et al. (1958)	Berkowitz et al. (1960)	Mesdjian (1969)	

Methionine sulfoximine	Johnson et al. (1965) Johnson and O'Leary (1965)	Proler and Kellaway (1962, 1965) Johnson et al. (1965) Wada and Ikeda (1966) Hrebicek and Kolousek (1968)	Proler and Kellaway (1962, 1965) Johnson et al. (1965) Wada and Ikeda (1966)	Lamar and Sellinger (1965) Folbergrova (1964) Rowe and Meister (1970) DeRobertis et al. (1967) Tews and Stone (1964) Warren and Schenker (1964) Hrebicek et al. (1971) Stransky (1969)	DeRobertis et al. (1967)
Ouabain		Bergmann et al. (1970) Lewin (1970) Lorenzo (1970)		Petsche and Rappelsberger (1970) Swanson and McIlwain (1965) Lewin (1971) Tower (1969, review)	Bignami et al. (1967) Bignami and Palladini (1966) Cornog et al. (1967)

decreased Cl⁻ in the penicillin solution, about the same change in membrane resistance occurred without an increase in the amplitude of excitatory synaptic potentials. Exchange with an equivalent penicillin-Van Harreveld's solution produced no further change in resistance but still increased the synaptic potentials, showing that these two effects were independent.

2. Drug spread

A second problem of topical drug application is spread of material to remote parts of the nervous system. This effect is very difficult to control, and the extent of spread may vary from experiment to experiment. Direct injection of drug into the brain may also result in diffusion away from the injection site, for example, into the ventricular system and thence in CSF to other remote brain areas (Gloor et al., 1967). This effect may be minimized by microinjections or extracellular microiontophoresis (Humphrey, 1968b; Lux et al., 1970; Walsh, 1971) which expose smaller cell populations to the agent in question; however, even with the microiontophoretic technique, there may be spread of drug over relatively large brain volumes in a short time (Herz et al., 1969). One of the consequences of spread is that the size of the epileptic neuronal aggregate (the acute focus) changes in time as drug penetrates the cortex, and spreads laterally in varying concentrations. Electrophysiological or biochemical studies must take this temporal factor into account in some way since it may affect results. An example of the difference in electrophysiological effects of a focal high concentration of penicillin as opposed to a more generalized brain exposure to a lower concentration of the drug is shown in Fig. 1. With focal topical application (A; 100,000 U/cc), typical paroxysmal interictal epilepiform events occur spontaneously and are accompanied by depolarizations and repetitive firing in neurons. In contrast, after an intramuscular penicillin injection of 300,000 U/kg, which results in a generalized low concentration of penicillin in brain and CSF, diffuse bursts of 4 to 5/sec spike-wave activity occur spontaneously (B, C; Prince and Farrell, 1969, and Prince, Farrell, Futamachi, and Gutnick, unpublished). The associated neuronal activity is quite different from that of A, consisting of rhythmic excitatory postsynaptic potential (EPSP)—inhibitory postsynaptic potential (IPSP) sequences during which the membrane potential increases and single spikes rather than spike bursts are generated (B). The contrast in electrographic features between A and B-C may be the result of differences in drug concentration as well as the nature and location of synaptic organization exposed to the agent.

Certain types of investigation are particularly vulnerable to the problem

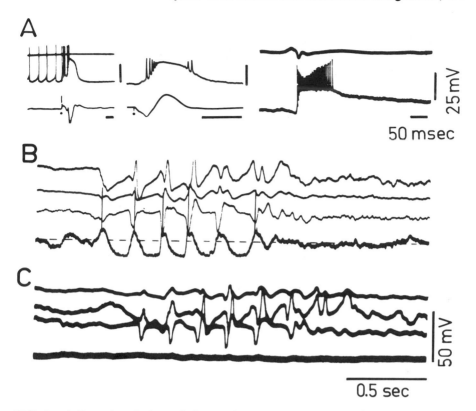

FIG. 1. *A:* Examples of triggered (dots) and spontaneous interictal epileptiform discharges from penicillin foci. Intracellular recordings show typical depolarization shifts and associated spike bursts. *B:* EEG activity (first three traces) and intracellular recording (lowest trace) during bursts of diffuse spike-wave discharges which occur spontaneously in unanesthetized cats after systemic penicillin administration. Microelectrode penetration at site of EEG recording in third trace. *C:* Same as *B* with microelectrode (lowest trace) in extracellular position after cell death to record field potential during another burst. *A,* modified from Prince (1968*b*); *B* and *C* from Prince, Farrell, Futamachi, and Gutnick (*unpublished data*).

of drug spread—for example, studies of projection phenomena and "mirror" foci where the assumption is made that an area of brain remote from the primary area of application is free of drug. This problem is magnified as the brain of the preparation becomes smaller. The controls for drug spread have not been rigorous in most experiments. Mixture of the convulsant agent with a fluorescent or other dye would allow for detection of gross contamination of adjacent areas; but this technique assumes that diffusion of drug and marker occur at the same rate, and that the marker can be detected with a sensitivity sufficient to control for even small concentrations of drug. These assumptions are not necessarily valid. One approach to this problem would be to use an isotopically labeled drug and record counts at the site of presumed noncontaminated brain as a control. In the case of the penicillin focus, it might be possible to use buffered penicillinase to protect the remote area being studied from the effects of penicillin (Gutnick and Prince, 1971). Of course, appropriate controls for the effect of topical penicillinase would then be required. Iatrogenic spread of drug can also occur, especially when agents active in minimal concentrations are used. Thus, drug may be spread by irrigating the focus with saline, or careless use of contaminated cortical recording electrodes or instruments. In some preparations it may be necessary to reapply the drug if the acute epileptogenic focus becomes inactive. In such instances, electrographic signs frequently indicate that more than one zone of epileptiform activity is present, making certain types of electrophysiological analysis more difficult.

3. Drug concentration

It is possible that the basic electrophysiological and/or biochemical lesions which are responsible for epileptogenesis in the case of a particular topical agent or metabolic antagonist are different at different drug concentrations, or that one drug may produce some effects which are unrelated to its action as an epileptogenic agent. These problems may make interpretation of electrophysiological, anatomical, or biochemical data difficult when it is not possible to correlate the findings with behavioral or electrographic signs of epileptiform activity. The use of the "simple" electrophysiological preparation for study of drug action is one case in point. Since penicillin can produce focal epileptiform activity when applied to the pial surface of cat cortex in concentrations as low as 1,000 to 5,000 U/cc (1.7 to 8.5 mM), actual tissue concentrations for producing focal epileptiform discharges must be much lower. It is difficult to know if the effects found when much higher concentrations of drug (e.g., 30,000 U/cc) are applied directly to cell membranes (e.g., Ayala et al., 1970a, 1971; Futamachi and Prince, 1971) are really those which induce epileptogenesis in the cortex. One approach to this problem in the case of penicillin is the possible use of penicillinase-inactivated drug as a control (Gutnick and Prince, 1971; Davidoff, 1972). In the case of both topical convulsants and metabolic antagonists, measurement of actual tissue concentrations of labeled drugs would be desirable wherever possible so that particular drug effects on metabolic and electrographic activities can be correlated with drug concentration.

4. Anesthesia

Anesthetics change the pattern of epileptiform activity produced by topical convulsant drugs and therefore must be considered as a variable in any experimental situation. The administration of pentobarbital in moderate doses suppresses the development of cortical ictal episodes (Sypert et al., 1970) and also may eliminate the peripheral myoclonic jerks which are associated with focal interictal discharges. The interictal discharges themselves are extremely resistant to high doses of intravenous barbiturates and in fact may persist against the background of a flat EEG produced by large amounts of intravenous pentobarbital. Since experiments with anesthetized animals present the problem of the effects of drug on electrical and metabolic events at all levels of the nervous system, as well as certain difficulties in maintaining constant levels from animal to animal or even at different times in the same experiment, it is important to perform at least some experiments in locally anesthetized preparations to control for such effects.

5. Acute locally anesthetized preparation

One important improvement in the preparation of locally anesthetized, immobilized animals has been the application of human anesthesia techniques and apparatus (de Jong et al., 1965). Using a small anesthesia machine with a copper kettle for delivering halothane mixed with nitrous oxide and oxygen, plus an infant-type face mask, it is not difficult to induce anesthesia rapidly in small animals. In practice, cats or rabbits are restrained and anesthesia given by face mask. As soon as the animal is relaxed, a cuffed endotracheal tube can be positioned with the aid of an infant-size laryngoscope, and anesthesia continued via the endotracheal route or a tracheotomy done directly. It is important to monitor heart sounds using an audio-amplifier and loudspeaker during halothane administration to detect bradicardia or arrythmias which may occur if too high a concentration is used. Animals may be immobilized with intravenous gallamine (initial dose 4 to 5 mg/kg), followed by cord or brainstem (Stefanis and Jasper, 1964; Ferguson and Jasper, 1971) transection. Following the surgical procedures, all pressure points and wound edges should be infiltrated with a long-acting local anesthetic (e.g., Zyljectin®, Abbott) and general anesthesia discontinued. Another approach which allows initial induction of anesthesia by the endotracheal route rather than by mask is as follows. The animal is given an intramuscular injection of succinylcholine (4 to 5 mg/kg) after all preparations for tracheal intubation and artificial respiration have been made. Within 1 min, neuromuscular blockade is effective, and intubation is performed rapidly while external artificial respiration is administered. The technique is not difficult but the investigator should have some proficiency at intubating anesthetized cats before attempting it. We have limited the paralyze-intubate-anesthetize technique to cats because rabbits and monkeys are more difficult to intubate. This procedure is also particularly useful in chronic or semi-chronic preparations where EEG or extracellular unit activity can be recorded without movements, even during induced convulsions. If no further succinylcholine (or gallamine triethiodide supplementation) is given, the animal will spontaneously recover respirations and gag response, and may be cautiously detubed after suctioning to remove accumulated secretions.

6. Animal maintenance

Since 8 to 12 hr or longer may elapse between the initial preparation and the termination of the experiment, careful attention to the physiological state of the animal is essential if stable conditions are to be maintained.

Temperature. The rectal or esophageal temperature should be monitored routinely, and a heating device used to maintain body temperature at 37 to 38°C. This may be done automatically by using a thermistor bridge and relay to control the heating device, and a thermistor to sense the animal's temperature. A similar feedback temperature control can be used to regulate the temperature of a cortical, spinal, or peripheral mineral oil pool.

Blood pressure. It is particularly useful to monitor femoral blood pressure in experiments where major operative procedures (e.g., neuraxis transection) are to be done, and also in acute unanesthetized preparations. In these instances, a sudden change in pressure may indicate some correctable and undesirable condition, e.g., accumulation of CO_2 due to atelectasis or an obstructed airway, shock due to inadequate fluid replacement, or appreciation of pain in the case of the acute preparation. Awareness that the animal is hypotensive may also save many hours of fruitless experimentation.

Respiration. In those experiments where artificial respiration is required, there is usually a tendency to overbreathe the animal, and, over hours, a profound respiratory alkalosis can result. Although an anesthetized cat normally has an end-expired CO_2 concentration of about 4 to 5%, in only a few minutes of overbreathing the CO_2 may be 2% or less. Parallel changes in arterial PCO_2 can have significant effects on the cerebral circulation and convulsive activity. It would be ideal to monitor blood gases directly during each experiment and regulate minute volume accordingly; however, facilities are not available for these determinations in most laboratories. It is possible to monitor continuously end-expired CO_2 using an infrared CO_2 analyzer and thus obtain a guideline for control of respirations which should be adequate except in cases where portions of the lungs are unaerated (e.g., atelectasis). In practice, a small volume and rapid rate may be required to limit respiratory pulsation. End-expired CO_2 can be maintained at 4% even during hyperventilation by respiring the animal with a mixture containing CO_2 (usually 1 to 2% is sufficient) via the anesthesia machine. The use of a bilateral pneumothorax to limit respiratory pulsations produces other problems. The absence of negative intrathoracic pressure and the small tidal volume give rise to atelectasis which can be controlled by occasional over-inflation and by submerging the respirator exhaust hose under a few centimeters of water. The exposed visceral pleura become dry unless the pleural cavity is occasionally irrigated with 1 or 2 cc of saline. Fluid loss from the exposed pleura and from rapid ventilation with dry air is much greater than in the anesthetized intact preparation. Four to 5 cc/kg/hr of a lactated Ringer's solution in 5% glucose given slowly intravenously or subcutaneously approximately replaces fluid and electrolyte losses. If adequate replacement is given, the animal will urinate during the course of the experiment.

Adequacy of local anesthesia. Animals maintained in good condition will generally remain asleep throughout the acute experiment as judged by slit-like pupils, a synchronized EEG, and the absence of acute blood pressure fluctuations. Noxious stimuli to unanesthetized areas will produce pupillary dilation, increase in blood pressure, and EEG desynchronization; these changes will signal the need for additional local anesthetic or conversion of the unanesthetized preparation to an anesthetized one by administration of small amounts of intravenous anesthetic. Generalized ictal episodes will also produce blood pressure changes and pupillary dilation which, in the absence of EEG recording, might be misinterpreted as arousal.

7. *Pulsation control for intracellular recordings*

Measures designed to limit respiratory and circulatory pulsations are usually not effective if the preparation itself is not in good condition, as, for example, in the case of an animal with low and unstable blood pressure or high pulse pressure, poor oxygenation, or brain hyperemia from exposure or elevated CO_2. The single most effective measure is continuous drainage of the spinal fluid established by opening the subarachnoid space at the cisterna magna or another site. In the deeply anesthetized preparation, this plus a wide craniectomy and some direct stabilization of the brain with agar or a small lucite pressor plate may be all that are necessary. The pressor plate should be placed while observing the superficial vessels with a dissecting microscope to avoid effects on local circulation. Other measures include axial suspension with elevation of the animal's thorax and abdomen above the experimental table, and bilateral pneumothorax. Controlled hyperventilation which lowers end-expired CO_2 to 3% may decrease vascular pulsations. When all else fails, it may be possible to eliminate pulsations by increasing the depth of anesthesia with pentobarbital. In some preparations, pulsations will make intracellular recordings impossible, in spite of the above maneuvers.

B. Intracellular recordings in acute cortical foci

Studies of intracellular activities in foci produced by topical drug application (Li, 1959; Matsumoto and Ajmone Marsan, 1964a,b; Matsumoto, 1964; Pollen and Ajmone Marsan, 1965; Pollen and Lux, 1966; Prince, 1966; 1968a,b, 1969a,b, 1971; Prince and Wilder, 1967; Prince and Gutnick, 1971, 1972; Prince et al., 1969; Matsumoto et al., 1969; Dichter and Spencer, 1969a,b; Ayala et al., 1970b; Hardy, 1970) have yielded valuable information about the cellular activities which underlie focal epileptiform discharges and the mechanisms which would tend to limit the spread of epileptogenic activity in the brain. Rather than dwell in detail upon the results of these studies, which have been recently reviewed (Ajmone Marsan, 1969; Prince, 1969b), we will consider certain aspects of the available data which illustrate the advantages and limitations of this powerful electrophysiological technique.

The outstanding characteristic of intracellular activity in chemically induced foci is the occurrence of large-amplitude, prolonged depolarizations (the paroxysmal depolarization shift or PDS of Matsumoto and Ajmone Marsan, 1964a) in the vast majority of neurons of the focus sampled by the microelectrode (Fig. 1A). Similar (though less marked) depolarizations occur coincident with surface epileptiform events in freeze foci (Goldensohn and Purpura, 1963) and chronic alumina cream foci (Prince and Futamachi, 1970). By using techniques of intracellular stimulation and recording, it has been possible to conclude that the PDS and the large hyperpolarization which usually follows this potential are derived in large part from excitatory and inhibitory synaptic potentials, respectively (Prince, 1968a,b; Dichter and Spencer, 1969a; Matsumoto et al., 1969). By using a bridge circuit for simultaneously stimulating and recording from single cells, it can be demonstrated that the PDS behaves like an excitatory synaptic potential in that it decreases and increases, respectively, in amplitude as the membrane potential of the neuron moves toward and away from the sodium equilibrium potential. In already depolarized neurons, it has been possible to pass sufficient depolarizing current through the electrode to reach a potential at which the PDS is either isopotential or actually inverted (Prince, 1968*b;* Matsumoto et al., 1969). These results must be interpreted cautiously, however, since they are obtained from injured neurons, and other factors such as a decrease in membrane resistance during intense depolarization (rectification) might also contribute to the decrease in PDS amplitude. Because of limitations in the amount of current which can be passed through the microelectrode, and the amount of direct depolarization which a cell will tolerate, it has not been possible to depolarize a "healthy" cell with a membrane potential of 50 or 60 mV sufficiently to examine in detail the reversal potential of the PDS. It is also possible that a component of the PDS could be nonsynaptic in nature [e.g., extracellular K^+ accumulation might make a contribution to cell depolarization (Lebovitz, 1970; Prince, 1971; Prince et al., 1972)]. The evidence for a synaptic origin of the hyperpolarization which follows the PDS is better. This potential has a reversal point negative to the resting membrane potential and may be inverted to a depolarizing event with relatively little hyperpolarizing current (Prince, 1968*a;* Ayala et al., 1969). It also may be inverted to a depolarizing potential by iontophoretic injection of Cl ion (Prince, 1968*a*), which shows that it is mediated by an increased Cl^- conductance and identifies it as an IPSP (Coombs et al., 1955; Lux, 1971).

Some of the limitations of the intracellular recording technique become apparent when one considers the possible origin of the PDS. Since similar "giant" synaptic potentials can occur in normal neurons during periods of intense synaptic drive (Sawa et al., 1963; Prince and Wilder, 1967), the recording of the PDS in a neuron is not evidence that the cell is behaving in an abnormal way because of exposure to a drug. In fact, the neurons in which the PDS is recorded appear to have no remarkable properties which would be unique to elements exposed to penicillin. When not involved in epileptogenesis, these neurons participate in normal spontaneous and evoked activities, and generate spikes and synaptic potentials which are indistinguishable from those of neurons of normal cortex. Their responses to intracellular current are similar to those of other neurons. On the basis of these findings, the cells of the focus appear "normal." This conclusion, however, should be qualified. For example, although IPSPs seem to be prominent in the penicillin focus (Prince, 1968*a*), the effects of penicillin on IPSPs in cortical neurons have not been examined quantitatively so that changes in inhibitory ionic mechanisms might still be present such as those that are produced by the action of NH_4^+ and other ions on motoneuron IPSPs (Lux and Schubert, 1969; Lux et al., 1970; Lux, 1971). Neither is it possible to make any quantitative statement about the effects of penicillin on the resting membrane potentials of cortical neurons because of the large variations which occur even in "normal" neurons as a result of the injury of impalement. A steady-state depolarization produced by the drug in large aggregates of neurons interconnected via recurrent excitatory pathways would be hard to detect and might give rise to epileptiform discharges in the population.

The intracellular technique itself has other limitations which make important elements of the "epileptic neuronal aggregate" inaccessible for study. There is a bias against obtaining adequate recordings from small interneurons which are presumably important in generating the PDS (Prince, 1966, 1968b; Matsumoto et al., 1969; Dichter and Spencer, 1969b). Also, intracellular recordings reflect activities "seen" by a microelectrode in the cell body (the presumed site of most successful penetrations), leaving open the possibility of abnormalities at distant sites on the same neuron (Prince, 1969b). For example, alteration in the function of presynaptic terminals not obvious in cortical intracellular recordings might produce a large change in the "gain" of the system because of resulting effects on excitation-secretion coupling. The results of studies of thalamocortical relay cells whose axons project into the area of the cortical penicillin focus indicate that just such an abnormality may be present (Gutnick and Prince, 1972). Bursts of spikes originating in axons and propagating orthodromically in the cortex would produce a powerful synaptic drive which would contribute to PDS generation.

Another area of the cell membrane whose activities cannot be adequately evaluated by intrasomatic recording is that of the distal dendritic tree (Rall, 1967). Some of the consequences of the relative electrical isolation of the soma from dendritic potentials are illustrated in studies of the effects of DC surface polarization on EEG potentials and intracellular activities in the penicillin focus. In Fig. 2, typical records of surface activities and simultaneous intracellular potentials from a pyramidal tract (PT) cell (depth 1,200 μ) during surface DC polarization are shown. The control response (A-1) to orthodromic (nVL) stimulation consists of a surface positive-negative wave (which is a complex of evoked response and triggered epileptiform event) and the associated intracellular PDS, followed by a hyperpolarization (IPSP). During polarization with weak surface cathodal and anodal currents (A-2 and B-1, respectively), there are very large changes in surface epileptiform events without significant alterations in antidromic spike height or the PDS. Small changes may occur in cellu-

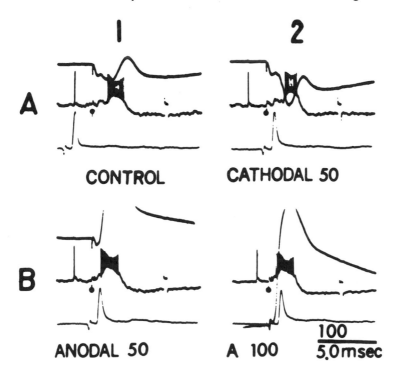

FIG. 2. Effects of surface DC polarization on intracellular (second and third traces) and EEG (top trace) activities in a penicillin focus. Bottom trace, expanded sweep of antidromic spike (PT cell); A1, responses during weak surface cathodal and anodal polarization; B2, responses during stronger surface anodal polarization. Antidromic spike heights 39 mV, 39 mV, and 38 mV during control (A1), cathodal 50 A (A-2), and anodal 50 μA (B-1) sweeps, respectively. Surface potentials: positivity down. Time calibrations in B2 for all frames: 100 msec for top two traces; 5 msec for third trace; 10 mV calibration pulse on microelectrode trace. From Prince, Futamachi, Gutnick, and Logan (*unpublished*).

lar activities with stronger polarization, when alterations in surface EEG potentials are even more dramatic (B-2). These results are similar to those reported by Purpura and McMurtry (1965) in normal cortex. They suggest that there is parallel synchronous activation of superficial and deep synaptic organizations in the epileptiform focus. The synaptic currents of the superficial (dendritic) organization generate EEG activity recorded from the pial surface and are profoundly affected by surface polarization. Deeper-lying synaptic activities which contribute to the generation of PDSs and control the output of the cell are influenced much less. The data also show that the contributions of superficial synaptic activities to generation of PDSs on deep-lying cell bodies are quite small, as are the contributions of PDS synaptic currents to the surface paroxysmal discharges. From these data, it is apparent that the intracellular recording technique is inadequate for studying superficial cortical synaptic activities or the overall distribution of synaptic currents through the cortex during epileptiform discharges. Sequential laminar analysis of extracellular field potentials is the dissecting tool of choice in dealing with such questions (Appendix II).

III. APPENDIX I: PREPARATION OF CONVULSANT DRUG SOLUTIONS

Assume that a penicillin solution of 10,000 U/cc was required to study the effects of the drug on neuromuscular transmission of the crayfish. The procedure would be as follows:

(1) Molecular weight Na penicillin G
$(C_6H_{17}NaN_2O_4S) = 356.38$

(2) 600 mg of Na penicillin G is equivalent to 10^6 units.

(3) Desired solution would contain 10^4 units or 6 mg Na penicillin/cc or 0.017 mmoles/cc $\left(\dfrac{6}{356.4}\right)$.

(4) Normal Van Harreveld's crayfish solution contains

NaCl	12 g/liter	=	205.3 mmoles/liter
KCl	0.4 g/liter	=	5.37 mmoles/liter
$MgCl_2 \cdot 6H_2O$	0.53 g/liter =		2.61 mmoles/liter
$CaCl_2 \cdot 2H_2O$	2.0 g/liter	=	13.55 mmoles/liter

(5) If an isotonic solution is required, 0.017 mmoles/cc of Na penicillin should be substituted for an equivalent amount of NaCl. Each cc of normal Van Harreveld's solution contains 0.205 mmoles of NaCl. The desired penicillin–Van Harreveld's solution would contain: NaCl 0.188 mmoles/cc (0.205–0.017) = 10.98 mg, Na penicillin 6 mg/cc, and other components as above.

(6) When mixed, the solution will have a pH of 5 to 7 and should be buffered to pH 7.2 to 7.5 with Tris. The concentration of the penicillin solution is 17 mM (0.017 mmoles/cc), and the concentration of Cl in the final solution is decreased by an equivalent amount. Since the total Cl concentration of normal Van Harreveld's solution is 243 mequiv/liter, the Cl concentration of the penicillin-Van Harreveld's solution will be decreased by 7% $\left(\dfrac{17}{243}\right)$.

Note that these values become very significant if more concentrated penicillin solutions are used. Thus, a solution containing 100,000 U/cc of Na penicillin dissolved in normal Van Harreveld's solution would be hypertonic by 170 mmoles/liter, whereas a solution prepared by substituting Na penicillin for NaCl would contain 170 mmoles less Cl^- than normal, or a replacement of 70% chloride.

IV. APPENDIX II: LAMINAR ANALYSIS OF CORTICAL POTENTIALS

The analysis of the antidromic cortical response from pyramidal stimulation by Humphrey (1968a) is an excellent example of the application of sequential laminar analysis.

As pointed out by Humphrey, the use of depth potential profiles to indicate the sites of "sources" and "sinks" of current flow is incorrect since current is proportional to the *voltage gradient* rather than the sign and magnitude of the recorded potential with respect to a reference point. An estimate of the sources and sinks of vertical extracellular current flow at selected times during a spontaneous or evoked event can be obtained by plotting the sites of maximum change in the vertical component of current, if it is assumed that changes in extracellular current density are due to transmembrane currents flowing at the same depth. Laminar plots of the transmembrane current flows at selected times during the course of the event are obtained by plotting the second differential of the depth-potential voltage profiles $\left[\frac{\delta^2 V}{\delta_z^2} \ (mV/mm^2)\right]$. See Humphrey (1968a) for more detailed discussion. An analysis of this type could be applied to epileptiform or evoked activity at any site.

V. APPENDIX III: PREPARATION OF MICROPIPETTES FOR UNIT RECORDING

A complete description of techniques for manufacturing, filling, and testing glass microelectrodes, as well as a discussion of their use for recording and stimulation, is provided by Frank and Becker (1964) and Burés (1967). Many methods for filling are available which may be adapted to the investigator's needs. One technique is described here.

(1) Cut Pyrex glass tubing (1 to 3 mm O.D.) in pieces to fit micropipette puller. Tubing with a lumen: wall ratio of at least 1:1 should be used.

(2) Clean in warm dichromate, filtered distilled water, and acetone, and dry in oven.

(3) Pull pipettes with a tip less than 1 μ and a long gradual taper (diameter 200 μ from tip approximately 20 μ) for intracellular recording. For extracellular recording, electrode tips should be broken to 1 to 3 μ. To accomplish this, mount the electrode in a holder on the mechanical stage of a microscope which is fitted with a calibrated grid in one ocular. Focus on the tip in the center of the field at about 100 × magnification. Move the stage to remove the electrode from the field. Fasten one end of a piece of clean 1 to 2-mm diameter glass tubing to the stage using modeling clay so that it is also in focus close to the center of the field, but oriented perpendicular to the microelectrode. Move the microelectrode tip into view so that it almost touches the glass rod. Tapping the stage gently will cause the rod to vibrate and break the electrode tip in a controlled manner. This may also be done after an electrode is filled in order to obtain a lower resistance tip.

(4) Secure electrodes with a rubber band to a thick glass rod, one end of which is embedded in a large rubber stopper. Then, completely emerse them, tips down, in a container of filtered absolute ethanol or methanol. Warm the alcohol slightly, and boil the electrodes for 10 to 15 min by applying suction to a glass tube penetrating the stopper. Do not use methanol when electrodes are to be subsequently filled with citrate because precipitation may occur.

(5) After electrodes appear to be filled, clamp the suction hose, and cool to room temperature.

(6) Immerse alcohol-filled electrodes into a container of filtered distilled H_2O and allow to stand for several hours.

(7) Fill electrodes with desired electrolyte. For intracellular recordings, 2 M K citrate, 0.6 M K_2SO_4, 3 M KCl or a mixture of 85% (by volume) of 1.5 M K citrate and 15% 3 M KCl may be used. Pure 3 M KCl is avoided if attenuation or inversion of inhibitory synaptic potentials would be undesirable. For extracellular recordings, 4 M NaCl may be used.

Filling is accomplished by (a) immersing holder in container of filtered electrolyte containing a few drops of ethylenediamine tetraacetate (to retard bacterial growth), or (b) backfilling each pipette using a fine gauge needle. Twenty-four to 48 hr is required for the electrolyte to diffuse completely into tips, as judged by resistance measurements.

(8) Microelectrodes should be stored in the refrigerator to retard bacterial growth and etching of tips, which is particularly rapid in warm citrate solutions. They may be stored immersed in electrolyte or in air, closed in a tight container with moist cotton gauze at its bottom. Electrodes are suitable for intracellular recordings from 2 to 3 days after filling; extracellular recording pipettes may be stored longer and still be adequate for use.

(9) Electrodes are tested prior to use by examining tips under the microscope to eliminate broken or clogged ones or tips with air bubbles, and by measuring resistance and current-carrying capacity (if electrode is to be used to stimulate neurons) as described by Frank and Becker (1964). Care must be taken not to test electrodes on a conventional DC ohmmeter because the current employed may produce polarization and irreversible changes in electrode properties. The use of a meter which uses an AC test current eliminates such effects.

Electrodes selected for intracellular recording generally have resistances of 20 to 40×10^6 Ω; extracellular electrodes filled with 4 M NaCl measure 1 to 5×10^6 Ω.

VI. APPENDIX IV: ELECTRODES FOR GROSS POTENTIAL RECORDING

For recording from cortical surface, a stable macroelectrode for AC or DC coupled recordings is manufactured by sealing (with dental wax) a sintered Ag-AgCl pellet or wire in a glass tube drawn to a course tip with a protruding cotton wick. The tube is filled with saline or agar-saline mixture. An identical Ag-AgCl pellet should be used as the reference electrode. Before recording from the animal is begun, the electrodes should be tested by placing them in a grounded dish of saline, and connecting them to the input of a high-gain differential DC amplifier to check for drift and high potential difference. Such wick electrodes are also useful for applying polarizing DC currents to the cortex.

Surface recordings can also be obtained using silver-ball electrodes made by heating silver wire (0.005 to 0.010 inch O.D.) in a flame to form a small ball and then chloriding the electrode in the dark with weak DC current in 0.9% NaCl as the anode against a large silver cathode.

Electrodes for stereotaxic depth stimulation and recording are conveniently made by first straightening pieces of enameled steel wire (0.015 to 0.020 inch O.D.) by stretching them slightly between two clamps. The wires are cut into desired lengths and one end sharpened with a fine carborundum disc using an electric drill so that 0.5 mm or less is exposed at the electrode tip. Two wires are glued side by side with Stoner Mudge (Mobile Chemical) or other lacquer so that the tip separation is about 1 to 2 mm. After two or three coats of tin lacquer are applied, electrodes are dried in room air and tested using a saline loop and an ohmmeter to rule out shorts between wires or leaky insulation. Concentric bipolar electrodes are made by preparing single wires and inserting them into lengths of hypodermic tubing (20 to 24 gauge) which are insulated by dipping in Epoxylite solution (Epoxylite Corp.) several times and baking at 250°C between coats. Insulation at the tip of the tubing and the wire can be removed by use of a dissecting microscope and electric drill with a fine grinding wheel. Care must be taken not to short the core wire to the hypodermic tubing, and electrodes should be tested with an ohmmeter before using.

VII. REFERENCES

Adler, M. W. (1965): Increased sensitivity to pentylenetetrazol and Flurothyl following cortical ablations in rats. *Journal of Pharmacology and Experimental Therapeutics*, 148:131–135.

Ajmone Marsan, C. (1966): Epilepsy. In: *Progress in Neurology and Psychiatry*, edited by E. A. Spiegel, vol. 21. Grune and Stratton, New York, pp. 195–260.

Ajmone Marsan, C. (1969): Acute effects of topical epileptogenic agents. In: *Basic Mechanisms of the Epilepsies*, edited by H. H. Jasper, A. A. Ward, Jr., and A. Pope. Little, Brown and Co., Boston, pp. 299–319.

Ajmone Marsan, C., and Abraham, K. (1963): Epilepsy. In: *Progress in Neurology and Psychiatry*, edited by E. A. Spiegel, vol. 18. Grune and Stratton, New York, pp. 244–267.

Ajmone Marsan, C., and Abraham, K. (1964): Epilepsy. In: *Progress in Neurology and Psychiatry*, edited by E. A. Spiegel. Grune and Stratton, New York, pp. 261–298.

Ajmone Marsan, C., and Abraham, K. (1965): Epilepsy. In: *Progress in Neurology and Psychiatry*, edited by E. A. Spiegel. Grune and Stratton, New York, pp. 286–351.

Angel, A., and Rogers, K. J. (1968): Convulsant action of polyphenols. *Nature*, 217:84–85.

Ayala, G. F., Lin, S., and Vasconetto, C. (1970a): Penicillin as epileptogenic agent: Its effect on an isolated neuron. *Science*, 167:1257–1260.

Ayala, G. F., Matsumoto, H., and Gumnit, R. J. (1970b): Excitability changes and inhibitory mechanisms in neocortical neurons during seizures. *Journal of Neurophysiology*, 33:73–85.

Ayala, G. F., Spencer, W. A., and Gumnit, R. J. (1971): Penicillin as an epileptogenic agent— effect on an isolated synapse. *Science,* 171:915–917.

Bach-y-Rita, G., Poncet, M., and Naquet, R. (1969): Morphology and spatio-temporal evolution of ictal discharges induced by cardiazol in the presence of various corticodiencephalic lesions in the cat. In: *The Physiopathogenesis of the Epilepsies,* edited by H. Gastaut, H. Jasper, J. Bancaud, and A. Waltregny. Charles C Thomas, Springfield, Ill., pp. 256–267.

Bain, J. A., and Williams, H. L. (1960): Concentrations of B_6 vitamers in tissues and tissue fluids. In: *Inhibition in the Nervous System and Gamma-Aminobutyric Acid,* edited by E. Roberts. Pergamon, New York, p. 275.

Baker, W. W., and Benedict, F. (1968): Analysis of local discharges induced by intrahippocampal microinjection of carbachol or diisopropylfluorophosphate (DFP). *International Journal of Neuropharmacology,* 7:135.

Baker, W. W., and Kratky, M. (1967): Changes in local excitability produced by intrahippocampal injections of thiosemicarbazide and GABA. *Archives Internationales de Pharmacodynamie et de Thérapie,* 170:81–92.

Baker, W. W., Kratky, M., and Benedict, F. (1965): Electrographic response to intrahippocampal injections of convulsant drugs. *Experimental Neurology,* 12:136–145.

Banna, N. R., and Jabbur, S. J. (1970): Increased transmitter release induced by convulsant phenols. *Brain Research,* 20:471–473.

Barlow, C. F. (1970): Regional permeability changes in experimental convulsive disorder. *Electroencephalography and Clinical Neurophysiology,* 29:323.

Benitez, D., Pscheidt, G. R., and Stone, W. E. (1954): Formation of ammonium ion in the cerebrum in fluoroacetate poisoning. *American Journal of Physiology,* 176:488–492.

Bergmann, F., Costin, A., Chaimovitz, M., and Zerachia, A. (1970): Seizure activity evoked by implantation of ouabain and related drugs into cortical and subcortical regions of the rabbit brain. *Neuropharmacology,* 9:441–449.

Berkowitz, E. C., Sundsten, J. W., and Sawyer, C. H. (1960): Electroencephalographic and behavioral changes in unrestrained rabbits during insulin hypoglycemia. *Neurology,* 10:355–364.

Bernard, P. J., Piette, Y., Delaunois, A. L., and DeSchaepdryver, A. F. (1969): Action of topically applied atropine, eserine, acetylcholine and nicotine on cortical epilepsy in the rabbit. *Archives Internationales de Pharmacodynamie et de Thérapie,* 177:486.

Bignami, A., and Palladini, G. (1966): Experimentally produced cerebral status spongiosus and continuous pseudorhythmic electroencephalographic discharges with a membrane-ATPase inhibitor in the rat. *Nature,* 209:413–414.

Bignami, A., Palladini, G., Appicciutoli, L., and Maccagnani, F. (1967): An experimental study of brain spongiosis. *Acta Neuropathologica* (Berlin), 3:119–126.

Bignami, A., Palladini, G., and Venturini, G. (1966): Effect of cardiazol on sodium-potassium-activated adenosine triphosphatase of the rat brain in vivo. *Brain Research,* 1:413–414.

Bishop, E. J. (1950): The strychnine spike as a physiological indicator of cortical maturity in the postnatal rabbit. *Electroencephalography and Clinical Neurophysiology,* 2:309–315.

Bonavita, V., Guarneri, R., and Monaco, P. (1964): Neurophysiological and neurochemical studies with the isonicotinoylhydrazone of pyridoxal 5-phosphate. *Journal of Neurochemistry,* 11:787–792.

Borys, H. K., and Esplin, D. W. (1969): Pentyl-enetetrazol and Renshaw-cell activity. *International Journal of Neuropharmacology,* 8:627–630.

Brenner, C., and Merritt, H. (1942): Effect of certain cholin derivation on electrical activity of the cortex. *Archives of Neurology and Psychiatry,* 48:382–395.

Bureš, J., Buresova, O., and Janebova, M. (1968): The effect of spreading depression in the thalamus, corpus striatum and hippocampus on the activity of a chemically induced focus of paroxysmal activity in the rat cerebral cortex. *Physiologia Bohemoslovaca,* 17:533–540.

Bureš, J., Petráň, M. and Zachar, J. (1967): *Electrophysiological Methods in Biological Research.* Academic Press, New York, pp. 208–227.

Butler, H. R., Manax, S. J., and Stavraky, G. W. (1964): Hexaflurodiethyl ether (Indoklon ®)

convulsions in corpus-callotomized white rats. *Canadian Journal of Physiology and Pharmacology*, 42:609–621.

Carter, S. H. and Stone, W. E. (1961): Effect of convulsants on brain glycogen in the mouse. *Journal of Neurochemistry*, 7:16–19.

Caveness, W. F. (1969): Ontogeny of focal seizures. In: *Basic Mechanisms of the Epilepsies*, edited by H. H. Jasper, A. A. Ward, Jr., and A. Pope. Little, Brown and Co. Boston, pp. 517–534.

Celesia, G. C., and Jasper, H. H. (1966): Acetylcholine released from cerebral cortex in relation to state of activation. *Neurology*, 16:1053–1063.

Chatfield, P. O., and Dempsey, E. W. (1942): Some effects of prostigmine and acetylcholine on cortical potentials. *American Journal of Physiology*, 135:633–640.

Coombs, J. S., Curtis, D. R., and Eccles, J. C. (1957): The interpretation of spike potentials of motoneurones. *Journal of Physiology*, 139:198–231.

Coombs, J. S., Eccles, J. C., and Fatt, P. (1955): The electrical properties of the motoneuron membrane. *Journal of Physiology*, 130:219–325.

Cornog, J. L., Jr., Gonatas, N. K., and Feierman, J. R. (1967): Effects of intracerebral injection of ouabain on the fine structure of rat cerebral cortex. *American Journal of Pathology*, 51:573–590.

Creutzfeldt, O. D. (1969): Neuronal mechanisms underlying the EEG. In: *Basic Mechanisms of the Epilepsies*, edited by H. H. Jasper, A. A. Ward, Jr., and A. Pope. Little, Brown and Co., Boston, pp. 397–420.

Creutzfeldt, O. D., and Meisch, J. J. (1963): Changes of cortical neuronal activity and EEG during hypoglycemia. *Electroencephalography and Clinical Neurophysiology*, 24(Suppl.): 158–171.

Creutzfeldt, O. D., Watanabe, S., and Lux, H. D. (1966): Relations between EEG phenomena and potentials of single cortical cells. II. Spontaneous and convulsoid activity. *Electroencephalography and Clinical Neurophysiology*, 20:19–37.

Crighel, E. (1968): Experimental data on the mechanism facilitating the passage of interictal spiking foci into focal and generalized seizures. *Epilepsia*, 9:55–70.

Crighel, E., and Stoica, E. (1961): Cercetari asupra focarului mescalinic sigmoidian. *Studii se Cercetari de Neurologie*, 6:547–556.

Crowell, R. M. (1970): Distant effects of a focal epileptogenic process. *Brain Research*, 18:137–154.

DaVanzo, J. P., Matthews, R. J., and Stafford, J. E. (1964a): Studies on the mechanism of action of aminooxyacetic acid. I. Reversal of aminooxyacetic acid-induced convulsions by various agents. *Toxicology and Applied Pharmacology*, 6:388–395.

DaVanzo, J. P., Matthews, R. J., Young, G. A., and Wingerson, F. (1964b): Studies on the mechanism of action of aminooxyacetic acid. II. Possible pyridoxin deficiency as a mechanism of action of aminooxyacetic acid toxicity. *Toxicology and Applied Pharmacology*, 6:396–401.

Davidoff, R. (1972): Penicillin and presynaptic inhibition in the amphibian spinal cord. *Brain Research*, 36:218–222.

Davidoff, R. A., Aprison, M. H., and Werman, R. (1969): The effects of strychnine on the inhibition of interneurons by glycine and γ-aminobutyric acid. *International Journal of Neuropharmacology*, 8:191–194.

deJong, R. H., Lutz, A., and Wagman, I. H. (1965): Use of halothane anesthesia for surgical preparation of the experimental animal. *Anesthesia and Analgesia Current Research*, 44:504–507.

DeRobertis, E., Sellinger, O. Z., Rodriguez de Lores Arnaiz, G., Alberici, M., and Zieher, L. M. (1967): Nerve endings in methionine sulphoximine convulsant rats, a neurochemical and ultrastructural study. *Journal of Neurochemistry*, 14:81–89.

Dichter, M., and Spencer, W. A. (1969a): Penicillin-induced interictal discharges from the cat hippocampus. I. Characteristics and topographical features. *Journal of Neurophysiology*, 32:649–662.

Dichter, M., and Spencer, W. A. (1969b): Penicillin-induced interictal discharges from the cat hippocampus. II. Mechanisms underlying origin and restriction. *Journal of Neurophysiology*, 32:663–687.

Domino, E. F. (1957): Pharmacological actions of a convulsant barbiturate. II. Effects compared with pentobarbital on cerebral cortex and some brain stem systems of the cat. *Journal of Pharmacology and Experimental Therapeutics*, 119:272–283.

Domino, E. F., Fox, K. E., and Brody, T. M. (1955): Pharmacological action of a convulsant barbiturate [sodium-5-ethyl-5-(1,3-dimethylbutyl) barbiturate]. I. Stimulant and depressant effects. *Journal of Pharmacology and Experimental Therapeutics*, 114:473–483.

Downes, H., Perry, R. S., Ostlund, R. E., and Karler, R. (1970): A study of the excitatory effects of barbiturates. *Journal of Pharmacology and Experimental Therapeutics*, 175: 692–699.

Downes, H., and Williams, J. K. (1969): Effects of a convulsant barbiturate on the spinal monosynaptic pathway. *Journal of Pharmacology and Experimental Therapeutics*, 168: 283–289.

Echlin, F. A. (1959): The supersensitivity of chronically "isolated" cortex as a mechanism in focal epilepsy. *Electroencephalography and Clinical Neurophysiology*, 11:697–722.

Epstein, M. H., and O'Connor, J. P. (1966): Effects of convulsive doses of penicillin on the metabolism of single neurons. *Experimental Neurology*, 15:172–179.

Esplin, D. W., and Zablocka, B. (1965): Central nervous system stimulants. In: *The Pharmacological Basis of Therapeutics* (*third edition*), edited by L. S. Goodman and A. Gilman. Macmillan, New York, pp. 345–353.

Esplin, D. W., and Zablocka-Esplin, B. (1969): Mechanisms of action of convulsants. In: *Basic Mechanisms of the Epilepsies*, edited by H. H. Jasper, A. A. Ward, Jr., and A. Pope. Little, Brown and Co., Boston, pp. 167–183.

Ferguson, J. H., and Jasper, H. H. (1971): Laminar DC studies of acetylcholine-activated epileptiform discharge in cerebral cortex. *Electroencephalography and Clinical Neurophysiology*, 30:377–390.

Ferngren, H. (1968): Further studies on chemically induced seizures and their antagonism by anticonvulsants during postnatal development in the mouse. *Acta Pharmacologica et Toxicologica*, 26:177–188.

Folbergrova, J. (1964): Free glutamine level in the rat brain in vivo after methionine sulphoximine administration. *Physiologica Bohemoslovaca*, 13:21–27.

Forster, F. M. (1945): Action of acetylcholine on motor cortex. Correlation of effects on acetylcholine and epilepsy. *Archives of Neurology and Psychiatry*, 54:391–394.

Frank, K., and Becker, M. C. (1964): Microelectrodes for recording and stimulation. In: *Physical Techniques in Biological Research*, Vol. V, *Electrophysiological Methods*, Part A, edited by W. L. Nastuk, Academic Press, New York and London, pp. 22–87.

Friedlander, W. J. (1967): Epilepsy. In: *Progress in Neurology and Psychiatry*, vol. 22, edited by E. A. Spiegel. Grune and Stratton, New York, p. 217–247.

Futamachi, K. J., and Prince, D. A. (1971): The effects of penicillin on crayfish neuromuscular junction. *Federation Proceedings*, 30:131.

Galindo, A. (1969): GABA picrotoxin interaction in the mammalian nervous system. *Brain Research*, 14:763–767.

Gammon, G. D., Gumnit, R., Damrin, R. P., and Kamrin, A. (1960): The effect of convulsant doses of analeptic agents upon the concentration of amino acids in brain tissue. In: *Inhibition in the Nervous System and Gamma-Aminobutyric Acid*, edited by E. Roberts. Pergamon, New York, p. 328.

Gastaut, H., Jasper, H., Bancaud, J., and Waltregny, A. (1969): *The Physiopathogenesis of the Epilepsies*. Charles C Thomas, Illinois.

Gastaut, H., Lyagoubi, S., Mesdjian, E., Saier, J., and Ouahchi, S. (1968a): Generalized epileptic seizures, induced by "non-convulsant" substances. Part I. Experimental study with special reference to insulin. *Epilepsia*, 9:311–316.

Gastaut, H., Saier, J., Mano, T., Santos, D., and Lyagoubi, S. (1968b): Generalized epileptic seizures, induced by "non-convulsant" substances. Part 2. Experimental study with special reference to ammonium chloride. *Epilepsia*, 9:317–327.

Giretti, M. L., Rucci, F. S., and LaRocca, M. (1969): Effects of lowered body temperature on hyperoxic seizures. *Electroencephalography and Clinical Neurophysiology,* 27:581–586.

Gloor, P., Hall, G., and Coceani, F. (1967): Differential epileptogenic action of penicillin on cortical and subcortical brain structures. *Electroencephalography and Clinical Neurophysiology,* 23:491.

Goldensohn, E. S., and Purpura, D. P. (1963): Intracellular potentials of cortical neurons during focal epileptogenic discharges. *Science,* 139:840–842.

Granpierre, R., Neverre, G., Rozier, J., Faltot, P., and Monkam, J. M. (1967): Sur le mecanisme et la prevention de la crise comitiale en atmosphere d'oxygène hyperbare chez le chat. *Comptes Rendus des Séances de la Société de Biologie et de Ses Filiales,* 161:782–787.

Grossman, S. P. (1963): Chemically induced epileptiform seizures in the cat. *Science,* 142: 409–411.

Grundfest, H. (1957): General problems of drug action on bioelectric phenomena. *Annals of the New York Academy of Sciences,* 66:537–591.

Grundfest, H. (1966a): Heterogeneity of excitable membrane: Electrophysiological and pharmacological evidence and some consequences. *Annals of the New York Academy of Sciences,* 137:901–949.

Grundfest, H. (1966b): Some determinants of repetitive electrogenesis and their role in the electrical activity of the central nervous system. In: *Comparative and Cellular Pathophysiology of Epilepsy,* edited by Z. Servit. Excerpta Medica Foundation, New York, pp. 19–42.

Gumnit, R. J., and Matsumoto, H. (1968): The DC field in the cortex beneath an epileptic focus. *Electroencephalography and Clinical Neurophysiology,* 24:291.

Gumnit, R. J., and Takahashi, T. (1965): Changes in direct current activity during experimental focal seizures. *Electroencephalography and Clinical Neurophysiology,* 19:63–74.

Gutnick, M. J., and Prince, D. A. (1971): Penicillinase and the convulsant action of penicillin. *Neurology,* 21:759–764.

Gutnick, M. J., and Prince, D. A. (1972): Thalamocortical relay neurons: antidromic invasion of spikes from a cortical epileptogenic focus. *Science,* 176:424–426.

Hardy, R. W. (1970): Unit activity in Premarin®-induced cortical epileptiform foci. *Epilepsia,* 11:179–186.

Hathway, D. E., Mallinson, A., and Akintonwa, D. A. A. (1965): Effects of dieldrin, picrotoxin and telodrin on the metabolism of ammonia in brain. *Biochemical Journal,* 94:676–686.

Herz, A., Ziegelgänsberger, W., and Färber, G. (1969): Microelectrophoretic studies concerning the spread of glutamic acid and GABA in brain tissue. *Experimental Brain Research,* 9:221–235.

Holubar, J. (1964): Primary (PCR) and direct (DCR) cortical responses of the penicillin focus in rats. *Physiologia Bohemslovaca,* 13:496–503.

Hrebicek, J., and Kolousek, J. (1968): Preparoxysmal changes of spontaneous and evoked electrical activity of the cat brain after administration of methionine sulphoximine. *Epilepsia,* 9:145–162.

Hrebicek, J., Kolousek, J., Wiedermann, M., and Charamza, O. (1971): Changes of the incorporation of (^{75}Se)methionine and of the electrical activity in various brain structures of the cat after administration of methionine sulphoximine. *Brain Research,* 28:109–117.

Humphrey, D. R. (1968a): Reanalysis of the antidromic cortical response. I. Potentials evoked by stimulation of the isolated pyramidal tract. *Electroencephalography and Clinical Neurophysiology,* 24:116–129.

Humphrey, D. R. (1968b): *Unpublished data,* cited in Ajmone Marsan (1969).

Hutter, O. F., and Warner, A. E. (1967): The pH sensitivity of the chloride conductance of frog skeletal muscle. *Journal of Physiology,* 189:403–425.

Ishida, R. (1967): Electroencephalographical studies on the seizure discharges induced by ammonium chloride in the rabbit. *Japanese Journal of Pharmacology,* 17:6–18.

Jasper, H. H., Ward, A. A., Jr., and Pope, A. (Editors) (1969): *Basic Mechanisms of the Epilepsies.* Little, Brown and Co., Boston.

Johnson, W. L., Goldring, S., and O'Leary, J. L. (1965): Behavioral, unit and slow potential changes in methionine sulfoximine seizures. *Electroencephalography and Clinical Neurophysiology,* 18:229–238.

Johnson, W. L., and O'Leary, J. L. (1965): Assay of convulsants using single unit activity. *Archives of Neurology,* 12:113–127.

Kandel, A., and Chemoweth, M. B. (1952): Metabolic disturbances produced by some fluorofatty acids: Relation to the pharmacologic activity of these compounds. *Journal of Pharmacology and Experimental Therapeutics,* 104:234–247.

Killam, K. F. (1957): Convulsant hydrazides. II. Comparison of electrical changes and enzyme inhibition induced by the administration of thiosemicarbazide. *Journal of Pharmacology and Experimental Therapeutics,* 119:263–271.

Killam, K. F., and Bain, J. A. (1957): Convulsant hydrazides. I. "in vitro" and "in vivo" inhibition of vitamin B_6 enzymes by convulsant hydrazides. *Journal of Pharmacology and Experimental Therapeutics,* 119:255–262.

Knoefel, P. K. (1945): Stimulation and depression of the central nervous system by derivatives of barbituric and thiobarbituric acids. *Journal of Pharmacology and Experimental Therapeutics,* 84:26–33.

Knyihar, E., Kiss, J., and Csillik, B. (1971): Thiosemicarbazide seizures—electron microscopic localization of ^{14}C-thiosemicarbazide in the rat hippocampal function. *Research Communications in Chemistry, Pathology, and Pharmacology,* 2:392–405.

Kopeloff, L. M., and Chusid, J. G. (1965): Pyridoxine and GABA as antagonists to drug-induced convulsions in monkey. *Journal of Applied Physiology,* 20:1337–1340.

Kowalski, M. K., Ashley, A., and Kydd, G. H. (1971): Inability of succinate to protect rats from the chronic effects of hyperbaric oxygen toxicity. *Aerospace Medicine,* 42:427–432.

Kreindler, A. (1965): Experimental epilepsy. *Progress in Brain Research,* 19:1–213.

Krnjevic, K. (1969): Neurotransmitters in normal and isolated cortex. In: *Basic Mechanisms of the Epilepsies,* edited by H. H. Jasper, A. A. Ward, Jr., and A. Pope. Little, Brown and Co., Boston, pp. 159–165.

Krnjevic, K., Reiffenstein, R. J., and Silver, A. (1970): Chemical sensitivity of neurons in long-isolated slabs of cat cerebral cortex. *Electroencephalography and Clinical Neurophysiology,* 29:269–282.

Lahiri, S., and Quastel, J. H. (1963): Fluoroacetate and the metabolism of ammonia in brain. *Biochemical Journal,* 89:157–163.

Lamar, C., Jr., and Sellinger, O. Z. (1965): The inhibition in vivo of cerebral glutamine synthetase and glutamine transferase by the convulsant methionine sulfoximine. *Biochemical Pharmacology,* 14:489–506.

Lebovitz, R. M. (1970): A theoretical examination of ionic interactions between neural and non-neural membranes. *Biophysical Journal,* 10:423–444.

Lewin, E. (1970): Epileptogenic foci induced with ouabain. *Electroencephalography and Clinical Neurophysiology,* 29:402–403.

Lewin, E. (1971): Epileptogenic cortical foci induced with ouabain. Sodium, potassium, water content, and sodium potassium activated ATPase activity. *Experimental Neurology,* 30:172–177.

Li, C. L. (1959): Cortical intracellular potentials and their responses to strychnine. *Journal of Neurophysiology,* 22:436–450.

Lorenzo, A. S. (1970): Experimental study of seizure mechanisms. *Electroencephalography and Clinical Neurophysiology,* 28:417–418.

Louis, S., Kutt, H., and McDowell, F. (1971): Modification of experimental seizures and anticonvulsant efficacy by peripheral stimulation. *Neurology,* 21:329–336.

Lux, H. D. (1971): Ammonium and chloride extrusion: Hyperpolarizing synaptic inhibition in spinal motoneurons. *Science,* 173:555–557.

Lux, H. D., Loracher, C., and Neher, E. (1970): The action of ammonium on postsynaptic inhibition of cat spinal motoneurons. *Experimental Brain Research,* 11:431–447.

Lux, H. D., and Schubert, P. (1969): Postsynaptic inhibition: Intracellular effects of various ions in spinal motoneurons. *Science,* 166:625–626.

Machek, J., and Fischer, J. (1966): Laminar analysis of the electric seizure activity elicited by electroshock and metrazole in the sensory motor cortex of the rabbit. In: *Comparative and Cellular Pathophysiology of Epilepsy*, edited by Z. Servit. *Excerpta Medica International Congress Series*, 124:139–143.

Marcus, E. M., Watson, C. W., and Goldman, P. L. (1966): Effects of steroids on cerebral cortical activity. *Archives of Neurology*, 15:521–532.

Marcus, E. M., Watson, C. W., and Simon, S. A. (1968): An experimental model of some varieties of petit mal epilepsy. *Epilepsia*, 9:233–248.

Matsumoto, H. (1964): Intracellular events during the activation of cortical epileptiform discharges. *Electroencephalography and Clinical Neurophysiology*, 17:294–307.

Matsumoto, H., and Ajmone Marsan, C. (1964a): Cortical cellular phenomena in experimental epilepsy: Interictal manifestations. *Experimental Neurology*, 9:286–304.

Matsumoto, H., and Ajmone Marsan, C. (1964b): Cortical cellular phenomena in experimental epilepsy – ictal manifestations. *Experimental Neurology*, 9:305–326.

Matsumoto, H., Ayala, G. F., and Gumnit, R. J. (1969): Neuronal behavior and triggering mechanism in cortical epileptic focus. *Journal of Neurophysiology*, 32:688–703.

McFarland, D., and Wainer, A. (1965): Convulsant properties of allyglycine. *Life Sciences*, 4:1587–1590.

Mchedlishvili, G. I., Ingvar, D. H., Barmidze, D. G., and Ekberg, R. (1970): Blood flow and vascular behavior in the cerebral cortex related to strychnine-induced spike activity. *Experimental Neurology*, 26:411–423.

McKhann, G. M., and Tower, D. B. (1961): Ammonia toxicity and cerebral oxidative metabolism. *American Journal of Physiology*, 200:420–424.

Merlis, J. K. (1962): Abnormal excitatory activity: Epilepsy. In: *Neural Physiology*, edited by R. G. Grenell. Harper and Row, New York, pp. 65–94.

Mesdjian, E. (1969): Hypoglycemic epilepsy: Preliminary biochemical data. In: *The Physiopathogenesis of the Epilepsies*, edited by H. Gastaut, H. Jasper, J. Bancaud, and A. Waltregny. Charles C Thomas, Springfield, Ill., pp. 125–127.

Mori, K., Mitani, H., and Fujita, M. (1971): Epileptogenic properties of diethyl ether on the cat central nervous system. *Electroencephalography and Clinical Neurophysiology*, 30:345–349.

Negishi, K., Bravo, M. C., and Verzeano, M. (1963): The action of convulsants on neuronal and gross wave activity in the thalamus and in the cortex. *Electroencephalography and Clinical Neurophysiology*, 24(Suppl.):90–96.

Ochs, S., Dowell, A. R., and Russell, I. S. (1962): Mescaline convulsive spikes triggered by direct cortical stimulation. *Electroencephalography and Clinical Neurophysiology*, 14:878–884.

Omer, V. S. (1971): Investigations into mechanisms responsible for seizures induced by chlorinated hydrocarbon insecticides: The role of brain ammonia and glutamine in convulsions in the rat and cocherel. *Journal of Neurochemistry*, 18:365–374.

Papy, J. J., and Naquet, R. (1971): Cerebral blood flow and seizures induced by Metrazol® in the baboon. *Clinics in Developmental Medicine*, 39:283–296.

Payan, H., Levine, S., and Strebel, R. (1966): Inhibition of experimental epilepsy by chemical stimulation of cerebellum. *Neurology*, 16:573–576.

Petsche, H., and Rappelsberger, P. (1970): Ouabain-induced status epilepticus as a model for the study of anticonvulsive drugs. *Pharmakopsychiatrie Neuropsychipharmakologie*, 3:151–161.

Pintillie, C., Mison-Crighel, N., and Badiu, G. (1967): Convulsive effect elicited by topical application of penicillin on glutamate-glutamine system of brain. *Nature* 214:1131–1132.

Pollen, D. A., and Ajmone Marsan, C. (1965): Cortical inhibitory post synaptic potentials and strychninization. *Journal of Neurophysiology*, 28:342–358.

Pollen, D. A., and Lux, H. D. (1966): Conductance changes during inhibitory post synaptic potentials in normal and strychninized cortical neurons. *Journal of Neurophysiology*, 29:369–381.

Porta, L., and Barbarani, V. (1969): Changes induced by hyperbaric oxygenation on the cerebral amines of the newborn animal. Protective action of MAO inhibiting drugs. *Medicina Experimentalis,* 19:293–300.

Prince, D. A. (1966): Modification of focal cortical epileptogenic discharge by afferent influences. *Epilepsia,* 7:181–201.

Prince, D. A. (1968a): Inhibition of "epileptic" neurons. *Experimental Neurology,* 21:307–321.

Prince, D. A. (1968b): The depolarization shift in "epileptic" neurons. *Experimental Neurology,* 21:467–485.

Prince, D. A. (1969a): Electrophysiology of "epileptic" neurons – spike generation. *Electroencephalography and Clinical Neurophysiology,* 26:476–487.

Prince, D. A. (1969b): Microelectrode studies of penicillin foci. In: *Basic Mechanisms of the Epilepsies,* edited by H. H. Jasper, A. A. Ward, Jr., and A. Pope. Little, Brown and Co., Boston, pp. 320–328.

Prince, D. A. (1971): Cortical cellular activities during cyclically occurring interictal epileptiform discharges. *Electroencephalography and Clinical Neurophysiology,* 31:469–484.

Prince, D. A., and Farrell, D. (1969): "Centrencephalic" spikewave discharges following parenteral penicillin injection in the cat. *Neurology,* 19:309–310.

Prince, D. A., and Futamachi, K. J. (1970): Intracellular recordings from chronic epileptogenic foci in the monkey. *Electroencephalography and Clinical Neurophysiology,* 29:496–510.

Prince, D. A., Futamachi, K. J., Logan, W., and Gutnick, M. (1969): Effects of DC polarization on cellular and EEG activities in cortical epileptogenic foci. *Physiologist,* 12:332.

Prince, D. A., and Gutnick, M. J. (1971): Cellular activities in epileptogenic foci of immature cortex. *Transactions of the American Neurological Association,* 96:88–91.

Prince, D. A., and Gutnick, M. (1972): Neuronal activities in epileptogenic foci of immature cortex. *Brain Research,* in press.

Prince, D. A., Lux, H. D., and Neher, E. (1972): Potassium activity in cat cortex measured with ion-sensitive microelectrodes. *Transactions of the American Neurological Association,* in press.

Prince, D. A., and Wilder, B. J. (1967): Control mechanisms in cortical epileptogenic foci. *Archives of Neurology,* 16:194–202.

Proler, M., and Kellaway, P. (1962): The methionine sulfoximine syndrome in the cat. *Epilepsia,* 3:117–130.

Proler, M. L., and Kellaway, P. (1965): Behavioral and convulsive phenomena induced in the cat by methionine sulfoximine: Ablation and electrographic studies. *Neurology,* 15:931–940.

Pscheidt, G. R., Benitez, D., Kirschner, L. B., and Stone, W. E. (1954): Effects of fluoroacetate poisoning on citrate, lacate and energy-rich phosphates in the cerebrum. *American Journal of Physiology,* 176:483–487.

Purpura, D. P., and McMurtry, J. G. (1965): Intracellular activities and evoked potential changes during polarization of motor cortex. *Journal of Neurophysiology,* 28:166–185.

Rall, W. (1967): Distinguishing theoretical synaptic potentials computed for different soma-dendritic distributions of synaptic input. *Journal of Neurophysiology,* 30:1072–1193.

Ralston, B. L. (1958): The mechanism of transition of interictal spiking foci into ictal seizure discharges. *Electroencephalography and Clinical Neurophysiology,* 10:217–232.

Ramwell, P. W., and Shaw, J. E. (1965): The effect of picrotoxin on motor activity and the electroencephalogram of mice. *British Journal of Pharmacology,* 24:651–658.

Roa, P. D., Tews, J. K., and Stone, W. E. (1964): A neurochemical study of thiosemicarbazide seizures and their inhibition by amino-oxyacetic acid. *Biochemical Pharmacology,* 13:477–487.

Roper, S., Diamond, J., and Yasargil, G. M. (1969): Does strychnine block inhibition postsynaptically? *Nature,* 223:1168–1169.

Rovit, R. L., and Swieciki, M. (1965): Some characteristics of multiple acute epileptogenic foci in cats. *Electroencephalography and Clinical Neurophysiology,* 18:608–616.

Rowe, W. B., and Meister, A. (1970): Identification of l-methionine-s-sulfoximine as the convulsant isomer of methionine sulfoximine. *Proceedings of the National Academy of Sciences*, 66:500–506.

Sakai, K., Yoshikawa, N., Kinoshita, Y., Oshika, H., and Nakai, K. (1964): Correlation between convulsive action and metabolism of Isoniazid. *Japanese Journal of Pharmacology*, 14:308–316.

Sawa, M., Maruyama, N., and Kaji, S. (1963): Intracellular potential during electrically induced seizures. *Electroencephalography and Clinical Neurophysiology*, 15:209–220.

Servit, Z. (1966): Comparative and cellular pathophysiology of epilepsy. *Excerpta Medica International Congress Series*, 124:1–359.

Servit, Z., and Strejckova, A. (1970): An electrographic epileptic focus in the fish forebrain. Conditions and pathways of propagation of focal and paroxysmal activity. *Brain Research*, 17:103–113.

Servit, Z., Strejckova, A., and Volanschi, D. (1968): An epileptogenic focus in the frog telencephalon. Pathways of propagation of focal activity. *Experimental Neurology*, 21: 383–396.

Shalit, M. N. (1965): The effect of metrazol on the hemodynamics and impedance of the cat's brain cortex. *Journal of Neuropathology and Experimental Neurology*, 24:75–84.

Sikdar, K., and Ghosh, J. J. (1964): Histological changes in structural constituents of spinal motoneurons after picrotoxin, strychnine and tetanus toxin administration. *Journal of Neurochemistry*, 11:545–549.

Speckman, E. J., and Caspers, H. (1969): Relations between EEG activity and postsynaptic potentials of spinal motoneurones during seizure discharges. *Electroencephalography and Clinical Neurophysiology*, 24:686–687.

Spehlmann, R., and Chang, C. M. (1969): Acetylcholine sensitivity of partially deafferented cortex. *Epilepsia*, 10:419.

Spehlmann, R., Daniels, J. C., and Chang, C. M. (1971): The effects of eserine and atropine on the epileptiform activity of chronically isolated cortex. *Epilepsia*, 12:123–132.

Stefanis, C., and Jasper, H. (1964): Intracellular microelectrode studies of antidromic responses in cortical pyramidal tract neurons. *Journal of Neurophysiology*, 27:828–854.

Stone, W. E. (1969): Action of convulsants: Neurochemical aspects. In: *Basic Mechanisms of the Epilepsies*, edited by H. H. Jasper, A. A. Ward, Jr., and A. Pope. Little, Brown and Co., Boston, pp. 184–193.

Stone, W. E. (1957): The role of acetylcholine in brain metabolism and function. *American Journal of Physical Medicine*, 36:222–255.

Stransky, Z. (1969): Time course of rat brain GABA levels following methionine sulphoximine treatment. *Nature*, 224:612–613.

Sugaya, E., Goldring, S., and O'Leary, J. L. (1964). Intracellular potentials associated with direct cortical response and seizure discharge in cat. *Electroencephalography and Clinical Neurophysiology*, 17:661–669.

Swanson, E. E. (1934): Short acting barbituric acid derivatives. *Proceedings of the Society for Experimental Biology and Medicine*, 31:963–964.

Swanson, E. E., and Chen, K. K. (1939): The aberrant action of sodium I: 3-dimethylbutyl-ethyl-barbiturate. *Quarterly Journal of Pharmacy and Pharmacology*, 12:657–660.

Swanson, P. D., and McIlwain, H. (1965): Inhibition of the sodium-ion-stimulated adenosine triphosphatase after treatment of isolated guinea pig cerebral cortex with ouabain and other agents. *Journal of Neurochemistry*, 12:877–891.

Sypert, G. W., Oakley, J., and Ward, A. A., Jr. (1970): Single-unit analysis of propagated seizures in neocortex. *Experimental Neurology*, 28:308–325.

Sze, P. Y., and Levell, R. A. (1970): A reexamination of the effect of thiosemicarbazide on brain GABA and glutamic decarboxylase in vivo. *Life Sciences*, 9:889–899.

Takeuchi, A., and Takeuchi, N. (1971): Anion interaction at the inhibitory post-synaptic membrane of the crayfish neuromuscular junction. *Journal of Physiology*, 212:337–351.

Tebecis, A. K., and Phillis, J. W. (1969): The use of convulsants in studying possible functions of amino acids in the toad spinal cord. *Comparative Biochemistry and Physiology*, 28: 1303–1315.

Tews, J. K. (1969): Pyridoxine deficiency and brain amino acids. *Annals of the New York Academy of Sciences*, 166:74–82.

Tews, J. K., Carter, S. H., Roa, P. D., and Stone, W. E. (1963): Free amino acids and related compounds in dog brain: Post-mortem and anoxic changes, effects of ammonium chloride infusion, and levels during seizures induced by picrotoxin and by pentylenetetrazol. *Journal of Neurochemistry*, 10:641–653.

Tews, J. K., and Stone, W. E. (1965): Free amino acids and related compounds in brain and other tissues: Effects of convulsant drugs. *Progress in Brain Research*, 16:135–163.

Tews, J. K., and Stone, W. E. (1964): Effects of methionine sulfoximine on levels of free amino acids and related substances in brain. *Biochemical Pharmacology*, 13:543.

Thompson, R. E., and Akers, T. K. (1970): Influence of sodium pentobarbital on mice poisoned by oxygen. *Aerospace Medicine*, 41:1025–1027.

Tokizane, T., and Sawyer, C. H. (1957): Sites of origin of hypoglycemic seizures in the rabbit. *Archives of Neurology and Psychiatry*, 77:259–266.

Torda, C. (1954): Effects of corticotropin and various convulsion-inducing agents on the P^{32} content of brain phospholipids, nucleoproteins and total acid-soluble phosphorus compounds. *American Journal of Physiology*, 177:179–182.

Tower, D. B. (1960): *Neurochemistry of Epilepsy*, Charles C Thomas, Springfield, Ill.

Tower, D. B. (1969): Neurochemical mechanisms. In: *Basic Mechanisms of the Epilepsies*, edited by H. H. Jasper, A. A. Ward, Jr., and A. Pope. Little, Brown and Co., Boston, pp. 611–646.

Uchida, T., and O'Brien, R. D. (1964a): The effects of hydrazines on rat brain 5-hydroxytryptamine, norepinephrine, and gamma-aminobutyric acid. *Biochemical Pharmacology*, 13: 725–730.

Uchida, T., and O'Brien, R. D. (1964b): The effects of hydrazines on pyridoxal phosphate in rat brain. *Biochemical Pharmacology*, 13:1143–1150.

Udvarhelyi, G. D., and Walker, A. E. (1965): Dissemination of acute focal seizures in the monkey. I. From cortical foci. *Archives of Neurology*, 12:333–356.

Usunoff, G., Atsev, E., and Tchavdarov, D. (1969): On the mechanisms of picrotoxin epileptic seizure (macro- and micro-electrode investigations). *Electroencephalography and Clinical Neurophysiology*, 27:444.

Van Meter, W. G., Owens, H. F., and Himwich, H. E. (1958): Cortical and rhinencephalic electrical potentials during hypoglycemia. *Archives of Neurology and Psychiatry*, 80:314–320.

Vastola, E. F., Homan, R., and Rosen, A. (1969): Inhibition of focal seizures by moderate hypothermia. A clinical and experimental study. *Archives of Neurology*, 20:430–439.

VonSchnakenburg, K., and Nolte, H. (1970): Histological studies of alterations in the rat brain under oxygen at high pressure. *Aerospace Medicine*, 41:1013–1017.

Wada, J. A., and Ikeda, H. (1966): Effect of atropine and eserine on the episodic behavioral and electrographic manifestations induced by methionine sulfoximine. *Experimental Neurology*, 16:450–463.

Wada, J. A., Terao, A., Scholtmeyer, H., and Trapp, W. G. (1970): Reversible audiogenic seizure susceptibility induced by hyperbaric oxygenation. *Experimental Neurology*, 29: 400–404.

Walsh, G. O. (1971): Penicillin iontophoresis in neocortex of cat—effects on the spontaneous and induced activity of single neurons. *Epilepsia*, 12:1–11.

Waltregny, A. (1969): Epilepsy and insulinic hypoglycemia: An experimental study. In: *The Physiopathogenesis of the Epilepsies*, edited by H. Gastaut, H. Jasper, J. Bancaud, and A. Waltregny. Charles C Thomas, Springfield, Ill., pp. 111–124.

Waltregny, A., and Mesdjian, E. (1969): Convulsive seizure and water intoxication: A polygraphic study. In: *The Physiopathogenesis of the Epilepsies*, edited by H. Gastaut, H. Jasper, J. Bancaud, and A. Waltregny. Charles C Thomas, Springfield, Ill., pp. 69–74.

Warren, K. S., and Schenker, S. (1964): Effects of an inhibitor of glutamine synthesis (methionine sulfoximine) on ammonia toxicity and metabolism. *Journal of Laboratory and Clinical Medicine*, 64:442–449.

Washizu, Y., Bonewell, G. W., and Terzuolo, C. A. (1961): Effect of strychnine upon the electrical activity of an isolated nerve cell. *Science*, 133:333–334.

Weir, F. W., Nemenzo, J. H., Bennett, S., and Meyers, F. H. (1964): A study of the mechanism of acute toxic effects of hydraxine, UDMH (1,1-dimethylhydrazine), MMH (methylhydrazine), and SDMH (1,2-dimethylhydrazine). *United States Air Force Technical Document Report Amrl*. TDR 64–26, 1–27.

4

Projection Phenomena and Secondary Epileptogenesis — Mirror Foci

B. J. Wilder

OUTLINE

I. INTRODUCTION

The choice of a model to study a pathological phenomenon of nature dictates that the model chosen must display certain characteristics which describe the phenomenon itself. A primary feature of focal cortical epilepsy is an abnormal electrical focus as recorded by the EEG which exhibits apparently autonomous epileptiform potentials which periodically alter their discharge features and change into paroxysms of sustained electrical seizure activity. This change would represent a second feature of focal cortical epilepsy. A third feature would be that the electrical seizure discharge would project and propagate to involve other areas of the brain including surrounding neuropil, contralateral cortex, and subcortical centers. Such a feature would result in a clinically recognizable alteration in behavior, i.e., a seizure, the fourth characteristic of human focal epilepsy. Ample clinical data attest to these four characteristics of focal epilepsy.

Some of the focal epilepsies, depending on their site of origin, have a fifth characteristic feature — that of inducing independent epileptiform alterations in distant areas of the brain. Clinicians who work primarily with epileptic patients and periodically examine their EEGs recognize that untreated or medically uncontrolled patients may become worse clinically and electroencephalographically with the passage of time even in the absence of anoxic, hypoxic, or other complicating factors. Secondary epileptic-like foci, both cortical and subcortical, develop and become autonomous or temporally independent in their discharge patterns from the original focus (Fischer-Williams and Cooper, 1963; Hughes, 1966, 1967; Takebayashi, 1966; Bancaud, 1967; Niedermeyer, 1968; Strobos, 1968). In other situations, the focal epileptic lesion may induce bilaterally synchronous EEG abnormalities from which the primary focus can only be separated by special diagnostic procedures (Bancaud, 1967; Stewart and Dreifuss, 1967).

The secondary focus subject to most investigations has been labeled the mirror focus because of its genesis in the cortex contralateral and homotopic to a primary epileptic lesion. In addition, secondary foci in subcortical cellular masses develop and have been investigated using physiological techniques.

A number of techniques have been used to study focal epilepsy. The application of various substances to the cortical surface results in alterations in EEG activity with the subsequent development of clinical seizures which are similar to those seen in the clinical situation. Alumina cream, cobalt, tungstic acid gel, cortical freezing, penicillin, tetanus toxin, strychnine, and a number of other metals and chemicals produce a focal cortical EEG lesion (see Chapters 1–3 and 5); however, the time span for development, the persistence of the focus, the genesis of secondary foci, and the spontaneous recurrent seizures vary with the agent used. With some exceptions, the electrical alterations recorded from cortical surface and from extra- and intracellular locations possess many similarities. The massive membrane depolarization of paroxysmal depolarization shift (Matsumoto and Ajmone Marsan, 1964*a,b*) has been recorded intracellularly from freeze lesions and those induced by alumina gel, cobalt, penicillin, and strychnine (Goldensohn, 1969). Other membrane phenomena such as aberrant spike initiation, fast prepotentials, propagated dendritic spikes, and axon spike generation have been described in the various models mentioned (Purpura, 1969; Ward, 1969). The artificially created cortical epileptic focus has been particularly suitable for study of the propagation of seizure discharge, the correlation of clinical seizure manifestations with site or origin, effect of drugs on seizure phenomena, and routes of propagation and projection of epileptiform abnormalities. Physiological studies of mirror and other secondary foci have utilized most of the agents mentioned for creation of the primary focus. However, the use of the primary lesion of the model systems mentioned in a study of microscopic, ultrastructural, enzymatic, or other neurobiochemical changes attendant to the epileptic process seems inappropriate with, perhaps, the exception of the freeze focus. All of the agents used produce nonspecific artifactual changes in the zone of the primary lesion depending on the particular epileptogenic agent selected. The use of the mirror focus model permits examination of an epileptic-like aggregate of neurons which is free of the contaminating effects of the agent used to create the primary lesion.

II. REVIEW AND CURRENT STATUS OF RESEARCH

A. Physiological data

1. Electroencephalographic and electrocorticographic data

For at least the last 35 years, investigators studying projection and propagation of EEG seizure discharge and clinical manifestations of seizures in experimental models have noted the spread of epileptiform discharge from a cortical focus to the contralateral homotopic cortex. Gozzano (1936) reported that the propagation of strychnine spikes from one cortex to a homologous area in the contralateral cortex was blocked by section of the corpus callosum. Erickson (1940) noted similarly that propagation of electrically induced seizure after-discharge to the contralateral cortex could be prevented by cutting the corpus callosum. Pacella et al. (1944), in studying focal seizures induced by alumina gel, observed one rhesus monkey that developed an independent, homotopic, contralateral EEG epileptic focus which they termed a mirror focus. Pope et al. (1947) noted independent epileptiform potentials in areas contralateral and homotopic to alumina lesions in monkeys; in one animal, the secondary focus persisted following corpus callosum section. Cure and Rasmussen (1950) reported similar findings in monkeys with alumina gel cortical foci. Morrell and Florenz (1958) observed the persistence of mirror foci in rabbits following ablation of an ethyl chloride-induced, primary, focal freeze epileptogenic lesion. Subsequently, Morrell (1959, 1960, 1961, 1964, 1969) and co-workers (1958, 1959, 1961) systematically studied and defined the physiological development of the mirror focus in several species of animals. These studies demonstrated that primary epileptic lesions created in certain areas of the cortex induced secondary lesions in the contralateral homologous cortex after varying time intervals, depending on the animal and epileptogenic agent used. The secondary focus initially has the characteristics of a projected, evoked discharge occurring after a time lapse consistent with a direct, evoked callosal response (Rutledge and Kennedy, 1961). The secondary focus subsequently becomes temporally independent of the primary focus in its epileptiform discharge characteristics. Section of the corpus callosum or major interhemispheric projection pathways prior to independency of the focus results in cessation of an epileptiform activity or projected discharges in the secondary focus. Similarly, isolation of the mirror focus from subcortical connections with the major interhemispheric projection pathway left intact prevents development of an autonomous secondary focus; however, projected abnormalities from the primary focus persist.

Thus, experimental physiological data indicate that the mirror focus requires two synaptic inputs for the development of independency, one direct via the major interhemispheric pathway and the other extracallosal and polysynaptic. At least two interhemispheric projection pathways, one direct via the corpus callosum and the other polysynaptic via the brainstem, have been demonstrated physiologically (Rutledge and Kennedy, 1961). Following the establishment of autonomous discharge, the secondary focus continues to generate epileptiform potentials for varying periods of time following isolation form the primary focus by interruption of the major interhemispheric pathway or by ablation of the primary lesion. Confirmation of these early studies has come from a number of investigators. Wilder and co-workers (1965, 1967, 1968, 1969, 1971) have used cortical freezing, alumina gel, penicillin, and cobalt in animals ranging from amphibians and reptiles to marsupials and higher mammals. Wada and Cornelius (1960), Guerrero-Figueroa et al. (1966), Holubar et al. (1966), Mutani (1967, 1968), Wada and Asakura (1968), and Westmoreland et al. (1970), and Chapter

21, to mention a few, have reported the development of an independent mirror foci following implantation of various focal cortical epileptogenic agents.

The development of independent secondary foci is not restricted to the homologous area of the contralateral cortex. Experimental data from many workers show that independent epileptic foci develop in areas which are richly innervated by efferents from a primary cortical epileptogenic lesion, regardless of the agent used to induce the original lesion. Wada (1958) described independent secondary foci developing in subcortical nuclear masses as a result of prolonged and sustained excitation from cortical epileptic foci. Suwa et al. (1954) reported the occurrence of independent spike activity in subcortical areas following repeated, electrically induced cortical seizures in animals. Wada and Cornelius (1960) produced alumina gel and freeze lesions in the peri-cruciate (sensory motor) cortex of cats and recorded from basal ganglia, thalamus, ipsilateral, and contralateral homologous areas of the cortex. Independent epileptogenic foci developed in all sites and persisted in subcortical structures following ablation of both the primary and cortical epileptic foci. Guerrero-Figueroa et al. (1964a,b, 1966), using alumina gel implants in the limbic system of experimental animals, further extended the physiological studies on secondary foci demonstrating their development in the amygdala, the septum, the hippocampus, and the hypothalamus.

Wilder and Schmidt (1965), in a chronic study of propagation of seizure discharge, made discrete alumina gel lesions in the sensory motor cortex of *Macaca mulatta* monkeys and noted preferential routes or propagation of seizure discharge to thalamus, basal ganglia, and reticular formation. All animals had focal motor and generalized seizures, and, after a period of 2 to 3 years, three animals with focal alumina gel implants without implanted cortical or subcortical electrodes were noted to develop a clinically different type of seizure, best described as tonic fits which persisted for 10 to 20 sec. Subsequent cortical and subcortical electrode implantation revealed the original primary focus and multiple autonomous subcortical foci (see Fig. 1). With the spontaneous occurrence of primarily subcortical electrical seizures, propagation was noted to proceed from various subcortical foci to all subcortical areas monitored, but not always to the cortex (Wilder et al., 1969). During tonic clinical seizures which occurred in one animal, polyspike discharges were recorded in the thalamus, basal ganglia, and reticular formation; however, an alerting type cortical EEG response was seen in recordings from bilateral cortical electrodes (Fig. 1). Similar EEG findings have been reported in patients with seizures of limbic system origin (Jasper, 1964; Freeman et al., 1970). Subsequent histological studies revealed pathological findings characteristic of the alumina gel focus (Stercova, 1966) at the primary lesion site and no consistent pathological changes in subcortical nuclei or contralateral cortex (Wilder et al., 1971).

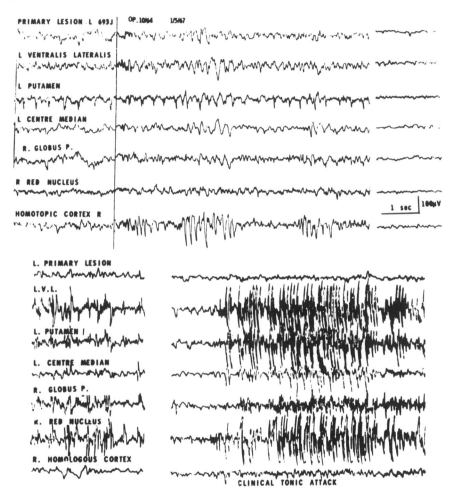

FIG. 1. Record from a rhesus monkey with primary alumina gel lesion in the left sensory motor cortex. Lesion was made 2 years and 7 months prior to recording. In the top record, active epileptiform discharge occurs at the mirror focus and in the left putamen. In the low left record, somewhat asynchronous epileptiform discharge occurs in right and left subcortical nuclei. No gross cortical abnormalities other than delta waves in the mirror focus are noted. In the right bottom record, tonic seizure discharge in the subcortical structures develops and produces a clinical tonic convulsion. The cortical surface electrodes show predominantly low-voltage fast activity.

2. Microelectrode recordings

In addition to corticographic and EEG data and depth recordings, extracellular and intracellular data have been obtained from dependent secondary foci. Ajmone Marsan (1963) reported on a microelectrode study of projected epileptiform discharges in the cortex contralateral to penicillin and strychnine foci. Animals were either studied under barbiturate anesthesia or as *cerveau isolé* preparations. Cellular activity within the primary focus was compared to that in the contralateral cortex. The findings differentiated primary focal from secondary projected discharges in that a smaller number of units were activated in the contralateral cortex and few units exhibited high-frequency burst discharge. In addition, inhibition of cellular discharge was a prominent feature in the projected focus. Ishijima and Walker (1969) reported microelectrode data from acute penicillin and chronic alumina gel foci and contralateral mirror foci. Data from the acute penicillin foci and contralateral secondary foci showed a much higher percentage of cells exhibiting burst activity in the primary focus. Also in this study, the dominant cellular response in the secondary focus was an arrest of firing during surface-recorded paroxysmal discharge. Many cells were seen whose background activity did not alter during surface epileptiform events. In the chronic animals, cellular activity in the mirror focus was to a much greater extent time-locked to ipsilateral surface-recorded paroxysmal activity, and a greater percent of the cells showed burst firing in association with surface discharge than in the previously described acute experiments. Some cells would change their firing characteristics during paroxysms of epileptiform activity recorded from the cortical surface.

Crowell (1970), in a study of cellular activity in the cortex contralateral to penicillin application and electrical stimulation, reported predominant arrest of cell discharge during surface paroxysmal discharges. Intracellular recording revealed long-lasting hyperpolarizing potentials during discharge arrest.

With the exception of the experiments of Ishijima and Walker (1969) on chronic foci, the above microelectrode studies were performed in models exhibiting projected discharge. This would correspond to the dependency stage of mirror focus development, and one might not expect changes in discharge patterns quantitatively similar to those in primary focus. Another important consideration is that most of the experiments described were performed with the animals under barbiturate anesthesia. One characteristic feature of projected discharges, particularly in the presence of barbiturate anesthesia, appears to be inhibitory in terms of cellular response.

Sypert et al. (1970), in a study of single-unit activity in cortex contralateral to repetitive electrical stimulation, have more clearly demonstrated the effect of barbiturate anesthesia on single-cell discharges. Furthermore, their study shows significant differences between projected paroxysmal discharges and propagated self-sustained seizure discharges. In barbiturate-anesthetized animals, the contralateral cellular response to repetitive electrical stimulation was primarily inhibitory with cessation of unit firing as reported in the above studies. In unanesthetized animals, almost all recorded units became involved in propagated ictal discharges. Characteristic ictal membrane changes of massive depolarization shift with high-frequency burst firing, failure of hyperpolarization, and cathodal inactivation were observed in a focus of neurons synaptically driven from a transcallosal site subject to electrical stimulation. These changes in cellular behavior contralateral and homotopic to the initiating stimulus are indistinguishable, both qualitatively and quantitatively, from those in a primary focus. Thus, an autonomous, independent, though transient, mirror focus developed as a result of massive synaptic bombardment. Wilder and Morrell (1967) recorded alterations in cellular firing patterns in independent mirror foci in the frog forebrain which are characteristic of interictal cellular activity seen in primary epileptic foci. This study, performed on the unanesthetized frog forebrain, revealed epileptogenic change of a quasi-permanent nature.

3. Excitability changes during epileptogenesis

Forsythe et al. (1969) studied alterations in cortical excitability as measured by responses to visual stimulation. Discrete, intracortical alumina gel lesions were made in the marginal gyrus of cats at the site where the largest visually evoked responses (VERs) could be recorded. Serial EEG recordings and single and computer-averaged VERs were obtained over an 18-month period. Within 15 to 30 days following alumina gel implantation, spontaneous epileptiform paroxysmal discharges (PDs) were recorded at the primary focus. Initial positive and negative components of the VER were enhanced in the primary focus and remained similar to control VERs in the contralateral cortex. During this initial period, projected PDs were recorded in the mirror focus. Between 30 and 45 days, spontaneous PDs occurred independently in the mirror focus, and single and averaged VERs became enhanced and equal in magnitude to those seen in the primary focus. After 45 days, the VERs in the mirror focus exceeded those recorded in the primary focus, and thereafter some diminution of the VERs occurred in the primary. After the 30- to 45-day period, strobic flash stimuli triggered epileptiform potentials bilaterally or unilaterally and independently in the primary and secondary foci. Often, photic stimuli

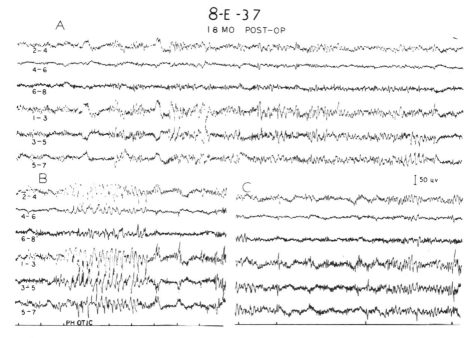

8-E -37

A

I 8 MO POST-OP

FIG. 2. *A:* Cat with marginal gyrus epileptic focus created by alumina gel 18 months earlier. Lesion size at time of sacrifice was approximately 2 to 3 mm in diameter and extended to corti cal layer IV. A gliotic scar surrounded the lesion. Electrodes 2, 4, 6, and 8 were arranged in an anterior-posterior fashion from the left pericruciate area to the occipital pole. The lesion was under electrode #4. Electrodes 1, 3, 5, and 7 were at homotopic points over the contra-lateral cortex. Note the spontaneous epileptic activity in the mirror focus. *B:* Photic stimu-lation at 1/sec stimulates electrical seizure in the mirror focus which spreads to the primary focus. *C:* Intermittent photic stimulation evokes markedly enhanced evoked responses at the mirror site.

triggered paroxysms of after-discharges which commenced bilaterally synchronously or in either focus before spreading to the contralateral side (see Fig. 2). Flash stimuli greater than 5/sec frequently induced electro-graphic and occasionally induced clinical seizures which were initiated electrically in either the primary or secondary focus. The decrease in amplitude of early components of the primary focus VER is probably as-sociated with gliosis and deafferentation secondary to the effects of alumina gel. Routine histological and Golgi studies of the primary and secondary foci revealed gliosis and loss of dendritic spines similar to findings reported by Westrum et al. (1964) and Wilder et al. (1971). Careful examination of Golgi sections failed to reveal consistent abnormalities in the region of the mirror focus. Some dendritic spine changes were noted and interpreted as being secondary to transcallosal degeneration.

The early period of heightened sensitivity of the primary focus occurring 15 to 20 days post-lesion corresponds to the dependency phase of secondary focus development. By the time a decrease in the VER occurred in the primary focus after 45 days, the mirror focus had become independent.

Experiments conducted by Goddard and co-workers (1969) are pertinent to any consideration of epileptogenic change secondary to excessive synaptic bombardment. Brief bursts of nonpolarizing electrical brain stimulation delivered daily at a constant intensity resulted in progressive changes in excitability leading to localized electrical seizures, focal seizures, and bilateral clonic convulsions with each successive period of stimulation. In the rat, optimal stimulus parameters were 50 μA peak to peak of 1-msec duration at a frequency of 60 Hz for 60 sec at daily intervals. More frequent stimulations retarded or prevented the effect. Stimulation within limbic structures resulted in convulsions within 15 days. A similar response was obtained in monkeys; however, a longer period was required and a larger current was used. Observation and parametric studies indicated that the effect which has been labeled "kindling" is due to electrical activation and not tissue damage. Changes induced by kindling are permanent, and experimental data indicate that the effects are mediated by synaptic mechanisms. Kindling in one area was shown to facilitate the development of secondary kindling in synaptically related regions. The analogy between secondary foci evoked by synaptic input from a primary focus and the kindling phenomenon is striking. In kindling, the stimulating electrode provides the synaptic drive.

B. Anatomical and histological correlates

Physiological studies have demonstrated the importance of the corpus callosum in the genesis of secondary foci. Following the establishment of an independent mirror focus, section of the corpus callosum or ablation of the primary lesion does not, for varying periods of time, significantly alter paroxysmal activity at the mirror site. The anatomical distribution of efferent projections from the primary focus to the mirror focus are pertinent to its evolution. Meyerson (1968) has shown in sheep cortex that callosal connections of bilateral homologous cortical fields are arranged in a point-to-point manner. Jacobsen (1965, 1966) demonstrated that axons of large pyramidal cells of the rat cortex bifurcate and then pass into the corpus callosum and project onto the striatum and thalamus, as originally suggested by Lorente de Nó (1922). Globus and Scheibel (1967) traced the termination of callosal fibers between homotopic visual association cortex to the oblique branches of apical dendrites of pyramidal cells. Jacobson and Marcus (1970) compared laminar distribution of fibers of corpus callosum by Fink-Heimer procedure for degenerating axons and axon terminals in the rat, cat, and primates. In the rat, terminal degeneration was heaviest in layers Ib+, II, and III, and lightest in IV. In the cat, layers III and IV showed intense terminal degeneration; degenerating terminals were lightest in V and VI. The monkey and chimpanzee differed, with layers Ib and II containing no degenerating terminals and layers III and IV showing heaviest degeneration. This study implies interspecies differences with regard to the role of the corpus callosum in transmission of epileptic discharges. Westmoreland et al. (1971), in a histochemical study of epileptogenesis in rats, found heavy degeneration of callosal fibers in layers V and VI. Histopathological changes in primary foci created with cobalt were restricted to the top three layers of the cortex. Also, sacrifice occurred at 21 days, somewhat late for fine-fiber degeneration.

These data indicate that callosal synaptic input in the species with contralateral cortices terminate in granular layers whereas in the rat's smooth cortex, the main callosal input is to supragranular layers. These anatomical differences should be considered in the selection of a model for either physiological or histochemical study of secondary epileptogenesis.

C. Biochemical data

1. RNA changes in secondary foci

Morrell (1961), in histological studies of the mirror focus, found nests of cells which stained heavily with methyl green pyronin, an RNA acid stain. This characteristic staining did not occur if sections were pretreated with ribonuclease. Later studies on histological sections from mirror foci were performed using more specific and reliable RNA stains, Azure B and gallo-cyanin (Morrell, 1964). Again, pretreatment with ribonuclease prevented uptake of the RNA stains. Dark-staining sclerotic cells similar to those found by Morrell in the mirror focus had previously been reported in human epileptic foci (Penfield and Humphreys, 1940) and later in experimental lesions (Stercova, 1966), and were equated with cortical injury and ciatrix formation. Subsequent studies on RNA turnover in mirror foci, using tritiated uridine, were done by Engel and Morrell (1970). Autoradiographic techniques were used to measure neuronal uptake of the radioactive precursor in an attempt to measure the rate of RNA synthesis. The uptake of tritiated uridine was markedly reduced in the dense cells showing increased staining with Azure B and Gallo-cyanin. Uptake of the radioactive precursor by other normal-appearing cells in the mirror focus was similar to that in control sections.

Westmoreland and co-workers (1971) measured RNA in the mirror focus by a histochemical technique which permitted a quantitative laminar analysis of these nucleic acids. RNA was reduced in all layers of the cortex. A decrease in RNA in the mirror focus is consistent with RNA studies which show that neuronal hyperactivity leads to depletion of the nucleic acid (Einarson and Krogh, 1955).

2. Membrane mechanisms and cationic transport in primary and secondary foci

Tower (1969), in discussing models for the study of biochemical mechanisms of epileptogenicity, placed particular emphasis on studies involving transport of cations across neuronal membranes. Defects in the mechanisms which maintain intracellular potassium and extrude excess sodium so the potential energy in the form of ionic gradients is available to support the controlled responses to incoming stimuli may play a central role in epileptic processes. Interference with the cation pump results in leakage of sodium and potassium down their concentration gradients, resulting in membrane depolarization, membrane instability, and the subsequent generation of spontaneous discharges which, if of sufficient intensity, spread locally and distantly producing a full-blown seizure (Tower, 1969).

During the past 10 years, ample evidence has accumulated to show that Na,K-ATPase plays an integral role in the active membrane transport system for sodium and potassium within the central nervous system. Ouabain significantly inhibits active transport of these cations at concentrations of 10^{-5} M by binding Na,K-ATPase (Albers et al., 1968). Thus, ouabain may be used as a model system for the study of defective membrane sodium and potassium transport mechanisms.

Recent studies utilizing freeze and mirror epileptic foci have revealed defects in the sodium and potassium transport mechanism at the synaptic membrane level. These data have been compared with studies performed on ouabain interference with cation transport. Lewin and McCrimmon (1967, 1968) studied the intralaminar distribution of Na,K-ATPase in freeze epileptogenic lesions and in mirror foci in the rat cortex (see Chapter 2). The animals were killed at 4, 8, and 24 hr after lesioning, and values for Na,K-ATPase were obtained. The techniques permitted sampling in each cortical layer. In the primary focus, significant elevations were found at 8 hr after lesioning. At 24 hr, values had returned to near normal in the primary; in the mirror focus, however, values were significantly increased above normal. The maximum Na,K-ATPase activity changed in the different cortical layers depending on the time of sacrifice—4, 8, or 24 hr. In the mirror focus, the 4-hr peak occurred in layer Vb; the 8-hr peak resembled the 4-hr peak of the primary focus (layer V); and the 24-hr level was elevated in layers I–III and V and VI above the primary focus and control samples. The 24-hr elevations were thought to coincide with the occurrence of independent epileptiform activity in the mirror focus.

The data were interpreted as indicating increased sodium-potassium transport at the synaptic membrane level. Earlier studies showed that Na,K-ATPase is largely restricted to neuronal structures (Cummins and Hyden, 1962). Subsequent studies by Lewin (1971) compared the effect of ouabain applied locally to the cortex with cortical freezing. Analyses for sodium, potassium, water content, and Na,K-ATPase were performed on the primary focus and contralateral cortex.

Escueta and Reilly (1971) and Escueta and Appel (1969, 1970a,b, 1972) have utilized a synaptic membrane model to study cation transport in primary freeze lesions and mirror foci. They have used the model for study of the diphenylhydantoin effect on sodium-potassium transport and of ouabain interference with cation transport, and have compared defects in cation transport in primary and secondary foci with normal controls.

The technique employs differential centrifugation for separation of synaptic membrane fractions (synaptosomes) containing vesicles, presynaptic terminals, and mitochondria from the synaptic membrane. Synaptosome metabolic activities are independent of neuron axonal and soma membrane. Synaptosomes accumulate potassium against a concentration gradient in vitro. This reaction depends on Na,K ATPase as evidenced by ouabain inhibition and requirements for ATP and sodium. Synaptosomes possess an energy-dependent transport system for sodium and are rich in Na,K-ATPase (Appel et al., 1969; Bradford, 1969; Escueta and Appel, 1972).

Synaptosomes isolated from primary and mirror foci showed no changes in baseline potassium. However, total potassium accumulation and ouabain inhibition were markedly decreased within synaptosomes of both primary and mirror foci. In the mirror focus, potassium uptake and ouabain inhibition were always present but were significantly decreased when compared to synaptosomes from controls. Studies on freeze lesions which did not develop epileptogenic discharge failed to show the above defects. Experiments were done on rats with lesions varying from 1 to 28 weeks. Abnormalities in sodium and potassium transport could be correlated with abnormal paroxysmal discharge in both primary and mirror foci. Alterations in synaptic activity as demonstrated by these studies on the mirror focus were associated with epileptic activity rather than structural damage.

3. Histochemical studies of secondary foci

Westmoreland and co-workers (1971) combined microchemical techniques with histological and EEG studies to investigate mirror foci in the rat cortex. Primary lesions were created by the topical application of cobalt. The intralaminar distribution of DNA, RNA, and ganglioside sialic acid were assayed in the mirror focus, and results were compared with similar nonepileptogenic control specimens and with cortex of rats subjected to coagulative lesions in the contralateral homotopic cortex.

Twenty-one days after cobalt application, persistent spike activity was seen in the contralateral homotopic cortical area ("mirror focus") associated with suppression of electrical activity at the site of the primary lesion. In contrast, animals subjected to a coagulative lesion showed a similar suppression of electrical activity at the site of injury, but no spike activity in the contralateral homotopic cortical area. Both the cobalt and coagulative lesions consisted of a 2-mm cup-shaped area of neuronal loss with astroglial proliferation. The cobalt lesion differed, however, in that it extended to variable depths in the cortex and showed an inflammatory response in the leptomeninges. In both experimental animals, coronal sections stained with Nauta's method showed abundant axonal degeneration surrounding the site of injury in addition to transcallosal axonal degeneration in layers V and VI of the contralateral homotopic cortical area.

In the area of secondary epileptogenesis induced by cobalt, DNA, an index of cellularity, showed no change in layers I through IV, but increased 18 to 35% in layers V and VI. A similar abnormality (11 to 37% DNA increase) was found in the homotopic cortex of animals subjected to contralateral coagulative lesions, suggesting that a mild proliferation of astroglia is associated with transcallosal axonal degeneration. However, RNA, an index of protein-synthesizing ribosomal organelles, was reduced by 25% in all cortical layers, whereas ganglioside sialic acid, an index of axodendritic arborization and synaptic mass (Wiegant, 1967), increased significantly in layers II through V, with a maximum elevation of 78% occurring in layer IV of the cobalt-induced mirror focus. In animals subjected to the coagulative lesions, RNA and ganglioside sialic acid levels in the homotopic area contralateral to the site of cortical injury were the same as in control areas of the cortex.

The results suggest that cortical lesions induced either by cobalt or coagulation result in transcallosal fiber degeneration and mild reactive astroglial proliferation in the homotopic cortical area contralateral to the site of injury, and this finding cannot be directly correlated with abnormal cortical epileptic activity. However, a pathologic diminution of protein-synthesizing ribosomal organelles in association with either an elaboration of synaptic contacts or a functional disturbance of ganglioside-related ion transport in neuronal membranes may correlate with the abnormal electrophysiological state of secondary epileptogenesis (G. Hanna and N. Bass, 1971, *personal communication*).

4. Amino acid and folate studies in primary and secondary foci

Saradshizhvili and co-workers (1970) have compared gamma-aminobutyric acid (GABA), glutamic acid, aspartic acid, and glutamine in primary cortical lesions and in dependent and independent mirror foci with normal cortex. Significant changes in the amino acid levels were found in primary foci and independent mirror foci when compared to normal cortex. No significant changes were noted in dependent mirror foci. Amino acid levels in independent mirror foci and primary foci were similar. Amino acid changes have recently been reported in human and experimental epileptic foci (van Gelder et al., 1971; van Gelder and Courtois, 1972). A decrease in GABA, aspartic acid, and glutamic acid, and an increase in glycine and taurine, were reported in human epileptogenic cortex (van Gelder, 1972). In experimental animals (cats with cortical epileptic lesions induced with cobalt), glutamic acid, aspartic acid, and GABA were decreased maximally at the focus and less so in contralateral homotopic and visual cortices, whereas glycine and glutamine were found to be increased. These studies were correlated with overall seizure activity and not with the development of secondary foci (van Gelder and Courtois, 1972).

Streiff et al. (1971) measured monoglutamic and polyglutamic acid in primary and mirror foci in cats and in a rhesus monkey with cobalt primary lesions in the cats and alumina gel lesion in the monkey. All animals had primary, independent mirror foci at the time of sacrifice which varied from 1 to 8 weeks in the cats and was 8 months in the monkey.

In the cats, monoglutamic acid was significantly elevated in both primary and mirror foci, ranging between two and three times greater than that in control cats. There were no significant differences in polyglutamic acid content between primary and mirror foci and control animals. In the monkey, the polyglutamate was 60 ng/mg and protein was 26 ng/mg in the primary and mirror foci, respectively, with control samples having 2.05

ng/mg of protein. There was no significant difference in monoglutamic acid content between primary and mirror foci and control samples, which ranged from 1 to 4 ng/mg of protein in the monkey.

The differences between the mono- and polyglutamic forms in the cats and monkey cannot be explained except possibly by the chronicity of the monkey primary and mirror foci (8 months post-lesion). Folate functions to transport or donate one-carbon fragments in synthetic reactions and is primarily involved in RNA and DNA metabolism (Stokstad and Koch, 1967). Folate could play a role in energy metabolism on the cortex in epileptic foci. The polyglutamate molecule traps seven glutamic acid molecules (Stokstad and Koch, 1967) and could be involved in the glutamate shunt; however, this mechanism of action has not been proven. Derangements in glutamate and GABA acid have been shown in human cortical and experimental foci (van Gelder et al., 1971; van Gelder and Courtois, 1972).

III. CHOICE OF A MODEL FOR STUDYING SECONDARY FOCI

A. Species differences

The choice of an animal model to study secondary epileptogenesis depends, to a great extent, upon the type of experiment planned and data to be collected. It has been my experience that a wide variety of animal species will develop secondary epileptic foci contralateral to an active primary epileptic foci created by any number of epileptogenic agents. Wilder et al. (1968) have studied the development of secondary foci in:

frogs (amphibian)	unconvoluted forebrain
caymans (reptile)	" "
opossums (marsupials)	" "
rabbits (rodents)	" "
rats (rodents) (*unpublished*)	" "
cats (*Carnivora*)	convoluted forebrain
dogs (*Carnivora*) (*unpublished*)	" "
squirrel monkey (old and new world primates)	unconvoluted forebrain
rhesus monkey (old and new world primates)	convoluted forebrain

In general, mirror foci develop more rapidly in animals low on the evolutionary scale and in animals with an unconvoluted forebrain. Servít presents data in Chapter 21 which is pertinent to epileptogenesis in submammalian species. Table 1 provides data on the rapidity of development of a secondary foci in several vertebrate models (Wilder et al., 1968). Stalmaster and Hanna (1972) report much earlier development following discrete cortical freezing lesions. The data presented clearly show that the time span for development of the secondary focus is related to the rapidity of development of the agent used to induce the primary focus. It has been our experience that the genesis of the secondary focus is influenced not only by the rapidity of development of the primary focus but also by the activity of the primary focus. The more active primary focus (in terms of PDs generated) results in the more rapid development of an independent secondary or mirror focus. Certainly, other factors influence the appearance of the secondary focus following creation of a primary lesion. The size and the cortical depth of the primary focus, the epileptogenic agent used, the animal chosen, the reinforcement with sensory stimulation, and the cortical site chosen are all factors which may influence the time course between creation of the primary focus and the development of the secondary focus. Sophistication of recording techniques may lead to earlier detection of the secondary focus. Stalmaster and Hanna (1972), using multiple corti-

TABLE 1. Time course for independent secondary epileptogenesis

Vertebrate model	Epileptogenic agent used to create primary focus	Time span for secondary focus development
		Less than
Amphibian — Frog	penicillin	60 min
Reptile — Cayman	penicillin	4 hr
Mammals		
Marsupial		
Opossum	penicillin	12 hr
Rodent		
Rat	penicillin	12 hr
Rabbit	cortical freeze	10 days
Carnivora[a]		
Cat (1)	cortical freeze	21 days
Cat (2)	alumina gel	45 days
Primates		
Squirrel monkey	alumina gel	3 months
Rhesus monkey	alumina gel	5 months

[a] See Table 2 for results using cobalt.

cal electrodes, noted extremely early development of mirror foci after cortical freezing.

The overall yield rate for independent secondary epileptogenic foci has been high in our experience. Following the development of a primary focus, mirror foci can be anticipated in over 80% of animals. Again, many factors are involved; however, a high yield rate occurs when models with an unconvoluted cortex are used. Primary epileptic foci in the marginal gyrus or temporal lobe cortex in the cat are followed by mirror foci development in over 80% of the animals in our experience.

For the investigator planning chronic, semiacute, or acute experiments designed to collect primarily physiological data, the cat is an excellent choice. Because of regional cortical differences in projection to the contralateral hemisphere, the site chosen for the creation of a primary focus is of importance. Kreindler (1970) has pointed out regional differences in the interhemispheric propagation of cortical epileptogenic foci. We would recommend using the marginal gyrus for the primary lesion. The subsequent development of the primary focus can be studied with photic stimulation. In this manner, excitability changes can be monitored and PDs triggered (Forsythe et al., 1969). The marginal gyrus is easily accessible surgically, and, should corpus callosum section be planned at a later time, it can be easily accomplished from the original craniotomy site or from the mirror focus side. Macro- and microelectrode studies can be performed on the primary and mirror foci in this preparation (see Chapter 8 for details). The cat historically has been the subject of most microelectrode studies.

Alternate locations for the creation of the primary focus are the pericruciate cortex or temporal cortex in the cat, and although operative techniques to approach these areas are more difficult, they are not prohibitively so. Chronic electrode implantation in the pericruciate region presents some problems, which have been solved in an elegant manner by Stalmaster and Hanna (1972). The pericruciate cortex can be stimulated by physiological stimuli applied to the contralateral limbs, as so well demonstrated by Stalmaster and Hanna.

Primary lesions can be readily made in hippocampus and amygdala by the use of stereotactic techniques (Guerrero-Figueroa et al., 1964a,b, 1966). Bipolar recording electrodes can be constructed from Teflon-coated, narrow-gauge stainless steel and implanted stereotactically into desired limbic and other subcortical nuclei.

The cat is again an excellent choice as a model to study biochemical alterations in mirror or secondary foci (Streiff et al., 1970; van Gelder and Courtois, 1972). However, in the majority of studies reported, the rat or the rabbit has been utilized (Morrell, 1964; Engel and Morrell, 1970;

Lewin and McCrimmon, 1970*a,b*, 1972; Westmoreland et al., 1971; Lewin, 1971; Escueta and Reilly, 1971). Precise techniques for biochemical determinations and techniques should be obtained from original articles or from the investigator himself.

The use of primates is particularly desirable when clinical, physiological, and biochemical correlations are of importance. The disadvantages are expense, maintenance, and handling. In the study of secondary epileptogenesis, the use of high-order primates is important because of inferences which may be made in relation to the human clinical situation. Techniques and experiments have been reported by Wilder and co-workers (1965, 1968, 1969).

The choice of the agent to induce the primary lesion may be of considerable importance depending on the data to be collected.

B. Techniques

Cortical freezing permits direct correlations of findings from primary and mirror foci. The use of metallic or other chemical agents has the disadvantage of the contaminating effect of the agent used. Malzone et al. (1971) have modified a cobalt technique described by Payan et al. (1965) and Fischer et al. (1967). Metallic cobalt powder is suspended in gelatin and subsequently treated with formalin. Pellets containing approximately 10 mg of powdered cobalt are then implanted on either pial surface, extradurally or on the inner calvarial table. Epileptic discharge develops either rapidly or in a slower, more sequential, fashion, depending on the locus of the cobalt. Table 2 gives the time course of development of primary and secondary epileptiform discharge characteristics using this technique.

Figure 3 illustrates the histology of the three lesions. The inner table implantation produces minimal cortical damage, restricted primarily to the upper layers of the cortex. This model is excellent for studying anticonvulsant drug effects on primary and secondary epileptogenesis. It also lends itself to biochemical studies on the mirror focus. The pial and extradural lesions induce rapid epileptogenesis and mirror focus formation and would be excellent for physiological studies because of the excessive epileptiform activity recorded at the mirror and primary sites. Recurrent clinical seizures occur with these techniques but rarely with the inner table implantation of the gelatin pellet. Use of the alumina gel model has obvious advantages in chronic long-term experiments in which clinical phenomena are to be observed along with physiological studies.

The method or technique used for the creation of the primary focus with any of the epileptogenic agents is often critical. Figure 3 illustrates

TABLE 2.   *Time courses of epileptic discharge characteristics using cobalt*

Epileptiform discharge characteristics	Time course (days post-surgery)		
	Locus of cobalt		
	Extradural[a]	Epidural[b]	Subdural[c]
Ipsilateral spikes	8.3 (6–11)	2.2 (1–3)	1.0 (1)
Dependent secondary spikes	12.0 (11–12)	4.4 (2–7)	1.5 (1–2)
Independent secondary spikes	18.6 (14–22)	6.4 (2–8)	2.0 (1–4)
Photic induced after-discharge	21.0 (16–27)	6.0 (2.8)	2.0 (1–4)
Bilateral polyspike-and-wave	22.3 (20–27)	7.2 (2–9)	1.5 (1–2)

Values given as mean (range in parentheses).
[a] Three animals.
[b] Five animals.
[c] Two animals.

the pathological changes which occur with similar amounts of cobalt implanted in different loci.   Stalmaster and Hanna (1972) have described a freezing technique which gives excellent reproduction of lesions in different animals.   This study on primary and secondary epileptogenesis secondary to cortical freezing can be used as a model of a well-designed and controlled experiment which is adaptable for electrophysiological, histological, and chemical studies of primary and mirror foci.   Their report gives more complete and precise physiological information on the genesis of primary and secondary foci following freeze lesions than do prior studies (see Chapter 2). In creating the freeze focus, we prefer using liquid nitrogen to cool a metallic instrument which is then applied to the pial or dural surface for a designated period of time.   The cortex is then flooded with saline to avoid tearing when the instrument is removed.   This technique permits replication of similar lesions in different animals.   Lesion size can be varied by changing sizes of instruments or by varying the time the instrument is left in contact with the cortical surface.

The synapse membrane model (Escueta and Appel, 1971) appears ideal for studies of membrane energy metabolism and cation transport in seizure states.   In addition to the studies reported above, the authors used this model to study diphenylhydantoin action.   Their data indicate that the primary site of diphenylhydantoin effect is the membrane sodium-potassium pump.   In epileptic foci, the drug appears to have a direct action on the synapse membrane which is independent of its action on membrane pump

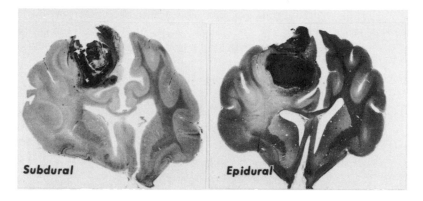

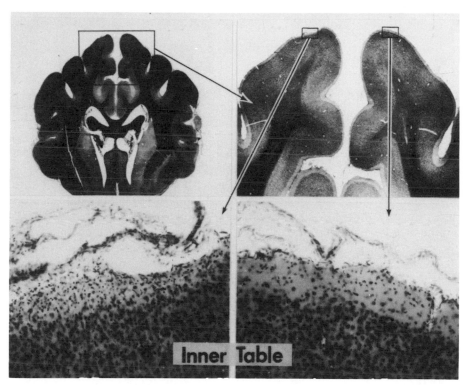

FIG. 3. *A:* Formalin-fixed cobalt gelatin pellets applied to cats' pial and dural surfaces. Marked tissue destruction resulted. However, these lesions induced an active independent mirror focus. The animals had clinical seizures. *B:* Inner calvarial table-placed cobalt pellet resulted in gliosis and some tissue destruction of molecular layer with cellular response in top two layers of cortex. A mild meningeal reaction occurred. The animal developed an active primary and independent mirror focus; however, no clinical seizures were noted.

activity. Diphenylhydantoin was shown to enhance synaptosome potassium influx in the presence of ouabain, provided that the sodium concentration was high (50 mM). Thus, the synapse membrane model appears to be suitable for many studies involving anticonvulsant and other drug action. These studies complement the ATPase studies of Lewin (1971), and Lewin and McCrimmon (1967, 1968).

The technique for lamina analysis of nucleic acids and lipoproteins used in the studies by Westmoreland et al. (1971) is particularly suitable for histochemical studies of epileptic foci and the cortex in general. Thus, the potentialities for qualitative and quantitative histochemical analyses of tissues and cells, definable by low- and high-power light microscopy, are now considerable. Baseline data on the histochemistry and cytochemistry of the nervous system are available (Adams, 1965; Friede, 1966). The application of some of these techniques in the study of primary and mirror foci have been reviewed.

IV. SUMMARY

The secondary epileptogenic or mirror focus has been shown to be an autonomous area of paroxysmal discharge which develops from continued synaptic activation from a primary epileptic lesion. As an electrical phenomenon, the independent mirror focus exists as an epileptic-like entity.

The advantages of using this model to study epileptic abnormalities are primarily those of studying an area uncontaminated by the agent used to create the primary lesion. The physiological and histochemical data presented indicate that certain changes of at least a quasi-permanent nature have occurred in the secondary focus. The exact nature of these changes and their significance are open for further research, both from biochemical and physiological approaches. The mirror focal phenomena in the experimental situation would appear to represent a true epileptic change.

The secondary focus seems particularly suited for research endeavors as described by Curtis in this volume (see Chapter 10). The application of biochemical and histochemical techniques, presented earlier, has yielded significant data concerning the mirror focus; however, the model is particularly well suited for extending such studies.

The primary disadvantage of using the mirror focus model is the uncertainty about if it is, in fact, pertinent to the clinical problem of epilepsy. The need for prospective long-term clinical studies to define the clinical significance of the electrical secondary focus phenomenon is apparent. A technical disadvantage is that the experimenter has to wait for the secondary focus to develop after the creation of the primary lesion. In biochemical studies, the location of the secondary focus must be carefully identified by electrical recording techniques so that tissue analyzed is indeed from the appropriate area (see Stalmaster and Hanna, 1972, for their precise recording techniques).

The secondary focus has repeatedly been said to result from repetitive synaptic activation. However, when metallic or chemical agents are used in the creation of the primary lesion, transfer of the inciting epileptogenic agent to the mirror site could occur. Transcallosal axoplasmic flow has not been ruled out. The use of cortical freezing to produce the primary lesion would seem to exclude such a possibility; however, biochemical changes induced by freezing might be transported to the mirror site by the axoplasmic route.

It is hoped that the phenomena of secondary epileptogenesis will serve as a stimulus for further investigation and that this chapter will provide background and technical information for devising appropriate experimental designs.

V. ACKNOWLEDGMENTS

This investigation was supported by a Veterans Administration Medical Research Grant, and by U.S. Public Health Service grants NB–06881 from the National Institute of Neurological Diseases and Stroke, RR–00421, and MO1 RR 0082 08.

VI. REFERENCES

Adams, C. W. (ed.) (1965): *Neurohistochemistry*. Elsevier, Amsterdam.
Albers, R., Koval, G., and Siegel, G. (1968): Studies on the interaction of ouabain and other cardioactive steroids with sodium-potassium activated adenosine triphosphatase. *Molecular Pharmacology*, 4:324.
Appel, S. H., Festoff, B. W., Autillo, L., and Escueta, A. V. (1969): Biochemical studies of synapses. III. Ionic activation of protein synthesis. *Journal of Biological Chemistry*, 244:3166–3172.
Bancaud, J. (1967): Multiple focal origin of certain cortical epilepsies. *Electroencephalography and Clinical Neurophysiology*, 23:581.
Bradford, H. P. (1969): Respiration *in vitro* of synaptosomes from mammalian cerebral cortex. *Journal of Neurochemistry*, 16:657–684.
Crowell, R. M. (1970): Distant effects of focal epileptogenic process. *Brain Research*, 18:137–154.

Cummins, J., and Hyden, H. (1962): Adenosine triphosphate and adenosine triphosphatases in neurons, glia, and neuronal membranes of the vestibular nucleus. *Biochemica Biophysica Acta*, 60:271.

Cure, C., and Rasmussen, T. (1950): Experimental epileptogenic lesions of the cerebral motor cortex and the insular cortex in monkeys. *Electroencephalography and Clinical Neurophysiology*, 2:254.

Einarson, L., and Krough, E. (1955): Variations in the basophilia of nerve cells associated with increased cell activity and functional stress. *Journal of Neurology, Neurosurgery, and Psychiatry*, 18:1–16.

Engel, J., Jr., and Morrell, F. (1970): Turnover of RNA in normal and secondary epileptogenic rabbit cortex. *Experimental Neurology*, 26:221–238.

Erickson, T. C. (1940): Spread of epileptic discharge: An experimental study of the afterdischarge induced by electrical stimulation of the cerebral cortex. *Archives of Neurology and Psychiatry*, 43:429–452.

Escueta, A. V., and Appel, S. H. (1969): Biochemical studies of synapses II. K transport. *Biochemistry*, 8:725–733.

Escueta, A. V., and Appel, S. H. (1970a): The effects of electrically induced seizures on potassium transport within isolated nerve terminals. *Neurology*, 20:392.

Escueta, A. V., and Appel, S. H. (1970b): Diphenylhydantoin and potassium transport in isolated nerve terminals. *Journal of Clinical Investigation*, 49:27a–28a.

Escueta, A. V., and Appel, S. H. (1972): Brain synapses: An *in vitro* model for the study of seizures. *Archives of Internal Medicine (in press)*.

Escueta, A. V., and Reilly, E. L. (1971): The effects of diphenylhydantoin on potassium transport within synaptic terminals of epileptic foci. *Neurology*, 21:418.

Fischer, J., Holubar, J., and Malik, V. (1967): A new method of producing chronic epileptogenic cortical foci in rats. *Physiologica Bohemoslovaka*, 16:272–277.

Fischer-Williams, M., and Cooper, R. A. (1963): Depth recording from the human brain in epilepsy. *Electroencephalography and Clinical Neurophysiology*, 15:568–587.

Forsythe, R. L., Wilder, B. J., and Schmidt, R. P. (1969): Evoked potential studies in experimental epilepsy. *Neurology*, 19:315.

Friede, R. L. (1966): *Topographic Brain Chemistry*, Academic Press, New York.

Globus, A., and Scheibel, A. B. (1967): Synaptic loci on parietal cortical neurons. Terminations of corpus callosum fibers. *Science*, 156:1127–1129.

Goddard, G., McIntyre, D., and Leech, C. (1969): A permanent change in brain function resulting from daily electrical stimulation. *Experimental Neurology*, 25:295–330.

Goldensohn, E. (1969): Experimental seizure mechanisms. In: *Basic Mechanisms of the Epilepsies*, edited by H. H. Jasper, A. A. Ward, Jr., and A. Pope. Little, Brown and Co., Boston, pp. 289–298.

Goldensohn, E., Perez, M., and Feier, J. (1965): Intracellular potentials and unit discharge patterns in primary and mirror epileptogenic foci. *Electroencephalography and Clinical Neurophysiology*, 18:519.

Gozzano, M. (1936): Biolektrische Erscheinungen bei der Reflexepilepsie. *Journal für Psychologie und Neurologie*, 47:24–39.

Guerrero-Figueroa, R., de Balbian, V. F., Barros, A., and Heath, R. G. (1964a): Cholinergic mechanism in subcortical mirror focus and effects of topical application of γ-aminobutyric acid and acetylcholine. *Epilepsia*, 5:140–155.

Guerrero-Figueroa, R., Barros, A., and Heath, R. G. (1964b): Experimental subcortical epileptiform focus. *Epilepsia*, 5:112–139.

Guerrero-Figueroa, R., Barros, A., Lester, B., and Heath, R. (1966): Electrophysiological studies of hippocampal epileptiform discharges during emotional states. *Acta Neurologica Latin America*, 12:6–28.

Holubar, J. Strejckova, A., and Servít, Z. (1966): Penicillin and mirror epileptogenic foci in the brain hemisphere of the frog. In: *Comparative and Cellular Pathophysiology of Epi-

lepsy, edited by Z. Servít. Excerpta Medica International Congress Series 124, Amsterdam, pp. 212–220.

Hughes, J. R. (1966): Bilateral EEG abnormalities on corresponding areas. *Epilepsia,* 7:44–52.

Hughes, J. R. (1967): EEG epileptiform abnormalities at different ages. *Epilepsia,* 8:95–104.

Ishijima, B., and Walker, A. E. (1969*a*): Single unit studies on acute and chronic epileptic foci, their surrounds, and their mirror foci in cats and monkeys. *Transactions of American Neurological Association,* 94:183–184.

Ishijima, B., and Walker, A. E. (1969*b*): Unit studies on transcallosal spread of epileptic activities in the cat's brain. *Electroencephalography and Clinical Neurophysiology,* 26:631.

Jacobsen, S. (1965): Intralaminar, interlaminar, callosal, and thalamocortical connections in frontal and parietal areas of the albino rat cerebral cortex. *Journal of Comprehensive Neurology,* 124:131–145.

Jacobsen, S. (1966): Electron microscopical localization of degenerating callosal axons. *Anatomical Record,* 154:362.

Jacobsen, S., and Marcus, E. (1970): The lamina distribution of fibers of the corpus callosum: A comparative study in the rat, cat, and rhesus monkey, and chimpanzee. *Brain Research,* 24:517–520.

Jasper, H. H. (1964): Some physiological mechanisms involved in epileptic automatisms. *Epilepsia,* 15:1–20.

Kreindler, A. (1970): Interhemispheric propagation of the cortical epileptogenic focus. *Revue Roumaine de Physiologie,* 7:103–113.

Lewin, E. (1971): Epileptogenic cortical foci induced with ouabain, sodium, potassium, water content, and sodium potassium-activated ATPase activity. *Experimental Neurology,* 30:172–177.

Lewin, E., and McCrimmon, A. (1967): ATP-ase activity in discharging cortical lesions induced by freezing. *Archives of Neurology,* 61:321.

Lewin, E., and McCrimmon, A. (1968): The intralaminar distribution of sodium-potassium activated ATP-ase activity in discharging cortical lesions induced by freezing. *Brain Research,* 8:291.

Lorente de No, R. (1922): La corteza cerebral del raton (primiera contrabución–la corteza acustica. *Trabajos Laboratorio Investigación Biologica Universidad Madrid,* 20:41–78.

Malzone, W. F., Wilder, B. J., and Mayersdorf, A. (1971): A method of modifying the rapidity of cobalt-induced epileptogenesis. American Epilepsy Society presentation, December 1971 *(manuscript in preparation).*

Matsumoto, H. (1964): Intracellular events during the activation of cortical epileptiform discharges. *Electroencephalography and Clinical Neurophysiology,* 17:294–307.

Matsumoto, H., and Ajmone Marsan, C. (1964*a*): Cortical cellular phenomena in experimental epilepsy: Interictal manifestations. *Experimental Neurology,* 9:286–304.

Matsumoto, H., and Ajmone Marsan, C. (1964*b*): Cortical cellular phenomena in experimental epilepsy: Ictal manifestations. *Experimental Neurology,* 9:305–326.

Mayersdorf, A., Wilder, B. J., Schmidt, R. P., Schimpff, R. D. (1971): Genesis of primary and secondary foci induced by metallic cobalt powder. *Electroencephalography and Clinical Neurophysiology,* 31:297.

Meyerson, B. A. (1968): Ontogeny of interhemispheric functions. *Acta Physiologica Scandinavica,* Suppl. 312.

Morrell, F. (1959): Experimental focal epilepsy in animals. AMA *Archives of Neurology,* 1:141–147.

Morrell, F. (1960): Secondary epileptogenic lesions. *Epilepsia,* 1:538–569.

Morrell, F. (1961): Lasting changes in synaptic organization produced by continuous neuronal bombardment. In: *CIOMS Symposium on Brain Mechanisms and Learning,* edited by A. Fessard. Blackwell, London, pp. 375–392.

Morrell, F. (1964): Modification of RNA as a result of neural activity. In: *Brain Function II.*

RNA and Brain Function, Memory, and Learning, edited by M. A. B. Brazier. University of California Press, Los Angeles, pp. 183–202.

Morrell, F. (1969): Physiology and histochemistry of the mirror focus. In: *Basic Mechanisms of the Epilepsies,* edited by H. H. Jasper, A. A. Ward, Jr., and A. Pope. Little, Brown and Co., Boston, pp. 357–370.

Morrell, F. and Baker, L. (1961): Effects of drugs on secondary epileptogenic lesions. *Neurology,* 11:651–664.

Morrell, F., and Florenz, A. (1958): Modifications of the freezing technique for producing experimental epileptogenic lesions. *Electroencephalography and Clinical Neurophysiology,* 10:187.

Morrell, F., Sandler, B., and Ross, G. (1959): The "mirror focus" as a model of neural learning. *Proceedings of XXI International Physiology Congress,* Buenos Aires, pp. 193. Excerpta Medica Foundation, Amsterdam.

Mutani, R. (1967): Experimental hippocampal epilepsy in the cat. *Epilepsia,* 8:223–240.

Mutani, R. (1968): Partial and generalized seizures induced by cobalt powder in the ventral amygdala of the cat. *Electroencephalography and Clinical Neurophysiology,* 25:83.

Niedermeyer, E. (1968): The occurrence of generalized (centrencephalic) and focal seizure patterns in the same patients. *The Johns Hopkins Medical Journal,* 122:11–25.

Pacella, B. L., Kopeloff, N., Barrera, S. E., and Kopeloff, L. M. (1944): Experimental production of focal epilepsy. *Archives of Neurology and Psychiatry,* 52:189–196.

Payan, H., Strebel, R., and Levine, S. (1965): Epileptogenic effect of extradural and extracranial cobalt. *Nature,* 208:792–793.

Penfield, W., and Humphreys, S. (1940): Epileptogenic lesions of the brain. *Archives of Neurology and Psychiatry,* 43:240–262.

Pope, A., Morris, A., Jasper, H., Elliott, K. A. C., and Penfield, W. (1947): Histochemical and action potential studies on epileptogenic areas of cerebral cortex in man and the monkey. *Association for Research in Nervous and Mental Diseases Proceedings,* 26:218–233.

Purpura, D. (1969): Stability and seizure susceptibility of immature brain. In: *Basic Mechanisms of the Epilepsies,* edited by H. H. Jasper, A. A. Ward, Jr., and A. Pope. Little, Brown and Co., Boston, pp. 481–505.

Rutledge, L. T., and Kennedy, T. T. (1961): Brain-stem and cortical interactions in the interhemispheric delayed response. *Experimental Neurology,* 4:470–483.

Saradzhizhvili, P., Vatrogon, F., and Okudzhava, V. (1970): Changes in levels of gamma aminobutyric, glutamic and aspartic acids and glutamine in the primary and "mirror foci" of epileptic activity. *Zhurnal Neuropatologi Psikhiatri imeni S. S. Korsakov,* 70:1771–1776.

Stalmaster, R. M., and Hanna, G. R. (1972): Epileptic phenomena of cortical freezing in the cat: Persistent multifocal effects of discrete superficial lesions. *Epilepsia (in press).*

Stercova, A. (1966): Dynamics of neurohistopathological change in epileptogenic focus produced by alumina cream in the rat. In: *Comparative and Cellular Pathophysiology of Epilepsy,* edited by Z. Servít. Excerpta Medica International Congress Series No. 124, pp. 247–257.

Stewart, L. E., and Dreifuss, F. E. (1967): Centrencephalic seizure discharges in focal hemispheral lesions. *Archives of Neurology,* 17:60–68.

Stokstad, E. L., and Koch, J. (1967): Folic acid metabolism. *Physiological Reviews,* 47:83–116.

Strobos, R. J., and Kavallinis, G. P. (1968): Changes in repeat EEGs in epileptics. *Neurology,* 18:622–633.

Suwa, N., Wada, J., and Furuya, O. (1954): On the neural mechanisms for the spread of convulsive impulse: Interrelation between cortico-subcortical structures and cerebellar structures in that connection. *Folia Psychiatry and Neurology (Japan),* 8:167.

Sypert, G. W., Oakley, J., and Ward, A. A., Jr. (1970): Single unit analysis of propagated seizures in neocortex. *Experimental Neurology,* 28:308–325.

Takebayashi, H., Komai, N., and Imamura, H. (1966): Depth EEG analysis of the epilepsies. *Confina Neurologica,* 27:144–148.

Tower, D. (1969): Neurochemical mechanisms. In: *Basic Mechanisms of the Epilepsies,* edited by H. H. Jasper, A. A. Ward, Jr., and A. Pope. Little, Brown and Co., Boston, pp. 611–638.

van Gelder, N. M., and Courtois, A. (1972): Changes in the concentrations of specific amino acids in cerebral cortex of cats with increasing severity of epilepsy induced by cobalt. *Brain Research (in press).*

van Gelder, N. M., Sherwin, A. L., and Rasmussen, T. (1971): An abnormality of secondary energy resources in epileptogenic human brain. *Epilepsia (in press).*

Wada, J., and Asakura, T. (1968): Auditory cerebral deafferentation and epileptogenicity. *Electroencephalography and Clinical Neurophysiology,* 24:287.

Wada, J., and Cornelius, L. (1960): Functional alterations of deep structures in cats and chronic initiative lesions. *Archives of Neurology,* 3:425–447.

Ward, A. A., Jr. (1969): The epileptic neuron: Chronic foci in animals and man. In: *Basic Mechanisms of the Epilepsies,* edited by H. H. Jasper, A. A. Ward, Jr., and A. Pope. Little, Brown and Co., Boston, pp. 273–288.

Westmoreland, B. F., Herman, M., Hanna, G., and Bass, N. (1971): Cobalt-induced secondary epileptogenesis in the cerebral cortex of the albino rat: A neurophysiologic, morphologic, and microchemical study. *Epilepsia,* 12:280.

Westrum, L. E., White, L. E., and Ward, A. A., Jr. (1964): Morphology of the experimental epileptic focus. *Journal of Neurosurgery,* 21:1033–1046.

Wiegant, H. (1967): The subcellular localization of gangliosides in the brain. *Journal of Neurochemistry,* 14:671–674.

Wilder, B. J., King, R. L., and Schmidt, R. P. (1968): Comparative study of secondary epileptogenesis. *Epilepsia,* 9:275–289.

Wilder, B. J., King, R. L., and Schmidt, R. P. (1969): Cortical and subcortical secondary epileptogenesis. *Neurology,* 19:643–652.

Wilder, B. J., and Morrell, F. (1967): Cellular behavior in secondary epileptic lesions. *Neurology,* 17:1193–1204.

Wilder, B. J., Schimpff, R. D., and Collins, G. H. (1972): Ultrastructure study of the chronic experimental epileptic focus. Proceedings, American Epilepsy Society annual meeting, *Epilepsia (in press). (manuscript in preparation.)*

Wilder, B. J., and Schmidt, R. P. (1965): Propagation of epileptic discharge from chronic neocortical foci in monkeys. *Epilepsia,* 6:297–309.

5

Experimental Models of Petit Mal Epilepsy

Elliott M. Marcus

OUTLINE

I. INTRODUCTION

It has long been recognized that seizure disorders fall into two general categories: those in which the initial sign of the seizure is the loss of consciousness (idiopathic, essential "generalized") and those in which the initial sign of the seizure is a focal phenomenon (motor, sensory, psychical) with the loss of consciousness and the tonic clonic convulsion as secondary phenomena (focal, secondary, partial, symptomatic, epileptiform). With the development of the electroencephalogram as a diagnostic tool in the evaluation of seizure disorders, this essential dichotomy was soon confirmed (Jasper and Kershman, 1941). Thus, from an electrical standpoint, focal seizures were found to be associated with a focal cortical discharge. Those seizures whose initial sign was the loss of consciousness (petit mal seizures and primary generalized convulsive seizures) were found to be associated with a bilateral, relatively synchronous and symmetrical, discharge which appeared to begin in a generalized manner without focal onset.

The most distinctive electroencephalographic pattern within the nonfocal group is the bilateral discharge of 2.5 to 3.5 cycles per second (cps) spike-wave complexes associated with the "absence" seizure of petit mal epilepsy. The discharge can usually be precipitated by hyperventilation and often by photic stimulation. Other patterns include the generalized polyspike—slow wave discharge of the myoclonic seizure and the generalized fast spike discharge of the tonic-clonic seizure.

A. Clinical aspects of the petit mal seizure

Our attention in this chapter will be directed to the petit mal seizure. It is perhaps best to begin by reviewing briefly the clinical phenomena of the petit mal seizure. The usual petit mal seizure consists of a short (5 to 30 sec) interruption of consciousness in which general postural tone is relatively well preserved. It is important to note that short bursts of spike-slow wave complexes (1 to 2 sec) in general do not have any definite clinical accompaniment; bursts of 6 to 20 sec duration are usually accompanied by some interruption of consciousness (Mirsky and Pragay, 1967; Geller and Geller, 1970; Goode et al., 1970). During this brief period, the patient is observed to stare, oblivious of stimuli introduced into his environment. He interrupts his ongoing activities. The interruption is relatively abrupt in onset and relatively abrupt in cessation. The patient's awareness and motor activities return promptly at the end of the electrical discharge. Memory is defective only for the period of the seizure. It is as though the patient, although physically present, is "absent" with regard to his higher cortical functions for the brief period of the seizure.

Minor motor phenomena usually accompany the petit mal seizure. Of these, the most characteristic are eyelid opening, eyelid myoclonus, and at times repetitive extraocular movements. Myoclonus of face and repetitive chewing may also occur. Some minor loss of postural tone in neck muscles may occur with dropping of the head onto the chest. Automatisms involving the hands may occur; at times these automatisms are appropriate to the environmental situation.

When examined more closely, it is found that the impairment of awareness, of response capacity, and of motor activity is a relative phenomenon occurring in variable degree. Thus patients are usually unaware of phrases or numbers which are provided as auditory or visual stimuli during the episode; some patients are aware of these same stimuli and can even repeat them during the episode or during questioning following the episode. Some patients are able to continue a familiar recitation during the petit mal seizure. Whether a response to a stimulus occurs during these brief seizures may in part depend on the intensity of the stimulus, and on the motivation and the past experience of the patient. There are no strict one-to-one correlations regarding the electroencephalogram and behavior; there are only relative degrees of correlation.

B. Possible experimental and theoretical approaches

The anatomical substrate (the location of pathological lesion) of the bilateral synchronous discharges and of the associated behavioral phenomena of the petit mal seizure remains uncertain. Several explanations based on different experimental models have been advanced.

A number of previous studies have attempted to answer the question of lesion location in terms of a centrencephalic hypothesis of location of lesion or disorder involving the nonspecific systems of thalamus or brainstem (Penfield and Jasper, 1954; Pollen, 1963; Guerrero-Figueroa, 1963; Weir, 1964). Other workers have approached this question from the standpoint of a focal, multifocal cortical, diffuse cortical, or diffuse cortical-subcortical location of lesion (Gibbs and Gibbs, 1952; Watson and Denny-Brown, 1953; Cohn, 1954; Ingvar, 1955; Petsche, 1962; Bancaud et al., 1965; Servit, 1966). These various approaches to this problem have been the subject of a number of recent reviews which have restated, reevaluated, or modified previous concepts regarding petit mal epilepsy (Marcus and Watson, 1966; Marcus et al., 1968*b;* Pollen, 1968; Ajmone Marsan, 1969; Gastaut, 1969; Gloor, 1969).

The centrencephalic hypothesis has been widely accepted. It is important to indicate that there is a certain logical simplicity in such a concept. Thus, since a single cortical focus of discharge is not present in this variety of seizure disorder, and since the discharge appears to begin all over the cortex at approximately the same time, it is logical to assume that some subcortical structure with diffuse connections must be driving the cerebral cortex of the two hemispheres in a bilateral manner. The centrencephalic concept[1] was, moreover, emerging at a time when Morison and Dempsey (1942) demonstrated that stimulation of the intralaminar system of the thalamus would produce a recruiting response over widespread areas of cortex in both cerebral hemispheres of the cat. The studies of Jasper and Droogleever-Fortuyn (1946) demonstrated that a stimulus-related 3 cps spike-and-wave pattern could be produced on stimulation of the midline nuclei or of the intralaminar system of thalamus. The studies of Hunter and Jasper (1949) demonstrated that stimulation of this area in the unanesthetized animal would produce arrest of movement, reproducing the behavioral components of the petit mal seizure. The later studies of Pollen

---

[1] It is important to note that the centrencephalic hypothesis has not remained a fixed static conception, but has evolved over the years from the initial suggestion that the seizures originated at a diencephalic or brainstem level to the later concept of the pathological process involving a system which included cerebral cortex as well as brainstem reticular formation and intralaminar system of thalamus.

(1963, 1964) have indicated that the spike of the thalamic-induced spike-and-wave corresponds to the recruiting response and is associated with excitatory postsynaptic potentials generated in superficial layers of cortex at axodendritic synapses. The long-duration surface-negative slow wave of the complex is the surface reflection of inhibitory postsynaptic potentials generated at synapses in the deeper cell layers. The nonspecific thalamic nuclei and the cortical elements involved in the recruiting response have been grouped together as the diffuse thalamo-cortical system, with the implication that a response occurs throughout all cortical areas. However, it is important to note that the original studies of Morison and Dempsey (1942) and Jasper (1949) indicated significant regional variability. In the monkey, the response is obtained primarily from frontal and parietal association areas (Starzl and Whitlock, 1952).[2]

From a technical standpoint, it is also important to note that the thalamic-induced spike-slow wave complex is dependent on conditions of arousal that are best obtained under conditions of relatively light anesthesia (Pollen et al., 1963).

The alternate experimental approach to the problem of petit mal epilepsy is based on the assumption that if the discharge appears to begin in a widespread manner over cerebral cortex of both hemispheres, perhaps the basic pathology is a lesion (structural or biochemical) which involves the cerebral cortex of the two hemispheres in a bilateral manner. There is some clinical basis for this hypothesis.

(1) A significant percentage of patients with classical, clinical petit mal "absences" and with the electrical pattern of synchronous 3 cps spike-slow wave may present, in addition, focal or multifocal clinical and electroencephalographic abnormalities. Gibbs and Gibbs (1952) found "focal larval petit mal" discharges in such classical cases during 30% of awake records and during 71% of sleep records. O'Brien et al. (1959) described focal or lateralized abnormalities in 35% of 100 such consecutive cases.

(2) The presumed interhemispheric synchrony of the bilateral spike-wave discharge is actually only a relative synchrony when subjected to

---

[2] In the studies of Jasper (1949) in the cat, frontal recruiting responses were predominantly obtained by stimulation of more rostral nuclei, and occipital responses by stimulation of more caudal thalamic areas. In addition, the effects were predominantly ipsilateral rather than bilaterally symmetrical. Moreover, the more recent studies in the cat by Velasco and Lindsley (1965) and by Clemente and Sterman (1967) suggest that the nonspecific nuclei do not have diffuse connections to many cortical areas but rather that information from these nuclei is sent to orbital frontal cortex via preoptic region (basal forebrain). From orbital frontal cortex, spread may then occur to other cortical areas via cortico-cortical association fiber systems. In these studies, the recruiting response could be produced by direct stimulation of basal forebrain or orbital frontal areas.

detailed cathode-ray oscilloscopic analysis. Both homologous and heterologous asynchrony occur in man with latencies of 5 to 20 msec (Cohn,
1954). Petsche (1962) found evidence of multiple, independent, bilateral
cortical generators of spike and of wave on toposcopic analysis of patients
with petit mal. McCulloch (1944) has estimated the speed of conduction
in "long" cortico-cortical association pathways to be approximately 50
m/sec (5 cm/msec). Such a conduction velocity would be consistent with
the frontal occipital or occipital-frontal "heterologous" asynchrony or the
interhemispheric "homologous" asynchrony of 5 to 20 msec found by Cohn
for the spike-wave complex.

(3) Simultaneous depth and surface recordings in man with petit mal
have yielded inconclusive data regarding the site of origin of both the spike
and slow wave components of the discharge (Hayne et al., 1949; Spiegel
et al., 1951; Williams, 1953).

In addition, a series of experimental observations suggest a significant
role of cerebral cortex in the generation of the spike-slow wave complex.

Thus, unilaterally isolated cortex is capable of producing a unilateral
3 cps spike-and-wave discharge in the absence of a subcortical generator or
pacemaker (Ingvar, 1955b; Echlin, 1959). An active rather than passive
cortical mechanism was also suggested by the observations of Starzl et al.
(1953) regarding pentylenetetrazol-induced seizures in the cat. The threshold for generalized spike-wave discharge was lower in the cortex (15 mg/kg)
than in subcortical structures (90 to 120 mg/kg); spike-wave discharge in
sensory motor cortex in the intermediate portion of the seizure was never
simultaneously associated with spike-wave activity in the medial thalamic
structures with diffuse projection. Threshold for discharge in isolated
cortex was similar to that in cortex of the intact preparation, suggesting
that subcortical structures were not facilitating cortical discharge.

With the emphasis on thalamocortical and reticulocortical relationships,
there had been a tendency to overlook the possible role of the corpus callosum in providing a pathway for synchronizing the discharge of the two
hemispheres.

Previous studies had indicated the role of the corpus callosum as regards the synchrony of the spontaneous paroxysmal bursts during deep
amobarbital (Amytal ®) narcosis in the dog brain (Swank, 1949). Bilateral
synchronous bursts of fast and slow wave forms have been noted following
bilateral section of subcortical-cortical fiber systems with preservation of
corpus callosum (Grafstein, 1959). With regard to bilateral discharge,
Swank (1949) demonstrated a high degree of interhemispheric synchrony of
"picrotoxin spikes" in frontal lobes isolated from thalamus but connected
by corpus callosum (under conditions of deep amobarbital narcosis). Dis-

ruption of interhemispheric synchrony of bilateral "strychnine spikes" was noted by Mattson and Bickford (1961) following section of corpus callosum. The report of Hursh (1945) indicating persistence of spike-slow wave synchrony after section of corpus callosum in human petit mal dealt only with partial section of this commissure without anatomical control. The effects of agenesis of the corpus callosum on the synchrony of bilateral electrical discharge in the human are also not yet clear. Various authors have arrived at conflicting conclusions (Goldensohn et al. 1941; Gastaut, 1959; Green and Russell, 1966; Fermaglich and O'Doherty, 1971.)

II. A MODEL OF PETIT MAL EPILEPSY EMPLOYING ACUTE BILATERAL EPILEPTOGENIC FOCI

A. Studies in the cat (adult)

Our initial studies (Marcus and Watson, 1964, 1966) demonstrated that bilateral epileptogenic foci in symmetrical cortical areas of the two cerebral hemispheres could interact to produce synchronous and symmetrical patterns of electrical discharge without the necessity of lesions in thalamus or brain stem.

All animals in this group were initially anesthetized with ether[3] to allow placement of the tracheal cannula and venous catheter. Gallamine triethiodide (Flaxedil ®) was then administered intravenously and artificial respiration by pump was begun. Body temperature was monitored and maintained in the range of 99 to 101°F. Following craniotomy and placement of silver ball electrodes for recording from pial surface, acute bilateral epileptogenic foci were produced.

In each experiment, these bilateral cortical epileptogenic foci were produced by the application of filter-paper tabs soaked with an acute convulsant agent [0.5 to 1% strychnine sulfate, or 1 to 2% conjugated estrogen (Premarin ®) (Marcus et al., 1966), or 10% pentylenetetrazol (Metrazol ®)] to relatively large, homologous areas of cerebral cortex (75–200 sq mm): the posterior sigmoid, the suprasylvian or the lateral gyri. In one animal, bilateral epileptogenic foci were produced by local freezing of cerebral cortex with dry ice.

An interaction of the bilateral foci rapidly occurred with the production

---

[3] For these acute experiments, barbiturate anesthetics such as pentobarbital (Nembutal ®) should not be employed. Such agents have established anticonvulsant effects with regard to cortical discharges. Repetitive discharges are reduced to single spike discharges.

of bilateral synchronous spike discharges which were often synchronized within 0 to 12 msec. Prolonged bilateral discharges of spikes, polyspikes, or spike-slow wave complexes soon developed. These discharges included prolonged bursts of $2\frac{1}{2}$ to 3 cps spike-slow wave complexes, in addition to spike-slow wave complexes of slower frequency (1 to 2 cps).

In a supplementary series of animals, screw electrodes were implanted in bone under ether anesthesia and bilateral foci were subsequently produced. Relevant behavioral concomitants of these bilateral discharges resembled some of the clinical phenomena observed in patients with idiopathic petit mal or grand mal seizures during similar bilateral discharges: bilateral facial muscle and forelimb myoclonus transient suspension or imperfect continuation of a repetitive act, and occasional generalized convulsive seizures.

Methods for the study of the mechanisms involved in the interaction of bilateral foci will be discussed in a later section.

B. Studies in the rhesus monkey (male *Macaca mulatta* of 3 to 6 kg)

It was evident to us that, although we were obtaining bilateral synchronous discharges with bilateral foci in the adult cat, the bursts of discharge were not the relatively well-regulated monomorphic $2\frac{1}{2}$ to 3 cps spike-slow wave which the clinical electroencephalographer would usually accept as characteristic of petit mal epilepsy. Rather, as noted also by Ajmone Marsan (1969), the $2\frac{1}{2}$ to 3 cps spike-slow wave complexes were occurring within the context of other types of synchronous discharge. Moreover, a similar lack of precise correlation was noted with regard to the behavioral effects.

Several approaches were considered: use of young kittens or use of an animal species more closely related to man, e.g., the monkey. Several factors led us to follow the second approach. Petit mal epilepsy occurs not in the infant, but in the older child and adolescent (age 4 to 15 years). The cerebral cortex and the callosal and association fiber systems of the relatively mature 3 to 6 kg monkey provide a much better approximation of this human stage than does the immature cerebral cortex of the young kitten. Moreover, it is evident that the bilateral discharges of the petit mal seizure are not equally distributed throughout all recording areas overlying cerebral cortex. Rather, the spike-slow wave discharges of petit mal epilepsy are most prominent in parasagittal frontal-central areas. The "larval" bilateral spike-slow wave discharges of petit mal epilepsy are often limited to the frontal-central area (Gibbs and Gibbs, 1952). Moreover, significant regional variations occur in the direct current potential changes as recorded by Chatrian (1968) during a petit mal seizure (most prominent, parasagittal premotor). The monkey was expected to provide a more appropriate species (and does in fact) than the cat for the study of a process which involves frontal, premotor, and motor cortex. The use of the monkey rather than the cat is recommended for investigators wishing to utilize a model of petit mal epilepsy.

C. Model of the electrical discharge of petit mal epilepsy

Our studies in the monkey (Marcus and Watson, 1968) employed standard acute epileptogenic foci produced by the application to cortex of 10×6-mm filter-paper tabs soaked in a 1% solution of conjugated estrogens. Male rhesus monkeys were prepared under conditions of ether–Flaxedil–artificial respiration. A significant interaction of these acute bilaterally symmetrical foci occurred. However, there were marked regional variations in the capacity for bilateral synchronous discharge. Persistent bilaterally synchronous and symmetrical patterns of discharge, including 1 to 4 cps spike or polyspike-slow wave complexes occurred with bilateral foci in frontal, precentral, and parietal areas. Consistent bilateral synchrony failed to develop with bilateral foci in striate occipital and middle-posterior portions of superior temporal gyrus. Somewhat better bilateral synchrony was obtained in preoccipital and anterior temporal areas. These regional variations in capacity for synchrony of bilateral discharge corresponded to the known regional variations in fiber density of the callosal system.

Within the frontal lobe area, particularly well regulated, bilaterally synchronous and symmetrical bursts of $2\frac{1}{2}$ to 4 cps spike-slow wave complexes resulted when bilateral foci were produced in the premotor areas. A significant degree of interhemispheric synchrony of the bilateral spike discharge was present (0 to 20 msec). As in the human case of petit mal epilepsy, the characteristic effect of a minor degree of hyperventilation in the precipitation or accentuation of bilateral bursts could be demonstrated (Fig. 1). Moreover, although the foci had been produced in the premotor area, when discharges were prolonged as with hyperventilation, the discharge often occurred in a generalized manner. [Hyperventilation, a minimal increase in depth of respiration for a standard 3-min period, was produced by increasing resistance on the open end of a T tube attached to a standard tracheostomy tube (one-quarter turn of screw clamp). This increase was insufficient to produce significant seizure discharges in the intact animal. Each animal served as its own control. Blood gas measurements have not been performed but would be of value in future experiments.]

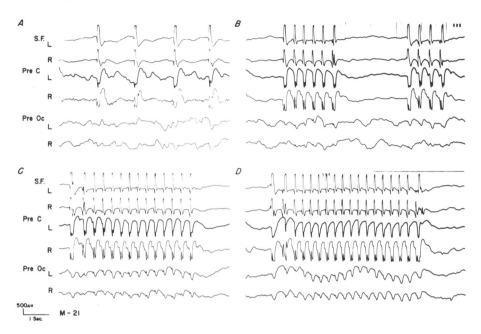

FIG. 1. Experimental 3 cps spike-wave discharges following production of bilateral epileptogenic foci in anterior premotor cortex of monkey. Repetitive bursts of synchronous and symmetrical $2\frac{1}{2}$ to 3 cps spike-wave complexes occurred frequently in this animal following a 3-min period of minor hyperventilation. Similar bursts occurred during periods of normal ventilation but were less frequent. A similar effect of hyperventilation is noted in the human patients with petit mal epilepsy. S.F., superior frontal-gyrus in prefrontal area; Pre C, precentral gyrus; Pre O, preoccipital area.

A: Just prior to hyperventilation; *B, C, D:* 2 to 3 min after beginning of hyperventilation. From Marcus and Watson (1968) with permission of the publisher.

D. Correlated electrical and behavioral model of petit mal epilepsy in the monkey

The clinical significance of any experimental model of the bilateral synchronous discharge of petit mal epilepsy is limited unless, as in the human, characteristic behavioral alterations are correlated with the electrical discharge. Since there was now available a model of the electrical discharge or petit mal epilepsy, we investigated the behavioral correlates of these bilateral synchronous discharges concentrating on the frontal lobe areas and using non-paralyzed monkeys (Marcus et al., 1968a,b). Under ether anesthesia,[4] screw electrodes were implanted in skull bone and insulated. Bilateral burr holes were placed in bone at desired sites of lesion. Bilateral epileptogenic foci were produced by application of a 1% solution of conjugated estrogen on 10 × 6-mm filter-paper tabs to pial surface following opening of dura. Application was relatively confined by a thick circular wall of Vaseline® gauze. (This was confirmed by adding Evans Blue to the solution in several animals and by the distinct differences in clinical seizure phenomena produced by changes in the anatomical location of the foci.)

Location of lesion at the time of surgery was determined using the following approximations. The junction of the sagittal and coronal sutures in the monkey is approximately 10 mm anterior to the central sulcus at the midline. The central sulcus at the midline also corresponds approximately to AP-O in the atlas of Snider and Lee (1961). In some instances, following opening of dura, the superior limb of the arcuate sulcus or the central sulcus could be visualized and employed as a landmark. The arcuate sulcus is, however, often variable in its course.

Following development of foci, dural closure, skin closure, and recovery from anesthesia, the animals' behavior and simultaneously displayed television monitor image of the electroencephalogram were photographed.

Bilateral foci in the *anterior premotor area*[5] (area 8 and adjacent area 6) at the rostral end of the superior limb of the arcuate sulcus (designated as Map Location A in Fig. 2) resulted in bilateral synchronous bursts of 3 cps spike-slow wave complexes. These bursts were associated with short staring spells resembling the absence seizure of petit mal epilepsy (Fig. 3). There was a variable interruption or arrest of motor activities and a variable alteration of response to visual and tactile stimuli. To a variable degree, myoclonic movements of eyelids, head or extraocular muscles also occurred.

If the foci were produced in the *posterior premotor area* (Map Location B), the electrical discharge had more prominent polyspike components. The associated seizure, although often involving an interruption of ongoing

---

[4] There are many disadvantages to the use of ether for such a long one-stage procedure. Our subsequent studies suggest that the procedure could be done more easily in one stage employing ketamine hydrochloride. Alternatively, a two-stage experiment could be performed, implanting electrodes and producing burr holes at the first stage under pentobarbital — then, 5 days later re-opening skin, opening dura, and producing epileptogenic foci under ketamine hydrochloride or ether (or halothane if equipment and experience are available).

[5] The designation anterior premotor refers to the center of the lesion 26 to 30 mm anterior to the central sulcus (at midline) and 5 to 8 mm lateral from midline: The designation posterior premotor refers to the center of the lesion 20 to 25 mm anterior to the central sulcus (at midline) and 5 to 8 mm lateral from midline.

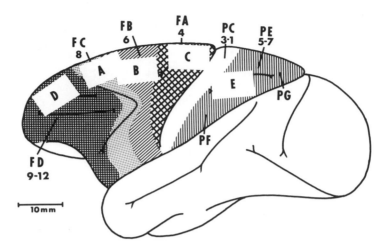

FIG. 2. Location of bilateral foci for behavioral correlation experiments. Map of lateral aspect of monkey cerebral hemisphere indicating location of 10 × 6-mm filter-paper tabs soaked in convulsant agent, 1% conjugated estrogen. Approximately cytoarchitectural designations based on several authors are superimposed. From Marcus et al. (1968a), with permission of the publisher.

motor activities, usually had prominent myoclonic phenomena involving face and forelimbs.

Control animals were also prepared with bilateral foci in precentral, anterior prefrontal, and parietal areas. These animals did not have absence seizures.

With bilateral foci in the *upper precentral area* (Map Location C), bilateral spikes occurred associated with bilateral myoclonic jerks of the lower extremities; progression to frequent generalized seizures soon occurred. Foci in the middle precentral area were associated with bilateral myoclonic jerks of upper extremities.

With bilateral foci in the *anterior prefrontal area* (Map Location D), although prolonged, localized polyspike discharge occurred, no definite alteration of behavior occurred.

In subsequent studies, adjacent areas have been studied employing bilateral foci; e.g., the area within the curve of the arcuate sulcus was found to have a relatively high threshold, and spike-slow wave discharges did not result unless the foci extended over the sulcus into Map Location A. Following these preliminary behavioral correlation studies, a more detailed analysis of the anterior premotor area was performed (Marcus et al., 1970).

It was possible to dissociate the eye movements in a predictable manner from the absence seizure; thus, foci involving the more posterior portion of

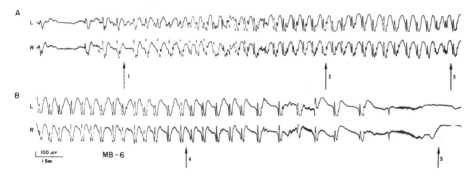

FIG. 3. Bilateral anterior premotor foci at Map Location A (1% conjugated estrogens). Correlation of behavior (absence seizure) with bilateral synchronous 2.5 to 3 cps spike-slow wave discharge. Bipolar recording from left and right premotor-precentral areas. Segments *A* and *B* are continuous. *Arrow 1:* Approximate onset of staring with eyes open and head fixed in relatively midline position. *Arrow 2:* Beaker of water introduced from animal's left into central visual field, then moved back and forth—animal looked down at beaker but failed to follow. Shortly thereafter, minor side-to-side myoclonic movements of head and eyes occurred. *Arrow 3:* Beaker of water placed to lips. Animal failed to orient head and failed to lick with tongue, even though lips were wet. No movements of hands occurred (compare to arrow 5). *Arrow 4:* Pencil introduced into central visual field then moved slowly back and forth, animal glanced slightly at object but failed to follow. *Arrow 5:* Beaker of water introduced from left. Animal looked at beaker, followed it back and forth and lifted both hands towards beaker. Beaker then placed to lips, animal oriented head down, licked water and brought hands up against bottom of beaker. At conclusion, animal licked lips with tongue. Shortly thereafter, an additional seizure occurred duplicating the correlations noted above. From Marcus et al. (1968a), with permission of the publisher.

Map Location A tended to produce greater side-to-side myoclonic movements of eyes. The bilateral discharges also tended to have somewhat greater polyspike components. Those foci involving the more anterior portions of Map Location A were associated with eye movements which were more restricted to eyelid opening and pupillary dilation. The pattern of discharge in these animals was a more selective spike-slow wave.

As additional animals were studied, it became apparent that this model of petit mal epilepsy could be employed in a consistent manner. However, it was evident that there was a considerable inter-animal variability in the degree of impairment of response to various stimuli, even when a standard location of bilateral foci was employed. The response of the animal during the seizure often appeared closely related to his interictal response; i.e., if an animal had attempted to push or kick away a beaker of water during the interictal period, he attempted to do so during the petit mal seizure as well, although in an imperfect manner. If the animal had attempted to take hold of the beaker with his hand and to bring the beaker to his mouth during the interictal period, he also attempted to do this during the petit mal seizure, although in an imperfect manner. Similar variations in the degree of impairment of awareness and of capacity for response have been noted in human petit mal epilepsy as discussed above. If one assumes that behavior such as arrest of movement or myoclonus is represented and re-represented at various levels of the neuraxis, then it is evident that simultaneous recordings from cortical and subcortical areas (e.g., mesencephalic and pontine reticular formation) might have been of value in providing a greater correlation with behavior.

III. DEVELOPMENT OF A CHRONIC MODEL OF PETIT MAL EPILEPSY: THE USE OF COBALT AS A CORTICAL EPILEPTOGENIC AGENT

A. Background

Acute topical convulsant agents such as strychnine or pentylenetetrazol produce an effect which begins within seconds to minutes of application but an effect which usually disappears within an hour of application. An agent such as penicillin produces a convulsant effect within 5 min, but the effect usually disappears within 4 to 7 hr. Conjugated estrogens also produce an epileptogenic effect within 5 min, but again the effect disappears in 3 to 6 hr. In recent experiments somewhat longer effects have been achieved, employing a 2% solution of conjugated estrogens rather than a 1% solution.

Human seizure disorders are chronic in the sense that seizures, be they petit mal, focal, or generalized convulsions, recur over a period of months and years. A chronic model of epilepsy represents a closer approximation to the human disease state. Such a chronic model is also desirable if studies of learned responses are to be performed. The attempts to develop a chronic model of focal epilepsy have been reviewed by Ward (1969). Aluminum hydroxide gel has been used successfully with regard to unilateral or bilateral foci in motor cortex of the rhesus monkey (Kopeloff et al., 1942, 1954, 1955). The effects of application to other cortical areas are less consistent, although Walker and Morello (1967) have presented a preliminary report of minor seizures resembling petit mal absences following unilateral injections of alumina cream into prefrontal areas. The study of Stamm and Pribram (1960) employed bilateral alumina cream in prefrontal areas (over principal sulcus anterior to the arcuate sulcus, an area of relatively high threshold). Spike discharges were recorded but no mention was made of clinical seizures. The illustrations do not indicate bilateral spike-slow wave discharges. The concern of the investigators was primarily with alterations in the learning capacity. Mutani and Fariello (1969) have recently confirmed the results of our earlier acute studies in the cat (Marcus and Watson, 1964, 1966a) through the use of chronic bilateral alumina cream foci in cat motor cortex.

From an experimental standpoint, there are several disadvantages to the use of alumina cream: for example, there is a significant latency prior to development of focal seizures as well as significant tissue destruction. The onset of focal seizures following application of the 133 sq mm disk to pial surface is 5 to 13 weeks. The latency of onset of focal motor seizures following multiple intracortical injections is variously estimated at 3 to 9 weeks (Kopeloff, 1955; Ward, 1969). The investigator, therefore, from a practical standpoint, would prefer an agent which has a relatively acute onset but a long duration of action.

In recent years, cobalt powder has been used as an effective convulsant agent (primarily in species other than the rhesus monkey) (Dow et al., 1962; Cereghino and Dow, 1970). In the rat, focal discharges begin at 5 to 8 days; clinical seizures begin during the second week and persist in a chronic manner. In the cat, focal discharges and focal seizures usually begin 24 to 48 hr after topical application of the cobalt powder and persist for 4 to 5 days.

Grimm et al. (1969) reported that in the squirrel monkey discharges began in 30 to 60 min. The intense period of discharge occurred at 4 to 12 hr. Discharge persisted for 48 to 96 hr. In four of nine monkeys, the focal discharge then reappeared after a period of days or weeks. A direct convulsant action as well as a secondary convulsant action due to histological response to the agent is thereby suggested.

Cobalt has *not* been extensively employed in the rhesus monkey. Chusid and Kopeloff (1962) initially reported that implantation of cobalt pellets in motor cortex had no significant epileptogenic effect. In a later report (1967), they did indicate an epileptogenic effect of motor cortex injections of cobalt powder in one of two monkeys. Apparently, seizures occurred as early as the second postoperative day and recurred for at least 3 months. (The actual duration is unclear from this report.)

Our recent experiments with cobalt powder as an epileptogenic agent in the rhesus monkey (Marcus et al., 1971) have employed a modification of the techniques of Grimm et al. (1969) and Cereghino and Dow (1970) (see methods below.) This agent has been proved useful for the production of unilateral foci in motor cortex. When the preparation was studied under conditions of gallamine triethiodide (Flaxedil®) and pump respirator, spike discharges began within 80 to 95 min of application of cobalt to pial surface. In chronic preparations prepared under short-acting nonbarbiturate anesthetics (ketamine hydrochloride), focal spike discharges began within 75 to 95 min of application. Clinical focal seizures began at 95 to 130 min and continued to recur for 72 hr. When pentobarbital anesthesia was employed for the procedure, onset of focal spike discharge was delayed until $2\frac{1}{2}$ to $5\frac{1}{2}$ hr after application. Clinical focal seizures occurred in a limited manner beginning at 5 to 7 hr and continuing for 24 hr. In occasional animals, a brief recurrence of clinical seizure activity was present at 4 to 5 days. Clinical seizures then disappeared although focal discharges continued to occur in the electroencephalogram. In two of five animals, however, clinical focal seizures began to recur in a chronic manner at 23 and 44 days.

B. Materials and methods; bilateral cobalt foci

The male rhesus monkey (*Macaca mulatta*) weighing 7 to 12 pounds was employed. The basic design involved the production of subacute-chronic bilateral foci in the anterior or posterior premotor cortex. These foci were produced by the application of cobalt powder (300 mesh). Approximately 60 mg of cobalt powder (previously dry sterilized) was coated onto a 10 × 10-mm square of gelfoam which had been moistened with Ringer's solution—so as to form a paste. The square was then applied (cobalt-paste side down) in a bilateral manner to the premotor area. The area of application was surrounded by a donut of Vaseline® gauze to limit spread of the agent.

Anesthesia was induced in one-stage procedures with pentobarbital (30 to 35 mg/kg, i.p.) or with repeated intramuscular administration of ketamine.[6] In some animals, a two-stage procedure was performed with placement of electrodes and burr holes under pentobarbital anesthesia as the first stage. Foci were then prepared 4 to 5 days later in a second short procedure employing ether or ketamine anesthesia. Such two-stage procedures were performed to minimize the anticonvulsant effects of barbiturate anesthesia.

Under aseptic conditions, 10 screw[7] electrodes for bipolar recording were implanted in bone at bilateral sites, overlying prefrontal, premotor,

---

[6] Ketamine has the advantage of being a rapid-onset, short-acting anesthetic agent which may be administered by the intramuscular or intravenous route without the necessity of endotracheal intubation (pharyngeal reflexes are well preserved).

[7] Stainless steel, machine-binding head screws ($\frac{2}{56}$ diameter and $\frac{5}{16}$ length) were inserted into the skull, binding head down after cutting a T-shaped craniectomy with a dental drill. The screws were then secured with stainless steel nuts.

precentral, inferior parietal, and occipital areas. (An additional ground electrode was also implanted.) Relatively accurate placements were obtained by using the approximations noted above in the procedure for the acute behavior correlation experiments. The electrodes were wired, insulated, and covered with dental acrylic after placements of burr holes over anterior premotor areas. The placement of these burr holes was determined by the desired location of the gelfoam squares. For bilateral anterior premotor foci, the center of the square was positioned approximately 28 to 30 mm anterior to the midline central sulcus (20 mm anterior to suture junction noted above) and 8 mm lateral from the midline. Usually it was possible to confirm the location by noting the location of the rostral end of the superior limb of the arcuate sulcus. While it is possible from a theoretical standpoint to confirm more precisely the placement of focus by means of local electrical stimulation of cerebral cortex to elicit selective eyelid opening and pupillary dilation, this is not practical since there is considerable variability in response obtained from frontal eyefields, particularly in relation to depth of anesthesia—a point stressed by Krieger et al. (1958), and Wagman et al. (1961), and very evident in our own experiments.

Following placement of the cobalt-coated gelfoam squares, the dura was closed with sutures and the skin was closed with surgical clips. The animal was then replaced in a long-term primate restraining chair and allowed to recover from anesthesia. Observations were then made continuously for 8 to 15 hr and then intermittently on a daily basis. Animals have been studied for periods up to 8 weeks.

Recording of EEG and behavior: Following recovery from anesthesia, the petit mal seizures were recorded. A television camera positioned over the pens of the EEG machine allowed display of six channels of the EEG on a television monitor placed next to the monkey. Both monkey and television monitor image were photographed on 16 mm film by a Bolex camera. Electrical activity was also recorded on a cathode-ray oscilloscope for more precise measurement of synchrony of bilateral discharge.

The animals' spontaneous behavior during these seizures was recorded with particular attention to eyelid opening and closing, and myoclonus of eyes, lids, face, and extremities. It was also noted if the animal interrupted his ongoing motor activities during the seizure. Responses to visual (beaker of water, food pellets, and plastic object), tactile (stick placed in hand and on shoulders), nociceptive (pin prick to face, hands, and shoulder), and auditory (whistle) stimuli were tested during ictal and interictal periods in a manner similar to the control periods. During interictal periods, intermittent photic stimulation (Grass, P.S. 1) at variable frequency was carried out to determine photosensitivity.

Termination: At periodic intervals following production of bilateral foci, animals were sacrificed to assay histological changes at the focus. Standard neuropathologic techniques (hematoxylin and eosin, Nissl and Nauta stains) were employed.

C. Preliminary acute studies employing bilateral cobalt foci

In a small number of animals, acute studies were performed to assay earliest onset of seizure discharges when anesthetic effects were minimized. For this purpose, animals were initially anesthetized with ether to allow placement of catheters within the trachea and saphenous vein. Appropriate pressure points were infiltrated with 1% procaine hydrochloride. The animal was immobilized with gallamine triethiodide and artificially ventilated. Burr holes were produced over premotor cortex. Screw electrodes were implanted in bone and insulated. Dura was then opened, foci produced as above, and dura closed. Recording of cortical electrical activity was performed using the EEG and the cathode-ray oscilloscope. Body temperature was monitored and maintained in physiological range (99 to 100°F). The effects of hyperventilation and photic stimulation were assayed using the methods discussed above. Animals were followed for periods up to 15 hr and then sacrificed to verify lesion and electrode location.

Well-developed, bilateral blunt spike discharges began 90 to 120 min after placement of the lesion. Initially these discharges consisted of single spikes. Grouped discharges of bilateral polyspikes and slow waves soon began to occur. With a minor degree of hyperventilation, these group discharges could be accentuated and prolonged generalized discharges could be produced. Intermittent discharges continued to occur for the duration of the experiments.

D. Chronic bilateral cobalt foci employing nonbarbiturate anesthetic ketamine hydrochloride

Bilateral spike discharges could be recorded 80 to 120 min after placement of the cobalt foci. With lesions in anterior premotor cortex (Map Location A), eyelid opening and upward movement of eyes was noted to accompany bilateral spike discharge at approximately $2\frac{1}{2}$ hr. Initial absence seizures could occur as early as $5\frac{1}{2}$ hr and continue at frequent intervals over a 72 to 96-hr period. In some animals, seizures ceased at 24 hr and recurred transiently at 72 hr. No additional clinical seizures occurred during the subsequent observation period of 7 weeks, although single bilateral or multifocal spikes could continue to occur for 2 to 3 weeks. In the animal shown in Figs. 4–6, exact time of onset of clinical seizures could

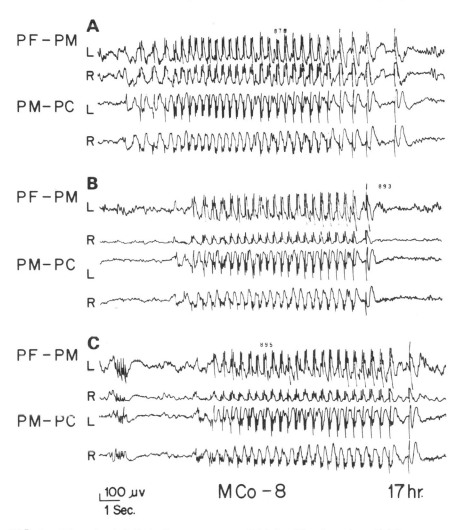

FIG. 4. Bilateral cobalt foci: Premotor cortex (17 hr). (Map Location, slightly more posterior than A, extends slightly into B location.) Repetitive seizures over a 6 min period are demonstrated. Each of the bursts of 3 cps spike-slow wave complexes was accompanied by an absence seizure. (Arrest of activity, eyelids open, staring.) All seizures in this animal over a total period of 20 min are demonstrated in Figs. 4–6. (Chronic preparation: rapid acting non-barbiturate anesthetic had been employed.) Bipolar recordings. PF, prefrontal; PM, premotor, PC = precentral.

not be ascertained. However, frequent generalized bursts of 3 cps spike-slow wave complexes, accompanied by clinical petit mal seizures, were noted when recordings were resumed 17 hr post-lesion. In this preparation, the foci had been produced somewhat more posteriorly than desired in the

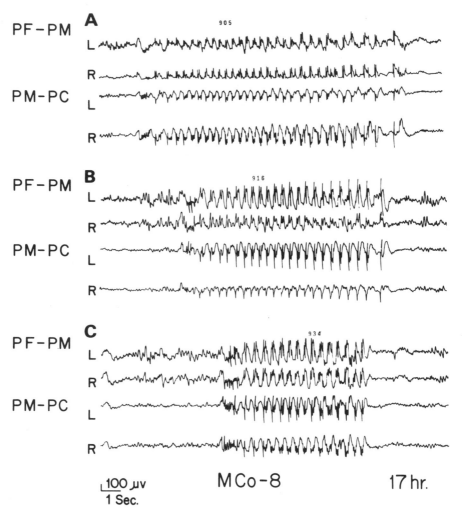

FIG. 5. Bilateral Cobalt foci: Premotor cortex (continuation of Fig. 4). Each of the bursts of spike-slow wave complexes was accompanied by an absence seizure.

premotor cortex (slightly posterior to Map Location A). · Single myoclonic jerks were soon noted to accompany the absence seizure and frequent generalized convulsive seizures occurred subsequently. These generalized seizures often began with multifocal adversive components and continued to occur for the next 5 days.

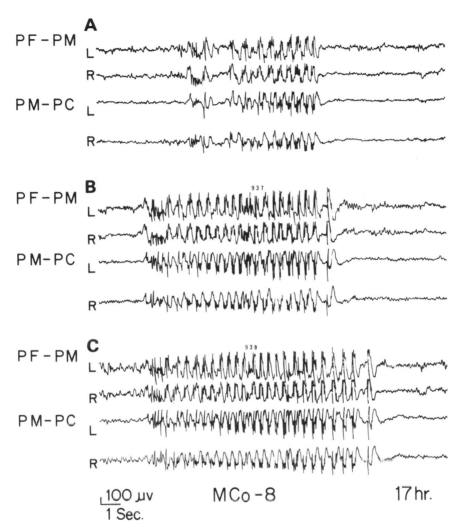

FIG. 6. Bilateral cobalt foci: Premotor cortex (continuation of Figs. 4 and 5). Each of the bursts of spike-slow wave complexes demonstrated was accompanied by an absence seizure which now included a single myoclonic jerk of the arms.

E. Chronic bilateral cobalt foci employing one-stage procedure under pentobarbital anesthesia

Onset of bilateral blunt-spike discharges was delayed until 3 to 6 hr after placement of lesions. Absence seizures began at 9 to 24 hr after placement of lesions and recurred until 30 hr. Seizures were not frequent when pentobarbital anesthesia was employed. No additional seizures were observed over a 17- to 18-day period of observation, except for minor recurrences at 4 to 5 days.

F. General conclusions concerning use of cobalt for production of bilateral foci

(1) Cobalt powder may be employed for the production of subacute bilateral foci in premotor cortex. Depending on the anesthetic agent employed, bilateral discharges may be noted within 80 to 120 min and absence seizures within $5\frac{1}{2}$ hr. The procedure outlined will result in a model of petit mal epilepsy which may be studied for periods up to 72 hr. A true chronic model does not result.

(2) When bilateral cobalt foci were employed, there was a general correlation between location of lesion (anterior vs. posterior premotor) and the behavioral components of the petit mal seizure (myoclonus of head, eyes, and arms; presence or absence of generalized seizures). However, we failed to obtain the much more discrete correlations noted with acute bilateral foci (produced with 1% conjugated estrogen).

(3) Similarly, the well-regulated, classical 3 cps spike-slow wave complex was less precisely obtained with the subacute bilateral foci produced with cobalt than with acute foci employed in our earlier experiments. It should, however, be noted that as we examined a larger number of animals with bilateral foci in the anterior premotor cortex, we found there are certain limits to the degree of behavioral–EEG correlation. Thus, the experimental absence seizure may be associated with a bilateral discharge of relatively pure, well-sustained, 3 cps spike-slow wave complexes. However, a similar absence seizure may also occur with a bilateral discharge that is composed primarily of 2 cps spike-slow wave complexes or of polyspikes and slow waves. What appears to be important for the behavioral aspect of the seizure is that a bilateral discharge involves the premotor cortex. (This, of course, presumes that the discharge continues for a period of at least 6 to 30 sec.)

IV. ANATOMICAL–PHYSIOLOGICAL RATIONALE: A REVIEW OF PREVIOUS DATA CONCERNING THE ANTERIOR PREMOTOR AREA OF THE RHESUS MONKEY

From an anatomical standpoint, the anterior premotor area (Map Location A) represents that section of the cortex at the rostral end of the superior limb of the arcuate sulcus. This corresponds to that area in the eye-movement studies of Smith (1944) which yielded eyelid-opening "awakening" and pupillary dilation on electrical stimulation. Our own studies on electrical stimulation of this area in lightly anesthetized animals indicate that selective eye opening and pupillary dilation may occur on stimulation. Moreover, these responses occur at a relatively low threshold compared to the voltages required for the production of eye movements in the other sectors of the frontal eye field below the superior limb of the arcuate sulcus (see Smith, 1944; Crosby et al., 1952). The relatively low threshold of this area for spreading seizure after-discharge had been previously noted in the studies of French et al. (1955). As we have already indicated, eyelid opening with pupillary dilation and eyelid myoclonus are often prominent during human petit mal seizures (a "blank stare").

We may assume that many of the behavioral phenomena of the petit mal seizure may be represented and re-represented at various levels of the neuraxis. Arrest of movement may occur on stimulation of caudate nucleus or intralaminar nuclei of the thalamus. [Our own unpublished studies (Watson and Marcus) indicate that arrest of movement may be induced in the midbrain or decerebrate preparation.] It is useful to review the anatomical connections of this cortical area. Much of the information about this area is derived from electrophysiological studies of evoked potentials. French et al. (1955) found a particularly dense collection of loci about this area (the superior limb of arcuate sulcus—"the frontal oculomotor area"), stimulation of which evoked potentials in the cephalic brain stem reticular formation. While behavioral arousal resulted from stimulation of these loci, the authors did point out that these particular cortical areas correspond to the "suppressor strips" (areas 4S, 2S, 8, 19, 24)—described previously in the studies of Dusser de Barenne and McCulloch (suppressor in the sense that movement was inhibited). McCulloch et al. (1946), using strychnine neuronography, described a pathway from area 4S to brainstem inhibitory area (paramedian lower pontine-medullary reticular formation). No response from area 8 could be found. Kuypers (1960; Animals 9 and 10), employing the Nauta technique (and utilizing large lesions primarily involving posterior premotor area), found fibers distributed to the medial pontine and medullary tegmentum. Astruc (1971), employing the Nauta-Gygax technique, has described abundant projections from area 8 to caudate, claustrum, and dorsolateral portion of putamen in addition to superior colliculus and pretectal areas. At a mesencephalic level, diffuse projections to central gray matter were also noted. At a pontine level, abundant fibers were found projecting to pontine nuclei with only a sparse projection to n. pontis centralis oralis.

The relationship of the specific cortical area to thalamic nuclei has been indicated in the retrograde degeneration studies of Akert (1964). Most of the area in question relates to the ventrolateral nucleus, the anterior portion (area 8) to dorsal median nucleus. The studies of Astruc (1971) also suggest a dense projection of area 8 to the intralaminar nuclei (n. paracentralis, centralis lateralis, and parafascicularis).

The relationship of this area to other cortical areas has also been described in detail employing the techniques of strychnine neuronography (McCulloch, 1944; Ward et al., 1946; Chusid et al., 1948). These studies suggested that area 6 projected widely in the ipsilateral hemisphere to areas 4, 1, 5, and 39 and in the contralateral hemisphere to areas 6, 4, 1, 5, and 39. Area 8 projected to areas 18 of the ipsilateral and contralateral hemisphere. More particularly (Chusid et al., 1948), the cortex buried in the posterior bank at the rostral end of the superior limb of the arcuate sulcus (an area where electrical stimulation produced pupillary dilation, eye opening, and lid blinking) had ipsilateral projections to areas 9, 6, 4, 1, 5, 7, 40, 39, 19, and 37, and to the lunate cortex of area 18.

These earlier studies also suggested that area 6 received afferent fibers from many cortical areas, e.g., 46, 5, 7, 41, 42, 23, and 24 (Ward et al., 1946). The concept of polysensory input (auditory, visual, and somatic) to the pre- and postarcuate frontal lobe areas of the monkey has also been elaborated in the studies of Bignall and Imbert (1969). These various physiological studies regarding widespread inputs to cortex in the pre- and postarcuate sulcus areas have been confirmed by recent anatomical studies employing the Nauta technique (Myers, 1967; Pandya and Kuypers, 1969).

These studies provide an anatomical and physiological background for the several reports of neglect of visual, tactile, and somatic sensory stimuli following unilateral or bilateral ablations of the cortex between the superior and inferior limbs of the arcuate sulcus. We have previously suggested (Marcus et al., 1968a) that the transient behavioral phenomena during the experimental petit mal seizures produced in our animals, with foci in Map Location A, in a sense resembled the more continuous behavioral alterations reported by Kennard (1939) and by Welch and Stuteville (1958) following ablation of this adjacent area of cortex within the curve of the arcuate sulcus. As we have indicated above, bilateral foci within the curve of the arcuate sulci have little effect. Pribram (1955) apparently failed to note any neglect of visual stimuli following bilateral cortical ablations of the frontal eye field in the baboon. (Ablations involved not only the area within the curve of the arcuate sulcus, but also the area superior to the arcuate sulcus corresponding to Map Location A.)

We have been unable to reproduce the neglect syndrome by limited unilateral ablations in the anterior premotor area. Moreover, small, unilateral cortical ablations within the curve of the arcuate sulcus also failed to result in the neglect syndrome (Marcus et al., 1970). The relationship, then, of the behavioral alteration produced by bilateral foci within the anterior premotor area to the previously reported neglect syndrome remains uncertain. The studies of Clark and Lashley (1947) have suggested that a more extensive ablation is required to produce the neglect syndrome (in addition to the area within the arcuate sulcus, much of the tissue medial and rostral, that is, within the anterior premotor area, must also be removed) or that a transverse lesion of the white matter of the cerebrum cutting the superior longitudinal fasciculus is required.

An animal model of another variety of bilateral synchronous discharge is available, the light-sensitive baboon *Papio papio* (See Naquet and Meldrum, this volume). It is of interest, and perhaps more than coincidental, that the bilateral discharges of polyspikes and of spike-slow wave discharges triggered by photic stimulation begin in frontal-central areas (pre-Rolandic) prior to their appearance in other cortical areas and prior to the discharge of subcortical areas (Naquet, 1968; Fischer-Williams et al., 1968). In more recent studies, Morrell and Naquet (1969) have recorded initial unit discharges in neurons of area 6. In our present experiments, we have not been able to trigger bilateral discharges by photic stimulation when acute or chronic bilateral foci were present in anterior or posterior premotor areas. The explanation for the lack of photosensitivity of the present experimental model is not clear at this time. The light-sensitive baboon may represent a somewhat more diffuse lesion than is present in our experimental model.

V. METHODS FOR THE STUDY OF THE MECHANISMS OF INTERACTION OF BILATERAL FOCI

The studies which have been described above would clearly suggest that a model of petit mal epilepsy may be developed in which the basic pathological lesion involves particular areas of cerebral cortex in a bilateral manner. In such a model, there is no necessity for lesions in the brainstem or diencephalon since these structures are intact.

It is possible to approach this model from a different standpoint and to inquire about the basic anatomical pathways involved in the interaction of bilateral foci. Do diencephalic and brainstem structures have a role in the synchrony of the bilateral cortical discharge found in this model?[8]   What is the role of the corpus callosum?

In our preliminary studies in the cat (Marcus and Watson, 1966), recordings from medial thalamic areas (n. centrum medianum, dorsomedial) indicated insignificant participation of these thalamic areas at the onset of the bilateral spike and spike-slow wave discharges.   Subcortical recordings do not provide direct answers to the question of the actual role of commissural pathways and subcortical structures in this interaction (also see discussion of Pollen, 1968).   We have, therefore, made use of several more direct anatomical methods.

A. Section of major commissures

Our initial studies were performed in the cat in relation to the acute studies described above.   Complete section of the corpus callosum was performed by suction under direct vision (using a 2.5 power binocular magnifier) after the medial surface of one hemisphere was retracted.   Animals were not included in this group unless there was retention of electrical activity and of seizure discharges in both hemispheres.   Bilateral synchrony was markedly disrupted.   The capacity for independent discharge was, however, retained in each hemisphere.

In the monkey, section of all major commissures (corpus callosum, anterior commissure, and hippocampal commissure) was performed by suction, employing glass micropipettes and with the aid of an operating-room microscope.   In the acute monkey preparation, the synchrony of discharge of bilateral foci was markedly disrupted (Marcus and Watson, 1968a,b). The capacity for prolonged independent discharge was, however, retained in each hemisphere.   With bilateral foci in high precentral area, alternate pathways for a coarse synchrony of slow discharge were noted.   Spikes occurring every 1 to 2 sec could be synchronized within 50 to 400 msec (compared to 0 to 20 msec in the intact monkey preparation or in the human patient with petit mal epilepsy).

A number of objections could be raised to such studies in the animal with acute section of commissures, e.g., depression of cortical activity due to operative procedure.   A series of monkeys was therefore prepared under aseptic conditions in which total section of major commissures was performed.   Approximately 6 to 18 days later, those animals who were other-

---

[8]It is important to note that in considering this question we are dealing only with the cortical electrical discharge of the petit mal seizure.   We assume that the behavioral components are obviously represented and re-represented at various levels of the neuraxis as discussed above.

wise intact from a neurological standpoint (with regard to absence of hemiparesis, of visual field defects, and of sensory neglect syndromes) were reoperated on as acute experiments with bilateral foci employing 1% conjugated estrogen. The results of the acute one-stage experiments cited above were completely confirmed.

B. Bilateral cortical callosal isolation

These results were in marked contrast to the high degree of synchrony between bilateral cortical foci obtained in the preparation in which large blocks of cerebral cortex in each hemisphere had been isolated from subcortical structures but remained connected via the corpus callosum (Fig. 7).

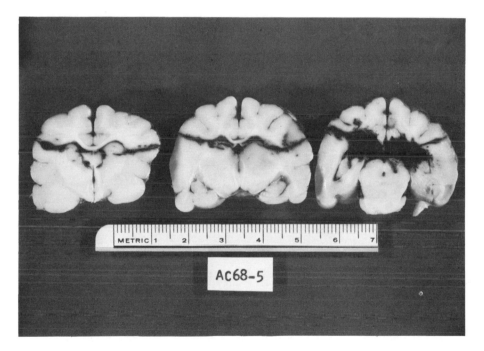

FIG. 7. Bilateral isolation of cerebral cortex and corpus callosum: The cortical callosal preparation. These coronal sections demonstrate the bilateral isolation of cerebral cortex in the cat. This was produced by dissection to the floor of each lateral ventricle at anterior and posterior poles. A curved spatula was then introduced into each lateral ventricle and cortex was undercut to pial surface. Pial blood supply remained intact. Cortex anterior and posterior to the isolation was then removed. In some animals, rostrum of corpus callosum, septum, and dorsal hippocampus were also ablated. A similar procedure may also be performed in the monkey.

This procedure is most easily performed in the cat (Marcus and Watson, 1966a). The procedure may be performed under conditions of ether–Flaxedil–respirator or under conditions of light anesthesia with pentobarbital. For a more detailed consideration of anesthetic effects, the reader is referred to Marcus and Watson (1966b). Dissection to the floor of each lateral ventricle at anterior and posterior poles was performed. A curved spatula was then introduced into each lateral ventricle, and cortex was undercut to pial surface. Pial blood supply remained intact. Cortex anterior and posterior to the isolation was usually removed. In some animals, rostrum of corpus callosum, septum, and dorsal hippocampus were also ablated. The animal was then studied as an acute preparation employing recording techniques described above.

Patterns of symmetrical spikes and repetitive 3 cps spike-wave complexes, often synchronized within 2 to 20 msec, followed the application of the convulsant agent to bilaterally isolated blocks of cortex (Fig. 8). This degree of synchronization was well within the limits of interhemispheric synchronization observed in man with petit mal.

The procedure can be performed in the monkey with essentially similar results (Marcus and Watson, 1968); however, there are a number of technical problems related, for example, to increased mass of cerebral cortex and of corpus callosum overlying the ventricular system. Therefore, a very small yield of successful preparations can be expected when the monkey is employed.

C. Other isolation procedures (thalamic ablation)

Similar results were obtained in the cat when bilateral cortical foci were produced in preparation subjected to ablation of the entire thalamus, hypothalamus, rostral mesencephalon, and dorsal hippocampus (Marcus and Watson, 1966a). The production of bilateral cortical foci in preparations with limited ablations of medial thalamus and adjacent rostral mesencephalon led to similar results.

D. Use of anatomical isolation methods to study other types of bilateral synchronous discharges

The methods which we have employed to investigate the interaction of bilateral foci may also be employed to assay mechanisms of action of various convulsant agents in producing bilateral synchronous discharges. Thus,

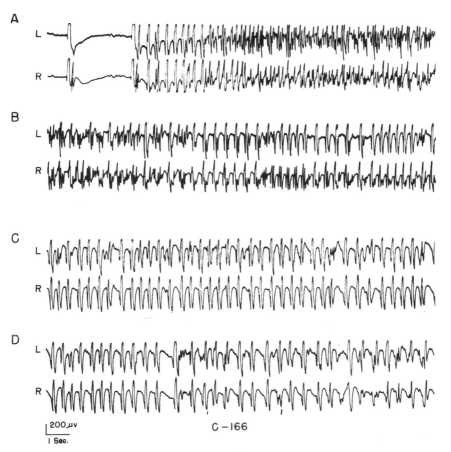

FIG. 8. Bilateral synchronous spike-slow wave discharges following the production of bilateral epileptogenic foci in the cortical callosal preparation (cat). Frequent prolonged bursts of 2 to 2½ cps spike-slow wave complexes occurred in the preparation in addition to polyspike-slow wave complexes. Recordings were obtained 10 hr after isolation and 80 min after production of bilateral foci in anterior-middle suprasylvian gyri. Pentobarbital anesthesia had been administered 12 hr previously (30 mg/kg i.p.). Segments are continuous except for a 2-min interval between B and C. From Marcus et al. (1968b), with permission of the publisher. A more detailed analysis of one degree of bilateral synchrony is provided in Marcus et al. (1968b) and Marcus and Watson (1966a).

it is possible to demonstrate that the synchrony of the bilateral cortical discharge produced with threshold amounts of pentylenetetrazol administered intravenously is dependent on the corpus callosum (Marcus et al., 1969; Marcus, 1972).

VI. SUMMARY

The clinical aspects of petit mal epilepsy are discussed, and various theoretical and experimental approaches to the pathophysiology of this disorder are considered. Several models of petit mal epilepsy in monkey and cat, employing the experimental design of bilateral cortical foci, are presented in detail.

It is demonstrated that it is possible to produce an experimental model of the electrical and behavioral characteristics of petit mal epilepsy in the monkey employing the design of bilateral cortical foci in the *anterior premotor areas*. These foci are produced by a variety of methods including acute topical agents such as conjugated estrogens and subacute agents such as cobalt powder.

Methods for investigating the synchrony of bilateral discharge produced by such foci are discussed, as well as the primary role of the corpus callosum in mediating the interaction of bilateral foci. In this model, it is demonstrated that the brainstem and diencephalic structures are not essential for the development of bilateral synchronous discharges.

Previous anatomical and physiological studies of the anterior premotor area are reviewed because of the importance in the experimental design of locating the bilateral foci within this area.

VII. ACKNOWLEDGMENTS

The suggestions of Dr. C. Wesley Watson and the technical assistance of Miss Evelyn Losh, Mr. Albert Fullerton, and Miss Renette Bowker are gratefully acknowledged.

This study was supported in part by U.S. Public Health Service research grant NB06937 from the National Institute of Neurological Diseases and Stroke, and by the institution grant from the National Institutes of Health to the New England Medical Center Hospital.

VIII. REFERENCES

Akert, K. (1946): Comparative anatomy of frontal cortex and thalamofrontal connections. In: *The Frontal Granular Cortex and Behavior*, edited by J. M. Warren and K. Akert. McGraw-Hill, New York, pp. 372–396.

Ajmone Marsan, C. (1969): Pathophysiology of the EEG pattern characteristic of petit mal epilepsy; a critical review of some of the experimental data. In: *The Physiopathogenesis of the Epilepsies,* edited by H. Gastaut et al. Charles C Thomas, Springfield, Ill., pp. 237–248.

Astruc, J. (1971): Corticofugal connections of area 8 (frontal eye field in *Macaca mulatta*). *Brain Research,* 33:241–756.

Bancaud, J., Talairach, J., Bonis, A., Schaub, C., Szikla, G., Morel, P., and Bordas-Ferer, M. (1965): *La Stéréo-Electroencéphalographic Dans L'Epilepsie.* Masson, Paris, p. 321.

Bignall, K. E., and Imbert, M. (1969): Polysensory and corticocortical projections to frontal lobe of squirrel and rhesus monkeys. *Electroencephalography and Clinical Neurophysiology,* 26:206–213.

Cereghino, J. J., and Dow, R. S. (1970): Effect of cobalt applied to the cerebellum on cobalt experimental epilepsy in the cat. *Epilepsia,* 11:413–421.

Chatrian, G. E., Somasundaram, M., and Tassinari, C. S. (1968): D.C. changes recorded transcranially during "typical" three per second spike and wave discharges in man. *Epilepsia,* 9:185–209.

Chusid, J. G., and Kopeloff, L. M. (1962): Epileptogenic effects of pure metals implanted in motor cortex of monkeys. *Journal of Applied Physiology,* 17:697–700.

Chusid, J. G., and Kopeloff, L. M. (1967): Epileptogenic effects of metal powder implants in motor cortex of monkeys. *International Journal of Neuropsychiatry,* 3:24–28.

Chusid, J. G., Sugar, O., and French, J. D. (1948): Corticocortical connections of the cerebral cortex lying within the arcuate and lunate sulci of the monkey (*Macaca mulatta*). *Journal of Neuropathology and Experimental Neurology,* 7:439–446.

Clark, G., and Lashley, K. S. (1947): Visual disturbances following frontal ablations in the monkey. *Anatomical Record,* 97:326.

Clemente, C. D., and Sterman, M. D. (1967): Basal forebrain mechanisms for internal inhibition and sleep. *Research Publications Association for Research in Nervous and Mental Disease,* 45:127–147.

Cohn, R. (1954): Spike-dome complex in the human electroencephalogram. *Archives of Neurology and Psychiatry,* 71:699–706.

Crosby, E. C., Yoss, R. E., and Henderson, J. W. (1952): The mammalian midbrain and isthmus regions, Part II, The fiber connections D: The pattern for eye movements on the frontal eye field and on discharge of specific portions of this field to and through midbrain levels. *Journal of Comparative Neurology,* 97:357–383.

Dow, R. S., Fernandez-Guardiola, A., and Manni, E. (1962): The influence of the cerebellum on experimental epilepsy. *Electroencephalography and Clinical Neurophysiology,* 14:383–398.

Echlin, F. A. (1959): The supersensitivity of chronically isolated cerebral cortex as a mechanism in focal epilepsy. *Electroencephalography and Clinical Neurophysiology,* 11:697–722.

Fermaglich, J., and O'Doherty, D. S. (1972): Agenesis of the corpus callosum: An Electroencephalographic Study. *Epilepsy,* 4th series, 13:345.

Fischer-Williams, M., Poncet, M., Riche, D., and Naquet, R. (1968): Light induced epilepsy in the baboon, *Papio papio:* Cortical and depth recordings. *Electroencephalography and Clinical Neurophysiology,* 25:557–569.

French, J. D., Hernandez-Peon, R., and Livingston, R. B. (1955): Projections from cortex to cephalic brain stem reticular formation in monkey. *Journal of Neurophysiology,* 18:74–95.

Gastaut, H. (1969): Introduction to the study of generalized epilepsies. In: *The Physiopathogenesis of the Epilepsies,* edited by H. Gastaut et al. Charles C Thomas, Springfield, Ill., pp. 11–16.

Gastaut, H., and Fischer-Williams, M. (1959): The physiopathology of epileptic seizures. In: *Handbook of Physiology,* edited by J. Field, Section 1, Vol. 1 (Neurophysiology). American Physiological Society, Washington, D.C., pp. 329–363.

Geller, M., and Geller, A. (1970): Brief amnestic effects of spike-wave discharges. *Neurology,* 20:1089–1095.

Gibbs, F. A., and Gibbs, E. L. (1952): *Atlas of Electroencephalography,* Vol. II, *Epilepsy.* Addison Wesley Press, Cambridge, Mass., p. 442.

Gloor, P. (1969): Neurophysiological bases of generalized seizures termed centrencephalic. In: *The Physiopathogenesis of the Epilepsies,* edited by H. Gastaut et al. Charles C Thomas, Springfield, Ill., pp. 209–236.

Goldensohn, D. N., Clardy, E. R., and Levine, K. (1941): Agenesis of the corpus callosum. *Journal of Nervous and Mental Disease,* 93:567–580.

Goode, D. J., Penry, J. K., and Dreifuss, F. E. (1970): Effects of paroxysmal spike-wave on continuous visual motor performance. *Epilepsia,* 11:241–254.

Grafstein, B. (1959): Organization of callosal connections in the suprasylvian gyrus of cat. *Journal of Neurophysiology,* 22:504–515.

Green, J. B., and Russell, D. J. (1966): Electroencephalographic asymmetry with midline cyst and deficient corpus callosum. *Neurology,* 16:541–545.

Grimm, R. J., Frazee, J. G., Bell, C. C., Kawasaki, T., and Dow, R. S. (1969): Quantitative studies in cobalt model epilepsy, The effect of cerebellar stimulation. *International Journal of Neurology,* 7:126–140.

Guerrero-Figueroa, R., Barros, A., DeBalbian-Vester, F., and Heath, R. G. (1963): Experimental "petit mal" in kittens. *Archives of Neurology,* 9:297–306.

Hayne, R. A., Belinson, L., and Gibbs, F. A. (1949): Electrical activity of subcortical areas in epilepsy. *Electroencephalography and Clinical Neurophysiology,* 1:437–445.

Hunter, J., and Jasper, H. H. (1949): Effects of thalamic stimulation in unanesthetized animals. *Electroencephalography and Clinical Neurophysiology,* 1:305–324.

Hursh, J. B. (1945): Origin of the spike wave pattern of petit mal epilepsy. *Archives of Neurology and Psychiatry,* 53:274–282.

Ingvar, D. H. (1955a): Reproduction of the three per second spike and wave EEG pattern by subcortical electrical stimulation in cats. *Acta Physiologica Scandinavica,* 33:137–150.

Ingvar, D. H. (1955b): Electrical activity of isolated cortex in the unanesthetized cat with intact brain stem. *Acta Physiologica Scandinavica,* 33:151–168.

Jasper, H. H. (1949): Diffuse projection system. The integrative action of the thalamic reticular system. *Electroencephalography and Clinical Neurophysiology,* 1:405–420.

Jasper, H. H., and Droogleever-Fortuyn, J. (1946): Experimental studies on the functional anatomy of petit mal epilepsy. *Research Publications Association for Research in Nervous and Mental Disease,* 26:272–298.

Jasper, H. H., and Kershman, J. (1941): Electroencephalographic classification of the epilepsies. *Archives of Neurology and Psychiatry,* 45:903.

Kennard, M. A. (1939): Alterations in response to visual stimuli following lesions of frontal lobe in monkeys. *Archives of Neurology and Psychiatry,* 41:1153–1164.

Kopeloff, L. M., Barrera, S. E., and Kopeloff, N. (1942): Recurrent convulsive seizures in animals produced by immunologic and chemical means. *American Journal of Psychiatry,* 98:881.

Kopeloff, L. M., Chusid, J. G., and Kopeloff, N. (1954): Chronic experimental epilepsy in *Macaca mulatta. Neurology,* 4:218–227.

Kopeloff, L. M., Chusid, J. C., and Kopeloff, N. (1955): Epilepsy in *Macaca mulatta* after cortical or intracerebral alumina. *Archives of Neurology and Psychiatry,* 74:523–526.

Krieger, H. P., Wagnan, I. H., and Bender, M. B. (1958): Changes in stage of consciousness and patterns of eye movements. *Journal of Neurophysiology,* 21:224–230.

Kuypers, H. G. J. M. (1960): Central cortical projections to motor and somato-sensory cell groups. *Brain,* 83:161–184.

Marcus, E. M. (1972): The electroencephalogram, seizures, sleep, coma and consciousness. In: *An Introduction to the Neurosciences,* edited by B. Curtis, S. Jacobson, and E. M. Marcus. W. B. Saunders, Philadelphia, pp. 710–752.

Marcus, E. M., Fullerton, A., Losh, E., and Bowker, R. (1972): Epileptogenic effects of cobalt in *Macaca mulatta:* Unilateral and bilateral cortical foci. *Epilepsia,* 4th series, 13:343–344.

Marcus, E. M., Jacobsen, S., Watson, C. W., Katzen, M., and Krolikowski, F. (1970): An experimental model of "petit mal epilepsy" in the monkey: additional studies of the anterior premotor area. *Transactions of American Neurological Association*, 95:297–281.

Marcus, E. M., and Watson, C. W. (1964): Bilateral epileptogenic foci in cat cerebral cortex: mechanisms of interaction in the intact, the bilateral cortical callosal and adiencephalic preparation. *Electroencephalography and Clinical Neurophysiology*, 17:454.

Marcus, E. M., and Watson, C. W. (1966a): Bilateral synchronous spike wave electrographic patterns in the cat: interaction of bilateral cortical foci in the intact, the bilateral cortical-callosal and adiencephalic preparation. *Archives of Neurology*, 14:601–610.

Marcus, E. M., and Watson, C. W. (1966b): Studies of the bilateral cortical callosal preparation. *Transactions of the American Neurological Association*, 91:291–293.

Marcus, E. M., and Watson, C. W. (1968): Bilateral symmetrical epileptogenic foci in monkey cerebral cortex: mechanisms of interaction and regional variations in capacity for synchronous spike slow wave discharges. *Archives of Neurology*, 19:99–116.

Marcus, E. M., Watson, C. W., and Goldman, P. L. (1966): Effects of steroids on cerebral electrical activity: epileptogenic effects of conjugated estrogens and related compounds in the cat and rabbit. *Archives of Neurology*, 15:521–532.

Marcus, E. M., Watson, C. W., and Jacobsen, S. (1969): Role of the corpus callosum in bilateral synchronous discharges induced by intravenous pentylenetetrazol. *Neurology*, 19:309.

Marcus, E. M., Watson, C. W., and Simon, S. (1968a): Behavioral correlates of acute bilateral symmetrical epileptogenic foci in monkey cerebral cortex. *Brain Research*, 9:370–373.

Marcus, E. M., Watson, C. W., and Simon, S. A. (1968b): An experimental model of some varieties of petit mal epilepsy. *Epilepsia*, 9:233–248.

Mattson, R. H., and Bickford, R. G. (1961): Firing patterns of strychnine spikes in the cortex of the cat. *Electroencephalography and Clinical Neurophysiology*, 13:144–145.

McCulloch, W. S. (1944): Cortico-cortical connections. In: *The Precentral Motor Cortex*, edited by P. C. Bucy. University of Illinois Press, Urbana, pp. 211–242.

McCulloch, W. S., Graff, C., and Magoun, H. W. (1946): A cortico-bulboreticular pathway from area 4S. *Journal of Neurophysiology*, 9:127–132.

Mirsky, A. F., and Pragay, E. B. (1967): The relation of EEG and performance in altered states of consciousness. *Research Publications Association for Research in Nervous and Mental Disease*, 45:514–534.

Morrell, F., Naquet, R., and Menini, C. (1969): Microphysiology of cortical single neurons in *Papio papio*. *Electroencephalography and Clinical Neurophysiology*, 27:708–709.

Morison, R. S., and Dempsey, E. W. (1942): A study of thalamocortical relations. *American Journal of Physiology*, 135:281–292.

Mutani, R., and Fariello, R. (1969): Effetti elettrocefalografiei e comportamentali di foci epilettogeni sperimentali cronici disposti in modo bilaterale e simmetrico sulla corteccia del gatto. *Rivista Di Neurologia*, 39:521–528.

Myers, R. E. (1967): Cerebral connectionism and brain function. In: *Brain Mechanisms Underlying Speech and Language*, edited by C. H. Millikan and F. L. Darley. Grune & Stratton, New York, pp. 61–72.

O'Brien, J. L., Goldensohn, E. S., and Hoefer, R. T. (1959): Electroencephalographic abnormalities in addition to bilaterally synchronous 3/sec spike and wave activity in petit mal. *Electroencephalography and Clinical Neurophysiology*, 13:747–761.

Pandya, D. N., and Kuypers, H. G. J. M. (1969): Cortico-cortical connections in the rhesus monkey. *Brain Research*, 13:13–36.

Penfield, W., and Jasper, H. (1954): *Epilepsy and the Functional Anatomy of the Human Brain*. Little Brown, Boston, p. 896.

Petsche, H. (1962): Pathophysiologic and klinik des petit mal. *Weiner Zeitschrift Fur Nervenheil-Kunde*, 19:345–442.

Pollen, D. A. (1968): Experimental spike and wave responses and petit mal epilepsy. *Epilepsia*, 9:221–232.

Pollen, D. A., Perot, P., and Reid, K. M. (1963): Experimental bilateral wave and spike from thalamic stimulation in relation to level of arousal. *Electroencephalography and Clinical Neurophysiology*, 15:1017–1028.

Pollen, D. A., Reid, K., and Perot, P. (1964): Micro-electrode studies of experimental 3/sec wave and spike in the cat. *Electroencephalography and Clinical Neurophysiology*, 17: 57–67.

Pribram, K. H. (1955): Lesions of "frontal eye fields" and delayed response of baboons. *Journal of Neurophysiology*, 18:105–112.

Servit, Z., Strejckova, A., and Fischer, J. (1966): Comparative physiology of the thalamic pacemaker of paroxysmal activity, extirpation of thalamus in the frog. In: *Comparative and Cellular Pathophysiology of Epilepsy*, edited by Z. Servit. Publishing House of Czechoslovak Academy of Sciences, Prague, pp. 270–276.

Smith, W. K. (1944): The frontal eye fields. In: *The Precentral Motor Cortex*, edited by P. C. Bucy. University of Illinois Press, Urbana, pp. 307–342.

Snider, R. S., and Lee, J. C. (1961): *A Sterotaxic Atlas of the Monkey Brain*. University of Chicago Press, Chicago.

Spiegel, E. A., Wycis, H. T., and Reyes, V. (1951): Diencephalic mechanisms in petit mal epilepsy. *Electroencephalography and Clinical Neurophysiology*, 3:473–475.

Stamm, J. S., and Pribram, K. H. (1960): Effects of epileptogenic lesions in frontal cortex on learning and retention in monkeys. *Journal of Neurophysiology*, 23:552–563.

Starzl, T. E., Niemer, W. T., Dell, M., and Foregrave, P. R. (1953): Cortical and subcortical electrical activity in experimental seizures induced by Metrazol. *Journal of Neuropathology and Experimental Neurology*, 12:262–276.

Starzl, T. E., and Whitlock, D. G. (1952): Diffuse thalamic projection system in the monkey. *Journal of Neurophysiology*, 15:449–468.

Swank, R. L. (1949): Synchronization of spontaneous electrical activity of cerebrum by barbiturate narcosis. *Journal of Neurophysiology*, 12:161–172.

Velasco, M., and Lindsley, D. B. (1965): Role of orbital cortex in regulation of the thalamocortical electrical activity. *Science*, 149:1375–1377.

Wagman, T. H., Krieger, H. P., Papatheodorou, C. A., and Bender, M. B. (1961): Eye movements elicited by surface and depth stimulation of frontal lobe of the macaque. *Journal of Comparative Neurology*, 117:179–188.

Walker, A. E., and Morello, G. (1967): Experimental petit mal. *Transactions of the American Neurological Association*, 92:57–61.

Ward, A. A. (1969): The epileptic neuron: Chronic foci in animals and man. In: *Basic Mechanisms of the Epilepsies*, edited by H. H. Jasper, A. A. Ward, Jr., and A. Pope. Little Brown, Boston, pp. 263–288.

Ward, A. A., Pededen, I. K., and Sugar, O. (1946): Cortico-cortical connections in the monkey with special reference to area 6. *Journal of Neurophysiology*, 9:453–461.

Watson, C. W., and Denny-Brown, D. (1953): Myoclonus epilepsy as a symptom of diffuse neuronal disease. *Archives of Neurology and Psychiatry*, 70:151–168.

Weir, B. (1964): Spike-wave from stimulation of reticular core. *Archives of Neurology*, 11: 209–218.

Welch, K., and Stuteville, P. (1958): Experimental production of unilateral neglect in monkeys. *Brain*, 81:341–347.

Williams, D. (1953): A study of thalamic and cortical rhythms in petit mal. *Brain*, 76:50–69.

6

Focal Electrical Stimulation

C. Ajmone Marsan

OUTLINE

I. INTRODUCTION

In the experimental approach to the study of epileptic disorders, repetitive electrical stimulation of more or less discrete regions of the central nervous system provides a most convenient, practical and relatively simple method for reproduction of the ictal phenomena of focal — or partial — epilepsy. This model represents one of the best examples of an acute, fully reversible condition which can be repeatedly reproduced with ease in otherwise normal neuronal structures. It is probably one of the earliest methods utilized in the experimental study of epilepsy (e.g., Fritsch and Hitzig, 1870; Ferrier, 1873; Luciani, 1878), and it continues to be widely employed by epileptologists throughout the world, although we owe to basic neurophysiologists much of the knowledge we presently possess concerning the mechanisms of its clinical and electrographic phenomenology.

This model is based on the observation (Adrian, 1936) that stimulation of various neuronal structures by means of repetitive electrical pulses of adequate parameters is capable of inducing a characteristic pattern of relatively long-lasting activity which is *self-sustained* (i.e., overlasts — and actually starts after — the end of the stimulating current) and is commonly referred to as *after-discharge* (AD). The prominent morphological and functional similarities between this phenomenon and the ictal episodes which occur spontaneously in epileptics, or which can be induced by a variety of known epileptogenic agents, make it an ideal experimental model for the investigation of a number of aspects in the field of seizure disorders.

II. SPECIFIC INDICATIONS FOR THE MODEL USE

For obvious reasons, this model is not suitable for the study of interictal epileptiform manifestations. In most situations, the neuronal structures to which the electrical stimulation is applied are anatomically and functionally normal, and, as a rule, their activity reverts to normality a few minutes after the application of the stimulus [although there are reports suggesting the possibility of development of autonomous epileptiform activity following repeated stimulations in the acute (see Erickson, 1940) and, especially, in chronic preparations (see Goddard et al., 1969)]. The model is, as already stated, an almost ideal one for the study of ictal episodes (or organized seizure activity) which can be reproduced at will in their full form or in a wide range of varieties. Depending on the parameters of stimulation and on the region to which this is applied, such ictal episodes may be purely electrical or may include all the peripheral manifestations which are appropriate to the topography and to the functional characteristics of the stimulated region. The model lends itself to the investigations of the mechanisms which might be at the basis of the development of an epileptic seizure, in spite of the obviously artificial nature of the events which, in this particular situation, lead to the AD. The same model permits a fairly accurate evaluation of what is commonly defined as "epileptic susceptibility": (1) in different species, (2) at different ontogenetic stages in any given species, and (3) at different levels and in various structures of the central nervous system. In each of these situations, the model also lends itself to the study of all those factors (e.g., systemic, functional, pharmacological, biochemical) which may modify the threshold for eliciting an AD and which should therefore be considered as potentially capable of modifying the susceptibility to seizures. Among these factors, one should also include the inhibitory or facilitatory effects exerted upon the structure involved by the epileptiform activation and resulting from the activation or elimination of certain specific structures or systems.

Inasmuch as, in this experimental model, both topography and "intensity" (see below) of the induced ictal episode can be controlled relatively well, it also becomes possible to study patterns and the extent of its spread to other central nervous system structures which had not been directly affected by the electrical stimulation. In fact, whereas most of these localized paroxysmal episodes are, as a rule, elicited in any given structure by its "direct" stimulation, it is also possible to study them in that same structure when the repetitive stimulation has been applied, elsewhere, to a neuronal aggregate connected to it or to its afferent pathway tract (Fields et al., 1949; Michishita, 1956, Kandel and Spencer, 1961; Blum, 1969; Crowell, 1970; Crowell and Ajmone Marsan, 1972). In this respect, the method of repetitive stimulation could also be considered as a useful electrophysiological tool to determine direct and synaptic connections and preferential paths between different structures. Finally, this method also finds practical applications in the study and surgical treatment of human epilepsy.

III. TECHNICAL CONSIDERATIONS

Technical details may vary in relation to the specific purposes of the experiment as outlined in the preceding section. The problems of monitoring and recording the peripheral manifestations of the induced ictal episode are not peculiar to this model. Actually, such problems are relatively simplified in comparison with those present in other experimental situations, by the possibility this model offers to control, and thus accurately predict, the incidence and time of occurrence of the seizure episodes. The same applies to the techniques of monitoring the central electrical correlates of such episodes. As in the case of most other models, gross electrodes (for both AC and DC recording) and micro-electrodes (for both extra- and intra-cellular pick-up) can be used individually or in association and in any number according to the specific question the investigator is asking of the experiment. The model is applicable to both acute and chronic preparations and, obviously, the type of electrodes and their application will have to be adjusted according to the type of preparation. Furthermore, in acute experiments, the presence and form of anesthesia will have to be considered since these are factors which are known to affect neuronal excitability. In the remainder of this chapter, emphasis is placed on the central electrical characteristics of the model rather than on its peripheral (e.g., motor, visceral, behavioral) manifestations, although many of the considerations implicitly apply to the latter as well.

IV. PARAMETERS OF STIMULATION

The crucial feature of an electrical stimulus for the production of ADs is its repetitive character (above a critical frequency). As a rule, a single electrical pulse, no matter how strong or long-lasting, is inadequate, and so are pulses repeated at a frequency of less than 5 to 6/sec. On the other hand, all the other individual parameters are much less crucial, the stimulation being generally effective within a relatively wide range of their variability. In early works, faradic stimulation was almost exclusively used and, in fact, this model is still occasionally referred to in the current French and Italian literature as "faradic epilepsy" (Moruzzi, 1939, 1950; Bremer, 1958). Indeed, in those times when sophisticated electronic equipment was not available, any source of alternating current at the common mainline frequency of 40 to 60 cps was perfectly suitable for the production of ADs. The main advantage of the modern electronic stimulators is that they allow a greater flexibility in the control of the various parameters, thus making it possible to achieve a more accurately quantitative evaluation of threshold values.

The use of constant-current stimulators or, at least, of devices which permit an exact assessment of current (rather than simply a voltage reading) is indispensable in studies which emphasize threshold characteristics, and is preferable in any case. When using stimulating current in the form of trains of repetitive, square (mono- or diphasic) pulses, the following parameters are commonly specified.

A. Peak current amplitude and polarity of each pulse

The peak current amplitude which is generally required for the production of an AD varies between 2.5 and 8 mA. Polarity is a relatively unimportant parameter in the case of monophasic pulses, and there are no remarkable differences of effects between mono- and diphasic pulses. The latter form of current, with the two pulses of opposite polarity separated by a brief interval, might be preferable in cases of experiments involving chronically repeated stimulations with implanted electrodes, when it becomes important to minimize brain damage (Lilly, 1961; see also Halpern, this volume).

B. Pulse duration

The above-mentioned fact that both faradic and 40 to 60 cps alternating currents are quite suitable for the elicitation of rhythmical, self-sustaining activity, also implies the effectiveness of stimulations with individual pulses of a relatively long duration. Indeed, also in the case of this parameter, one finds a rather wide range of effective values. Pulse durations of 0.5 to 10 msec are commonly used with satisfactory results. With shorter durations, it is generally difficult to elicit an AD, and with values of less than 0.2 msec its elicitation is practically impossible, even when the peak current amplitude is increased above the values given in the preceding section. The most consistent results are obtained with durations of 2 to 5 msec. Pulses longer than 10 msec are not necessarily more effective and are likely to cause either functional or anatomical damage, especially when the stimulating trains are repeatedly applied to the same structure.

C. Repetition rate (p/sec) in each train of pulses

The optimal frequency of stimulation for the production of self-sustained activity is between 25 and 60 p/sec. Lower frequencies are less constantly effective, and they are exceptionally so below 10 p/sec in intact or "normal" preparations. Higher frequencies (100 p/sec or over), while still being effective, appear less suitable for the production of long-lasting ADs.

D. Length of train of pulses

The optimal duration of each train is within 4 to 6 sec. In this parameter, as in the preceding ones, the range of useful values is relatively wide, although practical experience would indicate that it is rather difficult to elicit ADs with trains of repetitive pulses lasting less than 1.5 sec. On the other hand, the prolongation of the train beyond the optimal values tends to delay accordingly the onset of self-sustained activity without necessarily increasing its overall duration. Actually, with excessively long-lasting trains, the AD may start already while the stimulation is still going on, and the latter might even disrupt the regular rhythmicity of the discharge, accelerating its end or preventing its full development (Kreindler, 1965; Kreindler and Crighel, 1966).

E. Intervals between trains

This parameter becomes critical in those experiments – indeed the large majority – in which trains of stimulating pulses are applied repeatedly to the same structure in order to induce in it self-sustained activity over and over again. If a train of stimuli has been successful in eliciting such a form of activity, it is almost always impossible to elicit a second AD by applying another stimulating train to the same structure during, or immediately at the end of, the first paroxysmal episode. In fact, for a subsequent stimulation to be effective, it is necessary to delay its application to the same region for at least 15 sec after the end of the preceding AD. In practice, intervals of 2 to 3 min are considered more satisfactory, although longer intervals (up to 5 min or more) might be preferable, even in the case of supra-threshold stimuli, for securing the best effects. Intervals of 30 or more minutes become necessary whenever there is evidence that a previous stimulation has induced "spreading depression" (Pinsky and Burns, 1962; see also Leão, this volume). It should also be pointed out that, regardless of the duration of intervals between successive trains, their excessively repeated application to the same structure may modify the threshold for AD in that structure. As to the direction of such modification, both decreases and increases in threshold have been observed.

In this brief outline of stimulation parameters, their individual optimal values are approximative, and they have been provided mainly as a practical guide for the production of the experimental model under discussion. There are several reasons for this failure to specify quantitative values in a more accurate form. As repeatedly stated above, the optimal range for each parameter is rather extensive, both in the same and in different experimental conditions. Within certain limits, the effects of a change in the value of each individual parameter, even below or above the range which is considered optimal, can be compensated for — or corrected — by the appropriate modification of one or of several other parameters. As a rule, and especially in acute preparations, the AD does not behave as a morphologically stereotyped, all-or-none phenomenon (in chronic conditions the situation would be different, according to Berry, 1965). As a consequence, the effects of stimulation do not lend themselves to a totally satisfactory quantification. In such a situation, "threshold" becomes a relative concept and its accurate determination difficult to achieve.

Before elaborating on this important aspect, a brief description of the AD is necessary.

V. EPILEPTIFORM AFTER-DISCHARGE

The self-sustained activity, which can be elicited with appropriate repetitive stimulation of many structures within the central nervous system, has a complex pattern consisting of a variety of morphological features. Their description also reflects the different type of information provided by the different recording techniques. The records obtained by means of the traditional gross-electrode technique have been described and analyzed in great detail by Rosenblueth and Cannon (1941–2) in their classical study which should be consulted by anyone interested in this model (see also Jasper, 1954; Kreindler, 1965). In such records, the AD in its typical and fully developed form (see Fig. 3) is suggestively similar to a (local) miniature episode of "grand mal" seizure. In fact, its rhythmical characteristics, which generally become appreciable after a latent period of up to 1 to 2 sec from the end of the stimulating train, are initially those of the "tonic" stage, with low-voltage regular oscillations of an approximate frequency of 15 to 30 cps, progressively increasing in amplitude and decreasing in frequency to assume an overt "clonic" character in which large voltage oscillations occur at longer and longer intervals. The episode ends abruptly with the last one of such oscillations, the postictal stage being typically characterized by a marked depression of activity. The overall duration of the entire episode can be quite variable (10 to 90 sec or more), and the same is true for the postictal depression (2 to 15 sec or more). The sequence of phenomena in similarly typical ADs when recording with a DC technique or with intra- or extracellular micropipettes has been repeatedly analyzed and described

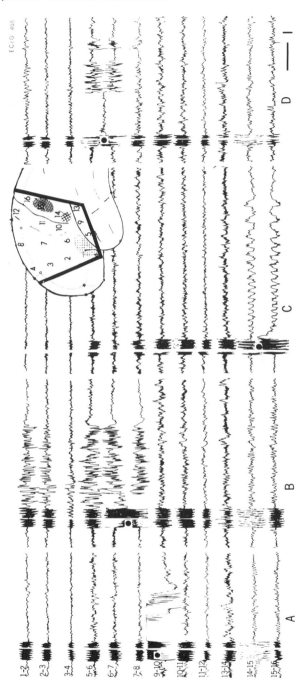

FIG. 1. Various patterns of larval and short-duration ADs. Epileptic patient with surgical exposure of cortex as indicated in brain outline with electrode position (electrodes 1 and 14 are close to cystic lesions and 15 is on an area of previously excised tissue). Parameters for the electrical stimulation in each of the four sections (A–D) are: diphasic pulses of 2.5 msec total duration, 4 mA peak-to-peak, 60/sec; train duration, 4 sec (portions of the stimulus artefact are deleted in the record). The black dot indicates the electrode closest to the stimulation site. Note long-lasting blocking of the amplifier in A and interlocking of pens in D; some artefacts and 60 cps interference at electrode 13. The AD remains well localized in A, C, and D but is relatively more widespread in B. No clinical correlates or subjective sensations noted with any of the ADs (see also Figs. 2 and 3). Calibrations: 2 sec, 500 μV.

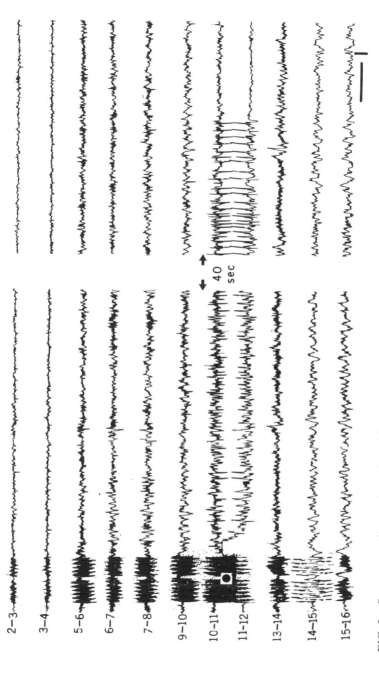

FIG. 2.   Same case and same electrode position as in Fig. 1.   Parameters of stimulation (close to electrode 11) as in Fig. 1, but intensity and train duration are decreased (2 mA, 2.5 sec).   In spite of this, a long-lasting AD (note deletion of 40 sec of record) was induced and this was accompanied by clinical phenomena (clonic flexion and extension of the fingers and metacarpo-phalangeal joints of the right hand).   Calibrations: 2 sec, 500 μV.

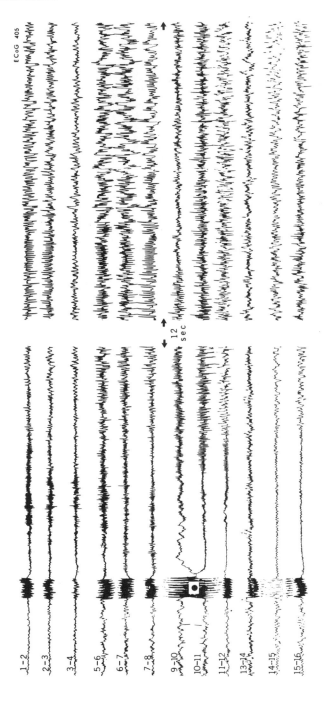

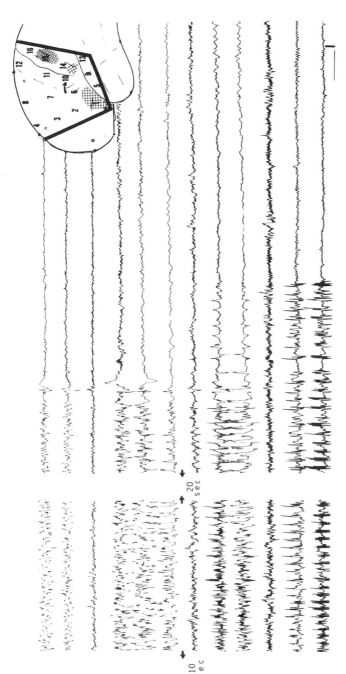

FIG. 3. Typical AD with rapid widespread distribution. Same case as in Figs. 1 and 2. Parameters of stimulation as in Fig. 1, except that train duration is decreased (about 1.5 sec). The long duration (note deletion of 42 sec of record) and diffuse distribution of self-sustained activity with this unusually brief stimulus train suggests a pathogically enhanced excitability of the stimulated and surrounding area (close to electrodes 10 and 11). Note quasi-simultaneous invasion of certain regions and a later invasion of others. The end of the AD occurs at different times in different regions. Postictal depression and slowing of activity can be observed. Clinical phenomena consisted of clonic movements of right upper and lower extremities, and later also, of the left arm. Calibrations: 2 sec, 500 μV.

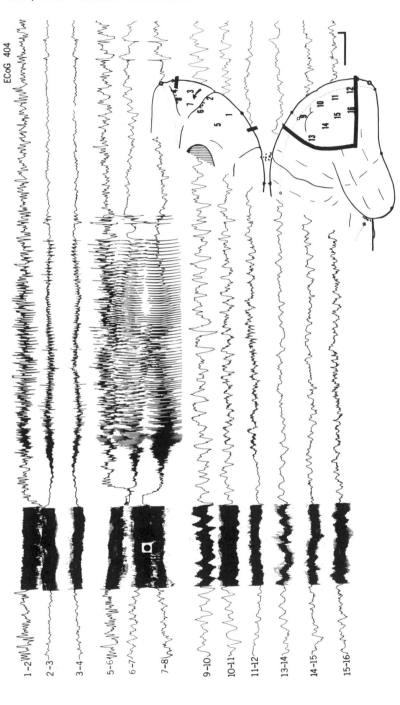

FIG. 4. Typical, relatively well-localized AD with tonic-clonic phases and brief postictal depression. Epileptic patient with surgical exposure of the occipital region as indicated in brain outline (lateral and mesial surfaces) with electrode position. Stimulation parameters as in Fig. 1 (see for additional explanations) except for intensity (6 mA) and train duration (2.5 sec). No clinical correlates or subjective sensations noted. Calibrations: 1 sec, 250 μV.

in a number of original papers to which the reader should refer (Baumgartner and Jung, 1955; Gerin, 1960; Kandel and Spencer, 1961; Gloor et al., 1962; Sawa et al., 1963; Sugaya et al., 1964; Glötzner and Grüsser, 1968; Sypert et al., 1970; Crowell and Ajmone Marsan, 1972).

In addition to the variabilities one often observes in the overall amplitude, frequency, and duration of a fully developed AD, it is also common to note considerable differences in these same parameters relative to each one of its two main stages, or, in the so-called "larval" forms of AD, the almost total absence of either stage (see Fig. 1*A, C*). These partial, or less typical, forms of self-sustained activity can be the result of an inadequate stimulation but are not infrequently observed following stimulation trains which are definitely supraliminal for a fully developed AD in another structure (compare Fig. 1 with Figs. 2 and 3) or in different experimental conditions (see below). It seems reasonable to state that, in general, the overall pattern and duration of an AD will depend on: (1) parameters of stimulation, (2) structure or region stimulated, (3) functional conditions of such structures, and (4) general systemic and specific experimental conditions.

Examples of various patterns of AD are illustrated in Figs. 1–4. Detailed descriptions of the same phenomenon in different structures can be found in a number of original articles in addition to those quoted above (Gastaut et al., 1952; Andy and Akert, 1955; Kreindler and Steriade, 1963; Elul, 1964; Machek and Fischer, 1966; Andy and Koshino, 1967; Peeler and Andy, 1967).

VI. THRESHOLD FOR ELICITATION OF AFTER-DISCHARGE

As already mentioned, and as the preceding illustrative examples indicate, the AD is not an all-or-none phenomenon. Its complex and variable morphological characteristics and the variability of its measurable parameters make it rather difficult to evaluate and quantify this particular type of self-sustained response to repetitive electrical stimulation and, consequently, to determine with accuracy the threshold value for the different parameters of the latter. Unquestionably, there are critical values for each of such parameters below which the stimulation is totally ineffective, with no traces of AD. Strictly speaking, a stimulation at such values should be considered as "threshold," simply because it can produce *some* form of self-sustained activity. However, among the various characteristics of this activity, its duration is the criterion most commonly used to determine the degree of development of an AD. Thus, as a more practical way to establish some type of threshold value, one should first determine with a supramaximal stimulation the longest duration of an AD that can be elicited in a given structure and under certain experimental conditions, and then progressively search for the lowest value for each individual parameter at which the stimulation is still capable of eliciting an AD of this maximal duration. The selection of "duration" for purposes of establishing threshold and, indirectly, to assess and quantify the "intensity" of the induced paroxysmal activity, is a reasonable, and probably the most practical, criterion among its various pattern characteristics, even though there are certain situations in which one might question its validity (compare, for instance, the two ADs in Fig. 1 where the one in *B* could be described as a better developed response than that in *C*, in spite of the longer duration of the latter; also compare Figs. 7 and 9*B* in Jasper et al., 1952, for a similar discrepancy).

A possibly preferable criterion for the assessment of threshold could be consideration of the duration, but exclusively of those ADs which are fully developed in their two main tonic-clonic stages. In either case, however, the measurement of this variable should take into consideration the possibility of a much earlier onset, i.e., of an AD beginning before the end of the stimulation train. This is a rather common occurrence, when excessively long-lasting trains are employed, and it might result in an underestimation of the total AD duration.

The work of Pinsky and Burns (1962) can be considered as one of the few studies in which the threshold for AD has been investigated systematically in fairly well-controlled—though somewhat unusual—conditions. [Among other works bearing more or less directly on the problem of AD threshold are those by Minz and Domino (1953), Andy et al. (1958), Berry (1965), and Straw (1968). Most of these studies analyze this aspect especially in relation to possible pharmacological effects or to CNS manipulations. Other papers in which the threshold of AD is related primarily to topographical factors will be mentioned in the next section.] Pinsky and Burns' experiments were performed in the absence of anesthesia but on isolated slabs of cerebral cortex (see also Halpern, this volume), and the ADs from which the data have been derived consisted of relatively simple, rhythmical self-sustained activity of the "clonic" type, with no fully developed tonic-clonic sequences. Duration was the criterion used for the assessment of stimulation, each individual parameter being tested in turn, while the others were kept constant. In these experimental conditions, the AD behaved as an all-or-none phenomenon with regard to: (1) strength of the stimulus (threshold range 2.5 to 4.3 V; average 3.4 mA); (2) pulse duration (threshold 0.3 to 0.4 msec); and (3) duration of the stimulus train (threshold 2 to 4 sec; longer trains would tend to delay the AD onset). In contrast, according to this same study, the AD duration would lose its all-or-none character with varying of the frequency of stimulation. The optimal frequency range was found to be between 32 and 64 p/sec. With lower frequencies, the AD duration would decrease (and no AD could be elicited with frequencies of 4 p/sec or lower), and it would equally decline for frequencies above this range.

According to Pinsky and Burns (1962), by increasing the strength or duration of the pulses, the number of excited neurons increases. Thus, for the production of an AD it would be necessary only to reach the excitation of a minimal number of elements; further increase in this number, however, would not affect the AD duration. Since the excitation must involve a critical minimum number of neurons, the same authors also attempted to determine the importance of the density of such a critical neuronal population. By the use of electrode discs of various diameters, or by varying the number of electrode contacts connected to the stimulator, it was possible to estimate the current (proportional to the applied current divided by the observed conductance) and to determine that the critical value required to induce an AD was no less when the area of stimulated cortex was large than when it was small. The conclusion from these findings was that for the development of an AD it is necessary to excite a minimum density of neurons per unit surface of the cortex.

The establishment of the threshold for AD was not the primary purpose of Gerin's (1960) interesting study. This, however, demonstrated certain early changes in neuronal activity, the occurrence or absence of which could determine whether a given stimulation would or would not lead to the development of self-sustained activity. Thus the efficiency of each of the above-mentioned individual parameters of stimulation could be predicted rather accurately already in the course of the stimulation, their minimal critical values being those at which the characteristic changes in neuronal activity began to appear. Such changes consisted mainly of a progressive decrease in the amplitude of the extracellularly recorded spikes with each subsequent stimulating pulse, and eventually in their disappearance. These findings were interpreted as indicative of a progressive building up of a marked depolarization of the neuronal membrane, a fact since then repeatedly confirmed by intracellular studies (see references above).

In earlier investigations (Jung, 1951; Toennis, 1951) based on the changes of cortical-surface electrical activity in the course of stimulation, the development of rhythmical bursts of epileptiform ADs with electrical pulses repeated at a critical frequency, had been attributed to the progressive lengthening and diminution or elimination — during the stimulation train—of a late component of the response to individual pulses. Such a relatively slow component (30 msec in duration) was called "bremswelle" (or "braking wave") and was considered an expression of neuronal defensive processes against seizure activity. In a subsequent study with extracellular micro-electrodes, Baumgartner and Jung (1955) could also show a pause in the neuronal spike firing, temporally related to presence and duration of this "braking" wave. Thus, from this and other investigations (see above; also Ajmone Marsan, 1961; Creutzfeldt, 1969), it would appear that the production of an AD by means of a train of repetitive electrical pulses will depend on those values of their parameters, which are adequate to decrease the polarization of neuronal membranes and to maintain it for some time at such critical low levels, either through direct excitation or by overcoming inhibitory processes which would otherwise oppose such depolarization. Once this critical depolarizing level is reached in the membrane of a certain number of elements,[1] repetitive firing of these takes place and continues in the absence of any triggering pulse; i.e., the activity becomes self-sustained and its successive phases and overall pattern will develop and be quite independent of the original stimulus. It is questionable if one needs to postulate a different repolarization rate between deeper and more superficial portions of the neurons, leading to the current flow from the latter to the former and, thus, to the development of such self-sustained activity (see Burns, 1953, 1954).

The brief preceding reference to some of these possible mechanisms was provided simply to make the concept of threshold more meaningful. A more thorough discussion of the pathophysiology of AD, which is outside the scope of this chapter, can be found in the above citations (see also Bremer, 1958; Von Euler et al., 1958; Gloor, 1962; Gloor et al., 1964; Zuckermann, 1971).

VII. REGIONAL FACTORS

The large majority of studies utilizing the model of local electrical stimulation have been performed on various areas of the neocortex and in rhinencephalic structures. The same model can be applied to other structures of the central nervous system with variable but, as a rule, less, or occasionally no success. Indeed, one finds already a rather wide range of

---

[1] According to V. Okujawa (*unpublished observation*), it is not possible to induce self-sustained activity with repetitive stimulation directly applied to the membrane of a *single* neuron.

variability in susceptibility to AD (or considerable differences in threshold) within the different neocortical regions and between neocortex and paleo-cortex or related structures. The latter (hippocampus, hippocampal gyrus, amygdala in particular) show probably the highest susceptibility to epilepti-form activity with this as well as with other models of elicitation (Kaada, 1951; Green and Naquet, 1957; Leclercq and Segal, 1965a,b; Segal and Leclercq, 1965). According to French et al. (1956), on the lateral surface of the neocortex of monkeys, the areas most prone to AD are the precentral motor area (especially for face and hand representation); the more anterior portions of the frontal lobe are relatively less susceptible, and the post-central and parietal regions even less so. Much higher threshold responses were found in the first temporal convolution and even higher in the second temporal gyrus where, in most instances, no AD could be elicited. The same was true for the cortex of the occipital lobe (see, however, Jasper et al., 1952). (Similar studies carried out in cats by Garner and French (1958), showed a higher susceptibility to AD in the para-auditory areas than in the sensory-motor cortex.)

In the mesial surface of the hemisphere, frontal, posterior parietal, and occipital areas were found to be generally refractory to the induction of self-sustained activity (see, however, Hughes and Mazurowski, 1964). This could be elicited from the remaining areas but, as a rule, with a rela-tively high threshold of stimulation. In the inferior surface, the anterior portions of the temporal lobe appeared to have a high susceptibility to ADs, while in its most posterior portions, in the basal occipital region, and in the orbital surface of the frontal lobe, no ADs could be produced. The findings of French et al. (1956) are schematically illustrated in Fig. 5.

The essentially valid results of the preceding experimental series had been, in part, already available in the original study of Rosenblueth and Cannon (1941–42) or were indirectly confirmed in subsequent investiga-tions (Leclercq and Segal, 1965a,b; Segal and Laclercq, 1965), primarily designed to study differences in the epileptic susceptibility within the corti-cal and limbic areas. In general, such studies show that ADs can indeed be elicited in all cortical areas, although the thresholds in the various re-gions may be quite different, with the difference being in the direction sug-gested by the experimental findings of French et al. (1956).

Repetitive stimulation of subcortical structures such as brainstem, thalamus, and basal ganglia, and of the cerebellum, with parameters which would be considered suprathreshold for neocortex and rhinencephalon, is less likely to yield an AD consistently. Most authors would agree with the original findings of Rosenblueth and Cannon on the negative results ob-tained by cerebellar stimulation. It is worth pointing out that the inapplica-

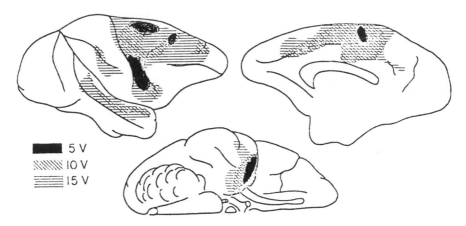

FIG. 5.   Different susceptibility to electrically induced ADs in the cortex of monkey.   Stimulation threshold in different areas as indicated by the three code patterns.   From French et al. (1956), with permission of the publisher.

bility of this model to the cerebellum is in keeping with the inapplicability to this same structure of most other models of experimental epilepsy.   Following repetitive stimulation of a variety of subcortical regions, the reported results are often contradictory.   The possibility of eliciting local ADs in any one of these regions was denied originally by Rosenblueth and Cannon. Such a possibility is, however, suggested by the results subsequently claimed by several authors (Ajmone Marsan and Stoll, 1951; Stoll et al., 1951; Michishita, 1956; Walker and Udvarhelyi, 1965a; Janzen et al., 1969). Yet, in spite of their positivity, the sporadicity of these results implicitly would seem to indicate a lesser susceptibility to seizure activity of these extra-cortical neuronal aggregates.   (For instance, Berman et al., 1953, describe in the rabbit a relatively discrete region in the mesencephalic reticular formation, stimulation of which would yield tonic-clonic convulsions at a rather low threshold; yet there is no report of local AD in this region.) This lesser susceptibility to AD is particularly evident in the data of Table 1, from the paper of Udvarhelyi and Walker (1965a).   In this table, a summary is given of the incidence of ADs in response to a large number of repetitive stimulations (with a wide range of strengths) applied to different cortical regions and to subcortical nuclear masses.

The very high threshold for—or the high incidence of failures to induce—ADs by means of a direct stimulation of basal ganglia, thalamus, and other brainstem structures is somewhat in contrast to the common observation that cortically (or even the occasional subcortically—see Walker and Udvarhelyi, 1965a) induced ADs almost always spread to these same

TABLE 1. *Response to electrical stimulation*

Structure stimulated	Total no. of electrical stimulations	No. of stimulations/no. of responses				
		1–2.5 V	2.6–5 V	5.1–10 V	10.1–20 V	20 V <
Frontal agranular cortex	125	*20/11*	87/62*	17/9	1/1	
Precentral motor face cortex	160	*61/50*	86/66	11/9	2/2	
Postcentral " " "	34	5/0	10/1	*14/7*	5/3†	
Anterior temporal cortex	62	*8/5*	35/19	12/6	7/2	
Cingulate gyrus	14		*10/4*	4/2		
Occipital cortex	25		*14/7*	8/6*	3/1	
Caudate nucleus	100	10/1	37/3	39/4	*14/10*	
Putamen	106	7/0	30/5	46/15	21/4	1/0†
Globus pallidus	42	5/0	7/0	15/1	10/1	5/0†
VA and VL	60	1/5	18/3	25/2	14/1	2/0†
VP	16	1/0	3/0	1/0	10/3	1/0†
MD	17		9/1	5/0	3/0	†
Amygdala	103	1/0	*60/37*	36/22	5/4	1/0
Hypothalamus	29	2/0	14/4	9/3	4/4	
Hippocampus	110	*9/5*	57/38	35/31*	9/4	
Substantia nigra	8		5/1	3/1		
Septum	10		7/0	1/1	2/0	
Fornix	11		3/2	6/1	2/0	
PRS	32		13/1	19/0	†	
Lt. cerebellum	13		8/0	5/0	†	
Vermis ant.	9	1/0	6/0	2/0	†	

*Over threshold value.
†Threshold is probably above 20 V.
‡Italics indicate threshold.
(From Udvarhelyi and Walker, 1965, with permission of the publisher.)

structures, which thus become involved, although indirectly, in the AD process (Ajmone Marsan and Stoll, 1951; Stoll et al., 1951; Jasper et al., 1952; French et al., 1956; Poggio et al., 1956; Walker et al., 1956; Udvarhelyi and Walker, 1965; Walker and Udvarhelyi, 1965b). This indicates that such structures can and do participate in epileptiform activation. Actually, this participation is not always a simply passive form of "driving," but can often assume the appearance of an autonomous phenomenon, morphologically and temporally independent from the original cortical process (see, e.g., Fig. 9B in Jasper et al., 1952). The anatomical substrate of the central nervous system, with its pre-established pathways and connections, is probably the most important factor in determining direction and distribution of spread of self-sustained activity from the primary site of stimulus application. It is nonetheless interesting to note that the cortically induced ADs spread preferentially to subcortical rather than to other cortical regions (possibly with the exception of a marked tendency in the case of certain areas of the cortex to spread to homologous areas of the contralateral hemisphere), regardless of the much lower threshold of the latter to direct stimulation. It is not inconceivable that the difficulty to induce ADs following local stimulation of most of the extracortical nuclei might be due not so much to a truly low susceptibility to epileptiform activation, but rather to inadequacy of the stimulation itself, i.e., to our failure to determine the right combination of its optimal parameters for the successful elicitation of an AD.

As already mentioned, this property of an AD to spread from the original site of stimulation and to invade surrounding regions and remote structures can be utilized for the study of preferential paths and connections between the various regions of the brain. When this is the main purpose of the model, it should be kept in mind that precautions are necessary to limit the extent of the stimulated regions or, at least, to monitor possible direct or secondary effects of the stimulation outside of such regions. Distribution and extent of the projected activity obviously reflect the size of the area primarily affected by the stimulation; hence, caution should always be exerted in any conclusion derived exclusively by this method on the existence of connections between any given discrete area and other structures.

The same property of the AD to spread also contributes significantly to the suitability of this experimental model for the investigation of additional aspects in the pathophysiology of epilepsy, i.e., patterns and pathways of spread in locally originated seizures, and mechanism of their occasional generalization. The above-mentioned studies (including the classical one of Rosenblueth and Cannon, as well as those by Andy et al., 1967; Erickson, 1940; Gloor, 1957; Green and Shimamoto, 1953; Green and Naquet, 1957; Konigsmark et al., 1958; and many others) provide much information on the anatomic topographical side of these specific problems.

As to the patterns which characterize the projected event, especially in relation to those features which might differentiate it from the local, primary AD, the following is worth mentioning. When monitored with gross electodes, an AD developing in a region at some distance from the stimulated site may be hardly distinguishable in its overall pattern and duration from that going on at the area close to the stimulating electrodes (see, e.g., Fig. 4). Its onset may be slightly delayed but it can also be quasi-simultaneous, and one often observes an almost perfect synchrony between individual oscillations of potential which characterize tonic and clonic phases of the paroxysmal episodes at the two locations. In other instances, however, there can be a considerable delay between the onset of the two episodes, and the distant AD might be shorter in duration or continue for several seconds after the primary one has ended. In still other cases, the distant AD will start at the end of the primary AD and behave in an autonomous way with morphological features totally different from those of the latter (see Fig. 9B in Jasper et al., 1952). As a rule, the phase of depressed activity characterizing the postictal stage is less prominent, briefer, or hardly appreciable in the case of the projected AD. More consistent differences between the two phenomena can be detected in microelectrode tracings (see Sawa et al., 1963, 1968; Sugaya et al., 1964; Crowell, 1970; Crowell and Ajmone Marsan, 1972). These differences can be summarized by saying that in the neocortex, excitatory phenomena are quite prominent in neurons directly activated by local stimulation, whereas inhibitory phenomena tend to characterize — especially in experiments under light barbiturate anesthesia — the behavior of neurons which participate in the secondary AD (see, however, Sypert et al., 1970).

VIII. APPLICATION OF THE MODEL TO HUMAN EPILEPSY

At variance with a number of other models, the model under discussion has the advantage of being applicable to man. This can be achieved in both acute and chronic conditions, i.e., in the course of surgical exposure of the brain (Walker et al., 1946; Penfield and Jasper, 1954; Pampiglione and Falconer, 1962), and when electrodes have been implanted (on the cortex or in depth) and left in place for some time (Bickford et al., 1953; Ribstein, 1960; Bancaud et al., 1965). There are no important differences in the application of this model between human and experimental situations: parameters of stimulation, gross threshold characteristics of the various structures, and morphological patterns of the induced AD are essentially similar. In practice, the main differences are found in the scope for the model application and in the fact that some of the neuronal aggregates to be stimulated in man are often abnormal and, in most instances, they could actually be considered as potentially "epileptic." The most common purpose for stimulating the brain of epileptic patients with repetitive pulses is to obtain additional confirmation of location and extent of their suspected foci, by the reproduction of clinical seizures with the same pattern as in their spontaneous attacks (Penfield and Jasper, 1954; Bancaud et al., 1968) and by the demonstration of a region with an unusually low threshold for AD. Analogous experimental situations suggestively confirm that in such patients the stimulated structures be expected to display a much higher susceptibility to epileptoform activity, and hence a much lower threshold for AD (see Walker et al., 1946). Indeed, it is easy to demonstrate that in epileptogenic foci induced by a variety of other models, ictal episodes can be readily evoked by repetitive electrical stimulation with parameters of such values that would be totally ineffective for normal structures (Walker and Johnson, 1948; see also Matsumoto and Ajmone Marsan, 1964).[2]

In these same patients, it is also a matter of routine to utilize brief trains of repetitive stimuli to localize better specific functions of the various cortical areas (Penfield, 1958). Since, in the course of this procedure, it is not exceptional to induce an AD (even though this was not the aim of the stimulation), it is important to monitor continuously the electrical activity. In fact, the failure of recognizing the occurrence of an AD following the stimulation of a given area could result in the wrong interpretation (and localization) of the effects of the subsequent stimulation of a different region.

IX. REFERENCES

Adrian, E. D. (1936): The spread of activity in the cerebral cortex. *Journal of Physiology,* 88:127–161.

Ajmone Marsan, C. (1961): Electrographic aspects of "epileptic" neuronal aggregates. *Epilepsia,* 2:22–38.

Ajmone Marsan, C., and Stoll, J., Jr. (1951): Subcortical connections of the temporal pole in relation to temporal lobe seizures. *Archives of Neurology and Psychiatry,* 66:669–686.

Andy, O. J., and Akert, K. (1955): Seizure patterns induced by electrical stimulation of hippocampal formation in the cat. *Journal of Neuropathology and Experimental Neurology,* 14:198–213.

Andy, O. J., Chinn, R., Allen, M. B., and Shawyer, E. F. (1958): Influence of mesencephalic and diencephalic stimulation on limbic system seizures. *Neurology,* 8:939–952.

Andy, O. J., and Koshino, K. (1967): Duration and frequency patterns of the after-discharge from septum and amygdala. *Electroencephalography and Clinical Neurophysiology,* 22: 167–173.

Andy, O. J., Mukawa, J., and Melvin, J. (1968): After discharge propagation between the amygdalae in the cat. *Journal of Nervous and Mental Diseases,* 147:85–90.

Bancaud, J., Talairach, J., Bonis, A., Schaub, C., Szikla, G., Morel, P., and Bordas-Ferer, M. (1965): *La Stéréo-Électroencéphalographie dans l'Épilepsie.* Masson, Paris.

Bancaud, J., Talairach, J., Bresson, M., and Morel, P. (1968): Accés épileptiques induits par stimulation du noyau amygdalien et de la corne d'Ammon. (Intéret de la stimulation dans la détermination des épilepsies temporales chez l'homme.) *Revue Neurologique,* 118:527–532.

Baumgartner, G., and Jung, R. (1955): Hemmungsphänomene an einzelnen corticalen Neuronen und ihre Bedeutung für die Bremsung convulsiver Entladungen. *Archivio di Scienze Biologiche* (Bologna), 39:474–486.

---

[2]There are cases of human focal epilepsy in which it is indeed possible to demonstrate an unusually low threshold for AD in the region of maximal interictal paroxysmal activity (compare the findings of Fig. 3 with those seen in Fig. 1) in the course of their surgical exploration. It should be pointed out, however, that such cases are rather infrequent. In our experience, cortical regional differences seem to be equally if not more important than the presence of a latent epileptogenic process for the determination of AD susceptibility to repetitive stimulation.

Bergmann, F., Costin, A., and Gutman, J. (1963): A low threshold convulsive area in the rabbit's mesencephalon. *Electroencephalography and Clinical Neurophysiology*, 15:683–690.

Berry, C. A. (1965): A study of cortical afterdischarge in the rabbit. *Archives Internationales de Pharmacodynamic et de Thérapie*, 159:197–209.

Bickford, C., Petersen, C., Dodge, W., Jr., and Sem-Jacobsen, W. (1953): Observations on depth stimulation of the human brain through implanted electrographic leads. *Proceedings of the Meetings of the Mayo Clinic*, 28:181–187.

Blum, B. (1969): A comparative study on hippocampal seizure discharges induced by direct and by indirect hippocampal stimulation in the cat and in the monkey. *Confinia Neurologica* (Basel), 31:316–326.

Bremer, F. (1958): Les processus d'excitation et d'inhibition dans les phénomènes épileptiques. In: *Bases Physiologiques et Aspects Cliniques de l'Epilepsie*, edited by T. Alajouanine. Masson, Paris.

Burns, B. D. (1953): Intracortical integration. *Electroencephalography and Clinical Neurophysiology*. Suppl. 4:72–81.

Burns, B. D. (1954): The production of after-bursts in isolated unanesthetized cerebral cortex. *Journal of Physiology*, 125:427–446.

Creutzfeldt, O. D. (1969): Neuronal mechanisms underlying the EEG. In: *Basic Mechanisms of the Epilepsies*, edited by H. H. Jasper, A. A. Ward, Jr., and A. Pope. Little Brown, Boston.

Crowell, R. M. (1970): Distant effects of a focal epileptogenic process. *Brain Research*, 18:137–154.

Crowell, R. M., and Ajmone Marsan, C. (1972): Topographical distribution and patterns of unit activity during electrically induced after-discharge. *Electroencephalography and Clinical Neurophysiology*, Suppl. (*in press*).

Elul, R. (1964): Regional differences in the hippocampus of the cat. 1. Specific discharge patterns of the dorsal and ventral hippocampus and their role in generalized seizures. *Electroencephalography and Clinical Neurophysiology*, 16:470–488.

Erickson, T. C. (1940): Spread of the epileptic discharge. An experimental study of the afterdischarge induced by electrical stimulation of the cerebral cortex. *Archives of Neurology and Psychiatry*, 43:429–452.

Ferrier, D. (1873): Experimental researches in cerebral physiology and pathology. *West Riding Lunatic Asylum Medical Report* (London), 3:1–50.

Fields, W. S., King, R. B., and O'Leary, J. L. (1949): Study of multiplied cortical response to repetitive stimulation in thalamus. *Journal of Neurophysiology*, 12:117–130.

French, J. D., Gernandt, B. E., and Livingston, R. B. (1956): Regional differences in seizure susceptibility in monkey cortex. *A.M.A. Archives of Neurology and Psychiatry*, 75:260–274.

Fritsch, G., and Hitzig, E. (1870): Ueber die elektrische Erregbarkeit des Grosshirns. *Archiv fur Anatomische Physiologische Wissenschaftliche Medizin*, 37:300–332.

Garner, J., and French, J. D. (1958): Regional differences in seizure susceptibility in cat cortex. *A.M.A. Archives of Neurology and Psychiatry*, 80:675–681.

Gastaut, H., Naquet, R., and Roger, A. (1952): Étude des postdécharges électriques provoquées par stimulation du complexe nucléaire amygdalien chez le rat. *Revue Neurologique*, 87:224–231.

Gerin, P. (1960): Microelectrode investigations on the mechanisms of the electrically induced epileptiform seizure ("afterdischarge"). *Archives Italiennes de Biologie*, 98:21–40.

Gloor, T. (1957): The pattern of conduction of amygdaloid seizure discharge. An experimental study in the cat. *Archives of Neurology and Psychiatry*, 77:247–258.

Gloor, P. (1962): Der neurophysiologische Mechanismus des epileptischen Anfalles. *Bulletin der Schweizerishchen Akademie der Medizinischen Wissenschaften*, 18:167–188.

Gloor, P., Sperti, L., and Vera, C. (1962): An analysis of hippocampal evoked responses and seizure discharges with extracellular microelectrode and DC-recordings. In: *Physiologie de l'Hippocampe*. CNRS, Paris.

Gloor, P., Sperti, L., and Vera, C. L. (1964): A consideration of feedback mechanisms in the genesis and maintenance of hippocampal seizure activity. *Epilepsia*, 5:213–238.

Glötzner, F., and Grusser, O. J. (1968): Membranpotential und Entladungsfolgen corticaler Zellen. EEG und corticales DC-Potential bei generalisierten Krampanfällen. *Archiv fur Psychiatrie und Nervenkrankheiten*, 210:313–339.

Goddard, G. V., McIntyre, D. C., and Leech, C. K. (1969): A permanent change in brain function resulting from daily electrical stimulation. *Experimental Neurology*, 25:295–330.

Green, J. D., and Naquet, R. (1957): Etude de la propagation locale et à distance des démarches épileptiques. *I Intl. Cong. Neurol. Sciences*, Brussels (Acta Medica Belgica, Brussels), 225–249.

Green, J. D., and Shimamoto, F. (1953): Hippocampal seizures and their propagation. *Archives of Neurology and Psychiatry*, 70:687–702.

Hughes, J. R., and Mazurowski, J. A. (1964): Studies on the supracallosal mesial cortex of unanesthetized, conscious mammals. II. Monkey. D. Vertex sharp waves and epileptiform activity. *Electroencephalography and Clinical Neurophysiology*, 16:561–574.

Janzen, R., Sauter, R., Winkel, K., and Kleim, J. (1969): Tierexperimentelle Studien zur Ausbreitung der epileptischen Erregung und zum Problem der Erregbarkeit (Anfallbereitschaft). *Deutsche Zeitscrift fur Nervenheilkunde*, 196:183–189.

Jasper, H. H. (1954): Electrophysiology and experimental epilepsy. In: *Epilepsy and the Functional Anatomy of the Human Brain*, edited by W. Penfield and H. Jasper. Little Brown, Boston.

Jasper, H. H., Ajmone Marsan, C., and Stoll, J. (1952): Corticofugal projections to the brain stem. *Archives of Neurology and Psychiatry*, 67:155–166.

Jung, R. (1952): Origine e propagazione di potenziali convulsivi cerebrali nelle ricerche sperimentali negli animali. *Rivista di Neurologica*, 21:347–357.

Kandel, E. R., and Spencer, W. A. (1961): Excitation and inhibition of single pyramidal cells during hippocampal seizure. *Experimental Neurology*, 4:162–179.

Kaada, B. R. (1951): Somato-motor autonomic and electrocorticographic responses to electrical stimulation of "rhinencephalic" and other structures in primates, cat and dog. *Acta Physiologica Scandinavica*, 24:Suppl. 83:1–285.

Konigsmark, B. W., Abdullah, A. F., and French, J. D. (1958): Cortical spread of after-discharge in the monkey. *Electroencephalography and Clinical Neurophysiology*, 10:687–696.

Kreindler, A. (1965): Experimental Epilepsy. (*Progress in Brain Research*, Vol. 19), Elsevier, Amsterdam.

Kreindler, A., and Crighel, E. (1966): The neocortical epileptic focus in the cat. A study of the mechanisms involved in the onset of convulsive activity. In: *Comparative and Cellular Pathophysiology of Epilepsy*, edited by Z. Servit. Excerpta Medica, Amsterdam.

Kreindler, A., and Steriade, M. (1963): Functional differentiation within the amygdaloid complex inferred from peculiarities of epileptic afterdischarges. *Electroencephalography and Clinical Neurophysiology*, 15:811–826.

Leclercq, B., and Segal, M. (1965a): Epileptogenic foci in rabbit brain. *Canadian Journal of Physiology and Pharmacology*, 43:251–256.

Leclercq, B., and Segal, M. (1965b): An investigation of centers susceptible to mechanically and electrically induced afterdischarge in the cat brain. *Canadian Journal of Physiology and Pharmacology*, 43:491–507.

Lilly, J. C. (1961): Injury and excitation by electric currents. In: *Electrical Stimulation of the Brain*, edited by D. E. Sheer. Univ. of Texas Press, Austin.

Luciani, L. (1878): Sulla patogenesi dell'epilessia. *Rivista Sperimentale di Freniatria e Medicina Legale*, 4:617–646.

Machek, J., and Fischer, J. (1966): Laminar analysis of the electric seizure activity elicited by electroshock and metrazol in the sensory motor cortex of the rabbit. In: *Comparative and Cellular Pathophysiology of Epilepsy*, edited by Z. Servit. Excerpta Medica, Amsterdam.

Matsumoto, H., and Ajmone Marsan, C. (1964): Cortical cellular phenomena in experimental epilepsy: ictal manifestations. *Experimental Neurology*, 9:305–326.

Michishita, C. (1956): On the paroxysmal cerebrocortical discharges evoked by repetitive electrical stimulation on the lateral geniculate body. *Folia Psychiatrica et Neurologica Japonica,* 10:83–116.

Minz, B., and Domino, E. F. (1953): Effects of epinephrine and norepinephrine on electrically induced seizures. *Journal of Pharmacology and Experimental Therapeutics,* 107:204–218.

Moruzzi, G. (1939): Contribution à l'électrophysiologie du cortex moteur: facilitation, after-discharge et épilepsie corticale. *Archives Internationales de Physiologie et de Biochimie,* 49:33–100.

Moruzzi, G. (1950): *L'Epilepsie Expérimentale.* Hermann, Paris.

Pampiglione, G., and Falconer, M. A. (1962): Phenomènes subjectifs et objectifs provoqués par la stimulation de l'hippocampe chez l'homme. In: *Physiologie de l'hippocampe.* CNRS, Paris, pp. 399–410.

Peeler, D. F., and Andy, O. J. (1967): Limbic system seizures in the kitten. *Electroencephalography and Clinical Neurophysiology,* 23:1–5.

Penfield, W. (1958): *The Excitable Cortex in Conscious Man.* (V Sherrington Lecture). Charles C Thomas, Springfield, Ill.

Penfield, W., and Jasper, H. H. (1954): *Epilepsy and the Functional Anatomy of the Human Brain.* Little Brown, Boston.

Pinsky, C., and Burns, D. B. (1962): Production of epileptiform afterdischarges in cat's cerebral cortex. *Journal of Neurophysiology,* 25:359–379.

Poggio, G. F., Walker, A. E., and Andy, O. J. (1956): The propagation of cortical after-discharge through subcortical structures. *Archives of Neurology and Psychiatry,* 75:350–361.

Ribstein, M. (1960): Exploration du cerveau humain par electrodes profondes. *Electroencephalography and Clinical Neurophysiology,* Suppl. 16:1–129.

Rosenblueth, A., and Cannon, W. B. (1941–42): Cortical responses to electrical stimulation. *American Journal of Physiology,* 135:690–741.

Sawa, M., Kaji, S., and Usuki, K. (1965): Intracellular phenomena in electrically induced seizures. *Electroencephalography and Clinical Neurophysiology,* 19:248–255.

Sawa, M., Maruyama, N., and Kaji, S. (1963): Intracellular potential during electrically induced seizures. *Electroencephalography and Clinical Neurophysiology,* 15:209–220.

Sawa, M., Nakamura, K., and Naito, H. (1968): Intracellular phenomena and spread of epileptic seizure discharges. *Electroencephalography and Clinical Neurophysiology,* 24: 146–154.

Segal, M., and Leclercq, B. (1965: Threshold studies and isoliminal mapping of electrically elicited afterdischarge in the cat brain. *Canadian Journal of Physiology and Pharmacology,* 43:685–697.

Stoll, J., Ajmone Marsan, C., and Jasper, H. H. (1951): Electrophysiological studies of subcortical connections of anterior temporal region in cat. *Journal of Neurophysiology,* 14: 305–316.

Straw, R. N. (1968): The effect of selected neuromuscular blocking agents and spinal cord transection on cortical after-discharge duration in the cat. *Electroencephalography and Clinical Neurophysiology,* 25:69–72.

Sugaya, E., Goldring, S., and O'Leary, J. L. (1964): Intracellular potentials associated with direct cortical response and seizure discharge in cat. *Electroencephalography and Clinical Neurophysiology,* 17:661–669.

Sypert, G. W. Oakley, J., and Ward, A. A., Jr. (1970): Single unit analysis of propagated seizures in neocortex. *Experimental Neurology,* 28:308–325.

Toennies, J. F. (1952): Controreazioni sinaptiche del fenomeno convulsivo: segnali di ritorno e capacità frenatrice. *Rivista di Neurologica,* 21:347–357.

Udavarhelyi, G. B., and Walker, A. E. (1965): Dissemination of acute focal seizures in the monkey. 1. From cortical foci. *Archives of Neurology,* 12:333–356.

Von Euler, C., Green, J. D., and Ricci, G. (1958): The role of hippocampal dendrites in evoked responses and after discharges. *Acta Physiologica Scandinavica,* 42:87–111.

Walker, A. F., and Johnson, H. C. (1948): Normal and pathological after-discharge from frontal cortex. *Research Publications of the Association for Research in Nervous and Mental Disease,* 27:460–475.

Walker, A. F., Marshall, C., and Beresford, E. N. (1946): Electrocorticographic characteristics of the cerebrum in posttraumatic epilepsy. *Research Publications of the Association for Research in Nervous and Mental Disease,* 26:502–515.

Walker, A. E., Poggio, G. F., and Andy, O. J. (1956): Structural spread of cortically-induced epileptic discharges. *Neurology* (Minneap.), 6:616–626.

Walker, A. E., and Udvarhelyi, G. B. (1965a): Dissemination of acute focal seizures in the monkey. II. From subcortical foci. *Archives of Neurology.* (Chicago), 12:357–380.

Walker, A. E., and Udvarhelyi, G. B. (1965b: The generalization of a seizure. *Journal of Nervous and Mental Diseases,* 140:252–271.

Zuckermann, E. C. (1971): Sequence of events leading to seizure activity at the level of a hippocampal epileptic pacemaker. *Experimental Neurology,* 32:413–430.

7

Spreading Depression

Aristides A. P. Leão

OUTLINE

I. INTRODUCTION

Spreading depression was identified as an artificially elicitable phenomenon in a study of "experimental epilepsy" in the cerebral cortex of the rabbit. The distinctive feature was a considerable, long-lasting depression of cortical "spontaneous" electrical activity and excitability, which slowly spread beyond the site of elicitation for greater and greater distances along the cortex—hence, the descriptive term "spreading depression" (Leão, 1944a). However, in its spread along the cortex, characteristics of the spread of epileptiform discharges were at once recognized; namely, it was self-sustained independently of a contribution through the connections of the cortex with other centers, and it proceeded to contiguous areas with little regard for functional or anatomical boundaries. Moreover, it was observed that during the depression of "spontaneous" electrical activity, an abnormal activity might develop in which epileptiform features or properties could always be recognized, and which, when intense, was in fact quite similar to cortical convulsive discharges. Later, unitary recordings obtained with microelectrodes (Grafstein, 1956) uncovered the occurrence of a brief burst of neuronal activity at the advancing front of spreading depression, further indicating the epileptiform nature of this phenomenon.

The foregoing and other observations provide evidence, which, treated as a whole, is sufficient to establish that fundamentally related mechanisms operate in spreading depression and cortical seizure marches. There is then in the phenomenon of spreading depression an opportunity for investigations into the basic mechanisms of the epilepsies. Indeed, although it is itself a very complex phenomenon, spreading depression (which henceforth will be denoted by SD) seems particularly useful to contribute to the elucidation of some of these mechanisms.

A valuable general account of SD was given by Marshall (1959); a review by Ochs (1962) contains additional data and a section on the use of SD in experimental psychology. The present chapter, except for section V, is restricted to SD in the mammalian cerebral cortex. Some remarks on the occurrence and propagation of the phenomenon are presented in section II, aspects relating to its elicitation are dealt with in section III, and some of its manifestations are considered separately in section IV. Finally, section V gives a summary of SD in preparations of isolated retina, in which it seems that various questions concerning fundamental mechanisms of the phenomenon can be most advantageously studied.

II. OCCURRENCE AND PROPAGATION OF SD

In this chapter, attention is focused on the occurrence of SD in the mammalian cerebral cortex. Since it has been suggested in the literature that the cortices of "lower" and "higher" mammals may be intrinsically different regarding the incidence of SD, it must be noted at the outset that this concept is without foundation. What is known is that SD is more readily elicited in the exposed cortex of the lissencephalic, generally small, mammals than in the cortex of the gyrencephalic animal, irrespective of the order to which the mammal belongs. Cortical SD is as readily elicited in the opossum, a marsupial whose neocortex is quite devoid of sulci or gyri, as in the marmoset, a primate who also possesses a smooth dorsolateral cortex, except for a deep Sylvian fissure. It seems equally certain that SD can occur only after a relatively advanced stage of maturation of the cortex has been reached during ontogenesis. It has been reported in rats, rabbits, and cats that it is not possible to elicit cortical SD until at least a few weeks after birth. However, in guinea pigs, who are born well along in development, cortical SD can be elicited immediately after birth (Bures, 1957; Schadé, 1959; Goldensohn et al., 1963).

There has been some controversy about whether SD occurs only in certain conditions of the cortical tissue. In my opinion, there can be no doubt that when SD is elicited at a limited region of the tissue, its subsequent spread over the surrounding regions meets with resistance, and proceeds only when this resistance fails. The underlying mechanisms are still conjectural, but what evidence there is indicates that SD "breaks through" a region only when, for some reason or another, the tissue, as a whole, is incapable of exercising the full range of its normal potentialities. That this may happen without any definite sign of impairment of functional performance is demonstrated by the production of learned responses involving cortex fully susceptible to SD (and that had previously sustained a series of SDs), observed in experimental studies of animal behavior in which SD was utilized to achieve a temporary, functional "decortication" in rats.

In rendering the cortical tissue susceptible to invasion of SD, exposure of its surface for experimental purposes is of first importance, as shown by Marshall and co-workers. These authors carried out a series of experiments to ascertain if the resulting dehydration and cooling of the tissue are involved in this effect. The temperature experiments (Marshall et al., 1951a) showed decisively that cooling of the cortical surface does indeed by itself render the tissue susceptible to invasion by SD. The dehydration experiments (Marshall, 1950), in which radical internal dehydration of the brain of cats was produced by intravenous administration of 90% sucrose, presented so many complications that a simple conclusion was not considered justified, even though cortical SD was found to spread fully in the dehydrated preparations. In contrast, experiments in which various solutions of different osmolarities were topically applied to the cortical surface of rabbits (Leão, 1963) indicate that hydration, not dehydration, is favorable to the incidence of SD. It is possible that other alterations of the ionic environment were dominant in Marshall's experiments, since some of these alterations are known to be most effective in decreasing tissue capability of opposing SD (Marshall et al., 1951*b;* Leão, 1963). In general, traumatic injury of the cortical tissue of any kind (including relatively slight mechanical damage from sustained moderate local pressure on its surface) also favors the incidence of SD.

Although SD does not as a rule propagate fully in the convoluted cortex of cats or macaque monkeys unless its surface has been exposed to the air for some time (on the order of hours), occasionally animals are encountered in which typical SDs extending widely across the sulci are observed immediately after exposure. These instances are of much interest because they indicate that the incidence of SD may be influenced by factors operative under physiological circumstances (e.g., humoral, metabolic, hormonal), as is the case with epileptic discharges. Also, in rabbits instances of departure from the usual susceptibility to SD can be noted, which are seemingly attributable to systemic conditions at the time the experiments were started. This is an aspect certainly worthy of further investigation.

The question of the conditions under which SD occurs is of considerable significance in the study of its propagation, a cardinal feature of the phenomenon, which is of special interest to the student of epilepsy. There is evidence that the upper cortical layers are dominant in the propagation, and that at any place, at the same time that SD spreads to contiguous superficial tissue along the cortex, it also spreads to contiguous deeper tissue, across the cortex (Leão, 1951; Muñoz-Martínez, 1970). The depth of penetration is variable (Phillis and Ochs, 1971). Although the spread along the cortex away from the site of origin is essentially uniform in all directions, considerable irregularities are always encountered which are related to differences in the conditions of the tissue in the various regions.

Regarding the mechanism of propagation, mention should be made of the hypothesis advanced by Grafstein (1956), which was based primarily on the fact that local application to the cortex of potassium chloride elicits SD. The postulate is that the brief burst of neuronal activity which occurs at the advancing front of SD leads to release of potassium into the interneuronal spaces in sufficient quantity to depolarize adjacent neurons; those which are thus activated in turn release potassium, which then excites a further set of neurons in the path of propagation, and so on, further and further away from the site of elicitation. Although a number of facts are not satisfactorily accounted for by this hypothesis alone, it deserves attention, and certainly can serve as a basis for further speculation and experiment. The blocking effect of calcium and magnesium on the propagation of SD was considered by Bures (1960) as evidence in its favor. The finding that potassium is lost from the cortex during SD (Krivánek and Bures, 1960; Brinley et al., 1960) is also compatible with this hypothesis, but, as pointed out by Grafstein (1963), the hypothesis is a difficult one to test experimentally, since release of potassium from neurons is likely to occur regardless of the mechanism of propagation. In this connection, it may be added that experiments in which saline solutions of different compositions were applied to the cortex showed that if a deficiency of chloride ions is produced in the neuronal environment, the speed of propagation of SD is increased. If, on the other hand, the concentration of chloride is raised above normal values (or if choline is substituted for sodium), the propagation of SD is blocked (Leão, 1963).

A mechanism of propagation similar to that proposed by Grafstein, but depending on the release of glutamic acid, has been suggested by Van Harreveld (1959). Recent experiments, however, have failed to confirm that SD is elicited when solutions of this compound are applied locally to the surface of the cortex (Do Carmo and Leão, 1972).

In relation to epilepsy, the similarity of the propagation of SD to that of the Jacksonian march in clinical seizures is often noted, but almost invariably with the reservation that motor seizures frequently propagate at much faster rates. A little consideration will show, however, that different rates of propagation of muscular manifestations do not necessarily mean different underlying cortical mechanisms. Let us assume that a cortical process, capable of initiating motor convulsions, spreads outward from the center of origin as a widening circle, and that this process, after having travelled over the cortex, reaches the precentral gyrus sideways, and invades it proceeding, say, in the direction from the central sulcus to the precentral sulcus. It is clear then that motor convulsions appearing in conformity with the sequence of representation may occur very rapidly, even if the rate of spread of the process is only a few millimeters per minute. This is not to be construed as implying that self-sustained convulsive discharges may not propagate at faster rates; our intention is merely to point out that processes propagating slowly may be operative in more instances than generally admitted.

In the case of migraine, the similarity between the time courses of the scotomas and SD is most striking. This was first noted by Milner (1958), who, on the evidence of observations made by Lashley (1941), suggested that migraine scotomas may be manifestations of cortical SD triggered in susceptible individuals (see also Basser, 1969). In fact, not only the rate of advance but also the fact that the scotomatous area may be totally blind or outlined by scintillations corresponds closely to the mode of occurrence of epileptiform activity during SD, as will be shown below.

III. ROUTINE ELICITATION OF SD

SD is generally elicited in anesthetized animals. A few barbiturates, urethane, and chloralose have been used for anesthesia, and although no notable differences were found, a systematic comparative study of the effects of these drugs has not been made. Owing to the long-lasting, rather even anesthesia produced, most workers have preferred the barbiturate dial, administered by intraperitoneal injection. In contrast to the drugs mentioned, ether has a distinct hindering action on the elicitation of SD (Leão, 1944a; Van Harreveld and Stamm, 1953b). With dial and other barbiturates, SD can be regularly elicited at very deep levels of anesthesia; with ether, the occurrence of the phenomenon is prevented with the inception of surgical anesthesia.

Several workers use, in acute experiments, animals that are immobilized by curarization and artificially ventilated. There can be no doubt that these preparations may yield valuable information, but it must be realized that the problem of ensuring that the animal is not subjected to undue suffering is not a simple one. That this aspect of such preparations must be thoroughly considered cannot be stressed too strongly. Bremer's *cerveau isolé* preparation has also been used to study SD in cats without the interference of a central depressant drug. It was from this preparation, in which the electrocorticogram exhibits permanently the same pattern of synchronized sleep as that observed under barbiturate narcosis, that Burns chose to cut his preparations of neurologically isolated slabs of cerebral cortex (see Burns, 1958). It was also in these slabs that the occurrence of a brief burst of neuronal discharges was first detected at the advancing front of SD by Grafstein (1956).

SD has also been recorded in waking animals by means of chronically implanted electrodes (Ochs et al., 1961; Johnson et al., 1965). The latter study, in which extradural electrodes were used, is of special interest in the present context, since it shows that the convulsive agent methionine sulfoximine gives rise to "spontaneous" recurrences of SD in the rabbit cortex.

Although cortical SD has been observed in neo-, paleo-, and archipallial areas of several species, experimental data have been obtained principally in the dorsolateral neopallial areas of the rabbit, rat, cat, and, to a lesser extent, the macaque monkey. In the dorsolateral areas of the rabbit and rat, it is possible as a rule to elicit typical SDs as soon as the dura is reflected. With ordinary care, useful experiments can be carried out for a few hours with the cortex exposed to the room air. In convoluted cortex, however, if surgical and other procedures have been properly carried out, SD in general is not propagated fully until exposure to the air has been prolonged for several hours (about 2 to 3 in the case of the cat). Earlier than this, SD can, as a rule, be elicited in a single gyrus, but it shows decrement in its propagation and vanishes before propagating far from the stimulated site. However, a condition of the cortex in which typical SDs can be regularly elicited is produced within some 15 to 20 min by placing over its surface a pool of Ringer's solution containing about 10 times the normal potassium concentration. This was shown by Marshall et al. (1951*b*), in whose experiments the potassium concentration was raised to 27 mequiv/liter (replacing sodium), but the present author has consistently obtained the effect with the potassium concentration raised to only 20 mequiv/liter. Such pretreatment with high-potassium Ringer's solution to render the cat cortex more susceptible to SD has been used by various workers (e.g., Freygang and Landau, 1955; Morlock et al., 1964).

Both electrical stimulation and local applications of potassium chloride are commonly employed for routine elicitation of SD. No study seems to have been made of optimal parameters for electrical stimulation, which is employed either in the form of a train of brief current pulses or of direct (galvanic) current. The trains of pulses (in general, 1 to 20 msec pulses at frequencies of 20 to 60/sec) are usually applied for 2 to 5 sec through wire electrodes placed 1.5 to 2 mm apart on the surface of the cortex. An intensity sub-threshold for the production of any after-discharge detectable in the conventional surface electrocorticogram is usually adequate for eliciting SD. It should be noted that with minimal effective values of the stimulus, several seconds may elapse following termination of the stimulation before any of the known manifestations of SD can be recorded. As to the use of direct current, since SD is regularly elicited at the cathode, the usual arrangement is to place this electrode on the surface of the cortex and to place the anode on some remote tissue (the neck muscles, for instance). The effectiveness of the cathode in eliciting SD was established in experiments in which the electrodes were connected to the surface of the tissue via a Ringer's solution bridge (Leão and Morison, 1945). Subsequently, several workers have reported the use of cathodal current applied for 1 to 3 sec through a silver-silver chloride wire electrode in direct contact with the surface of the cortex. This procedure may result in the tissue being rather severely injured by electrolytic effects (liberation of minute gas bubbles). Marshall (1959) has called attention to the possibility that the SD in this case is actually elicited by the injury. Local injury does indeed readily elicit SD. In this context, it may be added that under some circumstances a prick with a sharp-pointed needle will prove very convenient for elicitation of the phenomenon (in our laboratory we use a tungsten needle, 125μm in diameter).

As for potassium chloride, ordinarily a 1% solution is applied to cortical surface on pieces of filter paper or, preferably, loose cotton pledgets. It is not necessary to cover an area of more than some 2 to 3 mm². Potassium is a powerful SD-inducing agent, and applied in this way is often found to be effective in initiating SD when electrical means fail to do so. Marshall (1959) is correct in noting that a 1% solution of potassium chloride always causes SD; the phenomenon, however, remains local if the surrounding tissue resists its spread (see also Marshall et al., 1951b). Instead of repeated applications of a 1% solution, a single application of a 25% solution, or even of a small crystal of the salt, has been used to produce a continuing series of SDs, with intervals of a few minutes. The 25% solution has also been used in microinjections (0.5 to 1.0 μl) to elicit SD in subcortical structures, as shown in a study by Aquino-Cias and Bures (1966) who examined the effects of thalamic SD on discharges induced in the rat cortex by local application of pentylenetetrazol or electrical stimulation.

One point to be kept in mind is that all of the known modes of eliciting SD involve changes in the tissue of uncertain nature and extension. Because of this, unless one is concerned about the mechanisms of SD elicitation, it is best to take records of the phenomenon only after it has moved well away from the stimulated site, and is spreading over tissue not likely to have been involved in the initial stimulation.

The local events leading to the initiation of SD may be less complicated when the phenomenon is elicited in one area of the dorsolateral cortex by a train of electric shocks applied to the homologous area of the opposite cortex (Leão, 1944a). It has been shown that this mode of elicitation of cortical SD depends upon an intact corpus callosum. There is no reason to doubt that SD in this case is brought about by impulses transmitted by the fibers of that commissure (Leão and Morison, 1945). This is interesting because elicitation of SD by specific sensory afferent discharges of impulses has been observed only following activation by pentylenetetrazol (Van Harreveld and Stamm, 1955). The callosum-mediated stimulation of SD may be due to neuronal activity elicited in the area by impulses traveling in callosal fibers, either simply because this activity is more intense than in the case of sensory afferent discharges, or because of the different mode of termination of specific afferent and callosal fibers (see, e.g., Szentágothai, 1969). However, the possibility remains that antidromic impulses in callosal fibers that originate in the area are a significant factor.

As is well known, SD can be elicited by mechanical stimulation. This is usually produced by a few strokes on the cortical surface with the rounded end of a small glass rod, which cause slight compression of the tissue without visible structural damage. However, it may be well to remark that in some preparations the sensitivity to this form of stimulation may be so high as to risk unintentional mechanical elicitation of SD when, for example, electrodes are being placed on the surface of the cortex, or, more importantly, when solutions of drugs are being applied locally.

In our experiments on animals under barbiturate narcosis, we have ordinarily elicited cortical SDs at intervals of 20 min. The phenomenon can be elicited at intervals shorter than this, but generally a second SD cannot be elicited within the first 3 min or so after the first one, even if the strength of the stimulation is maximally raised. Nevertheless, after 20 min has elapsed, stimulation of the same strength again elicits SD; detailed examination of the "spontaneous" electrocorticogram usually shows that at that time the tissue cannot be considered to have fully recovered from SD. This is also indicated by the time required, following SD, for conditioned reflexes to reappear (Bures and Buresová, 1956), or for the glycogen content of the tissue to recover to normal values (Krivánek, 1958).

There is no doubt that useful experiments can be made with SDs elicited at intervals of 20 min or even less. However, the experimenter should keep in mind that when recovery is incomplete, the possibility exists of cumulative changes occurring which may have an influence, along with those changes resulting from exposure, or other operative procedures, on the manifestations and properties of SD during the course of the experiment.

IV. MANIFESTATIONS OF SD

During SD there is depression of cortical "spontaneous" activity, of responses to stimulation of specific sensory and other kinds of afferents of subcortical origin, of responses to ipsilateral and contralateral electrical stimulation of the cortex, and of local discharges induced by convulsive drugs or lesions. In view of the manner in which propagation and recovery proceed, it is obvious that depression of "spontaneous" activity is most favorably recorded with two electrodes placed on the cortical surface close to one another and at an approximately equal distance from the site of elicitation of SD. Depression of neuronal excitability can, however, be more accurately followed in records of discrete cortical responses, such as those evoked by single electrical shocks applied to, for example, sensory nerves or certain thalamic nuclei. In monopolar cathode-ray oscilloscope records, obtained with shocks applied in synchrony with the oscilloscope trace at intervals of 2 to 3 secs, the effects of SD on the different components of these responses are clearly displayed. Using microelectrodes, Morlock et al. (1964) and Phillis and Ochs (1971) recorded the "spontaneous" firing and the orthodromic or antidromic responses of individual cortical neurons during SD. Phillis and Ochs also recorded the responses induced by "pulses" of *l*-glutamate iontophoretically released from one of the barrels of a multi-barrel microelectrode. The records of the antidromic response show that the soma spike is completely abolished, but that a residual axon hillock and/or axon spike persists. In general, however, this response recovers within 1 min of SD invasion, whereas the neuronal excitability, as indicated by orthodromic and glutamate-induced responses, remains depressed for a further period of several minutes.

Turning to other manifestations, it may be well to consider first the electrical potential change with a duration of the order of minutes, now usually called the "slow potential change," which was found many years ago (Leão, 1947) to be associated with SD. Since SD without a slow potential change has never been found to occur in the cortex or any other neuronal aggregation, this rather well-defined and easily recorded change has come to be widely used simply to detect the presence of SD or to provide a suitable reference for timing other concurrent changes.

A. Slow potential change

As is well known, a steady potential difference between a point on the cortical surface and another anywhere on the body is normally present, although its value may drift in one direction or another in relation to certain states of physiological or pathological character. This potential difference is undoubtedly related to the potential gradient existing across cortical cell membranes, but the manner in which it is established is still far from certain. If the immediate interest is not in absolute values but rather in the measurement of transient changes associated with some local event, the only requirement as to the placement of the reference electrode in DC recordings is that the site be electrically stable during the change. If this condition is satisfied, any steady potential difference between the two leads may be counterbalanced, in setting a zero base line upon which the transient changes are measured. This is what is usually done in studies of the slow potential change of SD. However, it should be remembered that the possibility exists of a relation of that potential difference, or cortical polarity, to the incidence of SD (see Marshall et al., 1951a).

As an SD spreads along the cortex, the slow potential change and the depression of activity and excitability begin, in any region, at about the same time. A record of the slow potential change in the dorsolateral cortex of the rabbit is shown in Fig. 1. The most significant and constant feature is the negative wave. In many instances the small positive phase preceding it is not recorded, and the terminal positive phase, although usually present, is highly variable. Terminal positive phases of high amplitude and long duration, as the one shown in the figure, are as a rule present in SDs elicited soon after exposure of the cortex. However, as the experiment proceeds, and further SDs are elicited at intervals of 20 min or so, the slow potential change ordinarily undergoes a progressive alteration, consisting in an extension of the duration of the negative wave and a parallel reduction of the amplitude and duration of the terminal positive phase. Eventually, the amplitude of the negative wave also increases. This wave then usually

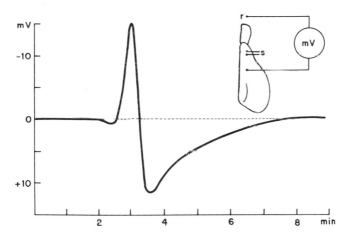

FIG. 1. Slow potential change, recorded from the surface of the dorsolateral cortex. Rabbit under dial. Electrodes arranged as shown in the inset (r, reference electrode, applied to nasal bone; s, stimulating electrodes). SD elicited by a 5-sec train of electric pulses, terminating at the start of the record.

presents a distinct break in its ascending course; the negative potential first rises rapidly to a certain value, and from there proceeds more slowly to its maximum. Occasionally, instead of a simple transition from a rapid to a slow rise, there may be, after the early rapid rise, a brief period of recess of the negative potential before the later slow rise starts on its course. In this case, the potential curve exhibits two maxima, the second one being generally of higher amplitude.

These alterations of the slow potential change are certainly related to the metabolic conditions of the tissue. Both hypoxemia (produced by reduction of the oxygen content in the inspired air) and hypoglycemia (produced by intravenous administration of insulin) extend the duration of the negative wave. The effect of hypoglycemia is characterized by a concomitant considerable increase in the amplitude of this wave (Martins Ferreira, 1955). Of much interest in this respect is the finding that acute interruption of the circulation, which prevents recovery of the original potential from the negativity (Leão, 1947), also prevents the development of the later, slow rise of the negative wave, referred to above (Leão and Martins Ferreira, 1959). This is illustrated in Fig. 2A, which shows records obtained from the hippocampus, but the same effect has been observed in the neocortex. On the other hand, if, with intact circulation, the concentration of potassium is locally increased, the later part of the negative wave is, as shown in Fig. 2B, greatly reduced (Leão and Martins Ferreira, 1965). A plausible interpretation seems to be that this is an effect of potassium on the metabolic processes responsible for the later rise of the negative potential.

Intracellular recordings have demonstrated that, as long inferred, a marked depolarization of cortical neurons occurs in correlation with the slow potential change of SD (Brozek, 1966; Collewijn and Van Harreveld, 1966; Goldensohn and Walsh, 1968). In the 13 recordings of Goldensohn and Walsh, the average resting potential was 61.5 mV, and the average depolarization during SD was 23 mV, with an average duration of 91 sec. (Goldensohn, 1969). Small and brief hyperpolarizations were also recorded, in several instances preceding and in a few cases following the depolarization. Depolarizations of the same order of magnitude and duration were recorded during SD in the so-called "idle" cells of the cat cortex by Karahashi and Goldring (1966).

The suggestion that pH-dependent blood-brain barrier processes are importantly involved in the generation of the slow potential change of SD (Tschirgi et al., 1957) has been subjected to examination by Rapoport and Marshall (1964). The results of their pH measurements, with glass membrane electrodes applied to the cortical surface, are incompatible with such

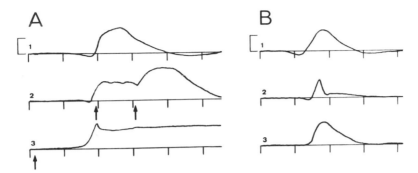

FIG. 2. Slow potential changes, recorded from the ventricular surface of Ammon's horn, exposed by removal of the overlying pallium. Rabbit under dial. Time marks, 1 min; amplitude calibrations, 10 mV, negativity upwards. *A* and *B* are two different experiments. The records (1–3) in each experiment are of three consecutive SDs, the intervals between them being about 20 min. SDs elicited by a prick with a sharp tungsten needle, except in *A*3. *A:* Effect of circulatory arrest (produced by arterial occlusion; see Leão and Morison, 1945). Exposed surface of Ammon's horn under a pool of mineral oil. (1) Control. Note break in ascending course of negative wave. (2) Arteries occluded at first arrow, shortly after onset of negative wave. Note that later, slow rise of this wave does not develop. Circulation reestablished at second arrow. (3) SD resulting from circulatory arrest. Arterial occlusion, at arrow, maintained until end of record. Note that subsequent to the rapid rise of negativity, neither the further slow rise nor recovery of the original potential occurs.

B: Effect of excess of potassium. (1) Control. Exposed surface of Ammon's horn under a pool of normal Ringer's solution (K+:3.3 mequiv/liter). (2) 16 min after pool of normal Ringer's solution was replaced by a pool of Ringer's solution containing 26.4 mequiv/liter of K+. (3) 19 min after reverting to pool of normal Ringer's solution.

a view. Although a small acidic change of about 0.03 pH units was usually recorded during the terminal positive phase, no significant pH change was detected during the negative wave.

B. Epileptiform activity

It has been noted above that a burst of neuronal activity lasting for a few seconds was found to occur at the advancing front of cortical SD by Grafstein (1956). The occurrence of this burst, in at least some of the cells examined, has been amply confirmed with extracellular unit recordings (Li and Salmoiraghi, 1963; Morlock et al., 1964; Muñoz-Martínez, 1970; Phillis and Ochs, 1971), as well as with intracellular recordings (Collewijn and Van Harreveld, 1966; Goldensohn and Walsh, 1968; Goldensohn, 1969). Even if these bursts do not occur in all cells, they are nevertheless a regular concomitant of SD. In time, the burst coincides with the onset of the negative wave of the slow potential change, and "spontaneously" active neurons typically cease firing for a few seconds just prior to it. During the burst, the spike amplitude decreases continuously until it is no longer detectable, as may be seen in Fig. 3. This example is of particular interest in the present context because it was taken from a study on relations between SD and experimentally produced seizure discharges. The intracellular records reproduced in the figure show the effect of SD on the paroxysmal depolarization shifts, accompanied by clusters of spikes, occurring in epileptogenic freezing lesion (Goldensohn, 1969). This early burst may be the only sign of abnormal neuronal firing recorded during SD. However, in many instances, within 1 min or so after its termination, epileptiform neuronal activity may again appear in the course of SD. When this happens, the mode in which the activity usually manifests itself is that characteristic of the later, "clonic" stage of convulsive seizure discharges.

It may be helpful to recall at this point some aspects of these discharges. In typical seizure marches, the discharges at the original and intermediate regions do not cease, whereas increasingly distant regions are successively affected; the "clonic" bursts proceed throughout the entire area affected

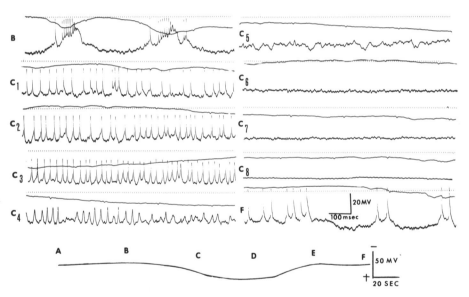

FIG. 3. Across bottom, *A–F* shows continuous DC recording of SD from cortical surface (anterior sigmoid gyrus, cat paralyzed with succinylcholine). Above are epochs from *B* and *C* portion of SD. *B:* Upper trace, EEG; lower trace, intracellular record using AC recording to show paroxysmal depolarization shifts of epileptogenic freezing lesion before SD arrives. $C_1 - C_8$ shows developing SD with elimination of depolarization shifts and progressive increase in firing rate until complete absence of surface and intracellular activity. *F:* Recovery. From Goldensohn (1969) with permission of the publisher.

in step with one another. Experimental studies (e.g., Rosenblueth and Cannon, 1942) have shown that the bursts are not perfectly synchronous throughout the total area. They originate in one place and are rapidly propagated to all others, there being no definite place of origin (i.e., no systematic pacemaker). It has also been found that during the "clonic" stage, properly timed single electrical shocks applied to the cortex or to sensory pathways may start a burst identical in every respect to the "spontaneously" occurring ones. It is possible to prolong for some time the duration of the "clonic" activity with a series of such shocks.

Now again with reference to SD, the activity in the episode under consideration varies greatly in intensity and complexity. Recorded from an electrode placed on the cortical surface, the activity consists, in its simplest form, of a series of discrete negative waves, of duration measured in tenths of a second, and of variable amplitude, commonly of a few millivolts, but occasionally reaching more than 10 mV. At any region, this abnormal activity ordinarily occurs during the early part of the terminal positive phase of the slow potential change, but it often begins when the potential is still passing from negative to positive. At the time of its beginning, therefore, the normal "spontaneous" activity is already quite depressed (Fig. 4). Since it occurs, at any region, only for a limited time, as SD spreads, the abnormal activity is present only over a band of tissue near the advancing front of the phenomenon. Behind this moving band (i.e., at the site of elicitation of SD and intermediate regions), there is only depression of activity. Inside the band, however, the tissue seems to be in a condition fundamentally of the same kind as that obtained during the "clonic" stage of seizures. Thus, the large waves just mentioned, similarly to the "clonic" bursts, originate in one place and are rapidly propagated to others around it. Again there is no definite place of origin, and waves identical to the "spontaneous" ones may be started by local cortical or afferent stimulation (Leão, 1944a). When the activity becomes more intense, the rate of recurrence of the waves increases, and faster ones (i.e., spikes) appear associated with them in various manners. In extreme cases, a full epileptiform "tonic-clonic" sequence develops.

Almost nothing is known about the factors involved in the appearance of this episode of activity during SD. It was observed that the activity in general becomes more intense when a series of SDs is elicited at intervals of 20 min or less (Leão, 1944a; Whieldon and Van Harreveld, 1950; Sloan and Jasper, 1950). Later, Van Harreveld and Stamm (1953a) reported that in curarized rabbits seizure activity is considerably intensified by administration of CO_2 (7 to 15%, in the air from the artificial respiration pump), and by topically applied solutions of acetylcholine or pilocarpine.

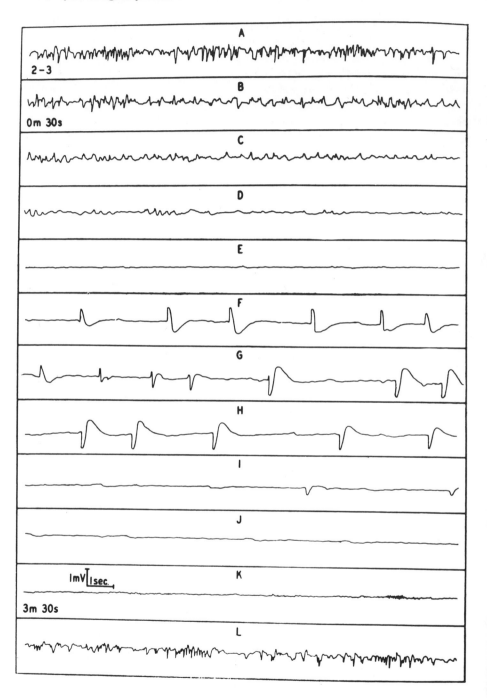

C. Electric impedance change

The increase of the impedance of the tissue starts at any region at about the same time as the negative wave of the slow voltage variation. The duration of the impedance increase is ordinarily of the order of 1.5 min. In studying this concomitant of SD, measurements of the alternating current impedance between two electrodes, with a Wheatstone bridge, as well as four-electrode techniques have been employed. The four-electrode method, with one pair of electrodes for a constant current supply and the second pair for potential measurement, obviates many of the difficulties caused by electrode polarization, and permits use of electrodes of much smaller dimensions than is possible in the method using two electrodes directly connected with a Wheatstone bridge or other impedance measuring device (for a valuable exposition on the determination of biological impedances, see Schwan, 1963).

In the earliest experiments, which were performed on the dorsolateral cortex of rabbits (Leão and Martins Ferreira, 1953), the alternating current impedance between an electrode placed on the cortical surface and a remote one was measured with a Wheatstone bridge over the frequency range from 50 to 10,000 cps. These experiments showed that the impedance increase accompanying SD is due mostly to an increase of resistance, but that there is also a capacitative alteration, which follows a time course different from that of the resistance change. Not only does the maximum of the capacity increase occur later than the maximum of resistance increase, but also, at frequencies approximately from 50 to 200 cps, a period of decrease of capacity appears preceding the increase.

As an example of a four-electrode arrangement, Freygang and Landau's (1955) experiments on the cortical resistivity increase during SD may be mentioned. A pool of Ringer's solution was built over the exposed cortex of cats, and brief pulses of voltage were applied through electrodes placed one in the pool and the other deep into the pharynx. The potential differ-

←

FIG. 4. Conventional electrocorticographic record of SD. Bipolar surface recording; distance between electrodes (numbered 2 and 3), approximately 2.5 mm. Upward deflection denotes negativity of electrode 2 with respect to electrode 3. Rabbit under dial. *A:* "Spontaneous" activity before elicitation of SD. *B–J:* Continuous record, starting when a SD, elicited 30 sec before at another site, reaches the recording site. The SD advances in the direction from electrode 2 to electrode 3. *F–H:* Epileptiform negative waves, recorded first from electrode 2 and then from electrode 3. *K:* Beginning of recovery of "spontaneous" activity, about 30 sec after *J. L:* 15 min later.

Although the purpose is to show the time of occurrence, it should be noted that because of their large amplitude and duration, as compared with the excursions of the "spontaneous" activity, the epileptiform negative waves are markedly distorted in these electrograms. From Leão (1944a) with permission of the publisher.

ence produced by the current pulses across the cortex was recorded from two glass micropipettes of 20- to 25-μm tip diameter. Since the current density is practically independent of the cortical resistance, this potential difference is proportional to the resistivity of that portion of the cortical tissue lying between the pipette tips.

Since membrane conductance is usually very low at low frequencies of applied current, there is good reason to admit, as suggested by Freygang and Landau (1955), that the increase of the tissue resistance during SD is related to a swelling of cells, with narrowing of the extracellular current path. Van Harreveld and associates considered that the relatively low value of the resistivity of cortical tissue is consonant with the presence of an appreciable extracellular space, and that the increase of resistance during SD can only be explained by a loss of extracellular electrolytes. They postulated that, as a consequence of a sudden increase in the sodium permeability of the cell membranes, sodium and chloride ions, as well as water, move into the intracellular compartment. A general account of the studies on impedance changes and electrolyte distribution in central nervous tissues carried out by these investigators, who resorted to histological methods in order to obtain supporting evidence for the postulated ion and water movements during SD, has been published by Van Harreveld (1966).

Further experimental work is needed, however, for an adequate analysis of cortical impedance measurements. The problems of such measurements and their interpretation are not simple, as evidenced, for instance, by the differences in the reported values for the resistivity of the cortex of the rabbit and cat (see Li et al., 1968). With regard to the application of the Maxwell equations for the resistance of suspensions to calculate the volume fraction occupied by cells, experiments on electrical analogs for tissues, such as those of Cole et al. (1969), are certainly of much interest.

D. Vascular reactions, P_{O_2}, and metabolism

Marked vasodilation and increase in blood flow in the pial vessels, associated with cortical SD, are easily observed with a low-power microscope in rabbits, (Leão, 1944b). These changes, which appear at the time that the slow potential and impedance changes occur, usually last for 2 to 4 min. As the arteries dilate, the rate of flow in the veins increases, and these vessels promptly become red with arterial blood.

Although it has been definitely established that circulatory changes are not an essential component of the mechanisms of the self-propagating phenomenon, these changes nevertheless deserve attention in relation to epilepsy. Indeed, they are very similar to those seen during seizures in the exposed cortex of epileptic patients, where, according to all available evidence, they are equally of an accessory character. The view generally held is that the increased blood flow is due to dilation of the vessels by substances formed in the tissue by the overactivity of the discharging cells. The fact that such changes occur during cortical SD, when no excessive neuronal discharges are manifested, shows that this view may be utterly wrong, and that to discard the vascular reactions as secondary after-effects may be to exclude a useful element of information on fundamental local events.

In direct observations of the pial vessels, the present author has consistently seen during cortical SD in the rat and cat the same changes as noted above for the rabbit. In the guinea pig, however, it was found that SD may be accompanied, under certain conditions not yet adequately studied, by a brief (1 to 1.5 min) period of intense arterial constriction and greatly reduced blood flow (Leão, 1954). Other workers have used thermoelectric methods to follow the changes of cortical blood flow during SD. Buresová (1957) used cooled thermocouples applied to the cortical surface, and recorded in the rat an increase, beginning as a rule, during the second minute after the onset of the slow potential change. In general, however, heated thermocouples have been used, and although there are reports of a variable change (e.g., Tschirgi et al., 1957), the occurrence, under ordinary conditions, of an increase in blood flow has been abundantly confirmed.

Data on blood flow are fundamental for the interpretation of the P_{O_2} changes that occur in the cortical tissue concomitantly with SD. Studies of these changes by means of the polarographic method, essentially as described by Davies and Brink (1942), have shown that a fall in cortical P_{O_2} may occur during the slow potential change (Van Harreveld and Stamm, 1952; Marshall, 1959; Lukyanova and Bures, 1967). This fall is currently generally interpreted as being caused by an increase in oxygen consumption. With the aid of a quantitative evaluation of records of the changes induced in the cortical P_{O_2} of the rat by brief periods of administration through the tracheal cannula of a mixture of 95% oxygen and 5% carbon dioxide, Lukyanova and Bures (1967) concluded that the increase in oxygen consumption occurs at the height of the negative wave and during the terminal positive phase of the slow potential change.

The increase in oxygen consumption agrees with other findings on metabolic changes associated with SD. Thus, Krivánek (1961) has shown that during the negative wave of the slow potential change there is an accumulation of lactic acid and a decrease in the content of glucose and creatine phosphate in the cortical tissue.

It may be added that the incorporation of labeled amino acids into cortical proteins has been found to be considerably inhibited during SD (Ruscak, 1964; Bennett and Edelman, 1969; Krivánek, 1970).

V. SD IN ISOLATED RETINA PREPARATIONS

Since isolated retina preparations seem eminently suited for *in vitro* experimentation on SD, it was considered pertinent to close this chapter with a discussion about them. Retinal SD, in these preparations, is similar to cortical SD in all fundamental respects, but is of special interest in that it is accompanied by visible optical changes. The original observations of Gouras (1958) were made on the retina of the toad, but a majority of the subsequent studies have been performed on the retina of the domestic chick. The avian retina, as the amphibian, retains the capacity to undergo SD for many hours after excision when kept in appropriate bathing solutions at body temperature or cooler. It is particularly favorable for many studies because of the lack of blood vessels within the retinal tissue.

Figure 5 shows the optical changes accompanying SD in the isolated chick retina. The preparation used is the posterior hemispheric segment of the eye, containing most of the retina, choroid, and sclera. As soon as the dissection was completed and the vitreous humor drawn off, the segment was immersed in the bathing solution, and, after the microphotograph at the upper left-hand corner of the figure was taken, SD was elicited by slightly pricking the retinal surface with a sharp tungsten needle. The milky appearance of the increasingly larger area invaded by SD is clearly seen in the other microphotographs.

Portions of the retina may be detached from the above-described preparation, and the pigment epithelium of the portions may be removed in order to obtain preparations consisting only of retinal tissue. Working with these preparations, Martins Ferreira and Oliveira Castro (1966) were able by means of microphotometric determinations to show that the optical changes accompanying SD are caused by variations in the amount of light scattered within the tissue, and that the magnitude of the variations is greatest in the inner plexiform layer.

In further investigations, with special optical techniques, Oliveira Castro and Martins Ferreira (1970) found that during SD the thickness of the retinal tissue preparations also changes, the change consisting typically in an initial decrease, with a duration of about 30 sec, followed by an increase of greater amplitude, lasting 15 to 20 min.

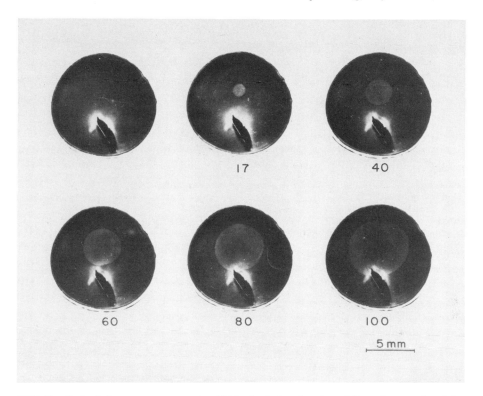

FIG. 5. Optical changes accompanying SD in the isolated retina. Microphotographs of the inner surface of the posterior hemispheric segment of the eye of the chick. The one at the upper left-hand corner of the figure was taken before elicitation of SD. The others, showing the changes (grayish circular areas), were taken after SD was elicited by slightly pricking the surface of the retina with a sharp tungsten needle. The numbers indicate the time the microphotograph was taken, in seconds after elicitation of SD. From Martins Ferreira and Oliveira Castro (1966) with permission of the publisher.

In these experiments, retinas of white Leghorn chicks, 1 to 20 days after hatching, were used, in which case the thickness of the retinal tissue preparations varies from 120 to 280 μm, depending on the region of the retina and the animal's age. These preparations are thus of much interest for biochemical and metabolic studies, not only because of their thinness, but also because cellular damage is extremely small in comparison with tissue slices cut from other parts of the brain.

Since the purpose of this section is only to provide an idea of the work that is possible with the isolated retina, other studies that have been performed on this material will not be considered. The reader interested in a general account is directed to Martins Ferreira and Oliveira Castro (1971).

VI. ACKNOWLEDGMENT

This investigation was supported by the BNDE (C. FUNTEC–74) and the CNPq, Rio de Janeiro, Brazil.

VII. REFERENCES

Aquino-Cias, J., and Bures, J. (1966): The effect of thalamic spreading depression on the epileptic discharge in rats. In: *Comparative and Cellular Pathophysiology of Epilepsy,* edited by Z. Servít. Excerpta Medica, Amsterdam, pp. 258–269.

Basser, L. S. (1969): The relation of migraine and epilepsy. *Brain,* 92:285–300.

Bennett, G. S., and Edelman, G. M. (1969): Amino acid incorporation into rat brain proteins during spreading cortical depression. *Science,* 163:393–395.

Brinley, F. J., Jr., Kandel, E. R., and Marshall, W. H. (1960): Potassium outflux from rabbit cortex during spreading depression. *Journal of Neurophysiology,* 23:246–256.

Brozek, G. (1966): Changes in the membrane potential of cortical cells during spreading depression. *Physiologia Bohemoslovenica,* 15:98–102.

Bures, J. (1957): The ontogenetic development of steady potential differences in the cerebral cortex in animals. *Electroencephalography and Clinical Neurophysiology,* 9:121–130.

Bures, J. (1960): Block of Leão's spreading cortical depression by bivalent cations. *Physiologia Bohemoslovenica,* 9:202–209.

Bures, J., and Buresová, O. (1956): A study on the metabolic nature and physiological manifestations of the spreading EEG depression of Leão. *Physiologia Bohemoslovenica,* 5(Suppl.): 4–6.

Buresová, O. (1957): Changes in cerebral circulation in rats during spreading EEG depression. *Physiologia Bohemoslovenica,* 6:1–11.

Burns, B. D. (1958): *The Mammalian Cerebral Cortex.* Edward Arnold, London.

Cole, K. S., Li, C.-L., and Bak, A. F. (1969): Electrical analogues for tissues. *Experimental Neurology,* 24:459–473.

Collewijn, H., and van Harreveld, A. (1966): Membrane potential of cerebral cortical cells during spreading depression and asphyxia. *Experimental Neurology,* 15:425–436.

Davies, P. W., and Brink, F. (1942): Microelectrodes for measuring local oxygen tension in animal tissues. *Review of Scientific Instruments,* 13:524–533.

Do Carmo, R., and Leão, A. A. P. (1972): On the relation of glutamic acid and some allied compounds to cortical spreading depression. *Brain Research,* 39:515–518.

Freygang, W. H., Jr., and Landau, W. M. (1955): Some relations between resistivity and electrical activity in the cerebral cortex of the cat. *Journal of Cellular and Comparative Physiology,* 45:377–392.

Goldensohn, E. S. (1969): Experimental seizure mechanisms; Discussion of Ward, A. A., Jr.: Epileptic neuron: Chronic foci in animals and man. In: *Basic Mechanisms of the Epilepsies,* edited by H. H. Jasper, A. A. Ward, Jr., and A. Pope. Little, Brown and Co., Boston, pp. 289–298.

Goldensohn, E. S., Shofer, R., and Purpura, D. P. (1963): Ontogenesis of focal discharges in epileptogenic lesions of cat neocortex. *Electroencephalography and Clinical Neurophysiology,* 15:153–154.

Goldensohn, E. S., and Walsh, G. (1968): Sequential functional changes in single cortical neurons during spreading depression. *Electroencephalography and Clinical Neurophysiology,* 24:290–291.

Gouras, P. (1958): Spreading depression of activity in amphibian retina. *American Journal of Physiology,* 195:28–32.

Grafstein, B. (1956): Mechanism of spreading cortical depression. *Journal of Neurophysiology,* 19:154–171.

Grafstein, B. (1963): Neuronal release of potassium during spreading depression. In: *Brain Function, Vol. I. Cortical Excitability and Steady Potentials; Relations of Basic Research to Space Biology,* edited by M. A. B. Brazier. University of California Press, Los Angeles, pp. 87–124.

Johnson, W. L., Goldring, S., and O'Leary, J. L. (1965): Behavioral, unit and slow potential changes in methionine sulfoximine seizures. *Electroencephalography and Clinical Neurophysiology,* 18:229–238.

Karahashi, Y., and Goldring, S. (1966): Intracellular potentials from "idle" cells in cerebral cortex of cat. *Electroencephalography and Clinical Neurophysiology,* 20:600–607.

Krivánek, J. (1958): Changes of brain glycogen in the spreading EEG-depression of Leão. *Journal of Neurochemistry,* 2:337–343.

Krivánek, J. (1961): Some metabolic changes accompanying Leão's spreading cortical depression in the rat. *Journal of Neurochemistry,* 6:183–189.

Krivánek, J. (1970): Effects of spreading cortical depression on the incorporation of (^{14}C)-leucine into proteins of rat brain. *Journal of Neurochemistry,* 17:531–538.

Krivánek, J., and Bures, J. (1960): Ion shifts during Leão's spreading cortical depression. *Physiologia Bohemoslovenica,* 9:494–503.

Lashley, K. S. (1941): Patterns of cerebral integration indicated by the scotomas of migraine. *Archives of Neurology and Psychiatry,* Chicago, 46:331–339.

Leáo, A. A. P. (1944a): Spreading depression of activity in the cerebral cortex. *Journal of Neurophysiology,* 7:359–390.

Leáo, A. A. P. (1944b): Pial circulation and spreading depression of activity in the cerebral cortex. *Journal of Neurophysiology,* 7:391–396.

Leáo, A. A. P. (1947): Further observations on the spreading depression of activity in the cerebral cortex. *Journal of Neurophysiology,* 10:409–414.

Leáo, A. A. P. (1951): The slow voltage variation of cortical spreading depression of activity. *Electroencephalography and Clinical Neurophysiology,* 3:315–321.

Leáo, A. A. P. (1954): Circulação na pia-mater e depressão alastrante da atividade do córtex cerebral. *Anais da Academia Brasileira de Ciências,* 26:XXII–XXIII.

Leáo, A. A. P. (1963): On the spread of spreading depression. In: *Brain Function, Volume I. Cortical Excitability and Steady Potentials; Relations of Basic Research to Space Biology,* edited by M. A. B. Brazier. University of California Press, Los Angeles, pp. 73–85.

Leáo, A. A. P., and Martins Ferreira, H. (1953): Alteração da impedância elétrica no decurso da depressão alastrante da atividade do córtex cerebral. *Anais da Academia Brasileira de Ciências,* 25:259–266.

Leáo, A. A. P., and Martins Ferreira, H. (1959): The negative voltage variations of spreading depression and circulatory arrest. *Abstracts of Communications, XXI. International Congress of Physiological Sciences (Buenos Aires),* p. 160.

Leáo, A. A. P., and Martins Ferreira, H. (1965): Efcito do potássio sôbre a variação lenta de voltagem da depressão alastrante. *Ciência e Cultura,* 17:279–280.

Leáo, A. A. P., and Morison, R. S. (1945): Propagation of spreading cortical depression. *Journal of Neurophysiology,* 8:33–45.

Li, C.-L., Bak, A. F., and Parker, L. O. (1968): Specific resistivity of the cerebral cortex and white matter. *Experimental Neurology,* 20:544–557.

Li, C.-L., and Salmoiraghi, G.-C. (1963): Cortical steady potential changes: extracellular microelectrode investigations. *Nature,* 198:858–859.

Lukyanová, L. D., and Bures, J. (1967): Changes in pO$_2$ due to spreading depression in the cortex and nucleus caudatus of the rat. *Physiologia Bohemoslovenica,* 16:449–455.

Marshall, W. H. (1950): The relation of dehydration of the brain to the spreading depression of Leão. *Electroencephalography and Clinical Neurophysiology,* 2:177–185.

Marshall, W. H. (1959): Spreading cortical depression of Leão. *Physiological Reviews,* 39:239–279.

Marshall, W. H., Essig, C. F., and Dubroff, S. J. (1951a): Relation of temperature of cerebral cortex to spreading depression of Leão. *Journal of Neurophysiology,* 14:153–166.

Marshall, W. H., Essig, C. F., and Witkin, L. B. (1951b): Spreading depression. *American Journal of Physiology,* 167:808.

Martins Ferreira, H. (1955): Variações lentas de voltagem durante a depressão alastrante. *Anais da Academia Brasileira de Ciências*, 27:XXIV–XXV.

Martins Ferreira, H., and Oliveira Castro, G. (1966): Light-scattering changes accompanying spreading depression in isolated retina. *Journal of Neurophysiology*, 29:715–726.

Martins Ferreira, H., and Oliveira Castro, G. (1971): Spreading depression in isolated chick retina. *Vision Research*, 11, *Suppl.* 3:171–184.

Milner, P. M. (1958): Note on a possible correspondence between the scotomas of migraine and spreading depression of Leão. *Electroencephalography and Clinical Neurophysiology*, 10:705.

Morlock, N. L., Mori, K., and Ward, A. A., Jr. (1964): A study of single cortical neurons during spreading depression. *Journal of Neurophysiology*, 27:1192–1198.

Muñoz-Martínez, E. J. (1970): Facilitation of cortical cell activity during spreading depression. *Journal of Neurobiology*, 2:47–60.

Ochs, S. (1962): The nature of spreading depression in neural networks. *International Review of Neurobiology*, 4:1–69.

Ochs, S., Hunt, K., and Booker, H. (1961): Spreading depression using chronically implanted electrodes. *American Journal of Physiology*, 200:1211–1214.

Oliveira Castro, G., and Martins Ferreira, H. (1970): Deformations and thickness variations accompanying spreading depression in the retina. *Journal of Neurophysiology*, 33:891–900.

Phillis, J. W., and Ochs, S. (1971): Excitation and depression of cortical neurons during spreading depression. *Experimental Brain Research*, 12:132–149.

Rapoport, S. I., and Marshall, W. H. (1964): Measurement of cortical pH in spreading cortical depression. *American Journal of Physiology*, 206:1177–1180.

Rosenblueth, A., and Cannon, W. B. (1942): Cortical responses to electric stimulation. *American Journal of Physiology*, 135:690–741.

Ruscák, M. (1964): Incorporation of 35S-methionine into proteins of the cerebral cortex in situ in rats during spreading EEG depression. *Physiologia Bohemoslovenica*, 13:16–20.

Schadé, J. P. (1959): Maturational aspects of EEG and of spreading depression in rabbit. *Journal of Neurophysiology*, 22:245–257.

Schwan, H. P. (1963): Determination of biological impedances. In: *Physical Techniques in Biological Research, Vol. VI, Part B*, edited by W. L. Nastuk. Academic Press, New York, pp. 323–407.

Sloan, N., and Jasper, H. (1950): The identity of spreading depression and "suppression." *Electroencephalography and Clinical Neurophysiology*, 2:59–78.

Szentágothai, J. (1969): Architecture of the cerebral cortex. In: *Basic Mechanisms of the Epilepsies*, edited by H. H. Jasper, A. A. Ward, Jr., and A. Pope. Little, Brown and Co., Boston, pp. 13–28.

Tschirgi, R. D., Inanaga, K., Taylor, J. L., Walker, R. M., and Sonnenschein, R. R. (1957): Changes in cortical pH and blood flow accompanying spreading cortical depression and convulsion. *American Journal of Physiology*, 190:557–562.

Van Harreveld, A. (1959): Compounds in brain extracts causing spreading depression of cerebral cortical activity and contraction of crustacean muscle. *Journal of Neurochemistry*, 3:300–315.

Van Harreveld, A. (1966): *Brain Tissue Electrolytes*. Butterworths, London.

Van Harreveld, A., and Stamm, J. S. (1952): Vascular concomitants of spreading cortical depression. *Journal of Neurophysiology*, 15:487–496.

Van Harreveld, A., and Stamm, J. S. (1953a): Spreading cortical convulsions and depressions. *Journal of Neurophysiology*, 16:352–366.

Van Harreveld, A., and Stamm, J. S. (1953b): Effect of pentobarbital and ether on the spreading cortical depression. *American Journal of Physiology*, 173:164–170.

Van Harreveld, A., and Stamm, J. S. (1955): Cortical responses to Metrazol ® and sensory stimulation in the rabbit. *Electroencephalography and Clinical Neurophysiology*, 7:363–370.

Whieldon, J. A., and van Harreveld, A. (1950): Cumulative effects of minimal cortical stimulations. *Electroencephalography and Clinical Neurophysiology*, 2:49–57.

8

Chronically Isolated Aggregates of Mammalian Cerebral Cortical Neurons Studied *In Situ*

Lawrence M. Halpern

OUTLINE

I. INTRODUCTION

Initial studies of the electrophysiological properties of surgically isolated or partially isolated neuronal subsystems were undertaken principally to investigate the origin of the rhythmic changes of potential recorded by the electroencephalograph and rapidly expanded to include studies of mechanisms basic to the epilepsies. Of particular interest to early investigators were two questions: Did cerebral cortex display autogenous electrical activity (Bremer, 1958), or did cerebral cortex display electrical activity only when driven from elsewhere in the brain (Burns, 1958)?

Spontaneous activity from isolated aggregates of nerve cells had been demonstrated by Adrian and his colleagues (Adrian, 1931; Adrian and Buytendijk, 1931) in isolated brainstem of goldfish, and in isolated optic, thoracic, and abdominal ganglia of *Dyticus marginalis,* a species of water beetle. Libet and Gerard (1939) were able to demonstrate spontaneous activity in isolated olfactory bulb of the frog. Investigations of this nature proceeded to the mammalian nervous system. As the choice of laboratory animals moved up the phylogenetic scale, electrophysiological analysis proceeded to suprasegmental levels. There were demonstrations of bursts of electrical activity which could be recorded from cerebral cortex after mesencephalic section of the brainstem (Bremer, 1935, 1936, 1938), and after cutting the thalamocortical radiation to a given area (Spiėgel, 1937; Bremer, 1938; Swank, 1949). Other investigators stressed the dependence of cortical activity on subcortical and reticular mechanisms (Dusser de Barenne and

McCulloch, 1941; Morison and Dempsey, 1943; Dempsey and Morison, 1942; Kennard, 1943; Obrador, 1943).

In 1949, Kristiansen and Curtois completely isolated a limited area of cerebral cortex in cat *in situ* in such a manner as to maintain pial circulation intact. Under these conditions, they recorded spontaneous electrical activity, activity induced by physostigmine and acetylcholine, and activity induced by direct electrical stimulation of the cortical surface. Spontaneous activity was recorded from the surface of the cortex both after deprivation of the thalamocortical radiation and after severance of all intracortical and subcortical connections. The spontaneous activity recorded resembled the normal alpha rhythm and supported the idea that the electroencephalographic activity recorded was an intrinsic property of cerebral cortex itself and not necessarily dependent upon the existence of intact subcortical or introcortical driving mechanisms. The electrical activity induced by electrical stimulation or by chemical means was indistinguishable from that induced by the same means in normal cortex. Local application of 5×10^{-3} g/ml of acetylcholine converted the rhythmic activity of the isolated slab to a series of rapid, high voltage spikes. These were described as being unlike typical strychnine spikes but similar to the spikes recorded in the vicinity of a cortical epileptogenic focus. It seemed clear even from the initial study that autogenous rhythms emanated from cerebral cortex and were somehow related to the abnormal rhythms recorded from the brains of epileptic patients. Thus, to the search for understanding the physiological basis for cortical electrogenesis was added a desire to understand the pathophysiological processes underlying the genesis of abnormal electrical activity recorded from cortex in human epilepsy and so characteristic as to be useful for diagnosis of that disease.

Simultaneously and independently, another technique was evolved for the study of acutely isolated cerebral cortex (Burns, 1949). Burns reported that isolated cortex studied in cat *in situ* under chloralose anesthesia did not produce spontaneous activity. In a larger series of experiments, Burns (1951) reported that slabs of neurologically isolated cortex could be prepared in decerebrate cats. This method allowed for experimentation with isolated cortex at a stage where the persistence of anesthetic utilized during the decerebration procedure was not a factor. In the latter preparation, as in the original one, the pial vasculature was the only remaining connection between the isolated cortex and the remainder of the animal. These acute preparations did not usually show spontaneous activity. Burns' method, which involved bilateral carotid clamping during the actual cutting of cortical connections, has been criticized because of the possibility that an undue degree of cortical hypoxia had occurred. Presumably, hypoxia influenced the results and might explain the failure of Burns and his collaborators to record spontaneous electrical activity shortly after surgery.

Echlin et al. (1952) observed low-voltage rhythmic activity from cerebral cortical slabs isolated from human cortex at the time of surgery, and found spontaneous activity which was frequently interrupted by paroxysmal spikes of large amplitude localized within the areas isolated and which could not be recorded from intact neighboring areas of cortex. Similarly, Henry and Scoville (1952) recorded observations from deafferented cortex in 25 patients.

Shortly after the early studies of electrical activity from neurally isolated cerebral cortex, investigators turned their attention to the changes in spontaneous and evoked cortical activity which occurred days, months, and years after initial cortical isolation (Echlin et al., 1952; Echlin and MacDonald, 1954; Spiegel and Szekeley, 1955; Grafstein and Sastry, 1957; Sharpless and Halpern, 1962). Although these studies of chronically isolated cortex are interesting, they suffer from the multiple defects of: technical differences in preparation of the cortex to be studied (i.e., hemisphere, gyrus, portion of gyrus); species differences (i.e., having been done in human, monkey, dog, and cat); and methods of study (e.g., acute vs. chronic). However, the basic description of temporally related augmentation of electrically and chemically evoked epileptiform activity from chronically isolated slabs has prompted other investigators to continue to study the model. Differences in surface activity, threshold and duration of after-discharge, presence or absence of cellular somatic activity, and sensitivity to neurohumoral transmitter and/or drug effects have been reported but are difficult to reconcile from the experimental literature to date.

II. RATIONALE

A. The occurrence of denervation supersensitivity

Denervation supersensitivity is a concept first used by Cannon and Rosenblueth (1949) to explain slowly developing permanent augmentation of physiological responses following injury to presynaptic neurons. Supersensitivity is well understood in peripheral structures, and it has been suggested that this phenomenon may play an important role in clinical disorders resulting from neural injury which are not adequately explained as "release" phenomenon due to sudden removal of inhibition. A body of evidence also exists which indicates that the central nervous system appears to become supersensitive to chemical or electrical stimulation following partial or total deafferentation of neurons by surgical or pharmacologic means. Certain abnormalities in the motor or sensory sphere, intellectual impairment, perceptual difficulties, pain behavior, and behavioral or emotional disorders have been attributed to denervation supersensitivity, particularly if these phenomena develop slowly after interruption of neural pathways and involve augmented responses to neural or chemical input.

Sensitization of an effector organ to a particular chemical substance following denervation is sometimes cited as evidence that the substance is involved in the normal transmission process across the neuroeffector junction. Thus, information about the kinds of drugs to which denervated cortex becomes sensitized may be useful in delineating the nature of the transmitting agents and receptor mechansims and may also provide information concerning the nature of the changes underlying the sensitization process itself. In addition, if denervation supersensitivity, regardless of the specific mechanism, is involved in the etiology of various neurological, behavioral, and pharmacologically induced disorders, then drugs which have selective effects on supersensitive central nervous tissue may prove useful in probing the nature of the disease process itself.

Epilepsy is the major disease process toward which studies of isolated neural subsystems have been directed. Deafferentation by degenerative metabolic, traumatic, or neoplastic means with development of denervation supersensitivity is now often considered as one possible mechanism for the development of cortical hyperexcitability in humans. Thus, the application of the isolated cortex technique to study processes involved in augmentation of electrical excitability following injury or partial isolation may provide information which may directly parallel some of the events occurring during the development of focal cortical epilepsy in humans.

III. TECHNIQUES

A. Choice of experimental preparations

Isolated neuronal subsystems have been studied *in situ* in such diverse species as goldfish, water beetle, frog, cat, monkey, and human. The choice of species by the investigator should be suitable for the study intended, and capable of being maintained in good physiological condition for the projected duration of the experiment. If it is intended that physiological monitoring be achieved under conditions of acute experimentation (e.g., with anesthesia, paralyzing agents, or mesencephalic section), then the behavioral repertoire of the species chosen is not problematic. If intact unanesthetized, unrestrained preparations are desired, they must be handled in such a manner that the animal's intrinsic behavior does not interfere with the execution of the experiments; for example, unrestrained monkeys have the annoying habit of interfering with connecting cables and implanted electrode arrays unless appropriate means are provided to prevent these occurrences. Cats tolerate electrode implants well and, with appropriate precautions, remain quiet for long periods of time.

For the most part, chronic experiments have been done in cats so that it is appropriate to describe the handling of these animals in some detail.

B. Presurgical conditioning

Cats from commercial sources vary in physical condition owing to factors such as infection, trauma, or malnutrition. Cats to be used for chronic surgical procedures should be isolated and observed prior to being housed in a colony with animals in whom cortical slabs have been constructed and are being allowed to age *in situ*. Cats surviving 6 weeks in holding or quarantine facilities and who demonstrate no respiratory problems prior to initial surgery generally survive surgery with no problems for periods up to 3 years. Furthermore, transmission of infectious disease to the rest of the colony is minimized.

If the animal is to be used in an unrestrained, unanesthetized state over a period of time, the investigator or his delegate should handle the animal as frequently as possible. Frightened, angry cats are extremely difficult to handle in chronic recording situations, whereas, handling and feeding generally domesticates and desensitizes an animal to the point where he becomes tractable for a variety of the techniques to be described below.

C. Anesthesia for initial surgery

The choice of anesthetic agent depends largely upon the interval between surgery and the first necessary physiological observation.

Pentobarbital or any other intermediate-duration barbiturate is unsuitable for preparations in which activity is to be recorded immediately after the surgery. The effect of pentobarbital, 35 mg/kg i.p., lasts approximately 2.5 hr. Excretion of the drug occurs more slowly, and electrophysiological activity may be altered for periods of a day or more. Signs of barbiturate activity can be observed in EEG records for periods up to 24 hours even after a single intravenous dose of sodium pentothal, an ultra-short-acting (20 min) barbiturate.

Ether anesthesia by inhalation provides a useful preparation within 2 to 4 hr after cessation of anesthesia; however, the sympathomimetic effect of ether tends to increase bleeding which may then be more difficult to control than bleeding encountered during surgery under barbiturate anesthesia. Ether tends to be a bit troublesome for extended surgery and requires considerable practice before consistent results are obtained.

Chloralose, 40 mg/kg i.p., is a long-duration anesthetic which produces convulsoid high-voltage spike activity in the EEG and which may interfere with data collection of spontaneous and electrically evoked activity of similar form.

Methoxyfluorane has been described as the inhalation anesthetic which produces the least effect on cortical neuronal activity; however, it is difficult to induce anesthesia with this agent.

Halothane, although expensive, has many advantages and has been used successfully in the author's laboratory for the past few years. Animals are smoothly induced on 5% halothane and oxygen at flow rates of 0.5 to 0.8 liter/min. After induction, animals may be maintained at 1.5 to 2% halothane and oxygen at constant level of anesthesia for several hours. Recovery is rapid and preparations may be used within 2 to 3 hr of cessation of anesthesia without observable effect on cortical unit activity or responses evoked by direct repetitive stimulation.

Induction of halothane is usually by mask using a closed anesthesia system and special halothane vaporizer. Cats may be held by hand or immobilized in a restraining bag. Following loss of consciousness, the animal is maintained at 5% halothane and oxygen for a few minutes. Anesthesia is then discontinued for a minute or two while a small endotracheal tube is fitted *per os* to allow for mechanical ventilation of the animal should respiratory failure ensue during anesthesia. Two percent cocaine or 10% lidocaine spray can be used to anesthetize the oropharynx locally and prevent gagging. A Miller No. 1 infant blade on a laryngoscope handle is used to guide the introduction of a No. 14–22 French endotracheal tube. Following ultimate cessation of halothane anesthesia and removal of the endotracheal tube, cats tend to regain consciousness within 30 min and experiments may begin 2 hr later.

A similar procedure is followed if halothane is to be used in an acute experiment except that tracheal cannulation is done surgically via the neck.

D. Local anesthetics

Procaine and lidocaine are local anesthetics, which, if used for infiltration anesthesia in usual doses, can temporarily reduce the local excitability of cortex because of their anticonvulsant actions.

E. Immobilizing agents

Gallamine triethiodide (Flaxedil®) has been shown to increase the excitability of cerebral cortex (Halpern and Black, 1968) and is not useful for isolated cortical slab or brain excitability studies for this reason. *d*-Tubocurarine or curare at intravenous doses of 450 μg/kg per hr provides neuromuscular paralysis without changes in cortical excitability.

Atropine or scopolamine may be used to prevent complications due to internal secretions but only if the investigator does not wish to use the preparation within the next week or two, since these anti-cholinergic agents slow cortical rhythms and persist for long duration.

F. Choice of head-holders

Having anesthetized the preparation, the problem now becomes one of securing a head rigidly enough so that a craniectomy may be accomplished carefully without damaging the cortical surface beneath the bone. Several kinds of head-holders are available. The Czermak type supports animals well by means of a palate bar and nasal clamp. This type of head-holder is rigid; it permits passive opening of the lower jaw, and yet allows for positive control of the position of the head. Since it is not a stereotaxic instrument, it allows free access to the entire cranial vault without the steric hindrance caused by the calibrated bars of the most usual kinds of stereotaxic head-holders. In addition, ear bars are not used to support the head and the chances of causing permanent ear damage are eliminated. Should it be necessary to do stereotaxic mapping or should the rigidity of the frame be necessary for holding electrodes during experimentation, then one must resort to a stereotaxic frame for surgery despite its disadvantages.

G. Acute vs. chronic preparations; the need for aseptic surgery

If the preparation of cerebral cortex which is to be isolated is intended for use soon after isolation, aseptic precautions are unnecessary. Thus, two types of preparations of cerebral cortex can be made available for study. In one, a slab of cortex is neurally isolated, the surgical wounds are carefully repaired, and the preparation is nursed to recovery and housed until some later time when an acute experiment is to be performed. The second type of preparation involves the surgical isolation of a portion of cerebral cortex with simultaneous implantation of electrodes for stimulation and recording of responses.

Since the chronically isolated slab represents a considerable expenditure of time in terms of preparation of electrodes, surgical techniques, and aftercare, our laboratory has chosen to follow aseptic procedures during all phases of preparative surgery for slabs intended for chronic experiments. Drapes, towels, gowns, surgical instruments, and accessories are autoclaved at 15 to 20 p.s.i. for periods of 20 to 30 min prior to use. Sharp instruments are wet-sterilized in 1:1,000 benzalkonium chloride solution. As in the general operating room, the sterile field is carefully built up around the surgically scrubbed cat's head and maintained through the conclusion of surgery.

H. Surgical instruments (see Appendix I)

I. Physiological instruments (see Appendix II)

J. Electrode fabrication

Stimulating and recording electrodes are constructed of 0.10-inch platinum wire beaded at one end in an oxygen flame. The wires are then insulated to the tip with polyethylene tubing (PE10) or flexible Teflon tubing equivalent. The electrodes are imbedded in a cortical stabilizer plate (Fig. 1), which is constructed of clear polyester resin. This material, with catalytic hardener added, is poured over the formed platinum beaded wires into a flexible mold of polyethylene. After it is cured for 24 hr, the electrode-bearing resinous plate is removed by flexing it from the mold. The electrode plate is then ground on fine emory paper until the platinum beads are 1-mm discs and the bottom of the electrode is clear and transparent. Electrodes are ultimately chlorided by passing current in an HCl, lead acetate, platinous chloride bath depositing platinum chloride as a nonpolarizable residue on the platinum discs prior to implantation.

Details of the head plug are illustrated (Fig. 1). Subminiature connectors (Cannon DD50S or equivalent) are press-fitted to the platinum leads in the electrode assembly. The bottom of the electrode assembly plug is carefully sealed with dental acrylic to avoid moisture-induced low-resistance shunting of the lead wires. The central post is a stainless steel screw made to scale. The head is knurled, and the bottom surface is polished. The bolt upon which the plug sits pulls the knurled edge up into the bone, adding further stability to the implants. Stainless steel lock washers may be used

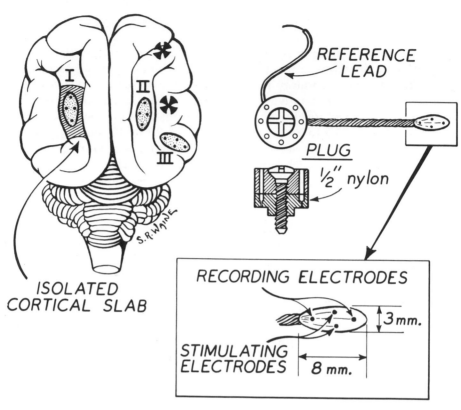

FIG. 1. Configuration of electrodes and sites of electrode implantation. Stimulating and recording electrodes are constructed of beaded platinum wire insulated with PE10 polyethylene tubing and cast into configurations shown in the recording electrodes insert. The cortical stabilizer in which the electrodes are embedded is made of clear, polyester Fiberglas resin. The delrin plug which is fabricated out of half-inch delrin rod contains subminiature connectors for stimulating and recording purposes. The bolts in the upper insert in the delrin plug and beneath it are fabricated to hold the delrin plug firmly on the post and hold the post firmly into bone. The reference lead is usually made of 0.010-inch Formvar-insulated type 316 stainless steel, further insulated by pulling it into polyethylene tubing (PE10). Roman numbers I and II indicate the site of implantation of electrodes over the isolated cortical slab (I). See text for method of isolation.

to stabilize the plug between the top screw insert and the bottom delrin nut. Reference leads may be of stainless steel, type 316, 0.010-inch Formvar-coated, pulled into polyethylene (PE10) sleeves, and may be used for ground or indifferent leads. The use of micro-electrodes is covered in Chapter 10 by Curtis.

K. Operative techniques for chronic electrode preparations

A midline incision is not used. Instead, a flap is made which allows the skin to be reflected to one side, thus exposing the cranial vault from ear to ear and from the supraorbital ridges, caudal to the external occipital protuberance. Once the skin is reflected, fascia and periosteum are divided in the midline enabling the large temporal muscles to be reflected bilaterally, uncovering the cranial vault as far temporally as possible. Subsequent to this procedure, a wide bilateral craniectomy is performed. Large amounts of bone are removed, thus exposing both hemispheres almost to the midline. A bridge of bone, 0.5 to 0.75 cm in width, is left to cover and protect the superior saggital sinus. The posterior margin of the craniectomy is the rostral surface of the bony tentorium while the anterior margin is the area in which diploe widens to encompass the frontal sinuses. Care must be taken not to enter the frontal sinuses, or infection of the cranial contents will result. The inferior margin of the bone opening extends laterally almost to the temporal pole. Upon conclusion of the craniectomy and after adequate hemostasis, erection of electrode supporting posts may be begun.

Notches are cut in the remaining midline bone in order to accommodate the width of the flat-headed screw to be used for supporting the electrode assembly (see Fig. 1). Extreme caution must be exercised to prevent injuries to superior saggital sinus. If this structure is injured, it is usually difficult if not impossible to achieve hemostasis. After the bone is notched bilaterally, bolts are positioned and locked into place with flat delrin nuts; in this manner, two rigid posts are constructed for supporting the electrode assembly. The electrodes, which have been previously sterilized in benzalkonium chloride, are rinsed in normal saline, mounted temporarily on the supporting posts, and molded into what is to become the form most suitable for permanent implantation. When the electrodes are suitably shaped, the course of their lead wires over bone is prepared in order that the lead wires may be subsequently attached to bone and rendered immovable. This is accomplished by anchoring folded lengths of 0.005-inch stainless steel wire to holes in the bone by means of small steel pins made from phonograph needles. In this manner, electrode wire can be firmly anchored with wire ties at a time when the electrodes are to be finally implanted.

When the wire ties have been prepared for future use, the electrode-mounting posts are permanently in place, and the electrode lead wires have been shaped so that the electrodes can be properly positioned on the surface of the cortex, the dura is incised and reflected bilaterally and hemostasis is achieved.

Neural isolation of left suprasylvian gyrus is done by the following method. The spatulate end of a Penfield No. 2 dissector or silver brain spatula, as described above, is inserted coronally to a depth of 5 to 7 mm into the cortex at the junction of the posterior downward convolution of the left suprasylvian gyrus and the straight portion of the gyrus. The dissector is then rotated 90° and advanced rostrally between the grey and white matter parallel to the surface of the gyrus at a depth of 3 to 4 mm for a total distance of 15 to 25 mm. The blunt leading edge of the blade can be directly visualized beneath the surface of the pia at the anterior margin of the undercut gyrus. To insure destruction of the largest number of subpial connections, a saline-moistened cotton ball is pressed gently on the surface of the pia, severing connections between the cotton ball and the blunt knife edge. The dissector is then rotated beneath the cortical surface in order that the superior margin of the gyrus may be isolated by pressing the cotton ball against the edge of the dissector in similar fashion. The dissector is then rotated until the other edge is seen through the pial surface, and, again, middle pressure of the cotton ball against the spatula blade is exerted. Thus, the posterior, anterior, superior, and lateral margins of the slab are isolated to the pia from beneath.

It is of critical importance to continue to observe the pial blood vessels to make sure that these are not occluded owing to upward pressure of the spatula during the subpial dissection procedures. With a little practice, this rather cavalier technique can achieve a viable cortical slab preparation. The previously shaped electrodes are then permanently bolted to the implanted mounting posts. Lead wires are anchored to bone by means of the previously attached wire ties. The cortical stabilizer plates are adjusted and seated squarely over the isolated slab and over its intact contralateral homolog. The spring tension of the electrode assembly can be easily judged by viewing the pial circulation directly through the transparent stabilizing plate. Thus it can be determined if the pial circulation is occluded because of downward pressure from the electrodes. Reference leads, one for grounding and one for use as an indifferent electrode, are anchored, one to bone over the frontal sinuses and one to bone on the external occipital protuberance. Dental acrylic cement is judiciously applied to points where wire and bone contact. This is done to minimize further artifact problems which can be caused by contraction of temporal muscle with concomitant movement of lead wires. When the dental cement is dry, the temporal muscles are wired together across the midline; they do not cover the plugs attached to the electrode assembly. Skin flap is replaced and the plugs exteriorized through a small incision just wide enough to pass the plug. Finally, the margin of the skin flap is repaired.

If the investigator does not intend to implant chronic electrodes of the type described, the initial surgical procedures are quite simple and straight-forward. Only a unilateral craniectomy is required at the time of initial surgery. Once the slab has been isolated, wet gelfilm is placed over the cortex and the dura sutured together, care being taken not to sew the muscle back so tightly that the pressure from the muscle occludes the blood vessels. The use of small pieces of gelfilm which dissolve and disappear in 6 to 8 weeks reduces the possibility of adhesions and allows redissection of the cortical slab at a later date without traumatizing the isolated cortical slab. The gelfilm may be removed earlier without difficulty.

L. Stimulation and recording

Chronic slabs intended for acute terminal study, require no special pre-cautions for stimulating; however, continued stimulation of animals with chronic electrodes over periods of months or years may require some special attention to stimulus parameters to maintain the tissue in good condition over long time periods.

Since one plans to stimulate the same site many hundreds of times during the course of an experiment, it is considered desirable to use paired, opposite-going, approximately square pulses in addition to the nonpolarizable electrodes (Fig. 2). It has been reported that this type of stimulation is less likely to produce tissue damage than monophasic pulse stimulation. Pulse durations of 0.5 msec with opposite polarity pulses separated by intervals of 0.5 msec may be used successfully. During stimulation, trains of pulse pairs are presented at 30 Hz for 2.5 sec. All parameters of stimulation may be held constant except peak current per pulse; the latter is determined by measuring voltage drop across a 1,000 Ω resistor in series with the stimulating electrodes or by use of a current probe, Tectronix 131 or equivalent, transformer coupled to the stimulator output. Current is varied systematically during the time course of an experiment. A step-wise attenuator providing approximately equilog increments of current may be incorporated into the stimulating circuit to allow simultaneous digital control of current output. Stimulus strength may be represented in two ways: in terms of peak current per pulse per threshold measurement, and in terms of the number of equilog increments of current over threshold, each increment being approximately 1.6 db. Comparison of stimulus strength in different animals in terms of peak current per pulse is not justifiable in every case since there is evidence that different proportions of the total current flow through the cortical tissue in different experiments. Expressed as a logarithm of the

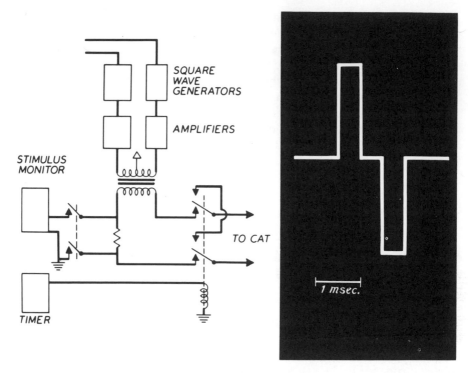

FIG. 2.   A method of obtaining paired, opposite-going square waves for stimulation of the -isolated cortex.   Square-wave generator output is amplified.   Stimulus isolation transformers are connected in series; 1,000 Ω resistor in series with the cat permits rapid current determination by measuring voltage drop across the resistor.   Relay at stimulating electrodes short-circuits stimulating electrodes between stimuli, aiding in rapid depolarization.   Parameters of stimulation are 0.5-msec pulses, 30 Hz, 2.5-sec duration.   Timer is used to control the duration of the stimulus burst.

proportion of threshold current, stimulus strength is independent of variations in shunt resistance among different cats at different experimental sessions.   See Fig. 3 for sample records.

M. Experimental design for after-discharge studies

There are essentially three parameters with which isolated cortical slab epileptiform after-discharge experiments are concerned: stimulus intensity, interstimulus interval, and the duration in seconds of epileptiform after-discharges resulting from suprathreshold stimulation of isolated intact

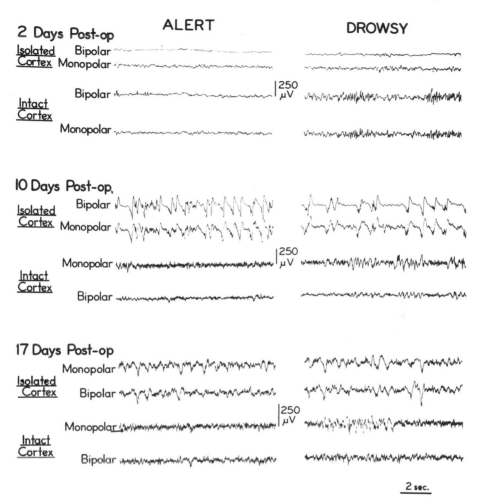

FIG. 3.   Spontaneous activity at various times after cortical isolation. Records obtained from one cat at successive recording sessions. Note the differences between activity recorded from isolated cortex and that from intact cortex.

cortical loci. The basic experimental design calls for alternating the presentation of stimuli to intact and isolated suprasylvian gyrus (Fig. 4). Once the threshold for epileptiform after-discharge has been determined for each side, presentation of suprathreshold stimuli proceeds at 10-min intervals. This usually results in serial presentation of increasing stimulus intensity

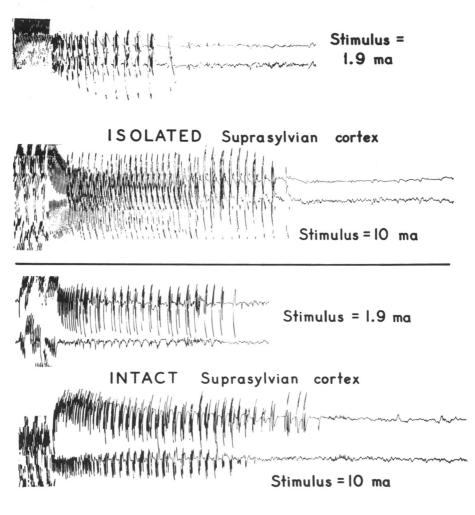

Stimulus =
1.9 ma

ISOLATED Suprasylvian cortex

Stimulus = 10 ma

Stimulus = 1.9 ma

INTACT Suprasylvian cortex

Stimulus = 10 ma

2 sec 250µV

FIG. 4. Comparison of the response of acutely isolated and normal intact cerebral cortex. The form of the response obtained from acutely isolated cortex is similar if not identical to the responses obtained from intact cortex. Increasing stimulus intensity to over 500% of threshold does not increase the duration of the response by more than a few seconds. The response of intact cortex to the 10-mA stimulus was one that did not produce any generalized seizure.

at each cortical location. These are repeated until five to ten after-discharges are obtained from each cortical site at each stimulus intensity (Tables 1 and 2).

TABLE 1. *Average durations of after-discharges obtained at a single experimental session*

Isolated cortex			Intact cortex		
Stimulus intensity (mA)	Time (sec)	SD	Stimulus intensity (mA)	Time (sec)	SD
1.4	57.2	72.5	2.6	11.3	7.1
1.6	40.5	33.2	3.0	13.0	6.2
1.9	64.9	44.9	3.5	15.6	4.3
2.2	99.4	57.0	4.1	14.1	4.0

Data obtained from one cat during a single experimental session. Averages are based on ten trials each. This table is primarily intended to illustrate the kind of quantitative data which may be obtained by using the experimental design outline in the text.

TABLE 2. *Mean durations of after-discharge taken for five cats tested at successive weekly intervals*

Week no.[a]	Cat no.[b]	Isolated cortex			Intact cortex		
		0[c]	1	2	0	1	2
1	S-38	0.6	7.4	7.4	1.8	1.8	7.6
	S-46	9.2	9.4	5.0	4.0	10.0	5.8
	S-50	3.0	5.0	14.2	1.0	7.4	7.8
	S-58	2.2	6.2	29.0	5.0	6.3	12.0
	S-64	5.2	7.4	7.4	0.4	5.4	1.0
	Mean	4.0	6.2	13.5		5.3	6.8
2	S-38	101.8	69.0	95.0	7.6	9.6	13.0
	S-46	4.0	8.4	35.8	1.2	7.4	10.1
	S-50	7.0	33.2	79.9	4.0	11.4	15.2
	S-58	3.0	6.8	9.8	3.2	7.6	15.6
	S-64	1.4	6.4	11.4	0.2	1.6	2.8
	Mean	23.4	36.3	46.4	3.2	7.5	11.3
3	S-38	2.0	71.6	127.2	9.4	13.6	16.0
	S-46	10.6	26.4	36.9	7.4	7.4	11.5
	S-50	3.0	14.8	46.1	3.0	20.2	16.0
	S-58	39.6	31.0	40.4	0.6	4.2	8.2
	S-64	79.6	78.2	100.4	3.0	6.2	21.2
	Mean	26.9	44.4	70.2	4.6	8.6	12.2

[a] Time after cortical isolation at which data were collected.
[b] Based on laboratory system for numbering animals.
[c] 0, 1, and 2 refer to method of scaling stimulus intensity as described in text.

IV. THE APPLICABILITY OF THE ISOLATED CORTICAL SLAB MODEL
TO SPECIFIC STUDIES

The morphology of isolated cortex has been described by Sastry (1957), Szentágothai (1965), Colonnier and Gray (1962), and others. These reports consist of a variety of light- and electron-microscopic investigations into the morphological changes of cortex following isolation. Histochemical studies have been reported by Hebb et al. (1963), demonstrating a reduction in acetylcholine and cholinesterase by histochemical methods. Green et al. (1970) reported a series of biochemical studies on enzyme activity in the isolated cortical slab. They studied such enzymes as succinic dehydrogenase, monoamine oxidase, acetylcholine esterase, acetylcholine acetylase, and the sodium-potassium-dependent ATPase. Drug studies in chronically isolated cortex have been reported by numerous investigators. The effects of antiepileptic drugs on electrically induced responses of acute and chronic isolated cerebral cortex in the cat were reported by Sanders and Gravlin (1968).

Isolated cortical slabs as a laboratory model of pathophysiologic conditions in human epilepsy have been studied by many of the investigators whose work is referenced in the bibliography (Pinsky and Burns, 1961; Krnjevic et al., 1965, 1970; Rutledge et al., 1967; Halpern and Ward, 1969; Spehlmann et al., 1970, 1971; Spehlmann, 1971).

V. LIMITATIONS OF THE ISOLATED CORTEX TECHNIQUE

A. Sources of error

The generation and use of chronically isolated cortical slab for continued study contains several pitfalls. The tissue itself is fragile and subject to anoxia, trauma and vascular occlusion by the electrode being used to study its electrical responses. The "fatigue" effect (Fig. 6) makes it difficult to get a hyperexcitable preparation with sufficiently uniform characteristics to be able to do statistically meaningful studies of reduction of after-discharge duration as a consequence of drug administration. Different physiological responses as a consequence of different modes of preparation and different species in which isolated cortical slabs are prepared make it difficult if not impossible to correlate studies done in one laboratory with those done in another. Isolated slabs have been prepared from half brain, full gyrus, or partial gyrus preparations. Consequently,

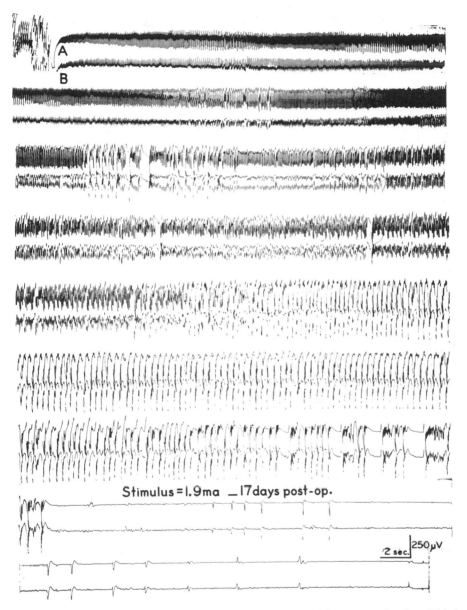

Stimulus = 1.9 ma — 17 days post-op.

2 sec. | 250 μV

FIG. 5. After-discharge from isolated cortex obtained on the 17th postoperative day. This is an example of the rather startling responses of which a chronically isolated slab of cortex is capable. The stimulus intensity is 1.9 mA, exactly the same as the stimulus intensity used to evoke the responses illustrated in Fig. 4. The average duration of 10 after-discharges obtained from this experimental session was well over 100 sec. Note the increased tonic portion of the response which now amounts to over half the duration of the response. *A* is a recording taken from isolated cortex to a point over frontal sinus. *B* is a bipolar recording. As a consequence of continued time after isolation, the after-discharge thus recorded gets longer and longer until, following a single suprathreshold stimulus, convulsive activity may be observed from a slab of cortex for hours and even days.

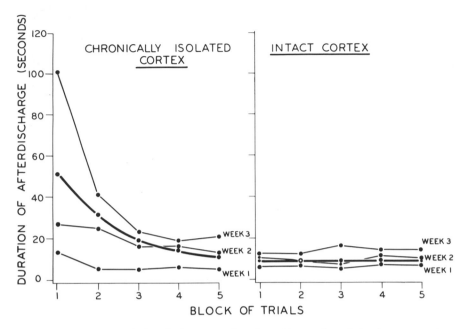

FIG. 6. The duration of after-discharge as a function of the number of stimulus presentations. The left-hand block represents changes in the average duration of after-discharge from isolated cortex of all cats tested within the first 3 postoperative weeks. The abscissa is the number of stimulus presentations. The ordinate is the duration of after-discharge in seconds. The three solid lines represent postoperative weeks as labeled. The right-hand block is a similar representation of the averages of after-discharges taken within the first 3 postoperative weeks as a function of presentation of stimuli. Abscissa and ordinate correspond to those from intact cortex. The degree of fatigue is of greater magnitude as, in isolated cortex, postoperative time increases. This effect is not seen in the average duration from intact cortex. The heavy line represents an exponential curve calculated by averaging all of the points from each presentation of stimulus. A similar curve appears in the schema for intact cortex.

differences in the reported behavior or even the presence or absence of single-unit discharges are rather difficult to reconcile because of these preparation differences.

B. Expectations

Under good conditions, one should be able to make uniform slabs of cortex capable of giving *reasonably* reproducible results. Using a standard method of preparing tissue, a standard electrode configuration, and standard stimulus parameters, one is able to come up with consistent responses. However, because of the natural variability of threshold and duration of responses, and the changes in threshold and duration of response as a consequence of repeated stimulation, one should not expect consistent statistical reliability as a criteria for reproducibility. Over a 6-week period, a chain of events that occur reliably allows one to observe the gradual increase in hyperexcitability or susceptibility to direct repetitive electrical stimulation of cortical surface (Fig. 5). Concomitantly over the first week a gradual reduction in number of extracellularly recorded spontaneous cells firing occurs until a point is reached at which spontaneous unit activity is virtually absent.

Methods for standardization and production of uniformly responding tissue do not exist, tending to make this model complicated and difficult to draw conclusions from in some cases. With reasonable caution and surgical skill, an investigator may reliably produce a series of cortical slabs from which similar but not identical changes may be recorded and described. The investigator should design his experiments with the peculiarities of the preparation in mind. Differences where they exist are apparent. Each particular step in the production and utilization of the model must be suspected of altering the output of the model from previous results. As indicated above, the presence or absence of local anesthetic or immobilizing agents, as well as anticonvulsants, alpha-adrenergic blocking drugs, catecholamine-depleting drugs, catecholamine-enhancing drugs, atropine-like or acetylcholine-like drugs, and serotonin depletors or enhancers may alter the epileptiform after-discharge duration, especially if these agents are used in acute preparations where the investigator does not have the ability to check the preparation repeatedly over days, weeks, and months to ascertain its characteristics.

The most interesting projected uses for the cortical slab preparation remain in the field of epilepsy, where detailed studies of the nature of the changes following disuse or deafferentation may provide valuable insights into the mechanism underlying deafferentation in focal cortical epilepsy. In addition, if denervation produces a supersensitivity to neurohumoral transmitters, which follows the characteristic supersensitivity to transmitters in other parts of the nervous system, then it should be possible to characterize neurohumoral transmitting materials as a consequence of their selective action and greater sensitivity of the neuronal aggregate preparation to their effects.

VI. APPENDIX I: SURGICAL INSTRUMENTS

Instrument trays, of course, vary greatly according to the needs, desires and skills of the individual. Basic surgical instrument subdivisions are as follows.

A. Skin set

For making and closing skin incisions, #3 scalpel handle with No. 10 blade, heavy dissecting scissors, tissue forceps, self-retaining retractor, periosteal elevator and needle drivers.

B. Bone set

Dental drill or equivalent, ⅜-inch trephine with removable center plug. A pair of large double action Fulton straight rongeurs, a pair of small double-action Stille angular rongeurs.

C. Dura set

No. 9 scalpel handle and No. 11 blade, small straight mouse-tooth forceps, small round mouse-tooth forceps, microneedle driver to be used with 6–0 ophthalmic suture needles for closing dura.

D. Instruments for cortical isolation

Blunt silver brain spatula, 7 mm wide, 17.5 cm long, 0.5 mm thick; other techniques involve broken pieces of razor blade and blunt wire hooks; automatic knife preparations used to make a stab wound and trace the margins of the knife to the pia subcortically have also been described.

E. General

Aspirator tip with fine suction tip and stylet for cleaning, aspirator pump, set of Penfield dissectors, numbers 1–4. A quantity of straight and curved 5-inch hemostats and a quantity of small towel clips, as well as a self-illuminating dissecting microscope, are also useful. No. 2 and no. 3 cotton pellets (dental), gelfilm, gelfoam, bone wax, gauze sponges; suture material: 6–0 silk, 3–0 chromic gut, 3–0 monofilament nylon.

VII. APPENDIX II: PHYSIOLOGICAL INSTRUMENTS

A. Recording

Ink-writer: Beckman Type R or equivalent, capable of writing EEGs, blood pressure, CO_2 output, and body temperature (six channels are required, eight channels of amplification are more useful); AC or AC-DC preamplifiers and cathode followers, Grass P511 or equivalent; Tectronix multibeam oscilloscope (Type

RM565); Grass oscilloscope camera; Bioelectric reflexor housing and camera mount; multichannel FM-modulated tape recorder such as Ampex FR100A or equivalent.

B. Stimulation equipment

Devices digitimer with gated pulse generator, relay unit and Mark 4 isolated stimulators (minimum of two required). Similarly, Tectronix 160 modules may be used with auxiliary isolation transformers or RF isolation links.

C. General

Infusion pump or suitable microdrip apparatus for continually infusing lactated Ringer's solution intravenously and administering drugs; Statham blood pressure transducer or equivalent for continuously monitoring arterial blood pressure; DC servo-regulated temperature monitor for recording and displaying body temperature and maintaining it within 0.5°C, histological equipment as necessary.

D. Calibration

Calibration may be done from the AC-DC preamplifiers so that ink-writer, oscilloscope, and tape recorder gains are all set to 200 μV/cm. Time-line calibration for the oscilloscope comes from the time-scale output of the Devices digitimer. Occasionally one may need frequency standards for operating rate meters or for direct comparison of oscilloscope traces. The crystal clock of the Devices digitimer is accurate at 0.01% (15 to 40°C).

VIII. ACKNOWLEDGMENTS

The preparation of this manuscript was partially supported by U.S. Public Health Service Research Grant MH12426 from the National Institutes of Mental Health. The author is indebted to D. Luisa Mayer for her invaluable assistance in the editorial work associated with the production of this manuscript.

IX. REFERENCES

Adrian, E. D. (1931): Potential changes in the isolated nervous system of *Dyticus marginalis*. *Journal of Physiology*, 72:132–151.
Adrian, E. D., and Buytendijk, F. J. J. (1931): Potential changes in the isolated brain stem of the goldfish. *Journal of Physiology*, 71:121–135.

Bremer, F. (1935): Cerveau "isolée" et physiologie du sommeil. *Comptes Rendus Séances de la Société de Biologie* (Paris), 118:1235–1241.

Bremer, F. (1936): Nouvelles récherches sur le méchanisme du sommeil. *Comptes Rendus Séances de la Société de Biologie* (Paris), 122:460–464.

Bremer, F. (1938): Effets de la déafférentiation complet d'une région de l'écorce cérébrale sur son activité électrique spontanée. *Comptes Rendus Séances de la Société de Biologie* (Paris), 127:355–358.

Bremer, F. (1958): Cerebral and cerebellar potentials. *Physiological Reviews*, 38:357–388.

Burns, B. D. (1949): Some properties of the cat's isolated cerebral cortex. *Journal of Physiology*, 110:9P.

Burns, B. D. (1951): Some properties of isolated cerebral cortex in the unanesthetized cat. *Journal of Physiology*, 112:156–175.

Burns, B. D. (1958): *The Mammalian Cerebral Cortex*. Monographs of the Physiological Society, No. 5, Arnold, London.

Cannon, W. B., and Rosenblueth, A. (1949): *The Supersensitivity of Denervated Structures: A Law of Denervation*. Macmillan, New York.

Colonnier, M. L., and Gray, E. G.: Degeneration in the cerebral cortex. In: *5th International Congress for Electron Microscopy*, edited by J. Breese and S. Sydney. Academic Press, New York.

Dempsey, E. W., and Morison, R. S. (1942): The interaction of certain spontaneous and induced cortical potentials. *American Journal of Physiology*, 135:301–315.

Dusser de Barenne, J. G., and McCulloch, W. S. (1941): Functional interdependence of sensory cortex and thalamus. *Journal of Neurophysiology*, 4:304–310.

Echlin, F. A., Arnett, V., and Zoll, J. (1952): Paroxysmal high voltage discharges from isolated and partially isolated human and animal cerebral cortex. *Electroencephalography and Clinical Neurophysiology*, 4:147–164.

Echlin, F. A., and MacDonald, J. (1954): The supersensitivity of chronically isolated and partially isolated cerebral cortex as a mechanism in focal cortical epilepsy. *Transactions of the American Neurological Association*, 79:75–79.

Grafstein, G., and Sastry, P. B. (1957): Some preliminary electrophysiological studies on chronic neuronally isolated cerebral cortex. *Electroencephalography and Clinical Neurophysiology*, 9:723–725.

Green, J. R., Halpern, L. M., and Van Niel, S. (1970): Alterations in the activity of selected enzymes in the chronic isolated cerebral cortex of cat. *Brain*, 93:57–64.

Halpern, L. M., and Black, R. G. (1968): Gallamine triethiodide facilitation of local cortical excitability compared with other neuromuscular blocking agents. *Journal of Pharmacology and Experimental Therapeutics*, 162:166–173.

Halpern, L. M., and Ward, A. A., Jr. (1969): The hyperexcitable neuron as a model for the laboratory analysis of anticonvulsant drugs. *Epilepsia*, 10:281–314.

Hebb, C. O., Krnjevic, K., and Silver, A. (1963): Effect of undercutting on the acetylcholinesterase and choline acetyltransferase activity in the cat's cerebral cortex. *Nature*, 198:692.

Henry, C. E., and Scoville, W. B. (1952): Suppression-burst activity from isolated cerebral cortex in man. *Electroencephalography and Clinical Neurophysiology*, 4:1–22.

Kennard, M. A. (1943): Effects on EEG of chronic lesions of basal ganglia, thalamus, and hypothalamus of monkeys. *Journal of Neurophysiology*, 6:405–415.

Kristiansen, K., and Courtois, G. (1949): Rhythmic electrical activity from isolated cerebral cortex. *Electroencephalography and Clinical Neurophysiology*, 1:265–272.

Krnjevic, K., Reiffenstein, R. J., and Silver, A. (1970): Chemical sensitivity of neurons in long-isolated slabs of cat cerebral cortex. *Electroencephalography and Clinical Neurophysiology*, 29:269–282.

Krnjevic, K., and Silver, A. (1965): A histochemical study of cholinergic fibres in the cerebral cortex. *Journal of Anatomy*, 99:711–759.

Libet, B., and Gerard, R. W. (1939): Control of the potential rhythm of the isolated frog brain. *Journal of Neurophysiology*, 2:153–169.

Lilly, J. C. (1960): Appendix: Injury and excitation of brain by electrical currents, In: *Electrical Studies on the Unanesthetized Brain*, edited by E. F. Ramey and D. S. O'Doherty. Hoeber, New York, pp. 96–105.

Morison, R. S., and Dempsey, E. W. (1943): Mechanism of thalamocortical augmentation and repetition. *American Journal of Physiology*, 138:297–308.

Obrador, S. (1943): Effect of hypothalamic lesions on electrical activity of cerebral cortex. *Journal of Neurophysiology*, 6:80–83.

Pinsky, C., and Burns, B. D. (1962): Production of epileptiform afterdischarges in cat's cerebral cortex. *Journal of Neurophysiology*, 25:359–379.

Rutledge, L. T., Ranck, J. B., Jr., and Duncan, J. A. (1967): Prevention of supersensitivity in partially isolated cerebral cortex. *Electroencephalography and Clinical Neurophysiology*, 23:256–262.

Sanders, H. D., and Gravlin, L. (1968): Effects of antiepileptic drugs on electrically-induced responses of acutely and chronically isolated cerebral cortex of the cat. *Epilepsia*, 9:341–353.

Sharpless, S. K., and Halpern, L. M. (1962): The electrical excitability of chronically isolated cortex studied by means of permanently implanted electrodes. *Electroencephalography and Clinical Neurophysiology*, 14:244–255.

Spehlmann, R. (1971): Acetylcholine and the epileptiform activity of chronically isolated cortex. II. Microelectrode studies. *Archives of Neurology*, 24:495–502.

Spehlmann, R., Chang, C. M., and Daniels, J. C. (1970): Excitability of partially deafferented cortex. I. Macroelectrode studies. II. Microelectrode studies. *Archives of Neurology*, 22:504–514.

Spehlmann, R., Daniels, M. B., and Chang, C. M. (1971): Acetylcholine and the epileptiform activity of chronically isolated cortex. I. Macroelectrode studies. *Archives of Neurology*, 24:401–408.

Spiegel, E. A. (1937): Comparative study of the thalamic, cerebral and cerebellar potentials. *American Journal of Physiology*, 118:569–579.

Spiegel, E. A., and Szckeley, E. G. (1955): Supersensitivity of the sensory cortex following partial deafferentation. *Electroencephalography and Clinical Neurophysiology*, 7:375–381.

Swank, R. L. (1949): Synchronization of spontaneous electrical activity of cerebrum by barbiturate narcosis. *Journal of Neurophysiology*, 12:161–172.

Szentágothai, J. (1965): The use of degeneration methods in the investigation of short neural connexions. In: *Degenerative Patterns in the Nervous System, Progress in Brain Research*, 14:1–32. Elsevier, New York.

9

Synaptic System Models

Don W. Esplin[*]

OUTLINE

[*] Associate of the Medical Research Council of Canada.

I. INTRODUCTION

The most practical and prudent course for anyone entering areas not fully explored is to have a map indicating the courses of roads and paths and the areas of uncharted wilderness. It is therefore appropriate to indicate for the subject under consideration, namely, synaptic system models, what we know and what we do not know, and also to indicate which areas we feel can presently be investigated and those in which we see at present no means for gaining substantial information.

It must be stated initially that we cannot list a substantial number of synaptic system models guaranteed to yield definitive information concerning the actions of antiepileptic drugs. Nevertheless, the list of models that have been employed in this endeavor is quite long—indeed, so long that the present discussion permits only selection of a few of the more prototypical models that have been of value in order to assess their utility. The most efficient means to accomplish this is to consider certain general criteria for selection of appropriate models and certain guidelines to be followed in the interpretation of results obtained from such models.

II. CRITERIA FOR SELECTION OF SYNAPTIC SYSTEM MODELS

An answer to the following question would be very useful in selecting an appropriate model for investigating actions of antiepileptic drugs: Do these agents exert their basic antiepileptic action on the abnormal neuron (the epileptogenic neuron), or do they prevent the manifestations of epilepsy by actions primarily upon normal neurons? It is clear that this crucial question cannot be answered prior to the selection of the model systems; information with regard to specific drugs will accumulate as additional models are investigated. Therefore, the problem must be approached in a different way. If the actions of antiepileptic agents are primarily upon abnormal neurons, then appropriate models will be difficult to find and to investigate. This statement can be made despite the variety of models of epileptogenic neurons that can be produced, as discussed in earlier chapters in this book. Such models have contributed greatly to our information concerning mechanisms of epilepsy; but as models for studying drug actions, including the most basic actions at the cellular level, they present enormous, but not wholly insurmountable, difficulties. Let us, therefore, take the easier course and assume that most antiepileptic drugs exert their beneficial actions on normal neurons. We should not totally disregard the alternate assumption but be prepared to test it when information from normal synaptic models suggests feasible and definitive experiments with epileptogenic neurons.

A good case can be made for the proposition that diphenylhydantoin exerts its antiepileptic actions primarily upon normal neurons. The studies of Toman and his associates (Toman and Goodman, 1948; Toman and Taylor, 1952), involving primarily electroshock seizure tests, provided clear evidence that the primary action of diphenylhydantoin was to prevent the spread of seizure discharge. It was subsequently shown (Esplin, 1957) that this agent blocks post-tetanic potentiation (PTP) in antiepileptic doses and is without other prominent effects upon two synaptic models, the spinal monosynaptic pathway and the stellate ganglion of the cat. The evaluation of more recent findings and the clinical observation that the drug often prevents the seizure without preventing the aura (see Toman, 1970) strongly indicate that it is not the discharge of the epileptogenic focus that is prevented by the drug, but excessive spread of activity from this discharge.

A weaker case can be made for phenobarbital. The principal evidence here is the similarity between diphenylhydantoin and phenobarbital in preventing the maximal electroshock seizure. On various other models, as will be described subsequently, the two agents can only rarely be shown to have similar actions. From present information, it is not profitable even to attempt to make a case for the other drugs effective against epilepsy.

The above at least partially supports the proposition that antiepileptic agents probably exert their action to a great extent upon normal neuronal systems, and, as a matter of practicality, the majority of our efforts, at least for some time into the future, must be concerned with such systems. Certainly, information will be obtained from a variety of synaptic models. It does not appear fruitful at present to quest after an ideal synaptic system model, but, clearly, certain models are going to be of more value than others. The utility of a particular model can be fully assessed only after it has been thoroughly studied and evaluated in relation to other models. Nevertheless, there are certain considerations that are useful beforehand in selecting the model and in designing the experiments to increase the probability of gaining fruitful results.

For the purposes of this discussion, several terms will be introduced and described in relation to the scheme of Fig. 1. Few drugs, if any at all, have a single action, and, as a consequence of that action, manifest a single effect. The spectrum of actions exerted by a drug is to a great extent a function of concentration (or dose); that is, a drug may appear to act rather selectively on one system at low dosage and yet exhibit greater and greater actions on a variety of other systems as dosage is increased. The two foregoing statements are as true of antiepileptic agents as of any other drugs. Now, considering the wide spectrum of actions that might be exerted by a given antiepileptic drug over a wide dosage range, it is evident that one or perhaps only a few of these actions may underlie its antiepileptic effect. Analysis of actions irrelevant to the antiepileptic effect may give information of little or no value. Therefore, an important, but not absolute, criterion for selection of a model is what may be termed "the criterion of dose correspondence."

For a given drug (X) at a dose or concentration (Y), we observe a particular effect or spectrum of effects (Z). If we consider the responsiveness of the entire nervous system to this drug, three compartments can be recognized, as depicted in the left-hand portion of Fig. 1. Some neural elements will be *insensitive* to the drug and some will be *sensitive* (that is, the drug will exert its characteristic actions on them), but the drug action here will be *irrelevant* to the studied effect of the drug. The third compartment comprises those elements that are sensitive to the drug and upon which the drug action underlies the characteristic effect. This *sensitive-relevant*

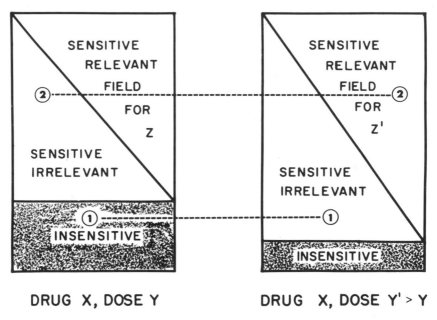

DRUG X, DOSE Y   DRUG X, DOSE Y' > Y

FIG. 1. Compartments of the responsiveness of the nervous system according to the model chosen and the dose of a given drug. Both schemes (left and right) represent three observable compartments of effects Z or Z' for a drug X at the dose Y on the left and the dose Y' on the right. Effects Z and Z' are different. Models 1 and 2 represent the neurons under study and their shift to different compartments.

compartment is termed the "field" for effect Z. In other words, if a model designed to represent specific characteristics is a subunit of some more complex whole, that whole is termed the field (see Esplin, 1968, for references to those who developed this concept and for further analyses of this in relation to drug actions).

The right-hand portion of Fig. 1 depicts the expected changes in the compartments mentioned if the dose of drug X is increased. Relating now the two sets of compartments, a few important conclusions can be drawn. Suppose that it is the analysis of effect Z that is of importance. A model, 1, is chosen and is found at dose Y to lie in the insensitive compartment. If the dose is increased, the insensitive compartment shrinks, and the model may now be in the sensitive-irrelevant compartment; but the action exerted on these sensitive neurons is that related to effect Z', not the one under study. Suppose now that model 2 is chosen and applied dose Y gives the effects, but these are not relevant to the characteristic action of the drug. Through disregard of the importance of dose correspondence criterion, the increase of the dose (Y') leads to an effect relevant to the action Z' which is not the subject of the studies. Similar examples of how changing dose can influence the results obtained from study of a model synaptic system can be imagined, and a specific example using diphenylhydantoin may be helpful. As mentioned above, this drug blocks PTP in the spinal monosynaptic pathway and in the stellate ganglion in doses known to be anticonvulsant in the cat. Thus, these synaptic models are sensitive to an action of diphenylhydantoin at the appropriate dose. The actions of the drug at these sites, however, is clearly irrelevant to the prevention of spread of seizure discharge through the brain. Therefore, the models selected may be with some assurance assigned to the sensitive-irrelevant compartment. As a further example, Tuttle and Preston (1963) confirmed the effects of diphenylhydantoin on PTP in the spinal cord. But these authors also employed doses of the drug that exceeded the anticonvulsant nontoxic range for the cat and observed depression of some polysynaptic inhibitory pathways in the brain. This effect is presumably unrelated to the antiepileptic effect of diphenylhydantoin (Z) but may be related to the signs of excitation (effect Z') seen with large doses of diphenylhydantoin.

The criteria discussed above must not be applied with absolute rigidity. Certainly, the accumulation of information about model systems necessary to characterize the field must be derived primarily from neurons in the sensitive compartments, and ultimately in the sensitive-relevant compartment. Nevertheless, information from models in the sensitive-irrelevant compartment and even in the insensitive compartment may yield valuable information concerning basic mechanisms of action at the cellular level. This aspect will be further amplified below.

III. CHARACTERISTICS OF SOME USEFUL SYNAPTIC SYSTEM MODELS

As mentioned throughout this chapter, our composite picture of the actions of a particular antiepileptic drug will be drawn from thorough studies of a variety of synaptic models. Each of the models presently available offers certain advantages and disadvantages. These can be partially categorized under the advantages that they possess.

Certain models are useful because they can be *easily investigated*. Accessibility of the synapse is an important consideration. Intracellular studies with microelectrodes contribute extremely valuable information; therefore, neurons that are easily impaled and can be held for considerable periods have definite advantages. Similarly, synaptic models that are easily maintained over long periods of time in stable conditions are useful. These advantages are possessed by peripheral synapses and especially by those that can be maintained in bath preparations *in vitro*.

The *ease with which the results can be interpreted* is also an important consideration. Of prime importance in this regard is that the model be well understood. The synaptic system under investigation should be isolated, that is, relatively free from indirect influences that might be secondary to actions of drugs on other neuronal systems. As described above, the sensitivity to the drug under investigation in the concentration relevant to the effect under investigation is a fundamental consideration. In analyses of synaptic function, much fundamental information can be gained if quantal aspects of synaptic transmission can be investigated.

Certain other conditions apply regarding the direct *relevance of the results obtained to actions of antiepileptic drugs*. It is generally considered that information obtained on synaptic models from the central nervous system is most directly relevant to the actions of centrally acting drugs. It is probably important that the synapse be capable of exhibiting complex patterns of neuronal activity, thus providing more aspects of neuronal function amenable to pharmacological manipulations. It is probably important also that the synapse have a variety of excitatory and inhibitory inputs, as an elaboration of the consideration mentioned just previously, to add diversity to the functions that may be manipulated by drugs.

On the assumption, discussed above, that antiepileptic drugs exert their actions upon normal neurons, then the synaptic models most relevant to actions of antiepileptic drugs are those involved in initiating, maintaining, terminating, or propagating the discharge of the epileptogenic neurons. Ultimately, synaptic models in these pathways, whether they be in the cortex, the temporal lobe, or the thalamus, must be investigated. For those drugs that appear to act primarily on the epileptogenic neuron, the most relevant model is obviously that abnormal neuron.

IV. SOME PROTOTYPICAL SYNAPTIC MODELS WITH SPECIAL REFERENCE TO THE SPINAL CORD

Although several structures of the peripheral nervous system or of the central nervous system of lower species have been used to study the effects of centrally acting drugs, including anticonvulsants and antiepileptics (Table 1), most of them lack the diversity of functions that could allow them to respond in various ways to drugs that have radically different actions. The studies on axons (which do not officially fall under the heading of this chapter), or on the neuromuscular junction, representing a simple relay between one terminal and one endplate, adequately illustrate these limitations.

TABLE 1. *Some simple models used in the studies of centrally acting drugs*

Model	Drugs studied	Reference
Axon	Antiepileptics Depressants Convulsants	Toman (1952) Morrell et al. (1958)
Neuromuscular junction	Antiepileptics Depressants	Raines and Standaert (1966) Quastel and Hackett (1971)
Aplysia ganglia	CO_2	Brown and Berman (1970) Brown et al. (1970) Walker and Brown (1970)
Autonomic ganglia	Antiepileptics Depressants	Esplin (1957) Brown and Quilliam (1964)

The various cells in *Aplysia* ganglia provide valuable information concerning membrane ionic conductances and transmitter action (see Tauc, 1967), yet the remoteness of these cells from the mammalian neurons on the phylogenetic scale calls for great caution in interpretation of the studies of centrally acting drugs in this simple synaptic system.

Autonomic ganglia represent the simplest synaptic system in mammals. However, they are complex enough to qualify as replacement models for central cholinergic synapses. The presence of two types of cholinergic receptors, nicotinic and muscarinic, as well as adrenergic receptors has been repeatedly verified (see Volle and Hancock, 1970; Libet, 1970). Basic synaptic phenomena such as facilitation or PTP elegantly described by Larrabee and Bronk (1947) have been exploited in drug studies.

With regard to more complex systems, the spinal cord provides synaptic models well suited for investigation of drug action. Various aspects of spinal synaptic transmission can be studied. The models are readily available and reasonably simple provided that sufficient knowledge of theoretical value and adequate practical skill in carrying out the techniques involved are acquired by the investigator. Therefore, the following section is designed to review some important spinal models from both technical and practical standpoints.

Adult cats of either sex are sufficiently suitable natural replacement models for studying subsystems such as neural pathways or nervous cells of the spinal cord.

Any chosen subsystem should be studied under conditions that greatly restrict influences from other parts of the nervous system and from drugs other than those being examined. This can be achieved to a reasonable extent if the experiments are carried out on unanesthetized spinal cats maintained in proper physiological state with regard to blood pressure, respiration, and temperature. Initially, the cat is anesthetized with ether in a special chamber. When the cat is under anesthetic, the tracheal cannula is promptly inserted, the spinal cord is transected at the atlanto-occipital junction, and the animal is immediately placed on a positive-pressure respirator. Ether is now discontinued. The carotid arteries are ligated and vertebral arteries occluded by an external clamp to further assure complete ischemia of the brain (absence of corneal and pupillary reflexes and pronounced dilation of pupils indicate the effectiveness of the decerebration). One of the carotid arteries is routinely cannulated and connected to a pressure gauge for continuous monitoring of mean arterial blood pressure. Experience from many experiments suggests that the optimum blood pressure for spinal cats should be 60 to 80 mm Hg, and no records should be taken when it drops to below 40 mm Hg for more than a few minutes (slow intravenous infusion of about 5 ml of 6% dextran solution is often helpful in elevating blood pressure). Very rigid control of the temperature of the preparation is required to maintain constant level of excitability of the cord. It is necessary to monitor the temperature by means of a subdural probe, which gives the true temperature of the spinal cord. Otherwise, it is reasonable to assume that the temperature of the preparation is intermediate between that recorded in the mineral oil covering the preparation and that of the animal. It is widely accepted that the spinal cord being used as a model should not be allowed to cool below 28°C. In addition, large variations in the temperature between 28 and 38°C greatly influence the excitability of the model, and records taken disregarding the temperature changes are misleading. The temperature of the cord should be kept steady with the variations not greater then ±1°C from that chosen. The normal temperature of the cat is considered to be 37°C.

Usually at the time when laminectomy is performed, the cat shows the previously mentioned signs of decerebration, and, at the end of the dissection of the spinal roots and peripheral nerves, anesthesia is virtually gone; therefore, the cat represents a spinal and unanesthetized model, and any design of the experiment leads to observations not obscured by the effects of an anesthetic or the neural supraspinal influences.

A laminectomy exposes the spinal cord from the insertion of the fifth lumbar dorsal root (DR-L$_5$) to the entry zone of the first sacral root (S$_1$). Two metal pins and a clamp are used to fix the animal to a rigid frame by the hips and the spinous process of the most cranial exposed vertebra. The skin of the back is retracted to form a "pool" which is filled with warm mineral oil. A midline incision, for the length of the laminectomy, is made in the dura. Then follows the identification and preparation of the spinal dorsal and ventral roots and the peripheral nerves. The stimulating and recording electrodes are fixed in the oil pool, and the appropriate cut roots and nerves are carefully placed on them. Attention is required at all times to keep the nerve-tissue elements sufficiently covered (submerged) by the oil.

When intracellular recordings are to be made, respiratory movements are reduced by performing a bilateral pneumothorax, and the spinal cord is firmly held in position by four metal bars which are pressed against the vertebral fragments on both sides of the cord, and fixed to the rigid frame. The small ligaments attaching the spinal cord to the dura are severed, and a section of the dura is isolated by transverse cuts above the insertion of the L$_6$ dorsal root and the entry zone of the L$_7$ root. The spinal cord is then rotated by gently pulling away this section of dura and pinning it to the back muscles. Rotation of the spinal cord changes the angle at which microelectrodes approach the ventral horn, and reduces the depth of tissue which must be penetrated before reaching the region where the motoneurons are located. Before the microelectrodes are inserted into the cord, the pia mater is also removed over the small space, carefully avoiding any damage to the blood vessels.

Animals require gallamine triethiodide (2 to 5 mg/kg) in order to abolish spontaneous movements and muscular twitching. Maintenance of the paralysis is almost always required throughout the entire experiment, and, therefore, the injections are repeated when necessary.

From the procedure described above, it seems clear that each of the experiments consists of three or four phases: (1) the period of stabilization which is allowed immediately after the end of surgery (1 hr), especially before the start of intracellular studies; (2) the control recording period; (3) the drug recording time; and, possibly, (4) the recovery to control if the drug is not long-acting.

The usual route of drug administration for experiments carried out on spinal animals is either systemic intravenous application through the cannulated brachial vein or close intra-arterial injection. The latter is of special importance if the drug has to be applied in very small doses in order to avoid massive side effects from systems other than the spinal cord. It is also practical when short duration of action directly on the neural tissue of the spinal cord is required. However, since this route involves ligation of several blood vessels (including those supplying the hind limbs), the peripheral nerves cannot be used for stimulating or recording. This technique is based on the one described by Holmstedt and Skoglund (1953). The cat must be eviscerated before laminectomy and the cannula inserted into the abdominal aorta for subsequent injections of a drug. Inserting the cannula requires temporary clamping of the aorta. The occlusion should not last longer than a few minutes if the interneurons (all extremely sensitive to anoxia) are included in experimental design.

The spinal unanesthetized cat serves as a good model to study spinal reflex activities, and in intracellular (motoneurons) and extracellular (interneurons) investigations. Reflex studies can be carried out via dorsal root (DR) stimulation (usually L_7 or S_1) and recording from the corresponding ventral root (VR). This arrangement gives general information about synaptic transmission. By stimulating DR, the mono- and polysynaptic discharges can be recorded from the electrode placed under the corresponding VR. The early monosynaptic spike (MSR) which represents the composite of the early synchronous discharge has a lower threshold for stimulation than the late polysynaptic component. The delay of the latter is clearly caused by several synapses interposed in the polysynaptic pathway. The stimulus applied to the whole dorsal root excites many afferent fibers and usually a quite complex waveform is recorded at the VR. DR-VR reflex studies are possibly the simplest way to show the selective effect of a drug on either discharge, since both are usually prominent. This excitatory reflex potential can be inhibited by applying the conditioning stimulus prior to the test to one of the adjacent DRs at the same side of the cord. In this way, a direct postsynaptic inhibition ("Lloyd inhibition") representing a good model for studying the inhibitory processes can be tested (see Fig. 2). In addition, when for several reasons extensive damage to the Ia fibers in

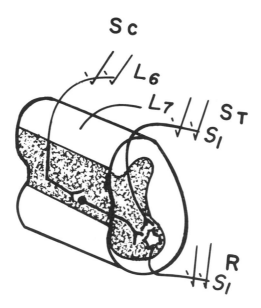

FIG. 2. Schematic representation of the lumbo-sacral section of spinal cord and placement of recording and stimulating electrodes. L_6, sixth lumbar DR with stimulating electrode—conditioning stimulus (S_c). S_1, first sacral DR with stimulating electrode test stimulus (S_T) and S_1-VR with recording electrode (R).

the periphery does not permit the conditioning and testing of specific pairs of muscle nerves, there is always the possibility that the central parts of these fibers within the DRs are still perfectly good to proceed with the experiment by studying the excitatory and inhibitory phenomena by way of DR-VR. Also, if the drug is applied by close intra-arterial injection to the lumbar part of the spinal cord, it is obvious from previous descriptions that only the spinal roots (lumbar) can be used for stimulating and recording. Consequently, where the recording is done through a microelectrode, identification of the motoneuron pool is clearly impossible.

Stimulation of a particular peripheral nerve from an extensor or flexor muscle or cutaneous branch allows the observation of the excitatory and inhibitory reflexes in the chosen pathways. Moreover, testing and conditioning at suitable intervals of appropriate pairs of peripheral nerves permits separate pursuit of postsynaptic direct, indirect, antidromic, and presynaptic inhibition (time courses and intensity) (see Fig. 3) in the spinal cord. Postsynaptic inhibition is mediated by an inhibitory transmitter released from terminals of interneurons, which acts on the postsynaptic membrane of the motoneuron. So-called "direct" pathways contain only one interneuron

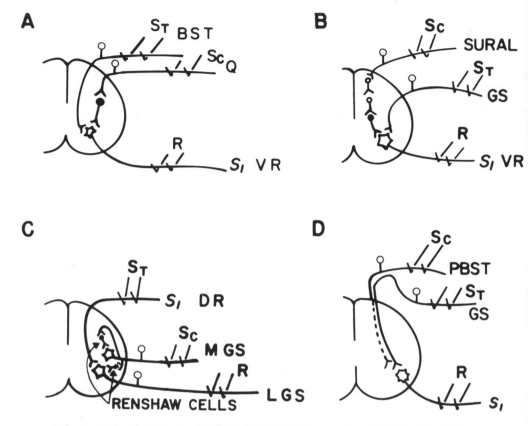

FIG. 3. As in Fig. 2. *A:* Testing direct inhibition between antagonistic muscles. BST, nerve to biceps semitendinosus muscle (flexor knee joint); Q, nerve to quadriceps muscle (extensor-knee joint). *B:* Testing polysynaptic inhibition from cutaneous nerve (sural) on the flexor muscle (GS, gastrocnemius nerve to triceps surae muscle). *C:* Testing antidromic inhibition (synergistic muscles). MGS, nerve to the medial head of triceps surae (TS); LGS, nerve to the lateral head of TS. *D:* Testing presynaptic inhibition. PBST, posterior branch of nerve to biceps semitendinosus muscle.

between the collateral of the group Ia afferent fiber and the motoneuron. This type of inhibition is also exerted by a variety of polysynaptic pathways as well as by recurrent pathways, such as that from motor axon collaterals via the Renshaw cell. The criteria for assessment of the anti-inhibitory action of drugs which alter the afferent drive has been established (Weakly et al., 1968). Although well-investigated drugs which increase inhibition are not available, it can be envisioned that such drugs might be of importance in the control of seizure activity (see Spencer and Kandel, 1969). Presynaptic inhibition has been described comparatively recently. Although not unequivocally proven, this inhibitory pathway contains at least two synapses according to the most generally accepted scheme. The inhibition is accomplished by axo-axonal connections between the terminals of afferent fibers. The inhibitory transmitter presumably causes reduction in the amount of excitatory transmitter released by depolarization of the terminals. The convulsive effects of picrotoxin were thought to be due to the reduction of presynaptic inhibition caused by this drug. However, mephenesine also depressed presynaptic inhibition without causing convulsions. Deeper knowledge of the physiological role of presynaptic inhibition is required before a definite link between the effects of drugs on this type of inhibition and their convulsive activity can be elucidated.

In summary, both MSR and polysynaptic discharges and phenomena such as inhibition or facilitation can be studied by way of DR-VR reflexes or in isolation while the peripheral nerves are used. Both methods may reveal the degree of selectivity of certain drugs on any of the above-mentioned processes.

Several antiepileptic drugs have been studied on the spinal mono-synaptic pathway by reflex recording techniques. Results of these studies have been summarized by Woodbury and Esplin (1959). It must be admitted, however, that the studies summarized in that review and the scattered information obtained since give very little basic information. Neither diphenylhydantoin nor trimethadione markedly affects the monosynaptic response.

The study of homosynaptic facilitation is possible by applying paired stimuli to the peripheral nerve. The first stimulus should be above threshold, and the second should be two times that maximal for MSR. When the intervals between stimuli fall to between 0.1 to 15 msec, the second response is always greater than the first. Any effect persisting longer than 15 msec is due to the interneuronal pathways and may be facilitatory or inhibitory to the second recorded response.

Testing of synaptic depression is analogous to measurement of the refractory period in nerve. Paired supramaximal stimuli are employed to the peripheral nerve or DR and recorded at the corresponding VR. The intervals between stimuli should begin at 100 msec and proceed to over 4 sec. Approximately 10 to 20 recorded responses at each time interval plotted as interval versus MSR amplitude result in a clear time course of synaptic depression. It is sufficient merely to have the pairs of pulses repeated every 8 sec to note marked depression of the amplitude at 100-msec intervals, moderate depression at 1 sec, and almost complete recovery to the control amplitude at the time interval over 4 sec. In the monosynaptic pathway, recovery of the motoneuron excitability is rather rapid (approximately 120 msec), whereas the recovery of presynaptic fibers requires more than 4 sec. Therefore, the time after stimulation when the monosynaptic spike returns to the control amplitude is essentially the time of *synaptic recovery,* which in turn is a composite of the recovery in the presynaptic fibers and that of motoneurons. By the above-described application of paired stimuli (but conditioning alternatively orthodromically or antidromically and recording at the VR), it is possible to plot time courses of the synaptic recovery for both presynaptic and postsynaptic composites (control curve) (see Fig. 4). In the study of drugs, it is important to ascertain if the drug affects (decrease or increase) the amplitude of the unconditioned monosynaptic spike. In the event of such an effect, the control curve for synaptic recovery cannot be directly compared with that of drug. It is necessary, therefore, to examine the general pattern of recovery at various levels of excitability by altering the temperature of the preparation, or by varying the level of afferent drive (change in the strength of applied stimulus or application of stimulus to the filaments of different sizes) in peripheral nerve or DR. The same principle applies to the other spinal cord models mentioned in this chapter.

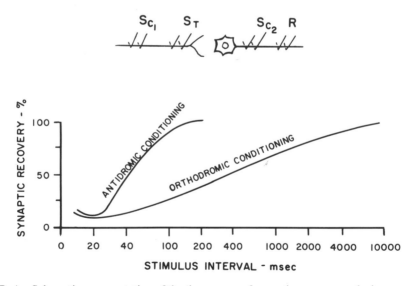

FIG. 4. Schematic representation of the time course of synaptic recovery and, above curves, electrode placements for its testing. S_{C_1}, orthodromic conditioning stimulation; S_{C_2}, antidromic conditioning stimulation. Synaptic recovery as percent amplitude of the control reflex spike recorded postsynaptically (R).

Repetitive synaptic activation in the spinal cord represents another example of a useful model to study. It leads to profound changes in both pre- and postsynaptic elements, and therefore might reflect an alteration in the release, mobilization, and replenishment of the neurotransmitter (possibly in the "readily releasable pool"). During stimulation of the muscle nerve for about 5 sec with frequencies of 3, 10, and up to 30 Hz, the amplitude of the monosynaptic spike falls steeply to a certain plateau. These effects during repetitive stimulation on the amplitude of the monosynaptic spike certainly suggest the above-mentioned assumptions concerning possible alterations in the transmitter turnover in the synapses involved. In addition, the level of the plateau and the rate of decline of the amplitudes of the observed spikes during repetitive stimulation are selectively changed by certain drugs. Trimethadione does not change the initial excitability, but the slope of the curve is steeper and the plateau is drastically lowered after this drug (Fig. 5) (Esplin, 1963).

PTP, a characteristic phenomenon of synaptic transmission, is a well-known example of the enhancement of release of the transmitter per volley for periods lasting up to several minutes, and leading to a considerable

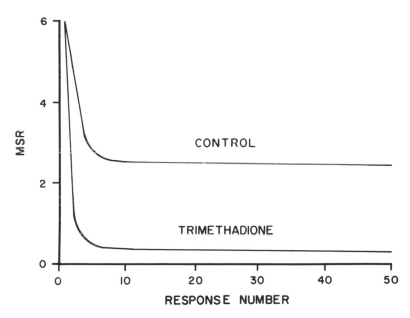

FIG. 5. Schematic representation of the changes in amplitude of the monosynaptic reflex spike (MSR) during repetitive stimulation at 20 Hz and after trimethadione (400 mg/kg) (modified from Esplin, 1963). *Ordinate:* MSR in arbitrary units. *Abscissa:* Number of responses in sequence from the beginning of the experiment.

increase in the MSR amplitude recorded at VR. The stimulation of the muscle nerve or DR for about 15 to 60 sec with a frequency of 50 to 500 Hz is followed by a several-fold increase of the control discharge. Figure 6 shows the time course of the observed changes in the MSR amplitude after applied tetanic stimulation of several different frequencies, and Fig. 7 shows the prominent blocking effect of diphenylhydantoin on PTP (Esplin, 1957).

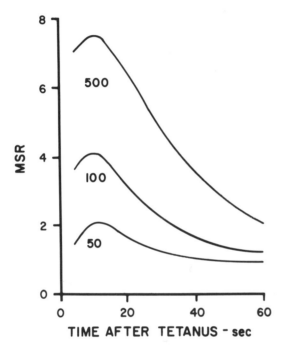

FIG. 6. Time course of the change in amplitude in MSR after very short 15-sec tetanization at three different frequencies, of the nerve to triceps surae. Recording at the VR. (Modified from Esplin, 1957.)

The *input-output relations* in a spinal synaptic system can be assessed by progressively increasing the strength of the stimulus applied to the muscle nerve or DR and then measuring the corresponding change in the recorded amplitude of the MSR at the VR (output). The changes of the stimulus strengths are recorded in volume at the entry of the dorsal root to the spinal cord. This incoming volley changes its amplitude with the change in the stimulus strength and is used to express the magnitude of *input*. In the spinal monosynaptic pathway, a certain fraction of the afferent fibers must be stimulated before any discharge from motoneurons can be recorded at the VR. Below this *critical input,* only excitatory postsynaptic potentials (EPSPs) are produced in the motoneurons. The EPSP must reach the firing

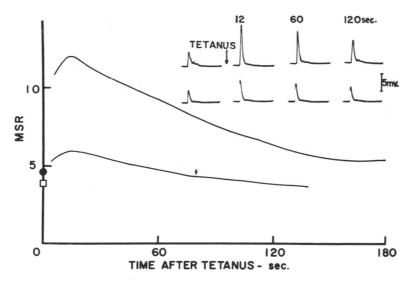

FIG. 7. Effect of diphenylhydantoin (40 mg/kg) on the spinal cord PTP. DR-VR preparation, tetanus 500 Hz for 15 sec. Upper right inset shows representative pre- and post-tetanic responses for control curves (*upper*, ●) and after diphenylhydantoin (*lower*, ☐). (Modified from Esplin, 1957.)

level in order to discharge a motoneuron. This depends on many factors; among the most important are the number of afferent fibers impinging upon the motoneuron and, consequently, the number of quanta of the transmitter released simultaneously after stimulation. An example of the relations between input and output in spinal synaptic systems (DR-VR, or peripheral nerve-VR) estimated at rest or taken during the peak of PTP is presented in Fig. 8. Input-output relations might therefore be used as controls to analyze the effects of drugs on the pool excitability (*critical input*) and the effects on the extent of the "total" pool discharge. These relations show several important features of discharges of synaptic populations.

About 100% input leads to the flattening (plateau) of the curve expressing output taken during the peak of PTP. By comparing the maximal output at rest and PTP, it can be concluded that the discharging motoneuron pool could be divided into the "maximum" discharge zone and that fraction of remaining neurons in the pool not discharged by a maximal volley at rest (subliminal fringe). Recently this relation was successfully used as a "standard curve" to determine the amount of transmitter release corresponding to the average amplitude of the MSR measured after tetanization in depletion studies (Esplin and Zablocka-Esplin, 1971). Such techniques have recently been described for characterizing parameters of transmitter

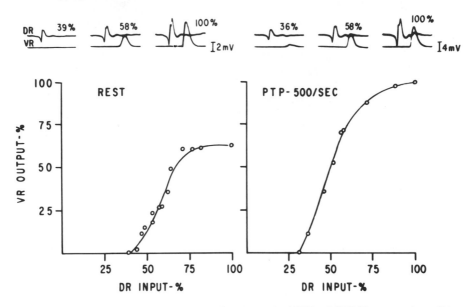

FIG. 8. Input-output relations at rest and at the peak of PTP. BST-VR preparation. Stimulation at rest 1 Hz with varied voltage applied to BST. Responses during PTP were taken at 1 Hz during the peak of PTP (20 to 40 sec) after tetanus of 60 sec at 500 Hz. *Inset: upper part,* volume recordings of the incoming volley (measurements of the negative deflection, *input*); *lower part,* corresponding MSR (*output*). (Modified from Esplin and Zablocka-Esplin, 1971.)

turnover in the spinal monosynaptic pathway (Esplin and Zablocka-Esplin, 1971; Zablocka-Esplin and Esplin, 1971), and these techniques may be suited to the investigation of the drugs. Furthermore, whereas the drugs mentioned do not affect the monosynaptic spike "at rest," diphenylhydantoin blocks PTP and trimethadione markedly decreases the response during repetitive stimulation. Therefore, studies with these drugs during or following a suitable period of tetanization may yield valuable information. The rationale behind this is that the number of active postsynaptic fibers (determining the amplitude of the monosynaptic reflex response) bears a relation to the number of active afferent fibers. The amount of transmitter released by each presynaptic volley bears, in turn, a relation to the number of active presynaptic fibers. Since in the spinal monosynaptic pathway each group Ia fiber, regardless of different diameters, releases the same amount of transmitter (Kuno and Miyahara, 1969), the input-output relation provides a means of expressing the amplitude of the spinal monosynaptic response in terms of the amount of transmitter released relative to that released at maximum input.

In addition to the models already described, there are subsystems in the spinal cord that make it possible to study single synapses (Esplin, 1968). Motoneurons of the ventral horn of the gray matter are sufficiently large to allow the insertion of microelectrodes, and antidromic stimulation of the chosen peripheral nerve allows for their identification. The activity of single cells may be recorded by means of fine electrodes (glass capillaries or metal microelectrodes). Either type of electrode can be used for extra-cellular recordings from cell bodies. Even though the extracellularly re-corded unit potentials are ordinarily rather small, the advantage of this pro-cedure is that the electrode does not need to penetrate the cell membrane, and the activity of even very small cells can be followed for sufficient time to study effects of drugs. Single-unit recordings with the aid of tungsten microelectrodes can be carried out, for instance, to study evoked and spon-taneous repetitive activity of Renshaw cells. Evoked activity of these cells is accomplished by orthodromic stimulation or antidromic stimulation of lumbar DR_7 or sacral DR_1, or of lumbar VR_7 or sacral VR_1 spinal ipsi-lateral roots. The synapse between the motoneuron collateral and the Renshaw cell is relatively easy to study by means of extracellular micro-electrodes. Characteristically, these cells respond by repetitive discharges to antidromic stimulation of efferent axons. Although a few depressants have been studied on this cholinergic synapse of nicotinic type, the ma-jority of drug studies have been with cholinergic and anticholinergic agents. It has not been exploited in the study of antiepileptic drugs. However, pentylenetetrazol was found by Borys and Esplin (1969) to have no effect on the patterns of Renshaw-cell discharges in doses twice those that pro-duce convulsions in the intact cat.

Intracellular studies are usually carried out on spinal motoneurons. This kind of transmembrane recording from single cells is a powerful electro-physiological tool. It allows an investigator to measure the value of the resting membrane potential, to record excitatory and inhibitory synaptic potentials and membrane resistance, and to estimate the firing threshold for the motoneurons under study. It is usually required for studies with drugs that the resting potential (V_m) of impaled motoneurons be at least -50 mV (normal $V_m = -70$), and the cell should be held for at least 5 min without any observable deviations from this value before the control records are taken and the drug applied.

A further advantage of the spinal models is that the motoneuron is easily impaled with microelectrodes and, in the majority of cases, can be held through control testing and that after drug administration. Intracellular studies can reveal the actions of drugs on presynaptic terminals (for example, the dynamics of the release of transmitter) or on the postsynaptic membrane (passive or active properties of it) (Weakly, 1969). A particular advantage of the spinal monosynaptic pathway is that this is the only central synapse at which quantal aspects of transmission can presently be analyzed. This technically difficult procedure was described by Kuno (1964, 1971). By dissection of natural bundles of small motor nerves (such as those to one head of the gastrocnemius muscle), some bundles can be found that contain very few spindle (group Ia) afferent fibers. Filaments are now selected that contain only one unit, with the appropriate latency, from one or more of the bundles stimulated peripherally. When such a dorsal root filament is found, all other relevant dorsal roots are cut. Thus peripheral stimulation activates only one afferent fiber entering the central nervous system. An impaled motoneuron that is innervated monosynaptically by the single fiber input behaves much like the magnesium-blocked neuromuscular junction. On the average, in an unanesthetized cat, each impulse releases approximately three quanta of transmitter. The distribution of response failures and evoked synaptic potentials follows the Poisson probability function, and can be analyzed by methods that are fully established (see Martin, 1966). These analyses enable one to determine drug action definitively at three potential sites: block of conduction in preterminal branches; effects on the terminal that reduce the probability of transmitter release; and decrease in the responsiveness of the postsynaptic membrane to one quantum of transmitter. No study of antiepileptic drugs with intracellular recording in this pathway has yet been reported. This is not surprising. All effective antiepileptic drugs are rather long-acting. If the criterion of dose correspondence is to be observed, this means that under optimum conditions one can obtain results at full dose levels from only one cell per preparation. Analysis of transmission from quantal aspects contains this substantial drawback coupled with the disadvantage that the dissections required prior to microelectrode impalement take many hours longer than simply setting up the basic spinal preparation.

Carbon dioxide is an anticonvulsant that has been compared with antiepileptic drugs in a variety of seizure tests (Woodbury and Esplin, 1959) and synaptic systems (Esplin, 1963; Esplin and Rosenstein, 1963). The analysis of quantal aspects of transmission, using the method of Kuno (1964, 1971) mentioned above, has given convincing evidence that the principle action of carbon dioxide in mammals is to block conduction in the preterminal afferent axons, presumably at the branch points in the spinal cord (Čapek et al., *in press*). This block, resulting in a decrease in the amount of excitatory transmitter released, fully accounts for the well-known depression of monosynaptic response brought about by this substance.

To accentuate the relevance of the spinal cord as a model system, it should be pointed out that the spinal cord is capable of intense self-sustained activity, which does not appear to be qualitatively different from that of supraspinal structures, as has been found in experimental (Esplin, 1959) as well as in rare clinical situations.

Various synapses in the central nervous system have been used as models for studying antiepileptic drugs, but information is so dispersed and scanty that it does not permit an evaluation of the model systems or a clear indication of definitive actions of the drug under investigation.

V. INTERPRETATION OF RESULTS OBTAINED FROM SYNAPTIC MODELS

It is apparent from the preceding discussion that no single model so far investigated will yield the information desired concerning site and mechanism of action of antiepileptic drugs. Some synaptic system models in the central nervous system may yield important clues concerning drug action (e.g., block of PTP by diphenylhydantoin), but the more intimate mechanisms by which this action is produced may best be investigated on more easily studied peripheral synapses. Going in the other direction, the question whether block of PTP by diphenylhydantoin is the mechanism by which the drug prevents seizure spread can only be investigated in complex pathways in the brain.

Clearly, therefore, our full knowledge of the actions of a particular antiepileptic drug will come from definitive information obtained from *hierarchies of models*. Such information will not only include electrophysiological experiments that are emphasized in this discussion, but will also require correlation of information obtained from electrophysiological studies with that from neurochemical and ultrastructural investigations.

VI. THE IMPORTANCE OF STUDYING
CENTRAL NERVOUS SYSTEM STIMULANTS

Precise data concerning the actions of antiepileptic drugs, the basic mechanisms of epilepsy, and the actions of central nervous system stimulants mutually complement each other. The drug that has been clearly of the most value as a laboratory tool in inducing chemical seizures for the purpose of testing antiepileptic drugs has been pentylenetetrazol. Antiinhibitory drugs are not valuable agents for inducing seizures to study antiepileptic agents, but knowledge of their actions will contribute to better understanding of mechanisms of inhibition and its role in epilepsy. The actions of both direct stimulants and of anti-inhibitory agents are discussed by Esplin and Zablocka-Esplin (1969). Only pentylenetetrazol will be briefly discussed here, although other convulsants that are antagonized by antiepileptic drugs would be equally deserving of investigation.

Pentylenetetrazol in low doses produces a minimal seizure that resembles some forms of petit mal epilepsy. The threshold for the pentylenetetrazol seizures is markedly elevated by trimethadione.

On a spinal monosynaptic pathway, the degree to which pentylenetetrazol and trimethadione can be titrated against one another is truly remarkable (Esplin and Curto, 1957; Lewin and Esplin, 1961). Studies with a variety of neuronal models have failed to give definitive clues to the basic action of pentylenetetrazol. In spinal synaptic systems, for example, the drug clearly excites some interneurons and will in large doses cause convulsions in spinal animals. In such doses, the drug causes a slight depression of the monosynaptic response, probably as a consequence of increased background activity (Lewin and Esplin, 1961). However, in the intracellular studies of motoneurons done by Borys (see Esplin and Zablocka-Esplin, 1969), no direct effects upon the motoneuron by pentylenetetrazol were detected.

VII. SOME KEY QUESTIONS TO WHICH ANSWERS SHOULD BE SOUGHT

There are many unresolved questions concerning the actions of antiepileptic drugs, but only a few crucial ones will be mentioned here. These questions are discussed in relation to the subject of synaptic system models, because they should be kept in mind in studies of different models. In fact, some of the questions are so crucial that it would be worthwhile to find models suitable to answer them.

One question that looms large in considering antiepileptic drugs is: How does the action of phenobarbital differ from that of non-antiepileptic barbiturates? Clinically and in seizure tests on animals, the antiepileptic effect of phenobarbital is clearly evident and that of the majority of other barbiturates, for example, pentobarbital, is clearly absent. It might be expected that phenobarbital, like diphenylhydantoin, would block PTP. However, studies of phenobarbital on the spinal cord by the author (largely unpublished, and discussed by Esplin, 1963) showed no direct effect of phenobarbital on PTP. The effects on other aspects of synaptic transmission were not different from those of pentobarbital. The author is not aware of any synaptic system model that has clearly shown a difference between the two types of barbiturates.

A question related to that posed above is: What are the similarities in action of diphenylhydantoin and phenobarbital? Both are effective in grand mal epilepsy, and both block spread of seizure discharge in maximal electroshock seizures in animals. More information about the similarities and differences in action of these two drugs would be of great value.

The striking action of trimethadione on transmission in the spinal mono-synaptic pathway is to reduce markedly transmission during repetitive stimulation (Esplin and Curto, 1957). It was suggested by Woodbury and Esplin (1959) that this action may underlie its antiepileptic effect. However, the question must now be asked: If the basic action of trimethadione is to terminate repetitive activity, why is it selective for petit mal epilepsy? In other words, why does trimethadione not terminate the repetitive activity of epileptogenic neurons in other types of epilepsy? Perhaps the described effect of trimethadione does not underlie its antiepileptic activity, or perhaps there are unique aspects of the thalamo-cortical relay system that make activity here particularly susceptible to the action of the drug.

Ethosuximide is a drug of great value in petit mal epilepsy; yet it has to date been very little studied on synaptic models. A very timely question therefore is: What are the actions of ethosuximide, as compared to those of trimethadione?

Phenacemide is a drug of interest because it is effective against psycho-motor epilepsy. Knowledge of the action of phenacemide would give valuable information concerning mechanisms of psychomotor epilepsy. It is therefore significant to ask: What are the actions of phenacemide as compared to other antiepileptic drugs?

The importance of studying convulsant drugs is emphasized in Section VI. The crucial question deserves reiteration: What are the basic actions of pentylenetetrazol?

VIII. SUMMARY

Some problems of interpreting results obtained from model systems have been briefly discussed, and some of the advantages and disadvantages of a few specific models have been mentioned. The scarcity of basic information concerning mechanisms of actions of antiepileptic drugs is evident throughout this chapter. This is especially emphasized in the preceding section that lists a few of the many crucial questions concerning antiepileptic drugs to which answers must be sought. Many models and many different types of approaches will undoubtedly be employed in obtaining answers to these questions. These answers will not only be of value in explaining the actions of antiepileptic drugs, but they will also contribute much useful information concerning basic mechanisms of epilepsy.

IX. ACKNOWLEDGMENTS

I would like to thank very much Dr. R. Čapek for substantial help in modifying the original manuscript. I am also grateful to other friends of my late husband for their advice, and for typing and preparing the figures.

Barbara Esplin

X. REFERENCES

Borys, H. K., and Esplin, D. W. (1969): Pentylenetetrazol and Renshaw cell activity. *International Journal of Neuropharmacology*, 8:627–630.

Brown, A. M., and Berman, P. R. (1970): Mechanism of excitation of *Aplysia* neurons by carbon dioxide. *Journal of General Physiology*, 56:543–558.

Brown, A. M., Walker, J. L., Jr., and Sutton, R. B. (1970): Increased chloride conductance as the proximate cause of hydrogen ion concentration effects in *Aplysia* neurons. *Journal of General Physiology*, 56:559–582.

Brown, D. A., and Quilliam, J. P. (1964): Observations of the mode of action of some central depressant drugs on transmission through the cat superior cervical ganglion. *British Journal of Pharmacology*, 23:257–272.

Čapek, R., Esplin, B. A., and Esplin, D. W. (*in press*): An intracellular study of the actions of carbon dioxide on the spinal monosynaptic pathway.

Esplin, D. W. (1957): Effects of diphenylhydantoin on synaptic transmission in cat spinal cord and stellate ganglion. *Journal of Pharmacology and Experimental Therapeutics*, 120:301–323.

Esplin, D. W. (1959): Spinal cord convulsions. *Archives of Neurology*, 1:485–490.

Esplin, D. W. (1963): Criteria for assessing effects of depressant drugs on spinal cord synaptic transmission, with examples of drug selectivity. *Archives Internationales de Pharmacodynamie et de Thérapie*, 143:479–497.

Esplin, D. W. (1968): A critical appraisal of electrophysiological techniques used to study drugs. In: *Importance of Fundamental Principles in Drug Evaluation*, edited by D. H. Tedeschi and R. E. Tedeschi. Raven Press, New York, pp. 361–381.

Esplin, D. W., and Curto, E. M. (1957): Effects of trimethadione on synaptic transmission in the spinal cord; antagonism of trimethadione and pentylenetetrazol. *Journal of Pharmacology and Experimental Therapeutics*, 121:457–467.

Esplin, D. W., and Rosenstein, R. (1963): Analysis of spinal depressant actions of carbon dioxide and acetazolamide. *Archives Internationales de Pharmacodynamie et de Thérapie,* 143:498–513.

Esplin, D. W., and Zablocka-Esplin, B. (1969): Mechanisms of action of convulsants. In: *Basic Mechanisms of the Epilepsies,* edited by H. H. Jasper, A. A. Ward, Jr., and A. Pope. Little, Brown and Co., Boston, pp. 167–193.

Esplin, D. W., and Zablocka-Esplin, B. (1971): Rates of transmitter turnover in spinal monosynaptic pathway investigated by electrophysiological techniques. *Journal of Neurophysiology,* 34:842–859.

Holmstedt, B., and Skoglund, C. R. (1953): The action on spinal reflexes of dimethylamido-ethoxy-phosphoryl cyanide, "Tabun," a cholinesterase inhibitor. *Acta Physiologica Scandinavica,* 29:(suppl. 10), 410–427.

Kuno, M. (1964): Quantal components of excitatory synaptic potentials in spinal motoneurones. *Journal of Physiology,* 175:81–99.

Kuno, M. (1971): Quantum aspects of central and ganglionic synaptic transmission in vertebrates. *Physiological Reviews,* 51:647–678.

Kuno, M., and Miyahara, J. T. (1969): Analysis of synaptic efficacy in spinal motoneurones from "quantum" aspects. *Journal of Physiology,* 201:479–493.

Larabee, M. G., and Bronk, D. W. (1947): Prolonged facilitation of synaptic excitation in sympathetic ganglia. *Journal of Neurophysiology,* 10:139–154.

Lewin, J., and Esplin, D. W. (1961): Analysis of the spinal excitatory action of pentylenetetrazol. *Journal of Pharmacology and Experimental Therapeutics,* 132:245–250.

Libet, B. (1970): Generation of slow inhibitory and excitatory postsynaptic potentials. *Federation Proceedings,* 29:1945–1956.

Martin, A. R. (1966): Quantal nature of synaptic transmission. *Physiological Reviews,* 46:51–66.

Morrell, F., Bradley, W., and Ptashne, M. (1958): Effect of diphenylhydantoin on peripheral nerve. *Neurology,* 8:140–144.

Quastel, D. M. J., and Hackett, J. T. (1971): Calcium: Is it required for transmitter secretion? *Science,* 172:1034–1036.

Raines, A., and Standaert, F. G. (1966): Pre- and postjunctional effects of diphenylhydantoin at the cat solcus neuromuscular junction. *Journal of Pharmacology and Experimental Therapeutics,* 153:361–366.

Spencer, W. A., and Kandel, E. R. (1969): Synaptic inhibition in seizures. In: *Basic Mechanisms of the Epilepsies,* edited by H. H. Jasper, A. A. Ward, Jr., and A. Pope. Little, Brown and Co., Boston, pp. 575–603.

Tauc, L. (1967): Transmission in invertebrate and vertebrate ganglia. *Physiological Reviews,* 47:521–593.

Toman, J. E. P. (1952): Neuropharmacology of peripheral nerve. *Pharmacological Reviews,* 4:168–218.

Toman, J. E. P. (1970): Drugs effective in convulsive disorders. In: *The Pharmacological Basis of Therapeutics,* edited by L. S. Goodman and A. Gilman. Macmillan, New York, pp. 204–225.

Toman, J. E. P., and Goodman, L. S. (1948): Anticonvulsants. *Physiological Reviews,* 28:409–432.

Toman, J. E. P., and Taylor, J. D. (1952): Mechanism of action and metabolism of anticonvulsants. *Epilepsia,* 1:31–48.

Tuttle, R. S., and Preston, J. B. (1963): The effects of diphenylhydantoin (Dilantin®) on segmental and suprasegmental facilitation and inhibition of segmental motoneurons in the cat. *Journal of Pharmacology and Experimental Therapeutics,* 141:84–91.

Volle, R. L., and Hancock, J. C. (1970): Transmission in sympathetic ganglia. *Federation Proceedings,* 29:1913–1918.

Walker, J. L., Jr., and Brown, A. M. (1970): Unified account of the variable effects of carbon dioxide on nerve cells. *Science,* 167:1502–1504.

Weakly, J. N. (1969): Effect of barbiturates on "quantal" synaptic transmission in spinal motoneurons. *Journal of Physiology,* 204:63–77.

Weakly, J. N., Esplin, D. W., and Zablocka, B. (1968): Criteria for assessing effects of drugs on postsynaptic inhibition. *Archives Internationales de Pharmacodynamie et de Thérapie,* 171:385.

Woodbury, D. M., and Esplin, D. W. (1959): Neuropharmacology and neurochemistry of anticonvulsant drugs. *Proceedings of the Association for Research in Nervous and Mental Disease,* 37:24–56.

Zablocka-Esplin, B. and Esplin, D. W. (1971): Persistent changes in transmission in spinal monosynaptic pathway after prolonged tetanization. *Journal of Neurophysiology,* 34:860–867.

10

Microelectrophoretic Studies
of Single Neurons

David R. Curtis

OUTLINE

INTRODUCTION

The technique of administering drugs from glass micropipettes by means of electrical currents was originally developed and used for a study of the chemical sensitivity of the muscle end plate (Nastuk, 1951; del Castillo and Katz, 1955), and was subsequently adapted for studying the pharmacology of single neurons in the central nervous system (Curtis, 1964; Curtis and Crawford, 1969). The major advantage of this method of investigation, so far as the central nervous system is concerned, is the ability to deliver small amounts of a drug close to a selected neuron, while simultaneously recording its behavior with an extra- or intracellular microelectrode.

Most neurons are innervated by many different afferent fibers, both excitatory and inhibitory, and, because of the geometrical complexity of any one cell and its immediately adjacent glial and neuronal environment, it is not possible to study the effects of drugs at individual synapses. Nevertheless, considerable use has been made of microelectrophoretic techniques in comparing the actions of compounds with those of transmitters, and in studying the pharmacology of synaptic excitation and inhibition (Curtis and Crawford, 1969). The methods used are thus directly applicable to *in vivo* studies of neuronal abnormalities in epileptic foci, for assessing the actions of convulsants and anticonvulsants, and even for initiating foci of abnormally active neurons. Furthermore, microelectrophoretic methods are of assistance in investigating the chemical sensitivity of cultured neurons *in vitro* (Crain, 1972).

II. MICROELECTROPHORETIC METHODS

A. Basic principles

The microelectrophoretic technique involves the controlled ejection of substances from relatively concentrated solutions within glass micropipettes having orifices usually less than 2 to 3 μ in diameter. An electrical current is passed between one electrode which contacts the solution within the pipette and another in contact with the bulk of the experimental tissue, which is usually the "indifferent" electrode of the recording system.

Since the majority of substances of pharmacological interest are well ionized in aqueous solution, the major factor determining the ejection from a micropipette is *iontophoresis:* ion movement along an electrical gradient according to charge, and at a rate determined by Faraday's law (see Curtis, 1964). Thus, as illustrated in Fig. 1, cations (C^+) can be ejected from the pipette orifice by making the solutions positive with respect to the external medium. The current which flows is called a *cationic* current; the reverse current, *anionic*, ejects anions from the orifice. A *retaining* current, of direction appropriate to the charge of the active ion in the solution, is used to control its diffusional and hydrostatic efflux from the pipette. Consequently a complementary ion (A^-) has to be chosen which does not interact with neuronal receptors.

A second factor, *electro-osmosis*, is also involved, particularly when the solution within the micropipette is of low ionic strength. Under these

MICROELECTROPHORESIS

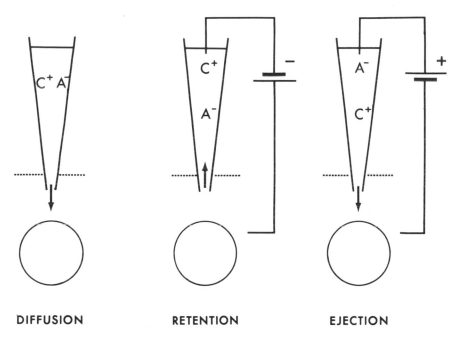

DIFFUSION   **RETENTION**   **EJECTION**

FIG. 1. Basic principle of microelectrophoresis. The diffusional efflux of an active cation (C^+) is reduced by a retaining current which enhances the efflux of an inactive anion (A^-) from a micropipette. The cation is ejected from the orifice by a cationic current, the solution within the pipette having been made positive to that outside.

conditions, the boundary potential between the glass wall and the solution becomes important, and the passage of current induces a bulk flow of the solution. The rate of electro-osmotic flow depends on the nature of the solution, its concentration, and the type of glass. In general, solutions in contact with Pyrex glass behave as if positively charged, and thus cationic currents enhance electro-osmotic flow (Curtis, 1964; Krnjević and Whittaker, 1965).

Since the types of glass micropipette used are usually identical with microelectrodes used for recording electrical responses from single neurons, the term *microelectrophoresis* thus encompasses *iontophoresis, electroosmosis,* and *microelectrodes.* A number of articles deal with practical and theoretical aspects of fluid-filled microelectrodes (Rush et al., 1968; Lavallée et al., 1969; Krischer, 1969*a,b;* Firth and de Felice, 1971).

B. Technical considerations

1. Types of micropipette and microelectrode

In investigations of the neuromuscular junction, drug-administering micropipettes and recording microelectrodes were maneuvered independently with different micromanipulators under visual control; indeed, such a procedure was essential in order to establish the relative sensitivity of different portions of the muscle fiber to acetylcholine. However, visual control and positioning of several micropipettes in the vicinity of a single neuron within the brain or spinal cord is clearly extremely difficult, and recording microelectrodes are, therefore, usually attached to drug-administering micropipettes for simultaneous movement by one micromanipulator.

Neurons from which electrical records are obtained can be identified by their position within the nervous system, their responses to orthodromic and antidromic stimulation, and by the electrophoretic deposition of a dye, intra- or extracellularly.

Extracellular recording. Electrophoretic drug administration has been combined with extracellular recording of action potentials by using two- to seven-barrel micropipettes arranged as in Fig. 2. The size of each barrel orifice should be less than 3 μm to limit tissue damage, and all orifices should be at the same level. One barrel, usually the central one, is filled with 3 to 4 M NaCl and is used as a recording microelectrode (Frank and Becker, 1964; Curtis, 1964; Salmoiraghi and Stefanis, 1967; Steiner, 1971; Krnjević, 1971).

The assistance of a skilled glass blower is advantageous for the initial preparation of multibarrel micropipettes, particularly to ensure that the

MICROELECTROPHORESIS —— EXTRACELLULAR RECORDING

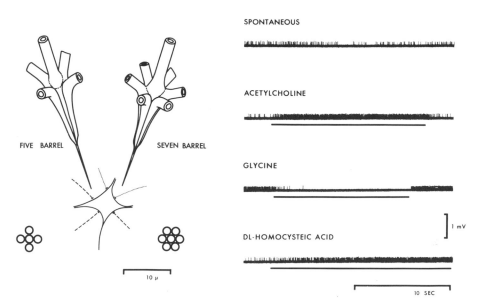

FIG. 2. The central barrels of five- or seven-barrel micropipettes, of total tip diameter 4 to 8 μm, are used to record extracellularly from neurons influenced by drugs administered electrophoretically from the other barrels. On the right are illustrated the spontaneous firing of a spinal Renshaw cell, excitation by acetylcholine (cation), DL-homocysteate (anion), and depression of firing by glycine (cation).

internal-external diameter ratio of the borosilicate glass tubing used is preserved and that adjacent barrels are fused together prior to pulling in a microelectrode puller (Curtis, 1964; Appendix). Other methods have been described in which pieces of glass tubing are assembled side by side, retained by adhesive within small metal rings, and during the pulling procedure one end is rotated by approximately 180° to facilitate fusion of adjacent barrels (Herz et al., 1965).

Intracellular recording. A number of compound micropipettes have been described which permit intracellular recording to be combined with extracellular drug administration. Thus, a study can be made of the action of one or more drugs on the membrane properties of an impaled neuron, properties which can be analyzed in detail by modifying the membrane potential and the intracellular content of ions (Eccles, 1964). A single- or a double-barrel (Coombs et al., 1955) recording microelectrode with a tip diameter less than 1 μm is attached to another single or multibarrel micropipette so that the tips are separated longitudinally or laterally: pencil or co-axial (concentric) pipettes (Tomita, 1956; Frank and Becker, 1964; Curtis, 1964; Spehlmann, 1969); twin pipettes (Krnjević and Schwartz, 1967; Werman et al., 1968; Krnjević, 1971); and parallel pipettes (Curtis, 1968; Phillis, 1970; Oliver, 1971). In the latter, as illustrated in Fig. 3, the two shafts are parallel or even slightly convergent, to prevent the separation of the tips during penetration of nervous tissue. All of these types of compound electrode can also be used for extracellular recording, the advantage being that the orifice of the recording electrode can be made smaller than,

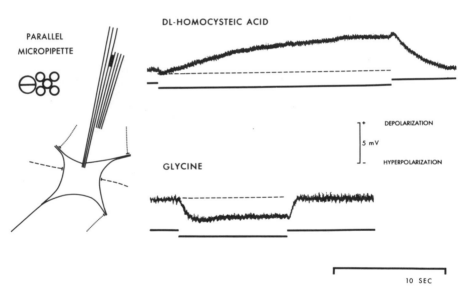

FIG. 3. The recording electrode of a pair of parallel micropipettes projects 30 to 60 μm beyond the openings of a five-barrel micropipette, and the shaft lies within the groove formed by two of these barrels, as shown in cross-section. The double-barrel electrode permits recording of intracellular responses together with the passage of current to modify the membrane potential of the impaled neuron, or of ions to alter intracellular ion concentrations. On the right are illustrated alterations in the resting membrane potential (−78 mV) of a motoneuron during the extracellular electrophoretic administration of DL-homocysteate and glycine.

and adjusted at different positions relative to, those of the drug-containing barrels, thus assisting the recording of potentials from small neurons (see Spehlmann, 1969).

Separate multibarrel micropipettes. Several investigations have made use of two multibarrel electrodes, either manipulated by different micro-manipulators or firmly attached together with preselected separation of the tips. The first type of experiment has proved useful in an analysis of the synaptic interconnections between neighboring groups of neurons; one multibarrel micropipette is used to excite and record from one type of cell, and the other to analyze the subsequent inhibition or excitation of the other type of cell (Crawford et al., 1966; Curtis and Felix, 1971). Double multi-barrel micropipettes, firmly attached together with different tip separations have been used in a study of the diffusion of amino acids in brain tissue (Herz et al., 1969).

2. Manufacture and testing of micropipettes

The making, filling, storage, and testing of micropipettes for micro-electrophoresis have been reported by a number of authors (Frank and Becker, 1964; Curtis, 1964; Salmoiraghi and Weight, 1967; Steiner, 1971; Krnjević, 1971). The following points require emphasis.

Scrupulous cleaning (alcohol, acid) of all glass and the strict avoidance of soaps and detergents are essential. Electrode "blanks" can be flushed with filtered, glass-distilled water (membrane filters, pore size 0.4 to $0.5\mu m$) and dried in a vacuum oven immediately before pulling and filling.

Extreme care should also be taken in the preparation of solutions, par-ticularly in choosing a suitable counter ion and in adjusting the pH for op-timal ionization according to the ionization constants (Perrin, 1965) of the dissolved substance. Although a high conductance of drug solutions is de-sirable, solutions of well-ionized compounds more concentrated than 0.2 M are rarely necessary. For extremely potent compounds, isotonic NaCl (165 mM) can be used to provide dilutions of 2, 5, or 10 mM of the active compound; the amount ejected by a particular current will be proportional to the dilution factor (McCance, 1969). Preparation of solutions in dilute NaCl may also be useful with poorly ionized compounds in order to facili-tate electro-osmotic ejection.

The solutions should be filtered or preferably centrifuged, since the presence of particulate matter interferes with the filling of dry micropipettes by centrifugation (Curtis, 1964) and with the subsequent passage of electro-phoretic currents. A rapid method of filling single or multibarrel micro-pipettes has been described (Tasaki et al., 1968) in which the pipettes are pulled containing a number of fibers of the same glass, and then filled from above, the fibers facilitating the flow of solution towards the tip.

The circuit described by Frank and Becker (1964) for measuring the electrical properties of microelectrodes by using brief voltage pulses is of considerable assistance for drug-filled micropipettes since resistances can be measured using different intensities and directions of current.

Microscopic examination of pipette tips before and after use is necessary to eliminate barrel breakage as a possible cause of the lack of action of a particular substance.

3. Electrical circuits

Conventional high-input impedance amplifiers are required for recording intracellular or extracellular responses (Burns, 1961; Fatt, 1961; Frank and Becker, 1964). Additional equipment is desirable for the measurement of membrane impedance changes using current pulses passed through the intracellular recording microelectrode, and for the conversion of extracellularly recorded action potentials into standard electrical pulses for on-line computation of firing frequencies, post-stimulus and interval histograms.

Each drug pipette requires polarizers for retaining and ejecting currents (Curtis, 1964; Salmoiraghi and Weight, 1967; Krnjević, 1971) connected to the solutions via a high resistance (50 to 100 MΩ) and either a nonpolarizable junction or, more simply, a clean silver wire. Suitable amplifiers or galvanometers are required for measuring electrophoretic currents which range from 1 to 500 nA (1 nA $= 10^{-9}$ A). It is convenient to be able to connect a voltage-measuring device to the drug barrels in order to measure their resistances *in situ,* and to set up retaining voltages of the correct polarity for each drug pipette (Curtis, 1964). A voltage of 0.5 V is usually adequate to control the efflux of compounds from pipettes having an internal diameter of 1 to 2 μm; occasionally this can be reduced or increased in the light of experimental observations, since theoretical predictions regarding the leakage of drugs from micropipettes have frequently proved to be incorrect. The diffusional efflux of acetylcholine from relatively large pipettes (100 μm) has been controlled by an ion-exchange gel (Kirkpatrick and Lomax, 1970).

A NaCl-filled barrel is sometimes used to pass a current equal to and opposite in polarity to the algebraic sum of all retaining and ejecting currents flowing in the other barrels (Salmoiraghi and Weight, 1967). In this way, no net current flows between the electrode and the tissue, thereby preventing electrotonic changes in neuron excitability. However, since tissue debris frequently caps and surrounds the tip of such relatively large micropipettes (Andersen and Curtis, 1964), it seems probable that ions delivered from the orifice of one barrel could be transferred into another by an electrophoretic current of the opposite direction, thus effectively reducing the rate of administration. Artifacts due to current alone are usually readily appreciated, and can be verified by passing inert ions of the appropriate type from other barrels.

4. Micromarking techniques

A number of methods are now available for staining or destroying tissue from which electrical records have been obtained for subsequent histological identification, the marking agent having been contained in one barrel of the electrode assembly. These range from the production of small tissue lesions (Galifret and Szabo, 1960; McCance and Phillis, 1965) to the extra- or intracellular deposition of dyes, including fast green FCF (Thomas and Wilson, 1965), trypan blue (Pohle and Matthies, 1966), methyl blue (Thomas and Wilson, 1966), Niagara sky blue 6B (Kaneko and Hashimoto, 1967), methylene blue (Sterc et al., 1968), Alcian blue 8G X (Lee et al., 1969), procion yellow M4RS (Stretton and Kravitz, 1968; Barrett and Graubard, 1970; Jankowska and Lindström, 1970), and pontamine sky blue 6BX (Hellon, 1971).

C. Advantages and disadvantages

The uses, advantages, and disadvantages of microelectrophoretic methods have been treated previously in considerable detail (Curtis, 1964; Salmoiraghi and Stefanis, 1967; Salmoiraghi and Weight, 1967; Steiner, 1971; Krnjević, 1971). The principles and methods of experimentation are relatively simple, but experience and considerable caution are necessary in the interpretation of changes in nerve cell activity resulting from the relatively localized administration of drugs.

A number of investigators have measured the rates of electrophoretic release, and so derived transport values relating current flow to rate of release (Krnjević, 1971; also Obata et al., 1970; Bradley and Candy, 1970; Begent and Born, 1970; Hoffer et al., 1971). Such figures, although of theoretical significance, are of little practical value since there are considerable differences in measured transport number for the same substance contained within different micropipettes, and for the same micropipette when the efflux into Ringer's solution is compared with that into brain tissue (Hoffer et al., 1971). The openings of micropipettes become partially, and often totally, blocked by tissue fragments, as indicated by fluctuations in electrical resistance as the pipettes are moved through nervous tissue, and the range of electrophoretic currents over which a linear output is achieved is probably very limited. When micropipettes do not behave as linear ohmic resistances, the apparent transport values of ions are reduced (Zieglgäns-berger et al., 1969), particularly when electrophoretic currents generate considerable electrical noise. Under such conditions, current presumably flows predominantly through or along the surface of the glass wall (see Firth and de Felice, 1971). Negative results must therefore be regarded with suspicion, unless confirmatory evidence can be obtained elsewhere in the nervous system that the particular agent studied can be administered electrophoretically. Any investigation of epileptogenic tissue should be preceded by an investigation of the identical but normal tissue, and such a procedure is certainly essential when evaluating possible alterations in the chemical sensitivity of nerve cells.

Many of the biological difficulties of microelectrophoretic experiments are common to any microelectrode investigation of surgically prepared, often paralyzed and artificially respired, anesthetized animals (see Curtis and Crawford, 1969). There is a sampling bias towards larger neurons (see Towe and Harding, 1970), particularly with intracellular microelectrodes, which may be of extreme importance in investigations of the cerebral cortex. Difficulties associated with the use of electrical currents, possible pH alterations in the tissues, and changes in tissue impedance associated with the addition of ions can usually be overcome by suitable control procedures (Curtis, 1964; Krnjević, 1971). On the other hand, estimates made of the concentrations attained in the vicinity of micropipette tips, and further away, can only be approximations, although a number of theoretical approaches are possible (del Castillo and Katz, 1955; Curtis, 1964; Jaeger, 1965; Waud, 1968). Even when substances are injected intracellularly, the concentrations attained are difficult to estimate because of the movement of ions and water through neuronal membrane.

More serious difficulties arise from the manner in which electrophoretically administered agents are distributed within the extracellular space. A number of factors will be involved, including the rate and duration of administration, the geometry and diffusion characteristics of the space, and the rate of inactivation of the substance (see Curtis, 1964). Clearly, concentrations will be much higher close to the pipette orifices than further away, and since the orifice of drug-ejecting micropipettes are usually very close to the recording electrodes—which in turn are usually in the vicinity of the soma of a neuron—dendritic membrane invariably will be exposed to lower concentrations than that of the soma. This situation raises problems in assessing interactions between agonists and antagonists, and in studying the pharmacology of synaptic events occurring predominantly on dendrites (Curtis et al., 1971). To some extent, concentrations at dendritic sites can be raised by increasing the rate of electrophoretic ejection, although the high perisomatic concentrations of a drug may result in relatively unspecific actions which possibly obscure effects on dendritic receptors. Separation of recording and drug-ejecting barrels may permit drugs to be selectively administered at dendritic sites, although it is unlikely that all of the dendrites of any one neuron will be uniformly affected by an administered agent. Moreover, separation of drug pipettes and recording electrodes probably increases the possibility that observed alterations in neuron properties may arise indirectly from drug action on blood vessels, glial cells, or neighboring neurons synaptically linked with the cell under observation. Such effects, which may complicate any microelectrophoretic investigation, can usually be excluded by demonstrating that neurons of a particular kind are consistently affected by a certain agent. Indirect effects as a result of excitation or inhibition of neighboring neurons frequently occur when tissue debris "caps" micropipettes, thus providing a barrier to the free diffusion of ejected substances to neurons from which relatively large extracellular action potentials are recorded. Under these conditions, alterations in the frequency of occurrence of smaller action potentials, from neurons "electrically" further from the recording microelectrode, precede changes in the firing rate of the cell of major interest, and voltage discriminators of the window type are useful in comparing the firing rates of several different cells. This type of effect is observed most commonly in nuclei where inhibitory interneurons lie close to more readily identified cell types, such as in the thalamus, cerebral cortex, olfactory bulb, and dorsal horn of the spinal cord (see Zieglgänsberger and Herz, 1971).

Problems associated with the investigation of dendritic regions of neurons are not confined to microelectrophoretic techniques, since a study of the ionic events associated with synaptic action at these sites is not possible using an intrasomatic recording electrode (Ginsborg, 1967; Diamond, 1968).

III. RELEVANCE TO MODELS OF EPILEPSY

Microelectrophoretic techniques can be used to study the properties of both neurons and glial cells which lead to paroxysmal neuronal firing, in relatively undisturbed *in vivo* conditions, both during and in the absence of such abnormal activity. Unfortunately, quantitative observations are difficult to make, certainly with the degree of precision and confidence which permit sophisticated statistical analyses, but comparisons can be made with normal tissue, often in the same experimental animal. Studies of the properties of cells within mirror foci (Wilder, 1972) may be particularly useful, since neuron identification is simplified by the absence of cell and axon damage usually associated with the methods used to initiate a primary focus (see Chapters 1–6).

A number of studies have been concerned with the electrophysiological properties of epileptic neurons in both primary and secondary foci using extra- and intracellular recording techniques (see Ward, 1969; Prince, 1969; Spencer and Kandel, 1969; Prince and Futamachi, 1970; Sypert et al., 1970; Ferguson and Jasper, 1971), and the following types of investigation are possible using such methods in combination with the local microelectrophoretic administration of pharmacologically active ions.

A. Single neuron biochemistry and biophysics

Abnormalities of intracellular metabolic processes may be associated with the initiation of paroxysmal discharges characteristic of neurons within epileptogenic foci. Preliminary investigations have shown that the *intracellular* injection of certain adenine dinucleotides and related compounds into spinal motoneurons produces a membrane depolarization, presumably because of interference with energy processes maintaining the distribution of ions across the neuronal membrane (Curtis et al., 1971). Thus, the direct intracellular administration of metabolic inhibitors and other agents, including enzymes, which may not necessarily gain access to this region after systemic administration, may provide information about intracellular enzymic and metabolic processes, and could assist a study of neuronal abnormalities associated with paroxysmal repetitive firing. A number of technical difficulties are involved, particularly the maintenance of stable membrane potentials with minimal evidence of physical damage to the membrane by the impaling microelectrode.

A related study concerns possible abnormalities of membrane ion permeability using the techniques of *intracellular* ion injection which have been so successfully exploited in analyses of the resting and synaptically activated membrane of motoneurons (Eccles, 1964). Considerable caution is required, however, in interpreting observations made on neurons of low and deteriorating resting potential, since a considerable proportion of the measured ion flux may occur at sites of damage to the membrane.

Seizures may result from systemic electrolyte disturbances (Millichap, 1969; Glaser, 1972), and the extracellular environment of a localized portion of the central nervous system may be modified microelectrophoretically to a greater extent than would be possible by changing plasma or CSF levels in an intact animal. Extracellular calcium levels have been reduced using chelating compounds (Curtis et al., 1960); potassium (Krnjević and Phillis, 1963), calcium and magnesium (Kato and Somjen, 1969), and ammonium (Lux et al., 1970) levels have been enhanced, but it seems improbable in view of the relatively low rates of microelectrophoretic ejection that significant changes can be achieved in extracellular sodium or chloride concentration.

B. Transmitter identification

The whole problem of the nature of transmitters within the nervous system is pertinent to epilepsy, since disturbances of transmitter synthesis, storage, release, action, and inactivation may lead to disordered activity of neurons. The subject is beyond the scope of this review (see Curtis and Crawford, 1969; Krnjević, 1969; Curtis, 1969; Curtis and Johnston, 1970; Phillis, 1970; Steiner, 1971), but microelectrophoretic techniques are essential for demonstrating that a suspected transmitter has a postsynaptic action on a given type of neuron identical to that of the synaptically released transmitter.

In view of the difficulty of establishing the precise relationship of a possible transmitter to particular nerve fibers and terminals with currently available chemical techniques, specific antagonists of transmitters have also proved of considerable assistance (see Curtis et al., 1971). Furthermore, it may be possible to investigate the effects of drugs which selectively interfere with the synthesis and inactivation of the transmitter, processes which again may be specific for a particular transmitter.

The excitation of cortical neurons by electrophoretically administered acetylcholine and the excitant amino acids, L-glutamate, L-aspartate, DL-homocysteate (the most potent commercially available excitant amino acid), and related compounds (Curtis and Watkins, 1965), provides a useful means of determining neuronal excitability in the absence of intracellular recording. Such a technique, which has proved useful in an analysis of cortical inhibition by providing a readily controlled background discharge upon which to measure the duration of synaptic inhibition (Crawford et al., 1963; Krnjević et al., 1966a; Curtis and Felix, 1971), and in measurement of changes in excitability associated with alterations of blood CO_2 levels (Krnjević et al., 1965) and spreading depression (Phillis and Ochs, 1971), should also prove of assistance in investigating the mode of action of anticonvulsants at the cellular level. Further elucidation of the mechanism of action of these substances will almost certainly require intracellular recording with direct measurement of membrane parameters, including resting, action and synaptic potentials, in association with extracellular and systemic administration of the anticonvulsant. It may then be possible to determine whether a particular substance has predominantly presynaptic, postsynaptic, or metabolic effects on the firing of neurons.

Since excitant and depressant amino acids, such as glutamate and gamma-aminobutyric acid (GABA), have effects only on neurons and not on nerve fibers, the electrophoretic administration of these substances can be used to study the origin of field potentials generated within nuclei or laminated structures, such as the cerebral cortex. Depolarization of cell bodies accentuates the potentials generated by inhibitory synaptic action (Krnjević et al., 1966b), and excessive amounts suppress neuronal activity (Curtis et al., 1960). In contrast, GABA reduces and may reverse potentials generated by the firing of neurons (Curtis et al., 1959).

C. Abnormal transmission mechanisms

There has been considerable speculation (see Ward, 1969; Sharpless, 1969) regarding the possibility that the hyperexcitability of epileptic neurons results from abnormal sensitivity to excitatory transmitters as a consequence of partial denervation, or from a lower efficiency of synaptic inhibitory mechanisms.

In the former situation, microelectrophoretic methods would seem applicable to an analysis of the chemical sensitivity of epileptic neurons, relative to those of normal tissue, although the two populations of neurons may not be strictly comparable since the experimental technique used to destroy afferent fibers may additionally disturb other properties of the tissue, and assumptions need to be made regarding the nature of the transmitters. Furthermore, dendritic receptors may not be readily accessible to microelectrophoretically administered compounds. Studies have been made using neurons of partially (Spehlmann, 1970) and totally (Krnjević et al., 1970a; Spehlmann, 1971) isolated cortical tissue which displays epileptiform activity: abnormal sensitivity to either acetylcholine or L-glutamate could not be demonstrated. Other putative transmitters should also be tested, but it seems possible that the effects of partial denervation are more subtly linked with the disposition of the remaining terminals and reinnervation by new terminals producing the same or other transmitters, rather than with an overall increase in the number of receptors to a particular transmitter.

Although the inhibition by surface stimulation of neurons in isolated cortical slabs has been reported to be "substantially preserved" (Krnjević et al., 1970b), and the cells appear to be as sensitive as normal cortical cells to GABA (Krnjević et al., 1970a; Spehlmann, 1970, 1971), it is doubtful whether such investigations have established that inhibitory mechanisms are completely normal in cortical tissue which displays paroxysmal electrical activity. There is a need for further investigation of different types of cortical inhibition, particularly those evoked by more physiological forms of stimuli, in both normal and epileptogenic cortices.

D. Initiation of a focus of excited cells

A number of methods have been used to produce foci of discharging neurons to serve as a model of epilepsy (see Ajmone Marsan, 1969; Ward, 1969; Chapters 1–6 of this volume). These methods usually involve irreversible cell damage, with or without gliosis, and the resultant chronic seizures may be paroxysmal or continuous. Several investigators (Biscoe and Straughan, 1966; P. Anderson, J. M. Crawford, and D. R. Curtis, *unpublished observations;* Stefanis, 1969) have observed that when hippocampal pyramidal cells are excited above a certain rate of discharge, by acetylcholine or an excitant amino acid, extracellular action potentials are replaced by slow negative-positive field potentials which progressively increase in amplitude. This effect may remain relatively localized and rapidly reverse when the administration of the excitant is terminated. However if chemical excitation continues, a self-sustained seizure-like activity occurs, during which rhythmic slow potentials can be recorded from the hippocampal surface (Stefanis, 1969). Eventually, the slow potentials cease abruptly to be replaced by a prolonged period during which the cells are insensitive to all excitants (postictal depression). Laminar analysis has shown that the phenomenon originates at the level of the bodies of pyramidal cells, and presumably the extracellularly recorded slow potentials reflect the membrane potentials of a number of such cells brought into synchronous rhythmic activity by the operation of collateral inhibitory feedback pathways (Stefanis, 1969). This technique thus provides a readily reproducible, but fully reversible, model of epilepsy, involving no organic tissue damage, of use particularly in studying methods of seizure propagation.

Extracellular positive potentials have also been observed to interrupt the chemically induced firing of neurons in the ventrobasal thalamus, and thus accentuate the spontaneous "spindle" type of discharge (Andersen and Curtis, 1964), but the phenomenon has not so far been reported to occur in normal cerebral cortex. Further investigation of the cerebral cortex, both normal and epileptic, seems warranted, perhaps using several micropipettes in order to excite a number of cells within a relatively small volume of tissue. It is possible that relatively small chronic epileptic foci could be established by administering toxic agents electrophoretically into various cortical layers, although the volume of tissue affected may be insufficient to initiate detectable experimental "epilepsy." Although intracortical penicillin has been used to establish such foci, the excitatory effects of electrophoretically administered penicillin on cortical neurons seem readily reversible (Walsh, 1971).

IV. APPENDIX

Although a variety of types and sizes of borosilicate glass tubing are available, tubing of the following sizes purchased from James A. Jobling & Co., Ltd., Wear Glass Works (Sunderland, England) is used routinely in the author's laboratory for single and for manufacturing multibarrel micropipettes: tubing, Pyrex borosilicate, precision bore 2.0 ± 0.05 mm, outer diameter 3.5 ± 0.25 mm. Tubing of slightly larger size (bore 2.2 ± 0.05 mm, outer diameter 3.75 ± 0.25 mm) is used for the center barrel of seven-barrel micropipettes. This glass is available in packets of 100 12-inch lengths.

Multibarrel micropipettes are available from the following firms:

B and D Glass and Instruments
104 Barkly Street
St. Kilda, Victoria 3182, Australia

Vancouver Scientific Glassblowing Co.
530 West 17 Avenue
Vancouver, British Columbia, Canada

Wesley Coe (Cambridge) Limited
Scotland Road
Cambridge, England

V. REFERENCES

Ajmone Marsan, C. (1969): Acute effects of topical epileptogenic agents. In: *Basic Mechanisms of the Epilepsies,* edited by H. H. Jasper, A. A. Ward, Jr., and A. Pope. Little, Brown & Company, Boston, pp. 299–319.
Andersen, P., and Curtis, D. R. (1964): The excitation of thalamic neurons by acetylcholine. *Acta Physiologica Scandinavica,* 61:85–99.

Barrett, J. N., and Graubard, K. (1970): Fluorescent staining of cat motoneurons *in vivo* with beveled micropipettes. *Brain Research*, 18:565–568.

Begent, N., and Born, G. V. R. (1970): Determination of the iontophoretic release of adenosine diphosphate from micropipettes. *British Journal of Pharmacology*, 40:592–593P.

Biscoe, T. J., and Straughan, D. W. (1966): Micro-electrophoretic studies of neurons in the cat hippocampus. *Journal of Physiology*, 183:341–359.

Bradley, P. B., and Candy, J. M. (1970): Iontophoretic release of acetylcholine, noradrenaline, 5-hydroxytryptamine and D-lysergic acid diethylamide from micropipettes. *British Journal of Pharmacology*, 40:194–201.

Burns, B. D. (1961): Use of extracellular microelectrodes. In: *Methods in Medical Research*, Vol. 9, edited by J. H. Quastel. Year Book Medical Publishers, Inc., Chicago, pp. 354–380.

Coombs, J. S., Eccles, J. C., and Fatt, P. (1955): The electrical properties of the motoneuron membrane. *Journal of Physiology*, 130:291–325.

Crain, S. M. (1972): This volume.

Crawford, J. M., Curtis, D. R., Voorhoeve, P. E., and Wilson, V. J. (1963): Strychnine and cortical inhibition. *Nature*, 200:845–846.

Crawford, J. M., Curtis, D. R., Voorhoeve, P. E., and Wilson, V. J. (1966): Acetylcholine sensitivity of cerebellar neurons in the cat. *Journal of Physiology*, 186:139–165.

Curtis, D. R. (1964): Microelectrophoresis. In: *Physical Techniques in Biological Research*, Vol. 5, edited by W. L. Nastuk. Academic Press, New York, pp. 144–190.

Curtis, D. R. (1968): A method for assembly of "parallel" micropipettes. *Electroencephalography and Clinical Neurophysiology*, 24:587–589.

Curtis, D. R. (1969): Central synaptic transmitters. In: *Basic Mechanisms of the Epilepsies*, edited by H. H. Jasper, A. A. Ward, Jr., and A. Pope. Little, Brown and Company, Boston, pp. 105–129.

Curtis, D. R., and Crawford, J. M. (1969): Central synaptic transmission—microelectrophoretic studies. *Annual Review of Pharmacology*, 9:209–240.

Curtis, D. R., Duggan, A. W., and Johnston, G. A. R. (1971): The specificity of strychnine as a glycine antagonist in the mammalian spinal cord. *Experimental Brain Research*, 12:547–565.

Curtis, D. R., and Felix, D. (1971): The effects of bicuculline upon synaptic inhibition in the cerebral and cerebellar cortices of the cat. *Brain Research*, 34:301–321.

Curtis, D. R., Felix, D., and Watkins, J. C. (1971): Effect of intracellular injection of pyridine nucleotides on electrical responses of spinal motoneurons. *Abstracts, III International Meeting, International Society of Neurochemistry*, 253.

Curtis, D. R., and Johnston, G. A. R. (1970): Amino acid transmitters. In: *Handbook of Neurochemistry*, Vol. 4, edited by A. Lajtha. Plenum Press, New York, pp. 115–134.

Curtis, D. R., Perrin, D. D., and Watkins, J. C. (1960): The excitation of spinal neurons by the iontophoretic application of agents which chelate calcium. *Journal of Neurochemistry*, 6:1–20.

Curtis, D. R., Phillis, J. W., and Watkins, J. C. (1959): The depression of spinal neurons by γ-amino-n-butyric acid and β-alanine. *Journal of Physiology*, 146:185–203.

Curtis, D. R., Phillis, J. W., and Watkins, J. C. (1960): The chemical excitation of spinal neurons by certain acidic amino acids. *Journal of Physiology*, 150:656–682.

Curtis, D. R., and Watkins, J. C. (1965): The pharmacology of amino acids related to gamma-aminobutyric acid. *Pharmacological Reviews*, 17:347–392.

del Castillo, J., and Katz, B. (1955): On the localization of acetylcholine receptors. *Journal of Physiology*, 128:157–181.

Diamond, J. (1968): The activation and distribution of GABA and L-glutamate receptors on goldfish Mauthner neurons: An analysis of dendritic remote inhibition. *Journal of Physiology*, 194:669–723.

Eccles, J. C. (1964): *Physiology of Synapses*. Springer-Verlag, Berlin.

Fatt, P. (1961): Intracellular microelectrodes. In: *Methods in Medical Research*, Vol. 9, edited by J. H. Quastel. Year Book Medical Publishers, Inc. Chicago, pp. 381–404.

Ferguson, J. H., and Jasper, H. H. (1971): Laminar DC studies of acetylcholine-activated epileptiform discharge in cerebral cortex. *Electroencephalography and Clinical Neurophysiology,* 30:377–390.

Firth, D. R., and de Felice, L. J. (1971): Electrical resistance and volume flow in glass microelectrodes. *Canadian Journal of Physiology and Pharmacology,* 49:436–447.

Frank, K., and Becker, M. C. (1964): Microelectrodes for recording and stimulation. In: *Physical Techniques in Biological Research,* edited by W. L. Nastuk. Academic Press, New York, pp. 22–87.

Galifret, Y., and Szabo, Th. (1960): Locating capillary microelectrode tips within nervous tissue. *Nature,* 188:1033–1034.

Ginsborg, B. L. (1967): Ion movements in junctional transmission. *Pharmacological Reviews,* 19:289–316.

Glaser, G. H. (1972): This volume.

Hellon, R. F. (1971): The marking of electrode tip positions in nervous tissue. *Journal of Physiology,* 214:12P.

Herz, A., Wickelmaier, M., and Nacimiento, A. (1965): Über die Herstellung von Mehrfachelektroden für die Mikroelektrophorese. *Pflügers Archiv für gesamter Physiology,* 284: 95–98.

Herz, A., Zieglgänsberger, W., and Färber, G. (1969): Microelectrophoretic studies concerning the spread of glutamic acid and GABA in brain tissue. *Experimental Brain Research,* 9:221–235.

Hoffer, B. J., Neff, N. H., and Siggins, G. R. (1971): Microiontophoretic release of norepinephrine from micropipettes. *Neuropharmacology,* 10:175–180.

Jaeger, J. C. (1965): Diffusion from constrictions. In: *Studies in Physiology, Presented to John C. Eccles,* edited by D. R. Curtis, and A. K. McIntyre. Springer-Verlag, Heidelberg, pp. 106–117.

Jankowska, E., and Lindström, S. (1970): Morphological identification of physiologically defined neurons in the cat spinal cord. *Brain Research,* 20:323–326.

Kaneko, A., and Hashimoto, H. (1967): Recording site of the single cone response determined by an electrode marking technique. *Vision Research,* 7:847–851.

Kato, G., and Somjen, G. G. (1969): Effects of micro-iontophoretic administration of magnesium and calcium on neurons in the central nervous system of cats. *Journal of Neurobiology,* 1:181–195.

Kirkpatrick, W. E., and Lomax, P. (1970): Temperature changes following iontophoretic injection of acetylcholine into the rostral hypothalamus of the rat. *Neuropharmacology,* 9:195–202.

Krischer, C. C. (1969a): Theoretical treatment of ohmic and rectifying properties of electrolyte micropipettes. *Zeitschrift für Naturforschung,* 24:151–155.

Krischer, C. C. (1969b): Current voltage measurements of electrolyte filled microelectrodes with ohmic and rectifying properties. *Zeitschrift für Naturforschung,* 24:156–161.

Krnjević, K. (1969): Neurotransmitters in normal and isolated cortex. In: *Basic Mechanisms of the Epilepsies,* edited by H. H. Jasper, A. A. Ward, Jr., and A. Pope. Little, Brown and Company, Boston, pp. 159–165.

Krnjević, K. (1971): Microiontophoresis. In: *Methods of Neurochemistry,* Vol. 1, edited by H. Fried. Marcel Dekker, Inc., New York, pp. 129–172.

Krnjević, K., and Phillis, J. W. (1963): Iontophoretic studies of neurons in the mammalian cerebral cortex. *Journal of Physiology,* 165:274–304.

Krnjević, K., Randić, M., and Siesjo, B. K. (1965): Cortical CO_2 tension and neuronal excitability. *Journal of Physiology,* 176:105–122.

Krnjević, K., Randić, M., and Straughan, D. W. (1966a): An inhibitory process in the cerebral cortex. *Journal of Physiology,* 184:16–48.

Krnjević, K., Randić, M., and Straughan, D. W. (1966b): Nature of a cortical inhibitory process. *Journal of Physiology,* 184:49–77.

Krnjević, K., Reiffenstein, R. J., and Silver, A. (1970a): Chemical sensitivity of neurons in long-isolated slabs of cat cerebral cortex. *Electroencephalography and Clinical Neurophysiology,* 29:269–282.

Krnjević, K., Reiffenstein, R. J., and Silver, A. (1970b): Inhibition and paroxysmal activity on long-isolated cortical slabs. *Electroencephalography and Clinical Neurophysiology*, 29: 283–294.

Krnjević, K., and Schwartz, S. (1967): The action of γ-aminobutyric acid on cortical neurones. *Experimental Brain Research*, 3:320–336.

Krnjević, K., and Whittaker, V. P. (1965): Excitation and depression of cortical neurons by brain fractions released from micropipettes. *Journal of Physiology*, 179:298–322.

Lavellée, M., Schanne, O. F., and Hébert, N. C., eds. (1969): *Glass Microelectrodes*. John Wiley and Sons, Inc., London.

Lee, B. B., Mandl, G., and Stean, J. P. B. (1969): Micro-electrode tip position marking in nervous tissue: A new dye method. *Electroencephalography and Clinical Neurophysiology*, 27:610–613.

Lux, H. D., Loracher, C., and Neher, E. (1970): The action of ammonium on postsynaptic inhibition of cat spinal motoneurons. *Experimental Brain Research*, 11:431–447.

McCance, I. (1969): The iontophoretic release of acetylcholine. *Australian Journal of Experimental Biology and Medical Science*, 47:P20–21.

McCance, I., and Phillis, J. W. (1965): The location of microelectrode tips in nervous tissues. *Experientia*, 21:108–109.

Millichap, J. G. (1969): Systemic electrolyte and neuroendocrine mechanisms. In: *Basic Mechanisms of the Epilepsies*, edited by H. H. Jasper, A. A. Ward, Jr., and A. Pope. Little, Brown and Company, Boston, pp. 709–726.

Nastuk, W. L. (1951): Membrane potential changes at a single muscle end-plate produced by acetylcholine. *Federation Proceedings*, 10:96.

Obata, K., Takeda, K., and Shinozaki, H. (1970): Electrophoretic release of γ-aminobutyric acid and glutamic acid from micropipettes. *Neuropharmacology*, 9:191–194.

Oliver, A. P. (1971): A simple rapid method for preparing parallel micropipette electrodes. *Electroencephalography and Clinical Neurophysiology*, 31:284–286.

Perrin, D. D. (1965): *Dissociation constants of organic bases in aqueous solution*. Butterworth, London.

Phillis, J. W. (1970): *The Pharmacology of Synapses. International Series of Monographs in Pure and Applied Biology, Division: Zoology*, Vol. 43. Pergamon Press, Oxford.

Phillis, J. W., and Ochs, S. (1971): Excitation and depression of cortical neurons during spreading depression. *Experimental Brain Research*, 12:132–149.

Pohle, W., and Matthies, H. (1966): Elektrophoretische Markierung von Nervenzellen bei extracellulärer Ableitung der Einzelzell Aktivität mit Vielfach Glasmikroelektroden. *Acta Biologica et Medica Germanica*, 17:721–726.

Prince, D. A. (1969): Microelectrode studies of penicillin foci. In: *Basic Mechanisms of the Epilepsies*, edited by H. H. Jasper, A. A. Ward, Jr., and A. Pope. Little, Brown and Company, Boston, pp. 320–328.

Prince, D. A., and Futamachi, K. J. (1970): Intracellular recordings from chronic epileptogenic foci in the monkey. *Electroencephalography and Clinical Neurophysiology*, 29:496–510.

Rush, S., Lepeschkin, E., and Brooks, H. O. (1968): Electrical and thermal properties of double-barreled ultra microelectrodes. *IEEE Transactions on Bio-Medical Engineering*, 15:80–93.

Salmoiraghi, G. C., and Stefanis, C. N. (1967): A critique of iontophoretic studies of central nervous system neurons. *International Review of Neurobiology*, 10:1–30.

Salmoiraghi, G. C., and Weight, F. (1967): Micromethods in neuropharmacology: An approach to the study of anesthetics. *Anesthesiology*, 28:54–64.

Sharpless, S. K. (1969): Isolated and deafferented neurons: disuse supersensitivity. In: *Basic Mechanisms of the Epilepsies*, edited by H. H. Jasper, A. A. Ward, Jr., and A. Pope. Little, Brown and Company, Boston, pp. 329–348.

Spehlmann, R. (1969): Multi-barreled coaxial micro-pipettes with independent control of the central recording barrel. *Electroencephalography and Clinical Neurophysiology*, 27:201–204.

Spehlmann, R. (1970): Excitability of partially deafferented cortex. II. Microelectrode studies. *Archives of Neurology*, 22:510–514.

Spehlmann, R. (1971): Acetylcholine and the epileptiform activity of chronically isolated cortex. II. Microelectrode studies. *Archives of Neurology*, 24:495–502.

Spencer, W. A., and Kandel, E. R. (1969): Synaptic inhibition in seizures. In: *Basic Mechanisms of the Epilepsies*, edited by H. H. Jasper, A. A. Ward, Jr., and A. Pope. Little, Brown and Company, Boston, pp. 575–603.

Stefanis, C. (1969): Discussion. In: *The Interneuron*, edited by M. A. Brazier. University of California Press, Los Angeles, pp. 442–447.

Steiner, F. A. (1971): *Neurotransmitter und Neuromodulatoren. Technik und Resultate der Mikroelektrophorese im Nervensystem.* Georg Thieme Verlag, Stuttgart.

Sterc, J., Pilny, J., Petsche, H., and Novakova, V. (1968): Zur Frage der Markierung einzelner Nervenzellen durch Mikroelektroden. *Experientia*, 24:305–307.

Stretton, A. O. W., and Kravitz, E. A. (1968): Neuronal geometry: Determination with a technique of intracellular dye injection. *Science*, 162:132–134.

Sypert, G. W., Oakley, J., and Ward, A. A., Jr. (1970): Single-unit analysis of propagated seizures in neocortex. *Experimental Neurology*, 28:308–325.

Tasaki, K., Tsukahara, Y., Ito, S., Wayner, M. J., and Yu, W. Y. (1968): A simple, direct and rapid method for filling microelectrodes. *Physiology and Behaviour*, 3:1009–1010.

Thomas, R. C., and Wilson, V. J. (1965): Precise localization of Renshaw cells with a new marking technique. *Nature*, 206:211–213.

Thomas, R. C., and Wilson, V. J. (1966): Marking single neurons by staining with intracellular recording microelectrodes. *Science*, 151:1538–1539.

Tomita, T. (1956): The nature of action potentials in the lateral eye of the horseshoe crab as revealed by simultaneous intra- and extracellular recordings. *Japanese Journal of Physiology*, 6:327–340.

Towe, A. L., and Harding, G. W. (1970): Extracellular microelectrode sampling bias. *Experimental Neurology*, 29:366–381.

Walsh, G. O. (1971): Penicillin iontophoresis in neocortex of cat: effects on the spontaneous and induced activity of single neurons. *Epilepsia*, 12:1–11.

Ward, A. A., Jr. (1969): The epileptic neuron: Chronic foci in animals and man. In: *Basic Mechanisms of the Epilepsies*, edited by H. H. Jasper, A. A. Ward, Jr., and A. Pope. Little, Brown and Company, Boston, pp. 263–288.

Waud, D. R. (1968): On diffusion from a point source. *Journal of Pharmacology and Experimental Therapeutics*, 159:123–128.

Werman, R., Davidoff, R. A., and Aprison, M. H. (1968): Inhibitory action of glycine on spinal neurons in the cat. *Journal of Neurophysiology*, 31:81–95.

Wilder, B. J. (1972): This volume.

Zieglgänsberger, W., and Herz, A. (1971): Changes of cutaneous receptive fields of spinocervical tract neurons and other dorsal horn neurons by microelectrophoretically administered amino acids. *Experimental Brain Research*, 13:111–126.

Zieglgänsberger, W., Herz, A., and Teschemacher, H. (1969): Electrophoretic release of tritium-labelled glutamic acid from micropipettes *in vitro*. *Brain Research*, 15:298–300.

11

Electrical Stimulation of Specified Subsystems of the Mammalian Brain, As Isolated Tissue Preparations

Henry McIlwain

OUTLINE

I. ORIENTATION AND RATIONALE

The localized character of epileptic phenomena, afflicting a brain which in many other respects is normal, directs investigation to sub-systems of the brain. Other contributors describe such regional studies made in the intact brain *in situ;* described here is the complementary technique of examining selected parts of the brain in isolation, as surviving tissue preparations *in vitro*.

Stimulation of isolated neural tissues is familiar from the use of frog sciatic nerve in elementary electrophysiology; handling of tissue slices is familiar from the elementary biochemical study of liver or kidney metabolism. Present studies do more than combine these two techniques, for chemical, anatomical, and electrophysiological factors interact with intriguing complexity in the mammalian brain. Consequently, there are many specific choices to be made in relation to the preparation of tissue and incubating media, as well as about what apparatus should be used for metabolic or electrophysiological study. Responses to be expected electrically include a rich variety of postsynaptic phenomena. Metabolic responses include those of energy metabolism, of neurotransmission, and also the slower, adaptive processes which give long-term adjustment of functioning. The scope of the subject is detailed in Table 1.

II. CHOICE AND PREPARATION OF TISSUE

Parts of the brain which have been successfully examined as tissue are included in Table 1. The bases for the choice may come from associated studies which direct attention to particular regions. This is especially true in applying the methods to study of particular types of epilepsy; also, biopsy samples may be available only from certain regions. If the investigator is studying general problems which would allow him to choose from any region of the brain, it is often to his advantage to study those regions fed by clearly defined neural input, such as those from the optic or olfactory tracts. By the use of small laboratory animals, it has proved feasible to observe both electrophysiological and metabolic consequences of conduction and of postsynaptic events from preparations of the order of a centimeter in maximal extent and weighing 20 to 60 mg.

It is critical to the technique of using isolated tissues that the preparations be sufficiently thin to allow supply of essential materials, and removal

TABLE 1. *Responses of isolated subsystems to electrical excitation*

Part of the brain	Metabolic responses	Electrical responses	Other observations	References
Subcortical white matter; corpus callosum	Respiration, glycolysis, inorganic phosphate phosphocreatine	Conducted impulses	With human tissues; on tract section	Bollard and McIlwain (1957) Kurokawa (1960) Yamamoto and McIlwain (1966)
Lateral olfactory tract	Respiration	Conduction: 10–12 m/sec	—	Yamamoto and McIlwain (1966)
Optic tract	—	Conduction: brief biphasic action potential; short latency and refractory period	—	Kawai and Yamamoto (1969)
Lateral olfactory tract— piriform cortex	Respiration, glycolysis, inorganic phosphate. K⁺, phosphocreatine; output of noradrenaline, serotonin	Pre- and post-synaptic in cortex; negative wave and unit discharges. Frequency-dependent attenuation; posttetanic potentiation	Actions of butobarbital, ether, scopolamine, γ-aminobutyrate, chlorpromazine	Yamamoto and McIlwain (1966) Campbell et al. (1967) Richards and Sercombe (1968) McIlwain and Snyder (1970)
Optic tract—superior colliculus	Serotonin output	Pre- and postsynaptic in brachium and colliculus; negative spike and wave discharges with relatively long and variable latency and refractory period	Some spontaneous and glutamate-induced firing; action of lysergic acid diethylamide	Kawai and Yamamoto (1969) Kawai (1970)
Medulla	Respiration, glycolysis, inorganic phosphate, phosphocreatine	—	—	Bollard and McIlwain (1957)
Hypothalamus	Serotonin output	—	Actions of Li⁺, ouabain, chlorpromazine	Chase et al. (1969)
Corpus striatum	Glutamate, γ-aminobutyrate, noradrenaline, serotonin	—	Tetrodotoxin, Li⁺, ouabain actions	Katz and Kopin (1969)

TABLE 1. (continued)

Hippocampus: dentate gyrus and associated structures	—	Negative spike and wave discharges. Rapid response from an electrically coupled synapse	Yamamoto and Kawai (1968) Yamamoto (1970)
		Low-Cl⁻ media induces seizure discharges; propagated	
Neocortex	Respiration, glycolysis, inorganic phosphate, cyclic AMP, phospho-creatine, Na^+, K^+, Ca^{++}, phospholipid incorporation; output of acetyl-choline, adenosine, γ-aminobutyrate, nora-drenaline, serotonin	Displacement and recovery of membrane potential; spike discharges; trans-mitted direct cortical response	McIlwain (1951, 1953) Anguiano and McIlwain (1951) McIlwain et al. (1952) Rowsell (1954) Greengard and McIlwain (1955) Brierley and McIlwain (1956) Li and McIlwain (1957) Cummins and McIlwain (1961) Srinivasan et al. (1969) Kakiuchi et al. (1969) Yamamoto and Kawai (1967) Pumphrey (1969) McIlwain and Pull (1972)
		With human tissues and neoplasms; induced gliosis; numerous drug interactions	

Preparations derived from the rat or guinea pig unless otherwise specified.

of metabolic products, by diffusion from or to the exposed surfaces of the tissue. Under ordinary conditions, this requires a tissue thickness of no greater than about 0.4 mm (or 0.5 mm in white-matter regions). These dimensions should be regarded merely as suggestions to be appraised by the investigator. At the exposed surfaces of the tissue preparation, metabolites exchange with a fluid chosen by the experimenter; for this exchange to be most effective, the fluid should be flowing or agitated. A limiting metabolite is commonly oxygen, which is supplied at tensions corresponding to 20 to 100% O_2 in a gas phase, according to tissue thickness: again, this is a matter to be appraised by the investigator in relation to his experimental system.

Many basic rules of handling tissues for metabolic studies are applicable to the present preparations (McIlwain and Rodnight, 1962). There should be minimal time between the interruption of the blood supply to the regions chosen and the placing of the derived tissue in oxygenated glucose salines at 37 to 38°C. An interval of no longer than 1 to 2 min should be aimed for, unless it can be demonstrated that no advantage accrues from brevity. In our experience, cooling the tissue during this interval is undesirable, although it may be done for a specific purpose, for example, during transport of biopsy material from operating room theater to laboratory, when a small closed container at 0 to 5°C has been used. In such cases, the effect of the cooling can be appraised by comparable cooling of tissue from a laboratory animal. Preparation of tissue of desired thickness from, for example, the neocortex is readily carried out with a narrow (1 mm) cutting blade and template (see McIlwain and Rodnight, 1962); however, several of the regions shown in Table 1 require separation from the brain by detailed dissection, or else by a simple preliminary dissection which then produces a block of tissue capable of being cut with blade and template (McIlwain and Snyder, 1970; Yamamoto, 1970). An example of the latter type is the superficial 0.3- to 0.4-mm tissue sample of the piriform lobe of the guinea pig which carries both the lateral olfactory tract and junctions of fibers of the tract with different cortical regions. A single cut with a fine scalpel about 1.5 mm medial to the surface of the lobe gives a block of tissue which may be laid on a cutting table, in order then to obtain the required region by blade and template.

III. MAINTENANCE AND STIMULATION OF TISSUE

Important items in tissue maintenance include the composition of incubating fluids and the apparatus which is to permit metabolic and/or electrical observation of the tissue (Harvey and McIlwain, 1969; McIlwain and

Bachelard, 1971). Initial studies may begin by using media based on ordinary bicarbonate-glucose salines, with only minor modifications for some known characteristics of cerebral tissues. A typical composition is (mM): NaCl, 120; KCl, 3.0; KH_2PO_4, 1.2; $MgSO_4$, 1.2; $CaCl_2$, 0.75; $NaHCO_3$, 25; and glucose, 10 — in equilibrium with O_2 containing 5% (v/v) CO_2. The Na, K, and Ca contents of the isolated tissues are closer to *in vivo* values when incubating fluids contain Ca at 0.75 mM rather than at the 2.8 mM concentration frequently employed.

Numerous additions to such fluids have been advocated for specific purposes; a tabulation and comment have been given by McIlwain and Rodnight (1962). It is not advisable to make additions without specific reason, since some additions can be deleterious. Most properties of isolated tissues depend on an adequate supply of metabolically derived energy and on the ion gradients which depend on such a supply (see McIlwain, 1969). It is thus advisable to establish the routine measurement of some chemical or metabolic characteristic of the tissue which can indicate its normal maintenance. For this purpose, respiratory or glycolytic rate, and K^+ or phosphocreatine content, may be measured in the tissue either during an experiment or at its completion. Values have been reported for ion content, distribution, and flux mainly in the neocortex of rodents (Harvey and McIlwain, 1969).

Apparatus and experimental arrangements needed for study of tissue constituents and respiration of the isolated preparations are described by McIlwain and Rodnight (1962), and Harvey and McIlwain (1969), and those for intra- and extracellular electrical recording by Gibson and McIlwain (1965), and Yamamoto and McIlwain (1966); see Appendix I. A superfusion system for maintaining isolated preparations, and following the output from them of neurotransmitters and tissue metabolites on excitation, is detailed by McIlwain and Snyder (1970); see Appendix II.

IV. ELECTRICAL RESPONSES TO EXCITATION

The electrical and metabolic responses to stimulation which occur in a given part of the brain have overlapping time sequences and much mutual dependence. They are often investigated separately in different experimental systems, but much advantage can come from their joint study and appraisal. Included in the present section are some electrical characteristics of responses which occur in tissue preparations, and experimental variations which can induce after-discharges and repetitive cell-firing.

A. Extracellular recording in normal media

Extracellular recording in normal media readily displays a great variety of types of responses from the different tissue preparations so far investigated. Figure 1, *A–C*, shows that the velocity of conduction along about 1 cm of the lateral olfactory tract of the guinea pig can be measured in a preparation from the piriform lobe maintained in isolation, and more com-

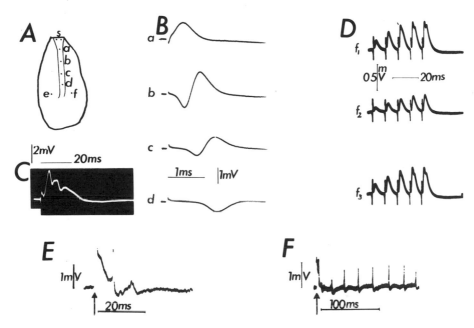

FIG. 1. Extracellular recordings of responses to stimulation of the lateral olfactory tract, piriform cortex, and neocortex of the guinea pig or rat (Yamamoto and McIlwain, 1966; Richards and McIlwain, 1967; Campbell et al., 1967).

A: A tissue preparation of the piriform lobe, indicating placements of stimulating electrodes (*s*) and recording electrodes (*a–f*); all electrodes were fine silver wires, ball-tipped at the surface of the tissue. *B:* Records from sites *a–d* after stimulation at *s*, showing conduction along the lateral olfactory tract. *C:* A surface response from the piriform cortex at *e* (surface-negative potential giving upward deflection as illustrated), showing the large negative wave with superimposed positive notches. *D:* Records from site *f* following stimulation at *s* and showing at f_1 recruitment of response to successive stimuli delivered at 5/sec, at f_2 diminished response to the same stimuli after 10-min exposure to 1mM phenobarbital, and at f_3 response restored after 15 min in saline in absence of the drug. *E:* Unit discharges from a neocortical preparation stimulated with surface electrodes and observed with a micropipette electrode, tip diameter 2 to 4 μm, about 2 mm distant and 200 μm below the cortical surface. *F:* Unit discharges observed as in *E*, from tissue in media in which sodium ethyl sulfonate partly replaced the normal chloride content. A single stimulus at the arrow (the 40th in a series applied at 1/sec) evoked a train of responses.

plex potentials can be observed in the adjacent cortex. These latter responses comprised a relatively slow negative wave, on which positive notches were superimposed. The responses increased in complexity as a result of repetitive stimuli delivered at the rate of a few per second (Fig. 1*D;* for more detailed depiction, see Yamamoto and McIlwain, 1966, and Campbell, 1967). They were more susceptible to phenobarbital or ether than were the conducted responses; these and other properties characterized the negative-wave complexes as being postsynaptic responses.

Within the preparations, unit discharges could be detected by micropipette electrodes of 2 to 4-μ tip diameter (Richards and McIlwain, 1967; Richards and Sercombe, 1968). Firing was more frequent after a conditioning shock, and repetitive stimuli were followed by repeated afterdischarges. After the stimuli, firing occurred at variable intervals; when the latency of such firing was plotted against the number of instances of firing at that latency in a given series of observations, a curve was obtained which matched the positive notches imposed on the negative wave, thereby suggesting their origin. The negative wave was abolished by high-frequency stimulation, but subsequently returned at increased amplitude in response to a standard stimulus (Yamamoto and McIlwain, 1966). Appreciable spontaneous activity was observed in some piriform preparations, affording either discharges in the absence of deliberate stimulation or rhythmic variation in response following standard stimuli. Some comparable observations made with neocortical and hippocampal systems are described in Section IV B.

Surface electrodes readily record transmission along the optic tracts, and a preparation is available (Fig. 2) which includes one of the tracts, the brachium of the contralateral superior colliculus, and the superior colliculus itself, from its outer surface to a depth of 0.35 to 0.55 mm. From the brachium, a simple, brief biphasic potential was recorded on stimulating the optic tract; the surface of superior colliculus afforded a brief positivity followed by a slow negative wave, greater in amplitude and some 20 msec in duration. The negative wave was concluded to be a field potential of the postsynaptic response (Kawai and Yamamoto, 1969). This wave was observed in over 100 preparations (more than 90% of those examined) and when tested with occasional stimuli delivered less frequently than 1/sec, characteristics of the response at the colliculus remained unchanged for over 1 hr.

Single-unit discharges were observed in the colliculus following stimulation of the optic tract, by insertion of glass capillary micropipettes, tip diameter 4 mm. Some of the discharges, with short latency and brief refractory periods, were presynaptic. Each insertion of a microelectrode to

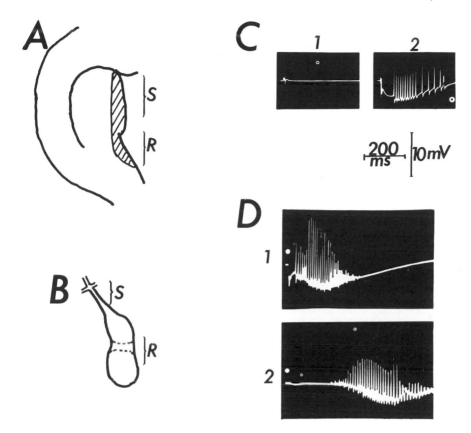

FIG. 2.   Two systems isolated from the guinea pig brain, showing the positions of stimulating (*S*) and recording (*R*) electrodes and responses (Yamamoto and Kawai, 1967, 1968).

A: A section of the hippocampus which includes parts of the dentate gyrus, alveus, stria oriens, and pyramidal cell layer. *B:* A preparation of the optic tract with contralateral brachium and superior colliculus. *C:* Response of the hippocampal preparation to stimulation in normal medium (*1*), and in medium containing propionate in place of chloride ions (*2*). *D:* Propagation of the after-discharge generated as in *C.* Distance of recording electrode from stimulating electrode, *1*, 1 mm; *2*, 5 mm.

the superior colliculus region of the preparation also detected the firing of at least one cell following stimulation of the optic tract.   Latency between stimulus and firing in these cases lasted milliseconds, often 10 msec but variable, and the firing was superimposed on a negative potential which corresponded to the negative wave obtainable by surface recording.   Paired stimuli showed much longer refractory periods postsynaptically than those observed presynaptically.

B. Modified media and intracellular recording

Many of the preparations shown in Table 1 have been the subject of intracellular recordings using micropipette electrodes with tips about 0.5 μm in diameter. Observations commenced with neocortical tissues of the guinea pig and cat (Li and McIlwain, 1957) which displayed resting membrane potentials, their displacement on stimulation, and occasional repetitive cell discharge. With specifically devised apparatus (Gibson and McIlwain, 1965), continuous recording of potentials was possible and the change in potentials with changed composition of incubating fluid could be measured. An average stable resting potential was −60 mV, modified in calculable fashion with changes in K^+ concentrations at the tissue surface.

Intracellular recording from hippocampal preparations, 0.3 mm in thickness and stimulated with bipolar silver electrodes 0.2 mm apart, has contributed to specification of the types of transmission occurring in the dentate gyrus (Yamamoto, 1970). Stimuli applied at the granule cell layer gave potentials which, observed extracellularly, were of variable latency and included a remarkably rapid discharge which was insensitive to a five-fold increase in Mg^{++} concentration, which would block other components of the response. Intracellular recordings gave resting potentials of −60 to −70 mV and showed responses to stimulation which featured a fast depolarization, rising from a flat base line and occurring 1.5 msec before the onset of the excitatory postsynaptic potential. These, together with other data, suggested that direct electrical coupling was occurring at synapses between mossy fibers and hippocampal neurons.

In hippocampal and in neocortical preparations, repetitive discharges have been induced by a simple modification of the normal incubating media (Richards and McIlwain, 1967; Yamamoto and Kawai, 1968). This was brought about in neocortical preparations by replacement of chloride by sodium methylsulfonate (Fig. 1) and in the hippocampal preparation by replacing chloride by bromate, sulfate, formate, acetate, or propionate (Fig. 2). Of these substitutions, that by propionate was innocuous in terms of the general behavior of the preparation and permitted repeated observations. The normal hippocampal response observed extracellularly was greatly altered when more than 70% of the chloride of bathing media was replaced by propionate. The immediate response to a stimulus was augmented, and it was followed by repetitive discharges. These became more frequent as chloride was further diminished and occurred with shorter latency.

The repetitive discharges were propagated through the dentate gyrus at velocities between 1 and 3 cm/sec, which varied with tissue treatment.

Findings were consistent with the participation of chloride ions in inhibitory mechanisms which normally limited cell discharge (see Eccles, 1964). Modification of chloride permeability or flux is thus a feasible mechanism for seizure discharges in pathological conditions, and the present isolated subsystems give a means for their study; *in vivo,* chloride concentrations cannot be so readily manipulated. A seizure discharge *in vivo* is unlikely to be secondary to changed chloride level in extracellular fluids generally but can be envisaged as secondary to changed metabolism of an inhibitory transmitter which acts by modifying chloride permeability.

V. METABOLIC RESPONSES TO STIMULATION

Indications of the metabolic responses observed on exciting isolated cerebral preparations are included in Table 1. One category of responses concerns cation movements and the major substrate utilization and energy metabolism of the tissues. These were appraised recently (McIlwain, 1969) and are given only incidental comment here. A second category concerns the release and metabolism of neurotransmitters and cognate substances. Less well documented but of much potential interest to the present theme are indications of longer-term changes.

The subject of neurotransmitter release on electrical stimulation of isolated preparations began with observations of the output of acetylcholine and noradrenaline from cortical preparations (Rowsell, 1954; Baldessarini and Kopin, 1966) and has been diversified to include the several agents and tissue preparations of Table 1. New opportunities were provided by studying the output of transmitters and cognate compounds in association with other electrophysiological or metabolic observation of the tissue. The olfactory tract-piriform cortex, and optic tract-superior colliculus, systems have been examined in this fashion (Figs. 3 and 4).

The superfusion apparatus employed previously (McIlwain and Snyder, 1970) enabled replicate tissue preparations, usually four, to be maintained under good metabolic conditions. The metabolic status and response of the tissue could be appraised during the experiment, for example, by measurement of lactate output (Figs. 3B and 4) and at the end of the experiment by analysis of the tissue. During preincubation periods, the tissues were exposed to the isotopically labeled compounds as specified. With commencement of superfusion, the excess of these and of any other reagents was removed; a small, gradually decreasing output of ^{3}H-glycine,

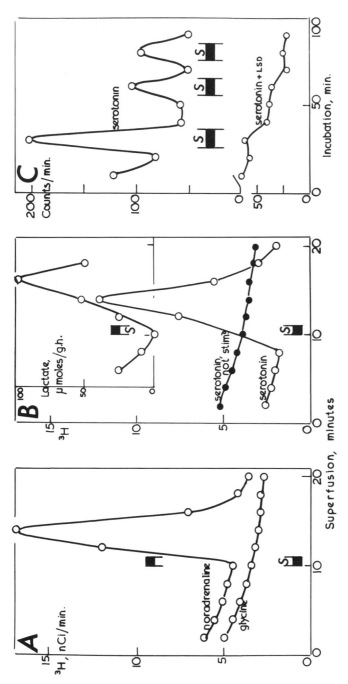

FIG. 3.: Output of serotonin and of noradrenaline from the lateral olfactory tract-piriform cortex system, and from the optic tract-brachium-superior colliculus system, as isolated tissue preparations (McIlwain and Snyder, 1970; Kawai, 1970).

A, B: The piriform system in a continuous-flow apparatus, with 2-min collections of superfusion fluid. This flowed over tissue previously incubated with [3H]-glycine, [3H]-noradrenaline, or [3H]-serotonin. During the 1-min periods (*S*), the same stimuli were applied in all experiments, except to the tissue marked as unstimulated. The inset in *B* shows the concomitant output of lactic acid from stimulated tissues. *C*: The optic tract system was previously exposed to [3H]-serotonin, with successive samples of incubating fluid changed every 10 min and subsequently analyzed. Stimuli were applied to the optic tract during the periods *S*. In the experiment reported by the lower line, the incubation medium contained 1 μM lysergic acid diethylamide with the serotonin. In *A–C*, separations and control experiments were carried out to specify the chemical identity of the output of [3H] compounds.

³H-noradrenaline, or ³H-serotonin remained. These responded differently to excitation: no change was found in the output of glycine, whereas output of noradrenaline and serotonin increased greatly. Much specificity was shown in such output when it was examined in different tissues or in the presence of different blocking agents, and some instances of this are given in Table 1.

The optic tract-brachium-superior colliculus preparation also assimilated ³H-serotonin during preincubation, and efflux of serotonin took place into successive batches of incubation fluid (Fig. 3*C*). By stimulation of the optic tract, output of ³H, demonstrated to be ³H-serotonin, increased two- to threefold. This increase could be prevented by section of the optic tract just before it reached the colliculus; output was also largely inhibited by the presence of lysergic acid diethylamide (Fig. 3*C*). Observation of electrical responses in the colliculus showed susceptibility to serotonin, and inhibition by lysergic acid diethylamide, at 1 μM (Kawai and Yamamoto, 1969).

Major changes in adenine derivatives occur on electrical excitation of the brain or of tissues isolated from it (see McIlwain, 1969, 1971). These changes have mainly been seen within the context of energy metabolism, but among them is a 10-fold increase in the cyclic AMP of isolated tissues (Kakiuchi et al., 1969). Knowing that neurohumoral agents, including noradrenaline, could increase cerebral cyclic AMP and were released on excitation, their action was examined; added noradrenaline was found not to reproduce but to act synergistically with electrical excitation. Synergism with noradrenaline was a property also of cerebral extracts and was found to be due to their content of adenosine; excitation was then found to release adenosine (Sattin and Rall, 1970; McIlwain and Pull, 1972).

¹⁴C-Adenine acted as precursor of adenine nucleotides in neocortical and piriform cortical preparations and proved to do so in a compartment amounting to about 3% of the total tissue volume (Santos et al., 1968; Shimizu et al., 1970). The release of ¹⁴C-adenine metabolites which took place on excitation was in temporal relation to changed glucose utilization and consisted of compounds which could all be regarded as derivatives of ¹⁴C-ATP (McIlwain and Pull, 1972; Fig. 4). The greatest increase on excitation was found in adenosine; its output increased with the frequency and duration of applied stimuli and was blocked by tetrodotoxin. Cyclic AMP, yielded by adenosine, has prompt effects on cell-firing in the cerebellum (Siggins et al., 1969) and also mediates long-term changes in cerebral systems (see McIlwain, 1971). It activates protein kinases in cerebral preparations, including histone kinases (Weller and Rodnight, 1970; Greengard and Kuo, 1970), which may be involved in derepressing deoxyribonucleic acid. Much is yet to be learned of how the stimulus-released

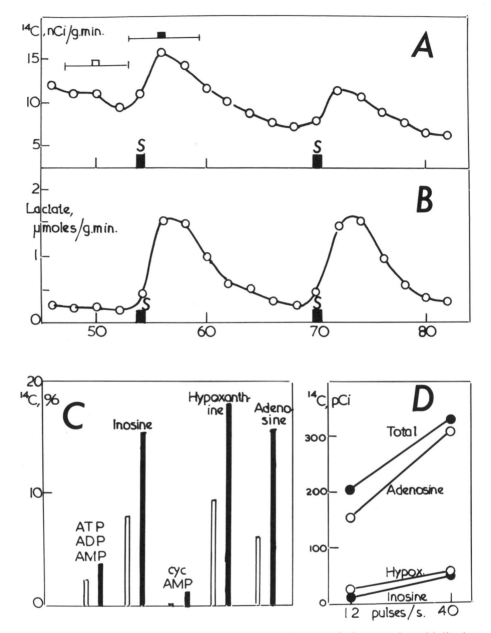

FIG. 4. Output of adenine derivatives from guinea pig neocortical preparations (McIlwain and Pull, 1971; Pull and McIlwain, 1972), preincubated in media containing ^{14}C-adenine.

A: The efflux from the tissue, which appeared in superfusion fluids, was augmented by electrical excitation (*S*) applied for 1-min periods (*S*). The samples I and II were pooled for chromatographic identification. *B:* The fluids of *A* were analyzed also for lactate and gave the rate of glycolysis by the tissue at the times shown. *C:* Chromatographic separation of the effluent samples I (before stimulation: open columns) and II (during and after stimulation: solid columns). *D:* Effluent ^{14}C compounds at two different frequencies of stimulation, each applied for 4 min.

adenosine participates in these series of events; synergism with neuro-transmitters in the production of cyclic AMP must contribute to localizing its site of action.

VI. APPRAISAL

Examining a cerebral subsystem in isolation allows the investigator to choose and specify the input to it, both chemical and electrical. Chemical input arrives at the tissue without meeting barriers other than those of the tissue cells. The tissue is available for analysis at chosen times; trauma of excision does not intervene between electrophysiological observation and sampling for chemical analyses. Electrical input can be arranged to come by a defined neural tract or by electrodes close to a chosen cell type.

Drug-development studies using such preparations as test systems can examine compounds which in an intact animal are toxic or have extraneous actions. Drug-evaluation studies with isolated subsystems of the brain are, in this sense, similar to chemotherapeutic screening programs which first test antimicrobial compounds for effect in microbial cultures, prior to exploring the active compounds in infected animals. Anti-seizure but toxic compounds will clearly not themselves be chosen as drugs but could be intermediary members of a series giving a new drug type. Other series of potential antiepileptics may have been judged unpromising because a given compound did not reach the relevant part of the brain; again, use of an isolated preparation allows continued examination of such series.

The major limitation to the use of isolated preparations comes, quite simply, from absence of the rest of the brain, and may be partly made good by examining other subsystems. This limitation is thus analagous to those accepted by investigators who examine an animal rather than a cohort, or a species rather than an ecological system. In contributing to the larger system, each subsystem remains recognizably itself but undergoes adaptation. It is thus propitious to future studies with cerebral subsystems that, as can be judged by Section V, they have been found suitable for observing adaptive phenomena and also for investigating some of the associated biochemical mechanisms.

VII. APPENDIX I: APPARATUS FOR RECORDING RESTING AND ACTION POTENTIALS IN MAMMALIAN TISSUES *IN VITRO*

The apparatus for recording resting and action potentials in mammalian tissues *in vitro* was developed by Gibson and McIlwain (1965), and its basic form is shown in Fig. 5. The incubating medium in the chamber (*a*) is maintained at 37°C by water

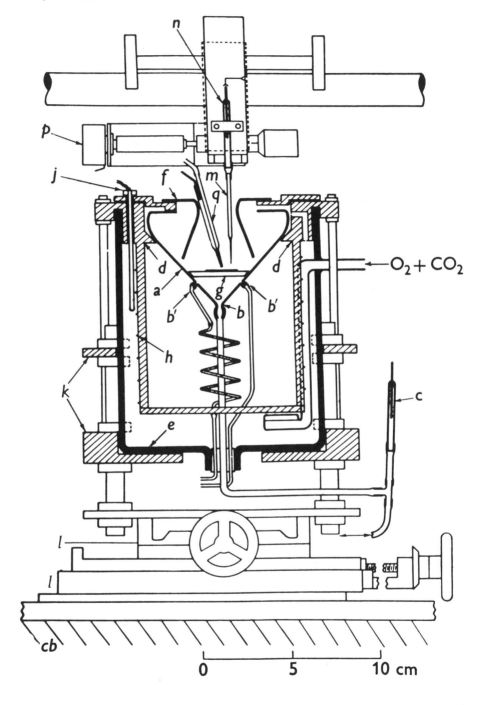

O₂ + CO₂

in the thermostat bath (*e*). The incoming gas (95% O_2, 5% CO_2) has passed through a flow-meter, and, after passing through the sintered-glass bubbler, it is moistened and warmed in its passage through the water in the thermostat bath; it is then guided across the moist surface of the tissue slice. This rests on a nylon and Perspex grid (*g*), and the gas passes out through the wide central opening about it.

The tissue is in immediate contact with about 5 ml of medium. Additional fluid can be added from a syringe by way of a tube connected to one opening (*b*) in the slice-chamber. The other openings (*b'* and *b*) are connected by fine tubing to a Watson-Marlow Flow Inducer, Type MHRV, enabling the incubating medium to be circulated at 1.25 ml/min. The thermostat bath is maintained by a heating coil (*h*) and control system consisting of the thermistor (*j*) which controls the current to the input of a transistorized DC amplifier, the output stage of which controls the current through the heating coil.

The Perspex and steel mounting (*k*) for the chamber forms a very rigid structure. The sliding lathe mounts (*l*) provide fine movement of the chamber system in a horizontal plane in two directions at right angles. Thus, it is only necessary to provide vertical movements for the recording microelectrode. The vertical movement portion of a micromanipulator is mounted on a horizontal brass bar supported at each end by vertical brass pillars. Vertical displacement of the microelectrode is recorded on one channel of a pen-recorder by means of a potentiometer (*p*) driven by the fine control of the micromanipulator. Movement of 130 μm (one revolution of the fine control) gives a pen movement of 12 mm.

Microelectrodes and micropipettes. The nonpolarizable electrodes (*c* and *n*) consist of silver chloride-coated silver wire sealed into a short length of glass tubing filled with 3% agar in saline solution. The microelectrodes are glass micropipettes filled with 2.7M KCl. Tips are <0.5μm, and DC resistances are 10 to 50 MΩ. The two nonpolarizable electrodes are connected to a cathode-follower probe mounted close to the micromanipulator. One side of the cathode follower is grounded to give single-sided operation. The probe forms part of a DC pre-amplifier, the output from which is fed to a cathode-ray oscilloscope and to one channel of a pen-recorder.

Fluids are applied to the surface of the tissue by a fine pipette, attached to a micrometer syringe. The pipette is drawn by hand, from microelectrode glass

---

FIG. 5. The tissue-chamber, thermostat, and electrode assembly of Gibson and McIlwain (1965). A conical glass tissue chamber (*a*) has three openings (*b*, *b'*, and *b'*), two for circulating fluid and one for the adjustment of fluid level and connection to the indifferent electrode *c*. The chamber is supported by a Perspex frame (*dd*) which fits onto the top of a glass thermostat bath (*e*). The baffle (*f*) deflects gas so that it passes over the moist surface of a tissue slice resting on a grid (*g*). A heating coil (*h*) is carried on a Perspex support and controlled by the thermistor (*j*). The Perspex and steel mounting for the chamber (*k*) is carried by the sliding lathe mounts (*l*), the lower of which is bolted to a steel plate fixed to the concrete block (*cb*). The microelectrode assembly (*n*) carries a glass microelectrode (*m*) flexibly attached to a nonpolarizable electrode which plugs into a socket mounted on a Perspex block. This block carries a grounded shield and is attached to the face of a micromanipulator to give vertical movements which are signaled by the potentiometer (*p*). The micro-injection pipette (*q*) is shown in position, but without its mounting, which is supported by a vertical pillar.

tubing, to a tip diameter of about 40 μm, and sealed with picene wax onto a bent hypodermic syringe needle. The micrometer syringe is fixed to a micromanipulator mounted near the chamber. Double-and triple-barreled pipettes are also made from similar tubing which was fused together before drawing. One barrel is fixed to the micrometer syringe as described above, and the other barrel(s) are attached by polyvinylchloride tubing to other micrometer syringe(s) placed near the chamber.

A binocular microscope (*bm*) is mounted independently on the base plate, and swung above the chamber when required, to view the tissue slice, pipette, and microelectrode. An eye-piece graticule enables horizontal distances between pipette and microelectrode to be measured.

Stimulation and extracellular recording. Stimulation and extracellular recording are carried out with silver electrodes, as described by Yamamoto and McIlwain (1966). The surface of the medium is lowered to the level of the nylon mesh in order to reduce short-circuiting of the potential by the medium. The stimulating electrode, consisting of a pair of ball-tipped silver wires (0.5-mm tip diameter, 1-mm tip distance), is placed at the chosen sites, e.g., on the frontal end of the lateral olfactory tract. Stimulation is carried out with rectangular pulses of 1- to 9-V potential and of 20- to 200-μsec duration. The recording electrode is also a ball-tipped silver wire. The potential is fed into a Tektronix oscilloscope (type 502) and photographed with a Cossor oscilloscope camera, model No. 1458.

VIII. APPENDIX II: A SUPERFUSION SYSTEM FOR METABOLIC STUDIES DURING TISSUE EXCITATION

A superfusion system for metabolic studies during tissue excitation, which enables four to seven samples of tissue to be studied simultaneously, was described by McIlwain and Snyder (1970). The samples are held in quick-transfer holders (Fig. 6*A*) which also carry electrodes by which electrical stimuli can be applied at chosen times. The holders are fitted to beakers carrying incubation solutions, and the beakers are sealed so that chosen gas atmospheres can be used. The beakers are held in an incubating bath (see McIlwain and Rodnight, 1962), which also carry distributors for the gas mixtures and for electrical stimuli.

The beakers also carry fine inflow and outflow tubes from a Technicon peristaltic pump, which supplies the flow of incubating solution at defined rates. Additions can be made to the solutions at chosen times, or the superfusing solution can be altered by transferring the inflow tubes to different bottles. The outflow tubes from the pump run to sample receivers, usually racks of test tubes, and the outflow is transferred from one tube to the next at measured intervals, usually of 1 or 2 min. The normal rate of flow of the pump is 3.2 ml/min; solutions require 2 min after leaving their bottles to reach the incubating beaker containing tissue, and 1 min after leaving the beaker to reach the sample tubes. Mixing does not occur during these intervals; the tubes are 0.8-mm internal diam., non-wettable, and of analytical grade.

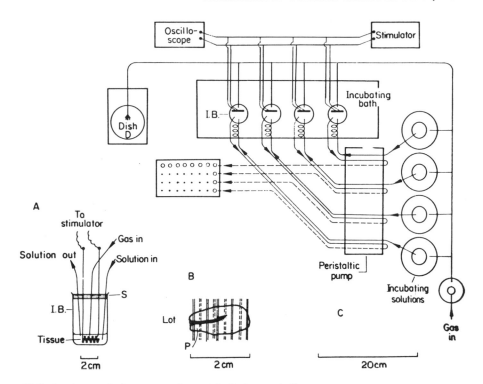

FIG. 6. A superfusion system for metabolic-tissue studies.

A: Tissue in transfer holder in incubation beaker (*I.B.*), which receives tubes bringing incubation solution and gas mixture, and removing incubation solution for sampling. The transfer holder, only part of which is shown, carries electrodes and is described by McIlwain and Rodnight (1962); the plastic seal (*S*) retains the chosen gas atmosphere during incubation; excess gas escapes at the holder. *B:* A sample of piriform lobe of the guinea pig which carries the lateral olfactory tract (*LOT*) between the electrodes of a quick-transfer holder; in some experiments, these electrodes were bared only at point *P*. For a fuller and more accurate drawing of the electrodes, see McIlwain and Rodnight (1962). *C:* Plan of incubating arrangements for four incubation-beakers *I.B.*, each with a tissue sample, receiving incubation solutions from separate reservoirs through a Technicon Autoanalyzer peristaltic pump and warming coils. The incubation solutions in their reservoirs and in the incubation bath receive the chosen gas mixture, usually 95% O_2–5% CO_2 (v/v). The pump also removes fluid from each incubation vessel to racks of sample tubes. The gas mixture is also supplied to the incubation solution in a crystallizing dish (*D*), in a small subsidiary bath at 38°C, and tissue samples are mounted in their transfer holders while floating in the bath *D*.

Electrical stimulation. The quick-transfer holders carry enameled silver wire which is bared at the portions at which it is to act as electrodes, giving the pattern of electrodes shown in Fig. 6*B*. Pulses of chosen frequency, potential, and duration are derived from a condenser-discharge stimulator and are applied to the electrodes as specified in individual experiments. Pulses are monitored throughout application by display on an oscilloscope, which is also used to demonstrate continuity of electrical connection at each electrode as it was operated from the stimulator. The potential gradients established in incubating fluids between electrodes of the characteristics used have been reported by McIlwain and Rodnight (1962). Pulses typically delivered at 5 to 50/sec are of exponential time-voltage relationship with time constants of 0.1 to 0.4 msec, of alternating polarity, and of 1 to 10 V in peak potential.

IX. REFERENCES

Anguiano, G., and McIlwain, H. (1951): Convulsive agents and the phosphates of brain examined *in vitro*. *British Journal of Pharmacology and Chemotherapy*, 6:448–453.

Baldessarini, R. J., and Kopin, I. J. (1966): Tritiated norepinephrine: Release from brain slices by electrical stimulation. *Science*, 152:1630–1631.

Bollard, B. M., and McIlwain, H. (1957): Metabolism and metabolic response to electrical pulses in white matter from the central nervous system. *Biochemical Journal*, 66:651–655.

Brierley, J. B., and McIlwain, H. (1956): Metabolic properties of cerebral tissues modified by neoplasia and by freezing. *Journal of Neurochemistry*, 1:109–118.

Campbell, W. J. (1967): Responses *in vitro* from the piriform cortex of the rat, and their susceptibility to centrally-acting drugs. *Journal of Neurochemistry*, 14:937–938.

Chase, T. N., Katz, R. I., and Kopin, I. J. (1969): Release of ^{3}H-serotonin from brain slices. *Journal of Neurochemistry*, 16:607–615.

Cummins, J. T., and McIlwain, H. (1961): Electrical pulses and the potassium and other ions of isolated cerebral tissues. *Biochemical Journal*, 79:330–341.

Gibson, I. M., and McIlwain, H. (1965): Continuous recording of changes in membrane potential in mammalian cerebral tissues *in vitro;* recovery after depolarization by added substances. *Journal of Physiology*, 176:261–283.

Greengard, P., and Kuo, J. F. (1970): On the mechanism of action of cyclic AMP. *Advances in Biochemical Psychopharmacology*, Vol. 3. Raven Press, New York, pp. 287–306.

Greengard, O., and McIlwain, H. (1955): Anticonvulsants and the metabolism of separated mammalian cerebral tissues. *Biochemical Journal*, 61:61–68.

Harvey, J. A., and McIlwain, H. (1969): Electrical phenomena and isolated tissues from the brain. In: *Handbook of Neurochemistry*, Vol. 2, edited by A. Lajtha. Plenum Press, New York, pp. 115–136.

Kakiuchi, S., Rall, T. W., and McIlwain, H. (1969): The effect of electrical stimulation upon the accumulation of adenosine 3',5'-phosphate in isolated cerebral tissue. *Journal of Neurochemistry*, 16:485–491.

Katz, R. I., and Kopin, I. J. (1969): Release of norepinephrine-^{3}H and serotonin-^{3}H evoked from brain slices by electrical-field stimulation—calcium dependency and the effects of lithium, ouabain and tetrodotoxin. *Biochemical Pharmacology*, 18:1935–1939.

Kawai, N. (1970): Release of 5-hydroxytryptamine from slices of superior colliculus by optic tract stimulation. *Neuropharmacology*, 9:395–397.

Kawai, N., and Yamamoto, C. (1969): Effects of 5-hydroxytryptamine, LSD and related compounds on electrical activities evoked *in vitro* in thin sections from the superior colliculus. *International Journal of Neuropharmacology*, 8:437–449.

Kurokawa, M. (1960): Metabolic consequences of localized application of electrical pulses to sections of cerebral white matter. *Journal of Neurochemistry*, 5:283–292.

Li, C.-L., and McIlwain, H. (1957): Maintenance of resting membrane potentials in slices of mammalian cerebral cortex and other tissues *in vitro*. *Journal of Physiology*, 139:178–190.

McIlwain, H. (1951): Metabolic response *in vitro* to electrical stimulation of sections of mammalian brain. *Biochemical Journal*, 49:382–393.

McIlwain, H. (1953): Substances which support respiration and metabolic response to electrical impulses in human cerebral tissues. *Journal of Neurology, Neurosurgery and Psychiatry*, 16:257–266.

McIlwain, H. (1969): Cerebral energy metabolism and membrane phenomena. In: *Basic Mechanisms of the Epilepsies*, edited by H. H. Jasper, A. A. Ward, and A. Pope. Little, Brown and Co., Boston, pp. 83–103.

McIlwain, H. (1971): Cyclic AMP and tissues of the brain. In: *Effects of Drugs on Cellular Control Mechanisms*, edited by B. R. Rabin. Macmillan, London, pp. 281–302.

McIlwain, H., Ayres, P. J. W., and Forda, O. (1952): Metabolic response to electrical stimulation in separated portions of human cerebral tissues. *Journal of Mental Science*, 98:265–272.

McIlwain, H., and Bachelard, H. S. (1971): *Biochemistry and the Central Nervous Systems*, 4th edition. Churchill, London.

McIlwain, H., and Pull, I. (1972): Release of adenine derivatives on electrical stimulation of superfused tissues from the brain. *Journal of Physiology*, 221:9–10P.

McIlwain, H., and Rodnight, R. (1962): *Practical Neurochemistry*. Churchill, London.

McIlwain, H., and Snyder, S. H. (1970): Stimulation of piriform and neocortical tissues in an *in vitro* flow-system: Metabolic properties and release of putative neurotransmitters. *Journal of Neurochemistry*, 17:521–530.

Pull, I., and McIlwain, H. (1972): Metabolism of ^{14}C-adenine and derivatives at cerebral tissues, superfused and electrically stimulated. *Biochemical Journal*, 126:965–973.

Pumphrey, A. M. (1969): Incorporation of ^{32}P-orthophosphate into brain-slice phospholipids and their precursors. *Biochemical Journal*, 112:61–70.

Richards, C. D., and McIlwain, H. (1967): Electrical responses in brain samples. *Nature*, 215:704–707.

Richards, C. D., and Sercombe, R. (1968): Electrical activity observed in guinea pig olfactory cortex maintained *in vitro*. *Journal of Physiology*, 197:667–683.

Rowsell, E. V. (1954): Applied electrical pulses and the ammonia and acetylcholine of isolated cerebral cortex slices. *Biochemical Journal*, 57:666–673.

Santos, J. N., Hempstead, K. W., Kopp, L. E., and Miech, R. P. (1968): Nucleotide metabolism in rat brain. *Journal of Neurochemistry*, 15:367–376.

Sattin, A., and Rall, T. W. (1970): The effect of adenosine and adenine nucleotides on the cyclic adenosine 3',5'-phosphate content of guinea pig cerebral cortex slices. *Molecular Pharmacology*, 6:13–23.

Shimizu, H., Creveling, C. R., and Daly, J. (1970): Stimulated formation of adenosine 3',5'-cyclic phosphate in cerebral cortex: Synergism between electrical activity and biogenic amines. *Proceedings of the National Academy of Sciences*, 65:1033–1040.

Siggins, G. R., Hoffer, B. J., and Bloom, F. E. (1969): Cyclic adenosine monophosphate: Possible mediator for norepinephrine effects on cerebellar Purkinje cells. *Science*, 165:1018–1020.

Srinivasan, V., Neal, M. J., and Mitchell, J. F. (1969): The effect of electrical stimulation and high potassium concentration on the efflux of ^{3}H-γ-aminobutyric acid from brain slices. *Journal of Neurochemistry*, 16:1235–1244.

Weller, M., and Rodnight, R. (1970): Stimulation by cyclic AMP of intrinsic protein kinase activity in ox brain membrane preparations. *Nature*, 225:187–188.

Yamamoto, C. (1970): Synaptic transmission between mossy fibre and hippocampal neurons studied *in vitro* in thin brain sections. *Proceedings of the Japan Academy*, 46:1041–1045.

Yamamoto, C., and Kawai, N. (1967): Origin of the direct cortical response as studied *in vitro* in thin cortical sections. *Experientia*, 23:821–822.

Yamamoto, C., and Kawai, N. (1968): Generation of the seizure discharge in thin sections from the guinea pig brain in chloride-free media *in vitro*. *Japanese Journal of Physiology*, 18:620–631.

Yamamoto, C., and McIlwain, H. (1966): Electrical activities in thin sections from the mammalian brain maintained in chemically defined media *in vitro*. *Journal of Neurochemistry*, 13:1333–1343.

12

Tissue Culture Models of Epileptiform Activity

Stanley M. Crain*

OUTLINE

*Kennedy Scholar at the Rose F. Kennedy Center for Research in Mental Retardation and Human Development, Albert Einstein College of Medicine, Bronx, New York

I. INTRODUCTION

The tissue culture method combines ontogenetic and microsurgical dissection of the mammalian brain so as to produce dramatic geometrical simplification while permitting sequential development of many significant types of organotypic CNS structures and functions. The feasibility of this model system is based upon demonstrations during the past decade, that small groups of embryonic mammalian CNS neurons possess intrinsic "self-organizing" properties even after isolation in culture at stages prior to the formation of synapses *in situ*. Microelectrode recordings in explants of fetal mammalian spinal cord, brainstem, and cerebral cortex tissues have shown that these neurons can still develop *in vitro* the capacity to generate complex patterned repetitive-spike or slow-wave discharges resembling the activity of synaptic networks of the central nervous system (Crain, 1966, 1970a). Arrays of CNS neurons growing in a culture chamber on a thin coverglass offer, therefore, a "window" not only for direct observation but also for flexible experimental manipulation of the intricate cellular networks of the *mammalian* brain.

Since these explanted CNS tissues often generate long-lasting, rhythmic, highly synchronized bioelectric discharges with strong mimicry of important components of normal as well as hyperexcitable EEG patterns (Crain, 1966), they provide a valuable model system for studies of mechanisms underlying epileptiform activity (Crain, 1969). Experiments can be carried out on the cultured CNS tissues under rigorously controlled physico-chemical conditions, and microelectrodes can be accurately positioned with respect to the neurons, under direct microscopic observation at high magnification, for long periods of study.

II. CULTURE TECHNIQUES

A. Slab explants

The procedure which has produced the most highly differentiated CNS cultures involves explanation of small fragments (ca. 1 mm^3) of embryonic tissue (e.g., fetal rodent brain or spinal cord; Fig. 1) onto collagen-coated coverglasses, and incubation at 35°C in Maximow depression-slide chambers, as "lying-drop" preparations (Bornstein, 1964; Peterson et al., 1965; Peterson and Crain, 1970; see also Moscona et al., 1965, for more general details and references regarding culture techniques). The explants are

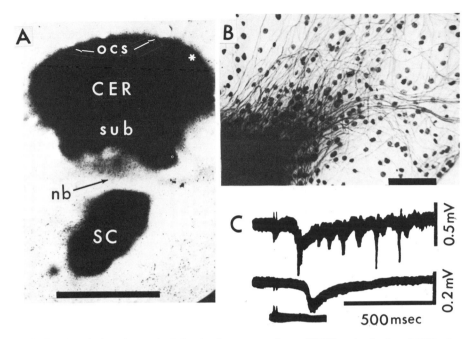

FIG. 1. Coupled explants of 15-day fetal mouse cerebrum (CER) and spinal cord (SC) after 2 weeks in culture. *A:* Low-power photomicrograph shows arrangement of explants to facilitate development of neuritic bridge (nb) between cord cross-section and subcortical region (sub) of cerebral slab. Original cortical (pial) surface (ocs) is at opposite edge of cerebral explant and shows characteristic crescent shape which it generally maintains for months *in vitro* (Bornstein, 1964). Focal recording electrodes can be positioned, in contact with the tissue, at regions near labels "ocs" and "CER", to obtain recordings analogous to those from superficial and deep cortical layers *in situ* (see Fig. 3). Distance of locus from "ocs" is referred to as "cortical depth" (see text). Scale: 1 mm. *B.* Higher-power view of "ocs" edge of cerebral explant (near *), showing numerous neurites which have emerged from the explant, along with glial cells, and grown onto the transparent collagen-coated coverglass (Bodian silver-impregnation). Scale: 50 μm. *C:* Electric stimulus applied to neurites located about 300 μm from "ocs" edge of cerebral explant (far beyond field of view in *B*) triggers complex repetitive discharge in the cerebral tissue (upper sweep; *cf.* Figs. 3 and 5) followed, after a still longer latency, by a simpler positive slow-wave response in the coupled spinal cord explant (*cf.* Figs. 4 and 6). *Note:* in this and all subsequent figures, time and amplitude calibrations, and specification of recording and stimulating sites, *apply to all succeeding records, until otherwise noted.* Upward deflection indicates negativity at active recording electrode, and onset of stimuli is indicated, where necessary, by sharp pulse (or arrow) or break in base line of 3rd sweep. From Crain and Bornstein (1964) and Crain et al. (1968b) with permission of the publisher.

cut so that one dimension is well under 1 mm, to facilitate diffusion of metabolites to and from the cells within the central region of the tissue. Dissection of embryonic CNS tissues and slicing to appropriate explant size require considerable skill to minimize surgical trauma to the extremely fragile structures. The culture medium is changed twice a week and generally contains mammalian serum in a balanced salt solution, with embryo extract or other special nutrients. Typical media used for culturing many of the CNS explants described in this review consists of human placental serum (25 to 40%) and Eagle's synthetic medium (25%) in Simms' balanced salt solution (BSS),[1] supplemented with 600 mg% glucose, and, in some cases, with rat or chick embryo extract and insulin. The total volume of medium is about 0.1 ml and the overlying air space about 2 ml. Care must be taken to ensure sterility during all of these experimental manipulations, especially since antibiotics are generally omitted to avoid possible noxious side-effects of these agents on neural tissues. Meticulous procedures are also necessary to minimize chemical impurities in the culture-chamber components and in the nutrient media, since CNS tissues are particularly sensitive to many chemical contaminants.

B. Dissociated cells

Methods have also been developed to dissociate embryonic tissues into suspensions of completely isolated cells, using various combinations of enzymatic and mechanical agitation procedures (Moscona, 1965). These techniques have recently begun to be successfully applied to CNS tissues so as to permit neuritic growth and synaptogenesis in cultures of such dissociated neurons (Meller et al., 1969; Shimada et al., 1969a,b). In some cases, the suspensions of cells have been cultured in flasks mounted on a rotating-shaker apparatus, which appears to facilitate more systematic reaggregation of the dissociated cells into organotypic arrays (ca. 1 mm^3) resembling laminated cortex *in situ* (De Long, 1970; Seeds, 1971). In other cases, the dissociated cells have been explanted onto collagen-coated coverglasses, and cultured in the usual Maximow slide chambers, to permit formation of a more graded series of reaggregates varying from two to a few hundred neurons per cluster (Bornstein and Model, 1972). In the latter experiments, 18-day fetal mouse cerebral neocortex or 13- to 14-day spinal cord and brainstem are dissociated by enzymatic treatment in 0.25% trypsin (in a Ca^{++}- and Mg^{++}-free physiological salt solution) and repeated pipetting. Suspensions of cells in concentrations of about 10^6 cells per ml of standard culture medium are explanted onto collagen films, using 0.05 to 0.1 ml per coverglass (22-mm diameter). This procedure produces cultures

---

[1]Composition of Simms' balanced salt solution (BSS), in mmoles per liter glass-distilled water: NaCl, 137; KCl, 2.7; $CaCl_2$, 1.0; $MgCl_2$, 1.0; Na_2HPO_4, 1.36; NaH_2PO_4, 0.15; $NaHCO_3$, 6.0; and glucose, 5.5.

containing many widely dispersed, small clusters of neurons and glial cells, connected by neuritic bridges and organized into complex synaptic networks (Crain and Bornstein, 1972; see Fig. 6 and Section IV C).

III. MICROELECTRODE RECORDING SYSTEMS

Cultures selected after serial microscopic examinations during days or weeks of incubation in Maximow slides are transferred to a micrurgical chamber for electrophysiologic study. For most studies, it is desirable to mount the micro-electrodes on micromanipulators so that the electrode tips can be directly observed, at high magnification, as they are positioned near, or inside of, the cultured neurons (Fig. 2). The culture coverglass is attached to the floor of a small glass-bottomed dish (with small clamps or grease), and a thin layer of fluid (0.2 to 1 ml) is generally used during recordings. This fluid overlay may be the original complex culture medium or a simpler physiological salt solution, e.g., Simms' BSS alone or supplemented with 10 to 20% serum (see footnote 1).

An inverted microscope, with a long working-distance condenser lens (10 to 20 mm), permits use of high-powered objectives close to the culture coverglass without serious restriction of the working space for manipulation of microelectrodes. The apparatus illustrated in Fig. 2 utilizes newly developed miniaturized magnetically coupled micromanipulators incorporated directly into a scaled micrurgical culture chamber (Baer and Crain, 1971). The microelectrodes can be precisely positioned, in three dimensions, by manual manipulation of magnets located on the *external* surface of the glass roof of the chamber (Fig. 2, EH and EV). Various conventional large micromanipulators can, of course, also be used by removing the glass roof of the chamber and introducing the electrodes directly into the culture (see reviews in Crain, 1970b, 1972a, which also include methods for similar micrurgical studies with upright microscopes). Provisions must then be made, however, to avoid excessive evaporation of the culture medium, especially when recordings are to be carried out at about 35°C for long periods.

Temperature can be conveniently maintained at 34 to 37°C by infrared lamps positioned about 2 feet from the chamber (and connected to variable-voltage supplies for intensity control). Small thermistor- (or thermocouple-) probes in the chamber can be used with monitoring or thermoregulating circuits. In open-chamber setups, partial enclosures may be constructed to maintain high humidity over the culture, without serious restrictions on micromanipulation procedures (Crain, 1970b, 1972a), or an overlay of mineral oil may be used (Kopac, 1959; Lieberman, 1967; Okun, 1972). The pH of the bicarbonate-buffered medium is maintained at about 7.4 by flowing 3 to 5% CO_2 through the chamber. It is convenient to construct a socket in the floor of the chamber, so that the culture dish can be plugged into position from below (Fig. 2). This permits rapid insertion or removal of cultures with minimal disturbance of complex microelectrode arrays, but requires a large

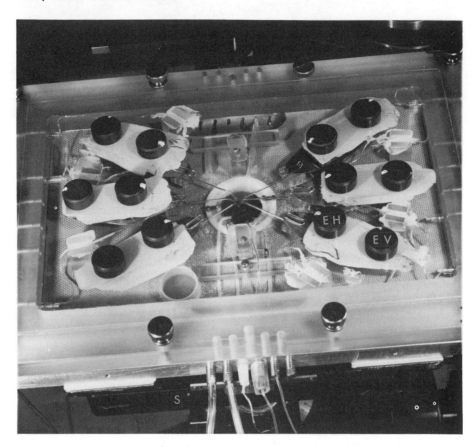

FIG. 2. Sealed micrurgical chamber with six miniature, magnetically coupled micromanipulators suspended from greased glass roof. Note pairs of external, manually operated control magnets (EH and EV), resting on glass roof, which are used to position micropipette electrodes (bent at right angle near tip) into central glass-bottomed culture dish. Entire array is mounted on mechanical stage (S) of inverted microscope (stage is positioned in three dimensions by standard rack and pinion controls). Microscope condenser lens and illuminator are normally located above central region of chamber (removed for clarity), and microscope objective lens is located below culture dish. Flexible insulated silver wires connect electrodes with sockets sealed into chamber wall. External couplings can then be readily made from these sockets to electronic recording and stimulating apparatus. Teflon tubes for perfusion of the culture dish, leads for bath electrodes, temperature probes, etc., are all sealed into the floor of the chamber (entering through gasketed holes in front edge of metal baseplate), and they are mounted so as to contact fluid in the peripheral region of the culture dish. From Crain (1972a) with permission of the publisher (see also Baer and Crain, 1971).

cut-out in the mechanical stage of the microscope. Stable bioelectric activity can generally be maintained for many hours in properly constructed, partly open, moist chambers (Crain, 1970b). The sealed chamber array (Fig. 2), however, permits far more rigorous control of the physico-chemical environment of the culture during electrophysiologic studies, and sterilized assemblies are now being developed for longitudinal bioelectric recordings over days or weeks, instead of the usual limit of less than 1 day (Crain, 1970c, 1972a).

Bioelectric activities of single neurons or small groups can be effectively recorded extracellularly with microelectrodes of 1- to 5-μm tip diameters. The electrode tips must be carefully positioned near or into the neural tissue so that they are located sufficiently close to the active cells without damaging the excitable membranes. Distances of a few microns are often critical, especially when the active neurons are covered by connective tissue or other short-circuiting membranes. Micropipettes filled with isotonic NaCl (or a more complete physiological salt solution) provide a reliable means of contacting the cultured cells. Use of these micro-salt-bridges avoids possible toxic effects of direct cell contacts with electrode metals, and stable electrode potentials can be obtained by inserting a chloridized silver wire into the pipette shaft (see Appendix; Frank and Becker, 1964; Kennard, 1958).

Pairs of electrodes are generally positioned (under direct visual control, at 100 to 400×) one against, or inside, the tissue and the other in the fluid nearby. A large chloridized silver wire in the periphery of the culture bath serves as a ground electrode. Bioelectric signals are recorded with differential, high input-impedance preamplifiers and a four-channel oscilloscope (passband generally from 0.2 cps to 10 kc). Small unity-gain probes, utilizing a field-effect transistor (FET) circuit as an impedance-lowering device, can be mounted close to the recording electrodes (Cechner et al., 1970). The output from these field-effect transistor units can then be fed into conventional high-gain preamplifiers which need not have high input impedance. Single-ended, rather than differential, recording is often adequate in cases where shielding from extraneous electric fields is optimal. Electric (square-wave) stimuli, from 0.1 to 0.5 msec in duration and up to 100 μA in strength, are applied locally through pairs of saline-filled pipettes with tips of about 10 μm diameter and 1 MΩ resistance. Stimulating currents of 1 to 10 μA are generally adequate if the cathodal electrode is properly positioned close to normally excitable neurons, unless excessive (shunting) connective tissue is present. R-F stimulus-isolation circuits are used to minimize shock artifacts. The stimulating current can be localized to individual neurons or small group of cells. Slight withdrawal of the stimulating electrode from contact with the excitable tissue results in sharp attenuation of all bioelectric responses that are mediated by neural pathways.

Methods for computer analysis of tape-recorded bioelectric activities obtained with extracellular microelectrodes in cultured neural tissues, e.g., interspike-interval and "cross-interval" histograms, have been recently described (Cechner et al., 1970; Cunningham et al., 1970; Schlapfer, 1969). These quantitative methods should be particularly valuable for analyses of organotypic CNS networks during long-term recordings with microelectrodes sealed into the culture chamber.

Similar micrurgical arrangements are used for intracellular recordings, using more finely tapered micropipettes, with tips of about 0.1 μm (30 to 100 MΩ when filled with 3 M KCl; for technical details, see Crain, 1972*a*). A serious obstacle to systematic intracellular studies of neurons in cultured tissues has been the frequent growth of thin layers of tough connective tissue over the explants (Crain, 1956; Hild and Tasaki, 1962; Cechner et al., 1970). These mechanical barriers often lead to tip breakage or to crude impalements by a pipette tip covered with fibrous tissue debris. In some cases, these fibrous layers can be selectively softened with proteolytic enzymes, e.g., trypsin or pronase, but this procedure involves the risk of serious disruption of the entire tissue culture array and its detachment from the collagen-coated coverglass. This problem appears to be less serious in dissociated cell cultures where much of the connective tissue is digested away *prior* to explantation (Scott et al., 1969; Fischbach, 1970; Varon and Raiborn, 1971). Piezoelectric or electromagnetic devices may be useful to produce microelectrode thrusts more suitable for reliable impalements in these explants.

Successful intracellular recordings of cultured neurons have been limited, so far, to microelectrodes positioned with conventional massive micromanipulators during short-term experiments in open chambers (*vide supra*). Attempts are now in progress to carry out similar intracellular studies in CNS cultures concomitant with, or at least directly following, long-term extracellular recordings in closed chambers with sealed-in magnetically coupled micromanipulators. This combined approach should facilitate analysis of the role of specific types of neuronal and glial cells in the generation of the complex organotypic discharge patterns of cultured CNS tissues. Neutralized input-capacity preamplifiers, with high input resistance and low grid current, facilitate reliable intracellular recordings of membrane resting and action potentials (Frank and Becker, 1964). For simultaneous recording and stimulation through a single micropipette, bridge circuits (e.g., Araki and Otani, 1955) have been used (Fischbach, 1970; Varon and Raiborn, 1971; Crain, 1972*a*).

IV. PROPERTIES OF ORGANOTYPIC BIOELECTRIC DISCHARGES IN CNS CULTURES

A. Ontogenetic development *in vitro*

Cerebral and other CNS tissues in culture constitute a particularly valuable model system for studies of the *development* of hyperexcitability properties of the CNS *in situ*. Since cultures of embryonic CNS tissues have shown far greater structural and functional integrity than explants from adult sources (Crain, 1966; *cf.* Kiernan and Pettit, 1971), various stages of CNS maturation are readily available for experimental study under controlled conditions *in vitro*. Explantation of CNS tissues prior to formation of synapses in the embryo provides, in particular, cellular arrays in which synaptogenesis and development of synaptic networks can be analyzed in depth.   Explants of fetal or newborn mouse cerebral neocortex, for example, show no signs of complex bioelectric activites during the first few days *in vitro*.   Simple spike potentials can be evoked with electric stimuli (Fig. 3*A*), but no evidence of transmission of impulses from one neuron to another has been detected in these immature tissues.   By 3 to 5 days in culture, however, evoked potentials with durations of the order of 400 msec may occur (Fig. 3*B*), with latencies of as much as 100 msec following the early spike response to a single stimulus.   Repetitive spike barrages often appear concomitant with these long-duration potentials.   The latter increase in amplitude and regularity during the following week *in vitro*, and their durations generally decrease below 100 msec (Fig. 3*C*). They often show characteristic negative polarity (Fig. 3*B, C:* upper sweeps) when recorded with a microelectrode located near the original pial surface of the cortex (Fig. 3*X*), whereas potentials recorded simultaneously from *deep* loci tend to be positive and even longer in latency and duration.   A sharp phase-reversal may occur at a critical "depth" of 200 to 400 μm. Facilitation of these complex evoked responses can be demonstrated with paired stimuli spaced at long test-intervals.   Small, oscillatory (15 to 20 per sec) potentials appear, at times, during the long-duration evoked response (Fig. 3*B*), and both components of the after-discharge may occur spontaneously (Crain, 1964, 1966, 1969; Crain and Bornstein, 1964; morphological correlates in Bornstein, 1964).   Strychnine and eserine, moreover, produce characteristic enhancement of these discharges, whereas procaine, xylocaine, and increased Mg^{++} can selectively block the complex bioelectric activities of cerebral explants at levels which still permit generation of propagated spike potentials (Crain et al., 1968a; see also Fig. 7 and Sections IV B and C).

Although intracellularly recorded postsynaptic potentials have not yet been obtained from cerebral tissue cultures, analysis of the extracellular data leaves little doubt that the complex bioelectric activities described above are mediated through synaptic networks. The characteristic negative and positive slow waves recorded from superficial and deep regions of the cerebral explants appear to be due to summated postsynaptic potentials that are predominantly excitatory and inhibitory, respectively. The negative evoked response recorded from superficial sites in cerebral explants shows marked similarities in temporal pattern to the prolonged excitatory postsynaptic potentials evoked in cortical neurons of the neonatal kitten *in situ* (Purpura et al., 1960) and to the responses evoked by local electric stimuli in neonatal rat cerebral cortex *in situ* (Armstrong-James and Williams, 1963). Furthermore, the positive evoked response recorded from deeper regions

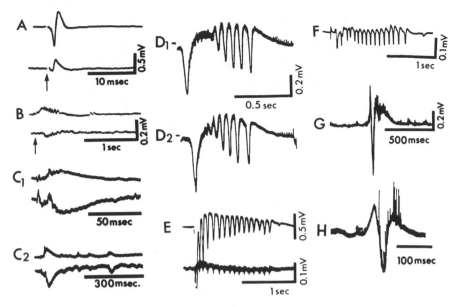

FIG. 3. Transition from simple to complex evoked responses and oscillatory after-discharges in cultured cerebral cortex tissue, during first 2 weeks after explantation from 1-day-old mouse. *A:* 3 days *in vitro*. Simultaneous records showing simple spikes evoked, at "cortical depths" (see Fig. 1) of 200 μm (upper sweep) and 400 μm, by stimulus applied near subcortical edge of explant (about 800 μm from original cortical surface). *B:* Early signs of complex response patterns recorded, at much slower sweep rates, in same culture and at same electrode loci as in *A*. Long-duration negativity arises gradually with a latency of about 100 msec after the early superficial spike (upper sweep); also note long-duration positivity which develops with a still longer latency after early deep spike (lower sweep). Arrow indicates onset of dual stimuli spaced 50 msec apart. Note that the second pair of stimuli, applied 1 second after first pair, is ineffective. C_1: 10 days *in vitro*. Simultaneous records of characteristic evoked potentials at "cortical depths" of 250 μm (upper sweep) and 650 μm to following single stimulus applied at depth of 700 μm (but 300 μm from deep recording site). Note 60-msec, negative evoked response in superficial region and positive response in deep zone which is similar, but of longer duration and greater latency. C_2: Same as C_1, but at slower sweep rate. Note that small-amplitude repetitive potentials at 10 to 20 per sec follow primary responses at both sites and are also of opposite polarities. *D, E:* 2 to 6 weeks *in vitro*. Repetitive oscillatory after-discharges evoked in two mouse cerebral explants by single stimulus applied several hundred micra from recording site. Lower record in *E* shows simultaneous recording from another region of explant (800 μm away). Note variation in latency of onset of repetitive discharge following initial, positive evoked potential ($D_{1,2}$). *F:* Characteristic repetitive after-discharge evoked in cerebral cortical slab in 5-day-old kitten, 3 days after neuronal isolation, *in situ*. Note similarity between this response pattern and those obtained from cerebral explants. *G:* Spontaneous discharge recorded in mouse cerebral explant (2 weeks *in vitro*). *H:* Characteristic paroxysmal abnormal wave recorded in epileptic cortex of adult monkey, *in situ*. Note similarity of the triphasic, initially negative complexes in *G* and *H*, with superimposed bursts of unit spikes. *A–E* and *G* from Crain (1964); *F* from Purpura and Housepian (1961); and *H* from Schmidt et al., (1959), with permission of the publishers.

in young cerebral explants shows a striking resemblance to the extraordinary long-lasting inhibitory postsynaptic potentials characteristic of immature neocortical neurons *in situ* (Purpura et al., 1965; Purpura, 1969, 1971). The duration of evoked responses in many of the cerebral explants also decreases during maturation in culture (*cf.* Fig. 3C vs. 3B), as occurs *in situ*. Extracellular microelectrode recordings from cerebral explants appear, then, to provide at least a crude monitor of neuronal PSP activities, but these data must be interpreted with caution pending correlative studies with intracellular electrodes. The onset of complex bioelectric activity in these mouse cerebral explants after 3 to 5 days *in vitro* is, moreover, consonant with the paucity of synaptic junctions observed in electron micrographs of the tissues at explantation and their abundance in 10-day cultures (Model et al., 1971).

B. Discharge patterns in long-term explants

1. Rhythmic oscillatory discharge sequences

Complex, rhythmic oscillatory after-discharges are quite prominent in many cerebral explants after 1 to 2 weeks *in vitro*. These stereotyped repetitive sequences generally consist of 3 to 12 large diphasic potentials, each lasting 25 to 50 msec and occurring at rates of 5 to 15 per sec (Figs. 3 and 4). A large, early evoked potential is often followed by a long delay prior to appearance of a repetitive series of predominantly positive potentials, which, in some cases, gradually increase in amplitude and then terminate abruptly (Figs. 1C, 3D, E, and 5A, C₂). The positive sharp waves often appear to be superimposed on a much longer lasting negativity, of the order of 1 sec in duration. Recordings at multiple sites indicate that these repetitive discharges are highly synchronized over large areas of the explant (Fig. 3E), and they may occur spontaneously (Fig. 5B, C₁) as well as in response to local stimulation of a few neurons, or even of a single neurite in the outgrowth zone of the explant (Fig. 1C). Analyses of the spontaneous discharge patterns in these and other types of cultured CNS tissues indicate that "pacemaker" neurons may generate spikes sporadically, or rhythmically, and these spontaneous impulses can then trigger widespread network discharges throughout the explant, depending upon the excitability threshold of the latter system (Corner and Crain, 1969, 1972; see also Crain, 1972b). These complex discharges last up to several seconds, and they may occur at regular intervals of the order of 1 to 10 sec, although activity patterns are often quite irregular. Some explants also show clear periodicity in the recurrence of phases of relative activity and inactivity, with cycle times ranging up to about 10 min. The tissue culture model is further strengthened by the demonstration that spontaneous patterned bioelectric discharges in spinal cord explants can trigger coordinated repetitive contractions of innervated skeletal muscle fibers (Fig. 4; Crain, 1970*b;* Crain et al., 1970).

The rhythmic oscillatory discharges in cerebral cultures show remarkable similarity to characteristic repetitive sequences evoked by single stimuli in slabs of neonatal kitten cerebral neocortex studied several days after

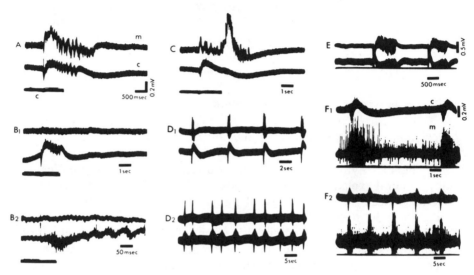

FIG. 4. Complex evoked and spontaneous discharges in coupled *fetal* rodent cord and *adult* rodent muscle explants (6- to 7-week cultures) after introduction of strychnine (10 μg/ml). *A:* Simultaneous recordings of complex oscillatory (ca. 10/sec) after-discharge evoked in mouse spinal cord (2nd sweep: c) and in mouse muscle (1st sweep: m) by single cord stimulus (3rd sweep: c). B_1: After replacement of strychnine by *d*-tubocurarine (10 μg/ml), entire cord-evoked muscle response disappears while characteristic repetitive discharge still occurs in cord. At faster sweep-rate (B_2), primary spike barrage in cord can be seen more clearly, followed by secondary oscillatory (15/sec) after-discharge. *C:* After return to normal medium, a complex repetitive discharge appears again in the muscle, lasting more than 4 sec following a cord stimulus which now evokes a simpler, but still long-lasting, response in the cord. *D:* Similar complex spontaneous discharges occurring rhythmically (at 3- to 5-sec intervals) and synchronously in another pair of coupled mouse cord and muscle explants under strychnine. *E:* Similar spontaneous discharges in coupled explants of *mouse cord* and *rat muscle* (*cf. A*). *F:* Similar spontaneous discharges in coupled explants of *rat* cord and *mouse* muscle. Note repetitive fibrillatory potentials continuing in muscle during intervals between synchronized cord and muscle discharges. (Muscle spikes have been retouched during first 4 sec of second sweep in F_1; spikes during remainder of this record are barely visible at this slow sweep rate, but their amplitude and temporal patterns are actually similar. In F_2, muscle spike bursts which occur synchronously with cord discharges have been reinforced; spikes also continue to occur, at lower frequency, during intervals between periodic discharges of cord and muscle, as in F_1.) From Crain et al. (1970) with permission of the publisher.

chronic neuronal isolation (Fig. 3F; Purpura and Housepian, 1961). Since the complex repetitive discharges in cerebral slabs *in situ* and *in vitro* display marked hyperexcitability properties (Purpura, 1969, and chapter 22 in this volume; Crain, 1969), these cultures may provide a valuable model system for analysis of mechanisms underlying altered behavior of CNS tissues under various conditions of neuronal isolation.

2. Epileptiform discharges

Discharges have been recorded, moreover, in some cerebral explants (Fig. 3G), which show remarkable mimicry of "paroxysmal abnormal waves" obtained with microelectrodes in epileptic cortex *in situ* (Fig. 3H; Schmidt et al., 1959). These epileptiform discharges often occur at relatively high repetition rates of about 1 to 3 per sec, whereas the longer lasting (10/sec) oscillatory sequences tend to be spaced by silent periods of about 3 to 15 sec (Crain, 1969). Spontaneous occurrence of epileptiform and other types of sustained "paroxysmal" activities in some of the cerebral explants may be related to uncontrolled parameters in the tissue culture environment. Depending upon age of the tissue, thickness of the fragment, growth patterns, and other factors, the central zone of many of these (free-hand-dissected) explants becomes necrotic due to relatively poor diffusion of nutrients and waste products to and from this region (Bunge et al., 1965; Peterson et al., 1965). Although healthy, organized tissues surrounding this necrotic core may be maintained for months *in vitro*, neurons at the edge of the degenerated zone may be in a state resembling conditions at an epileptogenic focus near a cortical glial scar *in situ*. Controlled production of miniature epileptogenic foci in cerebral explants by maintenance of physico-chemical gradients critically localized with respect to individual cells may provide a valuable model system to supplement studies of epileptic cortex *in situ*.

3. Effects of pharmacologic agents

Selective pharmacologic and immunologic agents, metabolic inhibitors, and enzymes can be introduced into the bathing medium to produce either acute or chronic alterations in the cultured cells. Diffusion barriers analogous to blood-brain barriers are often far less serious in these relatively unsheathed CNS tissues in culture. As noted above, strychnine leads to appearance of large slow waves in 1-week cerebral explants which increase in amplitude and decrease in duration during the following week *in vitro* (Crain and Bornstein, 1964), clearly resembling the changes in strychnine "sharp-waves" seen during ontogenetic development of mammalian cerebral cortex *in situ* (Bishop, 1950; Crain, 1952; Himwich, 1962). Strychnine may also cause polarity inversion of positive evoked potentials in cerebral explants leading to appearance of characteristic negative slow-waves of large amplitude and long duration. These phenomena can be interpreted as evidence of selective strychnine-blockage of inhibitory (hyperpolarizing) postsynaptic potentials, thereby unmasking excitatory (depolarizing) postsynaptic potential components (Crain, 1969). On the other hand, increasing the glycine or GABA concentration of the culture medium to 10 to 100 μg/ml rapidly and reversibly depresses spontaneous and evoked complex discharges in spinal cord explants (Crain, 1972c). Since glycine and GABA are likely to be functioning as transmitters at inhibitory synapses in the spinal cord (Werman et al., 1968; Curtis et al., 1968; Curtis and Felix, 1971), this evidence provides further support to the strychnine (and picrotoxin: Crain and Peterson, 1964) data suggesting inhibitory circuits in the cord cultures. Similar studies of the effects of glycine, GABA, and other postulated inhibitory mediators (and selective blocking agents) on *cerebral* explants may provide valuable data, especially in conjunction with correlative intracellular recordings, to clarify the mechanisms involved in these depressant effects, *in vitro* and *in situ*.

More drastic effects attributable to development of inhibitory circuits in CNS explants are observed, especially in older cultures, in cases where almost no signs of complex bioelectric activity can be detected in the normal culture medium. Even with large single or repetitive electric stimuli, the responses may be limited to brief spike potentials, often followed by a simple positive wave. Introduction of strychnine reveals, however, that these explants have, indeed, retained their capacity to generate elaborate, organotypic, synaptically mediated discharges, but that in normal culture media, inhibitory circuits effectively quench activation of these networks following initial generation of action potentials in some of the neurons. These observations in CNS cultures may be relevant to problems involved in restoration of function following denervation supersensitivity *in situ* (Crain, 1969) and to mechanisms associated with early embryonic behavior (Crain, 1972b).

Introduction of many other pharmacologic agents has also produced marked enhancement of various features of the complex evoked and spontaneous discharges in cerebral explants, mimicking, at times, epileptiform activities, e.g., acetylcholine, eserine, *d*-tubocurarine and caffeine (Crain, 1966, 1969). The sensitivity of the cultured CNS tissues to some of these alterations in the chemical environment appears, however, to vary widely, even among explants of the same group (see Section V). Therefore, although the CNS culture model may, indeed, be useful for direct studies of the mechanisms of action of many CNS excitants and depressants, especially in cases where experiments *in situ* are complicated by, for example, diffusion barriers or multiplicity of sites of action, standardized biological preparations suitable for quantitative analyses may often be quite difficult to obtain.

4. Complex interactions between coupled cerebral and brainstem explants

More complex tissue culture models can also be designed for studies of the effects of spinal cord, brainstem, or other subcortical tissues on cerebrum (Fig. 1). Rhythmic bioelectric discharges recorded in explants of fetal mouse medulla and cerebral cortex, after formation of neuritic connections *in vitro*, provide a particularly dramatic demonstration of the potentialities of this model system (Fig. 5). Spike barrages in the medulla explant can trigger characteristic oscillatory after-discharges in the cerebral tissue, and analysis of the complex temporal patterns suggests that *inhibitory* feedback mechanisms may develop between and within these explants (Crain et al., 1968*b*). Periodic generation of impulses in medulla "pacemaker" neurons appears to result not only in cerebral excitatory effects, but possibly also in sequential generation of inhibitory postsynaptic potentials in the cerebral explant (Fig. 5; note *positive* cerebral slow waves which often follow spike bursts in medulla). The medulla spike barrage may then be periodically self-quenched (possibly by local recurrent inhibitory networks), thereby attenuating the inhibitory activity to the cerebral explant. These remarks are, of course, highly speculative, but they provide a working hypothesis for further experiments on these complex heterogeneous neural networks, incorporating microelectrode recordings at multiple sites within each explant and correlative intracellular measurements in specific neurons (Crain et al., 1968*b*).

Coupling of pairs of cerebral explants may also provide a useful model for study of mechanisms underlying "mirror-foci" (see Wilder, Chapter 4).

C. Organotypic discharges in small neuronal reaggregates after complete dissociation

A most dramatic demonstration of intrinsic self-organizing properties of CNS neurons has recently been made utilizing small clusters of neurons, after reaggregation *in vitro* of trypsin-dissociated cells (see Section II B), obtained from 18-day fetal mouse cerebral neocortex or 13- to 14-day spinal

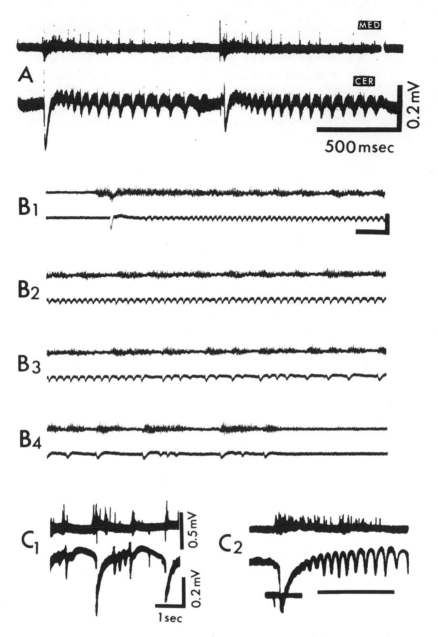

FIG. 5. Rhythmic repetitive discharges occurring synchronously between explants of fetal mouse cerebrum and medulla after formation of interneuronal connections in long-term culture (from 14-day fetus; 3 weeks *in vitro*). *A, B:* Spontaneous activities of medulla and cerebral explants recorded simultaneously in closed chamber with microelectrodes positioned by sealed-in magnetically coupled micromanipulators (see Fig. 2). Note sudden onset of each medullary spike-barrage (*A:* MED) followed closely by a complex cerebral oscillatory (ca.

cord and brainstem ("pre-synaptic" stages: *vide supra*). Microscopic observation immediately following explantation confirms that the cells have been completely dissociated prior to culture. Cytologic studies indicate development of characteristic neurons and glial cells, within the clusters as well as in the neuropil and neuritic bridges connecting many of the discrete clusters (Fig. 6*A*, *B*), and abundant axo-dendritic and axo-somatic synapses are observed in electron micrographs of these reaggregated neuronal networks (Bornstein and Model, 1972).

After 2 to 4 weeks *in vitro*, complex repetitive spike discharges can be recorded, spontaneously as well as in response to electric stimuli, from dozens of discrete neuronal clusters which become attached to the collagen-coated coverglass over an area of about 1 cm^2, and which appear to be connected to one another by complex neuritic bridges (Figs. 6*C*, *D* and 7). In the larger clusters containing dozens of neurons, characteristic long-lasting potentials are often observed in association with the spike barrages. The complex bioelectric potentials recorded in each cluster are clearly generated *within* the cell cluster, and they are not merely indications of impulses propagating along neurites passing through the cluster.

After introduction of strychnine (1 to 10 $\mu g/ml$), the amplitude of these slow waves and the duration and complexity of the discharge sequences arc greatly enhanced (Figs. 6*D* and 7*B*). All of the complex bioelectric activities are rapidly blocked, on the other hand, by raising the Mg^{++} concentration of the medium from 1 to 5 mM (Fig. 7C_1), although short-latency spike potentials can still be evoked (Fig. 7C_2). The sensitivity of the reaggregated CNS neurons to these pharmacologic agents is similar to that observed in larger intact CNS explants, and the data indicate that functional synaptic networks can develop even after this more traumatic dissociation procedure. Recent intracellular recordings of both excitatory and inhibitory postsynaptic potentials in similar arrays of dispersed chick embryo spinal cord neurons in culture (Fischbach, 1970; Dichter and Fischbach,

---

15/sec) discharge sequence (*A:* CER). B_{1-4}: Continuous recording of spontaneous discharges at same electrode loci as in *A*. Note rhythmic alterations in amplitude of medullary spike-burst patterns and synchronization with some of the cerebral discharges, as in *A*. C_1: Spontaneous discharges in another pair of medulla and cerebral explants, after coupling *in vitro*, recorded in an open moist-chamber with microelectrodes positioned by conventional large micromanipulators (see Section III). Note similarity between these records and those in *A* and *B* of rhythmic spike bursts in medulla and complex oscillatory discharges occurring synchronously in the cerebral explant. C_2: Simultaneous after-discharges evoked by single brief cerebral stimulus show same complex yet stereotyped patterns as recorded in sealed chamber (*cf.* C_2 and *A*). Records *A* and *B* from unpublished data of Crain and Baer; records $C_{1,2}$ from Fig. 7 in Crain et al. (1968*b*) which also includes photomicrograph of this culture (with permission of the publisher).

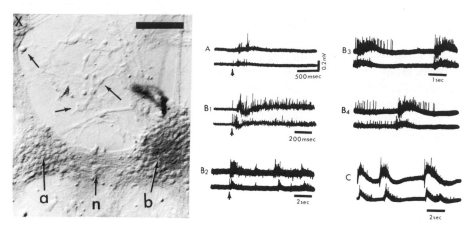

FIG. 6. Complex bioelectric discharges in cultured reaggregates of fetal mouse brainstem and spinal cord tissues, 2 weeks after dissociation. *X:* Photomicrograph showing two clusters of reaggregated cells (a,b) connected by neuritic bridge (n). Note neuron cell bodies within clusters and in looser array (arrows). Scale: 100 μm. *A:* Simultaneous microelectrode recordings of repetitive spike barrages and long-lasting negative slow-wave responses in two similar clusters of reaggregated neurons, but *3 mm* apart, elicited by single stimulus applied to intervening tissue. *B:* Under strychnine (10 μg/ml), evoked discharges are enhanced in amplitude, duration, and complexity ($B_{1,2}$), and similar potentials now occur spontaneously and *synchronously* between these distant regions of the neuronal network ($B_{3,4}$). *C:* Records of similar complex spontaneous discharges from two reaggregated clusters (about 3 mm apart) in another culture of dissociated brainstem and cord tissues, under strychnine. From Crain and Bornstein (1972) with permission of the publisher.

1971) provide still more direct evidence that trypsin-dissociated CNS cells can, indeed, recover *in vitro* and proceed to develop specialized synaptic relationships. In some of the reaggregates, moreover, especially of cerebral cortex cells, organotypic oscillatory (ca. 10 to 15 per sec) after-discharge patterns also occur, spontaneously as well as in response to stimuli (*cf.* Fig. 7B and Figs. 1, 3–5). These stereotyped, yet complex, repetitive discharge sequences have, therefore, been observed only in well-organized undissociated CNS explants. The spontaneous and evoked activities in the neuronal reaggregates are often clearly synchronized, even between clusters separated by distances greater than 3 mm (Figs. 6 and 7). The marked variation in latencies of the discharges between clusters reflect delays due to slow propagation of impulses in these fine-diameter neurites and to complex multi-synaptic transmission. Synchronization is greatly enhanced by strychnine, and even some of the small clusters containing only a few neuron perikarya then show patterned, long-lasting repetitive spike-bursts occurring synchronously with more complex discharges in larger clusters.

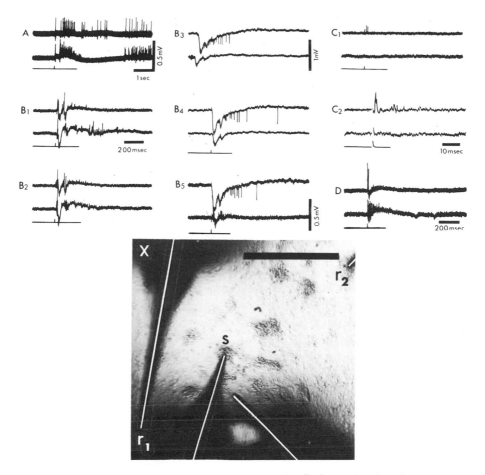

FIG. 7. Organotypic spike barrages and oscillatory after-discharges in cultured reaggregates of fetal mouse cerebral cortex, 2 weeks after complete cellular dissociation. *X:* Photomicrograph obtained during electrophysiologic recording from this culture. (White line through axis of each micropipette for clarity; r_1 not visible at this low magnification due to optical distortion produced by pipettes dipping into bath fluid.) Scale: 1 mm. *A:* Long-lasting intermittent bursts of repetitive spikes in two clusters of reaggregated neurons ($r_{1,2}$), 2 mm apart, evoked by single stimulus applied to intervening cluster (s). *B:* After introduction of strychnine (10 μg/ml), slow-wave components become greatly enhanced in amplitude and rhythmic positive potentials (ca. 15/sec) appear superimposed on a long lasting negativity ($B_{1,2}$; especially in lower sweeps). *B_3:* Similar repetitive sequences also occur spontaneously and synchronously between the two clusters. Note large amplitude of these slow waves and associated repetitive spike potentials. Also note sequential increase in amplitude of spikes during later stages of the spontaneous barrage sequence (upper sweep). This is even more evident in the discharges triggered shortly afterwards by single stimuli ($B_{4,5}$). Note the striking stereotyped, yet quite complex, pattern of these evoked and spontaneous discharges ($B_{3,4,5}$; upper sweeps). *C_1:* After increasing Mg++ concentration from 1 mM to 5 mM, all complex discharges are completely blocked, and only brief, short-latency spike potentials can be evoked (C_2). *D:* Restoration of complex discharges after return to 1 mM Mg++. From Crain and Bornstein (1972) with permission of the publisher.

Completely dissociated immature mammalian CNS neurons can, therefore, not only form synaptic connections after reaggregation in culture, but can also organize from a state of random dispersion into functional synaptic networks with complex organotypic properties indicating involvement of inhibitory as well as excitatory mechanisms. Since these dissociated neurons can now be studied with cytologic and bioelectric techniques during the *entire* period of regeneration and reaggregation in culture (Crain, 1972*a*), this method should greatly facilitate analysis of the role of each of the cells in these experimental networks in generating characteristic CNS discharge patterns. Cell fractionation procedures carried out prior to explantation of the dissociated CNS cells may, moreover, permit preparation of reaggregates containing pure populations of neurons or glial cells, or graded combinations of different cell types (e.g., Varon and Raiborn, 1969; see also Okun, 1972, regarding culture of isolated dorsal root ganglion cells after removal of Schwann and connective tissue cells during dissociation). This approach may be particularly useful in evaluating the functions of glial cells in relation to the development of organotypic synaptic networks.

V. LIMITATIONS OF CNS CULTURE MODELS

Tissue culture techniques are still not sufficiently standardized, especially with regard to development of complex CNS networks with characteristic synaptic functions, and microscopic observations of the living cultures are not yet adequate to evaluate the integrity of these interneuronal relationships. Potent "biochemical lesions" may occur which involve no detectable morphologic alterations, even at the electron-microscope level (*vide infra*). This is especially important to keep in mind in evaluating the functional significance of biochemical and cytological properties of cultured CNS tissues studied without correlative bioelectric tests on the same specimens. There are often serious variations between CNS cultures prepared under "standard" conditions even in a well-established laboratory, so that inferences about the functional integrity of *particular* explants based on bioelectric studies of this *type* of culture in another laboratory may be unwarranted extrapolations. No morphologic deficits have been detected, for example, during weeks of exposure of fetal cerebral cortex and spinal cord explants to xylocaine at concentrations which block (reversibly) generation of all nerve impulses and characteristic synaptically mediated discharges (Crain et al., 1968*a;* Model et al., 1971). Furthermore, sera obtained from animals with experimental allergic encephalomyelitis may produce rapid depression of complex bioelectric activities long before demyelinating or other structural efforts can be observed (Bornstein and Crain, 1965, 1971). The active antineuronal factor in these sera appears to be complement-dependent, and recent studies suggest that it may produce an immunopharmacologic blockade of specific CNS functions (Carnegie, 1971).

Even under optimal culture conditions, of course, CNS explants will generally develop some structural and functional deficits or abnormalities relative to their *in situ* counterparts. Separation of these small fragments of CNS tissue from their normal connections with other neurons undoubtedly leads to *alterations,* at least in neuronal excitability (Crain, 1969). Isolation in culture may, moreover, selectively damage or eliminate those types of neurons in a CNS explant which are more sensitive to mechanical trauma or to chemical deficiencies in the nutrient medium. Furthermore, even if synapses do form under a particular set of conditions *in vitro,* the resulting network may be significantly unbalanced as regards normal excitatory and inhibitory components; e.g., abnormal shifts towards inhibitory synaptic dominance may develop in older CNS explants (Section IV B; Crain, 1969). Altered chemosensitivity of some types of neuronal membranes may also be produced by chronic exposure, during maturation, to certain metabolites which may be present at relatively high (and presently uncontrolled) concentrations in routine tissue culture media, e.g., glycine and other amino acids involved in synaptic mediation. It is of interest, in this regard, that tolerance to *d*-tubocurarine appears to develop during chronic exposure of *in vitro*-coupled cord-muscle explants to this agent throughout the period when neuromuscular junctions are forming in culture (Crain and Peterson, 1971). Furthermore, current use of Maximow depression-slide chambers (see Section II A) involves marked alterations in the biochemical milieu during the 3- to 4-day period between feedings. Anabolites may dwindle and catabolites accumulate (including shifts to acid pH as CO_2 levels increase). Although these environmental fluctuations have been compatible with development and maintenance of "normal" CNS morphology in culture, they may be partly responsible for some of the variability in pharmacologic sensitivity noted above. In view of all these variables in the physico-chemical environment of CNS cultures, it is indeed remarkable that these isolated tissues show the degree of organotypic bioelectric properties described above, including characteristic sensitivity to at least some synapse-specific chemical tests, e.g., strychnine and Mg^{++}. Systematic pharmacologic studies are needed, however, using chambers permitting more rigorous long-term stability and control of the culture medium, to clarify the factors responsible for the aberrant sensitivity observed following many other experimental alterations of the chemical environment (see Section IV B).

In view of these present limitations in standardization of CNS explants, the burden of proof rests upon the investigator to determine the degree of organotypic function for each group of cultured CNS tissues, prepared by a particular set of culture techniques, utilizing bioelectric analyses carried out under well-defined physico-chemical conditions. These direct electrophysiologic studies will provide, then, a firm foundation for application of CNS cultures as a reproducible, experimental model system, with relevance to problems in epilepsy as well as other neurologic disorders.

VI. APPENDIX

Pyrex glass capillary tubing with an outer diameter of 0.8 mm and inner diameter of 0.6 mm has been convenient for construction of sharp-tapered micropipettes with tip orifices ranging from 1 to 10 μm. Smooth tips of desired tip diameter can be made automatically by careful control of the heat and weight applied to glass tubing mounted in a simple, vertical micropipette puller (with provision for application of relatively small weights). The shafts of the pipettes are bent at right angles, about 4 mm back from their tips (Fig. 2), by softening the glass with a small heating coil, under a dissecting microscope, and then applying gentle manual pressure to the shaftlet (with a needle suitably mounted with respect to the axis of the pipette). The pipettes are filled with isotonic saline by injection through a fine hypodermic needle (#31) inserted into the tapered region of the pipette (see Section III).

The silver electrode (0.25-mm diameter) is sealed into the pipette at the rear end to prevent evaporation of the saline bridge between the wire and the pipette tip. The resistance of these saline-filled micropipettes can be kept in the range of 1 to 5 MΩ (for 5- and 1-μm tips, respectively) by careful control of the taper near the pipette tip. Chloridized silver-core micropipettes, with 25-μm tips, have also been useful for recording both slow waves and spike potentials in CNS cultures (Crain and Bornstein, 1964; Crain and Peterson, 1964), but these microelectrodes have generally not been as stable and reliable as micro-salt-bridge pipettes (Frank and Becker, 1964). Platinum-black electrodes with still smaller tips (1 to 10 μm) have also been used with moderate success, especially for single-unit spike potentials, and they may be particularly convenient for long-term recordings under sterile conditions.

VII. ACKNOWLEDGMENTS

The author wishes to express appreciation to Dr. Murray B. Bornstein and Mrs. Edith R. Peterson (Department of Neurology, Albert Einstein College of Medicine) for their valuable cooperation in providing the cultures used for the physiologic studies described in this review. The work has been supported by grants from the National Institute of Neurological Diseases and Stroke (NS-06545 and NS-06735), the National Multiple Sclerosis Society (MS-760-A-1), and the Alfred P. Sloan Foundation.

VIII. REFERENCES

Araki, T., and Otani, T. (1955): Responses of single motoneurones to direct stimulation in toad's spinal cord. *Journal of Neurophysiology*, 18:472–485.

Armstrong-James, M. A., and Williams, T. D. (1963): Post-natal development of the direct cortical response in the rat. *Journal of Physiology*, 168:19–20.

Baer, S. C., and Crain, S. M. (1971): Magnetically coupled micromanipulator for use within a sealed chamber. *Journal of Applied Physiology*, 31:926–929.

Bishop, E. J. (1950): The strychnine spike as a physiological indicator of cortical maturity in the postnatal rabbit. *Electroencephalographic Clinical Neurophysiology*, 2:309–315.

Bornstein, M. B. (1964): Morphological development of neonatal mouse cerebral cortex in tissue culture. In: *Neurological and Electroencephalographic Correlative Studies in Infancy*, edited by P. Kellaway and I. Petersén. Grune and Stratton, New York, pp. 1–11.

Bornstein, M. B., and Crain, S. M. (1965): Functional studies of cultured mammalian CNS tissues as related to "demyelinative disorders." *Science*, 148:1242–1244.

Bornstein, M. B., and Crain, S. M. (1971): Lack of correlation between changes in bioelectric functions and myelin in cultured CNS tissues chronically exposed to sera from animals with EAE. *Journal of Neuropathology and Experimental Neurology*, 30:129P.

Bornstein, M. B., and Model, P. G. (1972): Development of neurons and synapses in cultures of dissociated spinal cord, brain stem and cerebrum of the embryo mouse. *Brain Research*, 37:287–293.

Bunge, R. P., Bunge, M. B., and Peterson, E. R. (1965): An electron-microscope study of cultured rat spinal cord. *Journal of Cell Biology*, 24:163–191.

Carnegie, P. R. (1971): Properties, structure and possible neuroreceptor role of the encephalitogenic protein of human brain. *Nature*, 229:25–27.

Cechner, R. L., Fleming, D. G., and Geller, H. M. (1970): Neurons in vitro: A tool for basic and applied research in neural electrodynamics. In: *Biomedical Engineering Systems*, edited by M. Clynes and J. H. Milsum. McGraw-Hill, New York, pp. 595–653.

Corner, M. A., and Crain, S. M. (1969): The development of spontaneous bioelectric activities and strychnine sensitivity during maturation in culture of embryonic chick and rodent central nervous tissues. *Archives Internationale Pharmacodynamica*, 182:404–406.

Corner, M. A., and Crain, S. M. (1972): Patterns of spontaneous bioelectric activity during maturation in culture of fetal rodent medulla and spinal cord tissues. *Journal of Neurobiology* 3:25–45.

Crain, S. M. (1952): Development of electrical activity in the cerebral cortex of the albino rat. *Proceedings of the Society for Experimental Biology and Medicine*, 81:49–51.

Crain, S. M. (1956): Resting and action potentials of cultured chick embryo spinal ganglion cells. *Journal of Comparative Neurology*, 104:285–330.

Crain, S. M. (1964): Development of bioelectric activity during growth of neonatal mouse cerebral cortex in tissue culture. In: *Neurological and Electroencephalographic Correlative Studies in Infancy*, edited by P. Kellaway and I. Petersén. Grune and Stratton, New York, pp. 12–26.

Crain, S. M. (1966): Development of "organotypic" bioelectric activities in central nervous tissues during maturation in culture. *International Review of Neurobiology*, 9:1–42.

Crain, S. M. (1969): Electrical activity of brain tissue developing in culture. In: *Basic*

Mechanisms of the Epilepsies, edited by H. H. Jasper, A. A. Ward, Jr., and A. Pope. Little, Brown and Co., Boston, pp. 506–516.

Crain, S. M. (1970a): Tissue culture studies of developing brain function. In: *Developmental Neurobiology,* edited by W. A. Himwich. Charles C Thomas, Springfield, Ill., pp. 165–196.

Crain, S. M. (1970b): Bioelectric interactions between cultured fetal rodent spinal cord and skeletal muscle after innervation *in vitro. Journal of Experimental Zoology,* 173:353–370.

Crain, S. M. (1970c): Long-term recordings from spinal cord explants in closed chamber with sealed-in manipulatable microelectrodes. *Journal of Cell Biology,* 47:43a.

Crain, S. M. (1972a): Microelectrode recording in brain tissue cultures. In: *Methods in Physiological Psychology,* Vol. 1, *Recording Techniques–Bioelectric Cellular Processes and Brain Potentials,* edited by R. F. Thompson and M. M. Patterson. Academic Press, New York *(in press).*

Crain, S. M. (1972b): Tissue culture models of developing brain functions. In: *Prenatal Ontogeny of Behavior and the Nervous System,* edited by G. Gottlieb. Univ. of Chicago Press, Chicago *(in press).*

Crain, S. M. (1972c): Depression of complex bioelectric activity of mouse spinal cord explants by glycine and γ-aminobutyric acid. *In Vitro,* 7:249.

Crain, S. M., Alfei, L., and Peterson, E. R. (1970): Neuromuscular transmission in cultures of adult human and rodent skeletal muscle after innervation *in vitro* by fetal rodent spinal cord. *Journal of Neurobiology,* 1:471–489.

Crain, S. M., and Bornstein, M. B. (1964): Bioelectric activity of neonatal mouse cerebral cortex during growth and differentiation in tissue culture. *Experimental Neurology,* 10: 425–450.

Crain, S. M., and Bornstein, M. B. (1972): Organotypic bioelectric activity in cultured reaggregates of dissociated rodent brain cells. *Science,* 176:182–184.

Crain, S. M., Bornstein, M. B., and Peterson, E. R. (1968a): Maturation of cultured embryonic CNS tissues during chronic exposure to agents which prevent bioelectric activity. *Brain Research,* 8:363–372.

Crain, S. M., and Peterson, E. R. (1964): Complex bioelectric activity in organized tissue cultures of spinal cord (human, rat and chick). *Journal of Cellular and Comparative Physiology,* 64:1–15.

Crain, S. M., and Peterson, E. R. (1971): Development of paired explants of fetal spinal cord and adult skeletal muscle during chronic exposure to curare and hemicholinium. *In Vitro,* 6:373.

Crain, S. M., Peterson, E. R., and Bornstein, M. B. (1968b): Formation of functional interneuronal connections between explants of various mammalian central nervous tissues during development *in vitro.* In: *Ciba Foundation Symposium, Growth of the Nervous System,* edited by G. E. W. Wolstenholme and M. O'Connor. Churchill, London, pp. 13–31.

Cunningham, A. W. B., Hamilton, A. E., King, M. F., Rojas-Corona, R. R., and Songster, G. F. (1970): Slow spontaneous signals from brain tissue culture. *Experientia,* 26:13–16.

Curtis, D. R., and Felix, D. (1971): GABA and prolonged spinal inhibition. *Nature, New Biology,* 231:187–188.

Curtis, D. R., Hösli, L., Johnston, G. A. R., and Johnston, I. H. (1968): The hyperpolarization of spinal motoneurones by glycine and related amino acids. *Experimental Brain Research,* 5:235–258.

DeLong, G. R. (1970): Histogenesis of fetal mouse isocortex and hippocampus in reaggregating cell cultures. *Developmental Biology,* 22:563–583.

Dichter, M., and Fischbach, G. D. (1971): Functional synapses in cell cultures of chick spinal cord and dorsal root ganglia. American Society for Cell Biology, 11th Annual Meeting, New Orleans, Abstract, p. 76.

Fischbach, G. D. (1970): Synaptic potentials recorded in cell cultures of nerve and muscle. *Science,* 169:1331–1333.

Frank, K., and Becker, M. C. (1964): Microelectrodes for recording and stimulation. In: *Physical Techniques in Biological Research,* Vol. V. *Electrophysiological Methods,* Part A, edited by W. L. Nastuk. Academic Press, New York, pp. 22–87.

Hild, W., and Tasaki, I. (1962): Morphological and physiological properties of neurons and glial cells in tissue culture. *Journal of Neurophysiology*, 25:277–304.

Himwich, W. A. (1962): Biochemical and neurophysiological development of the brain in the neonatal period. *International Review of Neurobiology*, 4:117–158.

Kennard, D. W. (1958): Glass microcapillary electrodes used for measuring potential in living tissues. In: *Electronic Apparatus for Biological Research*, edited by P. E. K. Donaldson. Butterworths, London, pp. 534–567.

Kiernan, J. A., and Pettit, D. R. (1971): Organ culture of the central nervous system of the adult rat. *Experimental Neurology*, 32:111–120.

Kopac, M. J. (1959): Micrurgical studies on living cells. In: *The Cell*, Vol. 1, edited by J. Brachet and A. E. Mirsky. Academic Press, New York, pp. 161–192.

Lieberman, M. (1967): Effects of cell density and low K on action potentials of cultured chick hearts. *Circulation Research*, 21:879–888.

Meller, K., Breipohl, W., Wagner, H. H., and Knuth, A. (1969): Die Differenzierung iso-lierter Nerven-und Gliazellen aus trypsiniertem Rückenmark von Hühnerembryonen in Gewebekulturen. *Zeitschrift für Zellforschung und Mikroskopische Anatomie*, 101:135–151.

Model, P. G., Bornstein, M. B., Crain, S. M., and Pappas, G. D. (1971): An electron micro-scopic study of the development of synapses in cultured fetal mouse cerebrum continuously exposed to xylocaine. *Journal of Cell Biology*, 49:362–371.

Moscona, A. A. (1965): Recombination of dissociated cells and the development of cell ag-gregates. In: *Cells and Tissues in Culture*, edited by E. N. Willmer. Academic Press, New York, pp. 489–529.

Moscona, A. A., Trowell, O. A., and Willmer, E. N. (1965): Methods. In: *Cells and Tissue in Culture*, Vol. 1, edited by E. N. Willmer. Academic Press, New York, pp. 19–98.

Okun, L. M. (1972): Isolated dorsal root ganglion neurons in culture: cytological maturation and extension of electrically active processes. *Journal of Neurobiology*, 3:111–151.

Peterson, E. R., and Crain, S. M. (1970): Innervation in cultures of fetal rodent skeletal muscle by organotypic explants of spinal cord from different animals. *Zeitschrift für Zell-forschung und Mikroskopische Anatomie*, 106:1–21.

Peterson, E. R., Crain, S. M., and Murray, M. R. (1965): Differentiation and prolonged maintenance of bioelectrically active spinal cord cultures (rat, chick and human). *Zeit-schrift für Zellforschung und Mikroskopische Anatomie*, 66:130–154.

Purpura, D. P. (1969): Stability and seizure susceptibility of immature brain. In: *Basic Mechanisms of the Epilepsies*, edited by H. H. Jasper, A. A. Ward, Jr., and A. Pope. Little, Brown and Co., Boston, pp. 481–505.

Purpura, D. P. (1971): Synaptogenesis in mammalian cortex: Problems and perspectives. In: *Brain Development and Behavior*, edited by M. B. Sterman, D. J. McGinty and A. M. Adinolfi. Academic Press, New York, pp. 23–41.

Purpura, D. P., Carmichael, M. W., and Housepian, E. M. (1960): Physiological and anatomi-cal studies of development of superficial axodendritic synaptic pathways in neocortex. *Ex-perimental Neurology*, 2:324–347.

Purpura, D. P., and Housepian, E. M. (1961): Morphological and physiological properties of chronically isolated immature neocortex. *Experimental Neurology*, 4:377–401.

Purpura, D. P., Shofer, R. J., and Scarff, T. (1965): Properties of synaptic activities and spike potentials of neurons in immature neocortex. *Journal of Neurophysiology*, 28:925–942.

Schlapfer, W. T. (1969): Bioelectric activity of neurons in tissue: Synaptic interactions and effects of environmental changes. Ph.D. Thesis, Univ. of California, Berkeley.

Schmidt, R. P., Thomas, L. B., and Ward, A. A. (1959): The hyperexcitable neurone. Micro-electrode studies of chronic epileptic foci in monkey. *Journal of Neurophysiology*, 22:285–296.

Scott, B. S., Engelbert, V. E., and Fisher, K. C. (1969): Morphological and electrophysiological characteristics of dissociated chick embryonic spinal ganglion cells in culture. *Experimental Neurology*, 23:230–248.

Seeds, N. W. (1971): Biochemical differentiation in reaggregating brain cell culture. *Proceedings of the National Academy of Sciences,* 68:1858–1861.

Shimada, Y., Fischman, D. A., and Moscona, A. A. (1969a): Formation of neuromuscular junctions in embryonic cell cultures. *Proceedings of the National Academy of Sciences,* 62:715–721.

Shimada, Y., Fischman, D. A., and Moscona, A. A. (1969b): The development of nerve-muscle junctions in monolayer cultures of embryonic spinal cord and skeletal muscle cells. *Journal of Cell Biology,* 43:382–387.

Varon, S., and Raiborn, C. W. (1969): Dissociation, fractionation, and culture of embryonic brain cells. *Brain Research,* 12:180–199.

Varon, S., and Raiborn, C. W. (1971): Excitability and conduction in neurons of dissociated ganglionic cell cultures. *Brain Research,* 30:83–98.

Werman, R., Davidoff, R. A., and Aprison, M. H. (1968): Inhibitory action of glycine on spinal neurons in the cat. *Journal of Neurophysiology,* 31:81–95.

13

Experimental Derangements of Extracellular Ionic Environment

Gilbert H. Glaser

OUTLINE

I. INTRODUCTION

  Changes in ionic concentration in extracellular spaces of the brain may be one of the basic precipitating causes of seizures (Tower, 1960, 1969; Glaser, 1964; Hillman, 1970). Shifts from the normal ionic gradients between intracellular and extracellular components in brain occur during seizure activity induced by a variety of methods (Tower, 1960, 1969). Also, such changes, which alter the ratios of intracellular and extracellular ionic concentrations (particularly sodium and potassium), may be primary factors in producing the hyperexcitable state in neurons in an already existing epileptogenic focus. To investigate these influences, an experimental model has been developed in our laboratory that utilizes a technique of localized intraventricular perfusion. Because of the highly selective and efficient blood-brain and blood-cerebrospinal fluid (CSF) barriers for ions, such as sodium and potassium, and the apparently ready exchange between CSF and brain for the same ions, we considered that the maintenance by perfusion of a constant change of ionic concentration in the CSF for a relatively long period of time would be a more effective method of experimentation than single intraventricular injections which we had used initially (Glaser and Wolf, 1963). By this method we hoped to simulate closely the perfusion of isolated neuronal structures with an artificial fluid, and to acquire relevant data about the action of extracellular ions, as well as other pharmacologically active substances, on cerebral neuronal activity.

  The maintenance of a constant concentration in a fluid, which is constantly diluted with new, naturally produced CSF, and which is rapidly cleared of abnormally high concentrations of ions into the blood, requires active perfusion at controlled flow and limited to a small region of brain. For many reasons, we decided that the most suitable region for such a study would be the dorsal hippocampus: it has a low convulsive threshold, the basal and apical dendritic layers are clearly delineated, and it can be perfused along its alvear surface, beneath which lie the basal dendrites of the hippocampal pyramids. Consequently, a technique has been developed to perfuse locally the inferior horn of the lateral ventricle just above the dorsal hippocampus (Zuckermann and Glaser, 1968a,b, 1970a,b). This procedure is a variant of the method used by other workers who have utilized a more generalized perfusion of the ventricles, for example, from lateral ventricle to the cisterna magna (Pappenheimer et al., 1962; Feldberg, 1963; Bradbury and Davson, 1965; Cserr, 1965; Katzman et al., 1965; Bradbury and Štulcová, 1970). The basic method of acute intraventricular injections and ventricular perfusions is presented by Feldberg (1963), together with studies indicating the extent of penetration through the ventricular walls into cerebral tissue, especially grey matter, of substances such as histamine, bromphenol blue, and acetazolamide.

In our studies we have used cats implanted chronically with intraventricular cannulae and various types of intracerebral electrodes. The technique of using chronic animals has the advantage of obviating the interference by anesthetics and acute brain trauma at the time of the perfusion experiments, and, with care, the technique allows repeated testing of the same animal for many months.

Most of our experiments with this model have been devoted to a study of effects of perfusion of CSF with increased potassium concentrations, in order to evaluate the possible significance of K^+ accumulation of extracellular spaces of brain as a precipitating factor in epileptogenic activity. Some studies also have been performed with increased or decreased concentrations of calcium (Ca^{++}). When data are extrapolated from studies of peripheral axons, neuromuscular junctions, or neuronal perikarya of more primitive animals, it seems clear that the extracellular K^+ concentration exerts a significant influence on the membrane potential of central neurons and, by implication, on their reactivity to presynaptic volleys of stimuli. Extensive studies of the genesis of spreading depression (Marshall, 1959), for example, have demonstrated the ability of highly concentrated K^+ solutions to produce steady depolarization of central neurons; other investigations have demonstrated the possibility of inducing seizure activity by simple intraventricular injections of K^+ (Feldberg and Sherwood, 1957; John et al., 1959). The basic condition, however, for an accurate analysis of the action of K^+ or any other ion on cerebral neurons would seem to depend on a change of its extracellular concentration kept at a steady level throughout the experiment at ranges close to those found in physiological or even pathophysiological situations. Rigorous blood-brain and blood-CSF barriers exist that essentially exclude vascular delivery of K^+. Moreover, there is rapid equilibrium between CSF and interstitial fluid, so that the imposition of an altered steady-state concentration of K^+ in CSF will be followed after a short delay by an equivalent alteration in K^+ concentration in extracellular spaces of subjacent cerebral tissue (Pappenheimer et al., 1962; Katzman et al., 1964, 1965; Bradbury and Davson, 1965; Cserr, 1965; Bradbury and Štulcová, 1970). Because numerous mechanisms act to clear both CSF and extracellular spaces of abnormally high concentrations of K^+, influx of the ion into the CSF must be maintained by constant perfusion at a high rate of an artificial CSF in order to counterbalance the efflux and to keep a steady state. Because the clearance from CSF is apparently directly proportional to the total surface area of the pathway along which the CSF flows, a satisfactory perfusion under such experimental conditions would be limited to a very small area of ependymal or arachnoidal surface. We believe that for these investigative purposes the technique of perfusing over the dorsal hippocampus or even the neocortex (Glaser and Zuckermann, 1968) is preferable to those which deposit or circulate the active substance within the neuronal parenchyma itself (Wagner and DeGroot, 1963; Bronzino et al., 1972). In spite of the obvious advantage of the highly localized action of such a stimulation, the mechanical effects of this type of implantation or irrigation produce destruction of tissue, making it more difficult to interpret the results, especially since any normal or near-normal exchanges among blood, CSF, extracellular spaces, neuroglia, and neurons would be more greatly altered. In our method, we consider the possible diffusion of K^+ in significant amounts outside the perfused area to be of less importance, since we are interested in the events taking place in the structures directly beneath the area of perfusion where equilibrium with the CSF takes place. If the active substance to be used in the experiments is a normal component of CSF and is rapidly cleared from extracellular spaces and CSF, the diffusion around the perfused area can have only minimal effects on distant structures. Of course, the situation could be different if the active substance is a pharmacological agent which is not cleared from CSF and continuously accumulates around the perfused area. Even under these circumstances, however, with the use of such drugs as ouabain and pentylenetetrazol, the results obtained with our method show a sharply localized change of neuronal activity just beneath the area of perfusion.

II. METHODS

A. Implantation of cannulae and electrodes

Our investigations have been carried out using cats. Monkeys also would make satisfactory experimental animals and have been used in chronic CSF perfusion studies (Katzman et al., 1964). The perfusion cannulae are 22-gauge stainless steel tubes, fixed stereotaxically into the inferior horn of each lateral ventricle at coordinates A3–3.5 (Snider and Niemer, 1961), the region in which the horn is considered largest. Two cannulae are implanted into each horn using a special holder, one at L4.5–L5 and the other at L7. To determine that the tips are actually in the ventricular cavity and patent, the following procedure is used. A cannula with an attached length of polyethylene tubing is fixed into the cisterna magna. When the ventricular cannulae are inserted to a height considered just at the surface of the inferior horn, they are connected to a water manometer, filled to a pressure of 25 to 30 cm of water with normal artificial CSF, and the cisternal tubing is fixed at −5 to −6 cm below the zero line. When the tips of the cannulae are actually in the ventricle, a rapid decrease in the pressure registered by the manometer occurs, and, after 1 to 2 sec, perfusion fluid flows out of the cisternal cannulae outflow. If these phenomena fail to occur, the ventricular cannulae are inserted more deeply, in steps of 0.3 mm, until the outflow appears. In our experience, for cats weighing 2.3 to 3.2 kg and with a bregma at coordinates A17–18.5 mm, localization using the coordinates of the Snider and Niemer Atlas (1961) has been highly satisfactory. Supplementary cannulae also can be fixed by a similar technique into the lateral ventricle at the level of the foramen of Monroe.

For general macroelectrode recording and stimulation, stainless steel electrodes of 50 to 100 μm diameter are constructed and implanted in various locations in hippocampus and other brain regions. For example, in some experiments to study hippocampal evoked responses, in order to record from both apical and basal dendritic layers, the electrodes are constructed in pairs with a horizontal separation of 0.1 to 0.3 mm and a vertical separation between the tips of 0.8 to 0.9 mm. Four to eight pairs are implanted stereotaxically in field Ca-1 of each dorsal hippocampus. The interhippocampal response is checked during the insertion of the electrode, clear responses with opposite polarity in each electrode of a pair being the sign of a correct position. Stimulation electrodes are 250 μm stainless steel wires inserted at the level of the alvear surface.

For other recording purposes, Teflon-coated stainless steel wires 100 μm in diameter are attached in pairs to the outer surface of the perfusion cannulae. The electrodes attached to the cannulae are 1 to 1.5 mm longer at the lower tip than the cannulae in order to reach the hippocampal surface beneath the perfusion area. Implantations are also made in various cortical areas such as the gyrus ectosylvius, gyrus suprasylvius, gyrus sygmoideous, or on the superior wall of the inferior horn. Various locations in the brainstem down to the medulla are implanted in different experiments.

The electrodes are fixed through Amphenol connectors to an Amphenol plug fixed on the skull with dental cement. At the termination of implantation, the cannula from the cisterna magna is withdrawn; the neck musculature is then sutured, and each ventricular cannula is sealed with exact-fitting stainless steel stylets.

Experiments have also been carried out utilizing DC recording of slow potential shifts in dorsal hippocampus. For these experiments, the implantation of stimulation and recording electrodes (AC) in field Ca-1 of hippocampus is as already described. The DC recording electrodes are glass pipettes with 50-μm tips, filled with saline and 1% agar and connected to sockets through a silver-silver chloride wire. When tested before implantation, electrodes with a drift larger than 2 μV/min are rejected. They are implanted usually 50 μm apart alternately in the basal and apical dendritic layers, using the pattern of interhippocampal response as a test for correct implantation. Teflon-coated, stainless steel electrodes for AC recording also are attached to the DC guides in order to achieve both AC and DC recordings from the region as close together as possible.

In all experiments, care was taken to avoid significant edema, brain damage, or mechanical distortion of tissue during electrode implantation. Use of adrenocortical steroid and mannitol proved to be helpful in the control of cerebral edema. Many variations were used in the spatial relationships between the perfused area and the localization of stimulating and recording electrodes. Those reproduced in Fig. 1 have been used most often.

B. Preparation of experimental epileptogenic foci

An experimental model utilizing chronic, latent epileptogenic foci also has been utilized in certain perfusion experiments (Zuckermann and Glaser, 1970b). The basic preparations are similar to those described above: two cannulae are implanted in the inferior horn of the lateral ventricle for constant perfusion over a region of the dorsal hippocampus. An array of eight electrodes for recording purposes is implanted in the underlying region of the hippocampus, and another eight in the homotopic points of the contra-

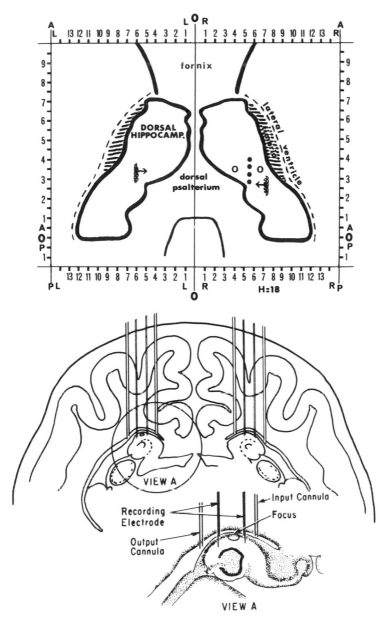

FIG. 1. *Top:* Horizontal section through the dorsal hippocampus of cat (viewed from above), showing the usual location of recording and stimulating electrodes and of perfusion cannulae. Large dots, recording electrodes; arrows, stimulating electrodes; open circles, perfusion cannulae. Coordinates after Snider and Niemer (1961). *Bottom:* Frontal coronal section of cat brain at stereotaxic coordinate A 3.4 (Snider and Niemer, 1961) to show the relationships among perfusing cannulae, recording electrodes, and a latent epileptogenic focus. From Zuckermann and Glaser (1970*b*) with permission of the publisher.

lateral hippocampus. The chronic focus is placed in the middle of the perfused area by injecting either 3 to 5 mg of cobalt powder or 0.03 to 0.05 ml of alumina cream (see Chapter 1). The amount of irritative material is determined empirically as that amount capable of producing a sub-threshold focus, activated only by supplementary stimulation; this amount is, of course, smaller than that generally used for producing an active discharging focus. A diagram of this experimental preparation is shown in Fig. 1*B* (view A).

C. Method of perfusion and perfusion fluid

After the implantations, the animals are allowed to recover for a period of 14 to 24 days before any experiments are carried out. Although we initially attempted to carry out perfusion and recording experiments with the animal unrestrained, we have found it more appropriate and effective to place the cat in a specially constructed box which restrains it comfortably in a normal lying position and allows movement of the head only. All experiments are carried out in this way with the animals confined but relatively unrestrained and usually in a naturally awake state of consciousness; some studies may involve animals that are drowsy or asleep. Anesthesia is not used.

The perfusions are performed with a Harvard infusion pump connected by polyethylene tubing fitted to the implanted cannulae in the inferior ventricular horn. Both inflow and outflow pressures are established and monitored by a transducer connected to one channel of a polygraph, and with a water manometer in parallel with the pump. The outflow cannula is connected to a collecting tube and monitored by a drop counter. Negative pressure in the test system can be adjusted to keep the rate and pressure of the perfusion within relatively constant limits. Generally, the pressure of the inflow system is kept between 15 and 30 cm of CSF. The perfusion can be performed at different speeds but usually at 0.05 to 0.08, 0.1, or 0.3 to 0.5 ml per minute. Before reaching the inflow cannula, the artificial CSF circulates through a thermostatically controlled bath to keep the temperature of the perfusion fluid at 37.5 to 38.5°C at the cerebral inflow level.

The composition of the artificial CSF for perfusion is similar to that used by previous workers with slight modifications: (in μequiv/ml) Na, 152; K, 2.7; Ca, 2.2; Mg, 1.2; Cl, 133; HCO_3, 25; and H_2PO_4, 0.6. Most of the experimental studies have been carried out with the solutions of artificial CSF containing increased concentrations of K^+, balanced by an equivalent decrease in Na^+, to keep the total osmolarity constant. The normal concentration of potassium is 2.7 μequiv/ml and this is increased in various experiments, usually two to four times, to 5.4 to 10.8 μequiv/ml (rarely to 16 μequiv/ml). At these higher concentrations, we have not considered it necessary to use sulfate in place of chloride, since the changes produced by water penetration into neurons apparently occur at higher levels of CSF potassium (27 μequiv/ml). The pH of perfusion fluids is usually set at 7.35 to 7.45. We have performed some experiments with high calcium CSF, calcium-free CSF, and with CSF to which L-glutamate (5 to 50 μequiv/ml) has been added, and with ouabain.

An experimental perfusion session usually begins with the perfusion of normal artificial CSF for a period of 30 to 60 min, followed by a change in the perfusion to an artificial CSF with a higher K^+ concentration, and finally back to normal artificial CSF. Initially, this basic procedure is varied in relation to duration of individual perfusions, pause between perfusion, pressure of perfusions, and total number of different perfusions performed, in order to study and exclude all possible hazardous effects. Usually, an experimental session is repeated 4 to 10 days after a previous one, to minimize any long-lasting effects. In total, five to twelve perfusions can be performed with each animal over a 2- to 6-month period without any significant, untoward changes.

Experiments in which ouabain is added to the perfusion fluid are carried out utilizing concentrations of 10^{-7} to 10^{-4} M ouabain in the artificial CSF. Ouabain also can be infused in known amounts of 2 to 20 μg into the inferior horns with one of the perfusion cannulae.

The effluent samples of perfusate are collected during the perfusion for analysis of concentrations of the various ions.

D. Recording and stimulating methods

Electrophysiologic recordings are performed with either a Grass electroencephalograph or polygraph and are monitored oscilloscopically. Background electroencephalographic activity and responses to stimuli amplified through the polygraph (time constant, 0.45 sec; high-frequency filter at 3 KC), were also recorded on magnetic tape (Honeywell 7600). Responses to stimuli were displayed also on a Tektronix storage oscilloscope and analyzed with computer of averaging transients. However, under the conditions of these experiments, we find the averaged response is less illustrative than analysis of independent responses. For DC recordings, a low-level DC preamplifier (7P1A) is utilized in the polygraph.

To investigate the excitability of hippocampal neurons during perfusion, trains of single stimuli are delivered to the dorsal hippocampus before any perfusion and during perfusion with artificial normal CSF and hyperpotassium CSF. The single stimuli are delivered by a Grass S88 stimulator through an isolation unit. Biphasic and monophasic square waves are used at a frequency of one every 2.5 sec to one every 5 sec, in trains of 10 stimuli; the duration of each wave was 0.1 to 1 msec. The intensity is adjusted before perfusion to produce a threshold motor response, usually a small jerk of the contralateral ear, whiskers, or periorbital musculature. Thereafter, this stimulus intensity is kept constant. Stimulation is either bipolar (between two hippocampal electrodes) or monopolar (using as cathode one of the dorsal hippocampal electrodes at coordinates anterior 3.5 to 4.0 and lateral 5.0 to 7.0, or anterior 1.0 to 0.0 and lateral 9.0 to 11.0, and a large indifferent electrode on the animal's back). During perfusion with increased K^+ concentrations, the trains of single stimuli are started 15 to 20 min earlier than when perfusing with normal CSF, i.e., during the latent period before any expected onset of a spontaneous seizure. Each train is followed by another, 2 to 4 min later, and usually 12 series represent the maximal total stimulation delivered in any one experimental session.

The local hippocampal and interhippocampal responses (LHR and IHR) to these stimulations are rechecked after the animal has recovered for 3 weeks, and animals with constant responses in at least three pairs of electrodes are selected for further experiments. In each experimental session, the LHR and IHR were determined at intensities from threshold to four times threshold before any perfusion. After perfusion with artificial normal CSF is started, the LHR and IHR are studied at a constant intensity of stimulation, usually threshold, threshold $\times$ 1.5, or threshold $\times$ 2. Perfusions with increased K^+ concentration are then performed, and single stimuli of identical intensity are delivered at suitable intervals. Each perfusion lasts no more than 30 min at a rate of 0.1 ml/min, with a pause of 30 to 40 min between perfusions. When seizure activity is induced, the perfusion is discontinued and restarted after the usual pause.

At the end of experiments, the animal is anesthetized with pentobarbital, and electrolytic lesions marking positions are made by passing a DC current through each electrode. The animal is then sacrificed by intracardiac perfusion with saline and 10% formalin. The brain is sectioned, and alternate 15- to 20-μm slices are stained with thionine, hematoxylin and eosin, Weils' stain, and Gomori's iron stain to verify electrode placement and to examine for pathological changes.

E. Postmortem brain examinations

Postmortem brain examinations confirm the location of the cannulae in the inferior horns of the lateral ventricles, and of the electrodes in various positions of the brain. We have seen no indications of significant inflammatory reaction involving ependymal or subependymal layers. Any pathologic changes are limited mainly to tissue damage caused by the insertion of cannulae and electrodes and the persistence in the brain of these foreign elements. Depending on the length of time between the surgical implantation and the death of the animal, various stages of tissue reaction are observed. Some capillary proliferation, microglial cell infiltration, and increasing numbers of fibroblasts are seen along the electrode and cannula tracks. There is no evidence of edema. Myelin stains show minimal, degenerating myelin immediately adjacent to the cannula or electrode tracks. Fragmentation or almost disappearance of ependyma has been noted in the experiments involving ouabain perfusion, and in these cases there was a greater number of polymorphonuclear and mononuclear leukocytes in the reactive areas of tissue.

III. RESULTS FROM SERIES OF EXPERIMENTS UTILIZING THE HIPPOCAMPAL PERFUSION MODEL

A. General behavior during perfusions: induced clinical seizure activity (Glaser and Zuckermann, 1968; Zuckermann and Glaser, 1968a)

The animals adapt well to the relatively mild restraints imposed by the boxes, settling down quickly. When the perfusion is with normal artificial CSF or even with an increased K^+ concentration below that producing seizure activity, the animals behave during the perfusion as before it, remaining alert, investigating changes in the environment, and purring when patted. Sometimes during prolonged confinement they fall asleep, as in the absence of any perfusion, but are aroused easily by sudden stimuli. Immediately after liberation from the box, they behave normally.

When the perfusion fluid contains an increased K^+ concentration and seizures are induced, the behavior of the animal changes according to the intensity of the convulsive activity. Usually, no evident behavioral or autonomic changes are noticed during very brief localized electrical hippocampal seizure activity. However, when the discharge lasts more than 15 to 30 sec and spreads to contralateral hippocampus, the animals exhibit characteristic signs of hippocampal seizure phenomena: respiratory, pupillary, and salivary changes as well as minor aggressive movements. Often hyperpnea and tachypnea herald an imminent convulsion. Just prior to greater seizure activity, the animals begin licking their lips, sniffing, and exhibiting focal muscular twitches in and about the face. Clonic and tonic convulsive activities appear when the paroxysmal discharges become generalized. After the experimental perfusion, the behavior is normal when only two or three brief unilateral hippocampal seizures have been induced. When the epileptic activity has been more intense (as with prolonged perfusions), the postictal behavior remains altered for the following 24 to 48 hr with anorexia, lethargy, and general motor instability, all of which, however, gradually return to normal. Occasionally, persistence of aggressive behavior is noted during this period. In general, experiments can be repeated at intervals of 3 to 4 days but usually, if generalized seizures have occurred, the animals are placed in test situations at intervals of 5 to 7 days. In this way, most animals can be kept for as long as 6 months.

B. Perfusion with normal CSF

Observations now have been made of several hundred perfusions with normal artificial CSF. In no instance has there been any occurrence of clinical seizure activity, or evidence of paroxysmal discharge in the electroencephalogram. In addition, perfusion with normal CSF has produced no seizure activity under any of the following special experimental situations: (1) when the perfusion lasted for a long time (e.g., 2 hr); (2) when the perfusion with normal CSF was alternated in the same experimental session with a high K^+ CSF, which had previously produced seizures; (3) when the pH of the solution was changed between 7.1 and 8.1; (4) when the temperature of the perfusion varied between 24 and 40°C; (5) when the perfusion pressure was increased from the usual 15 to 30 cm of water to 60 to 90 cm of water (however, with an increase of pressure above 120 to 130 cm of water, marked depression of EEG activity, and signs of brainstem compression were noted); and (6) when the rate of perfusion was increased to an average of 0.7 to 0.9 ml/min.

C. Hippocampal epileptic activity induced by localized ventricular perfusion with high-potassium CSF (Zuckermann and Glaser, 1968a)

Localized paroxysmal discharges appear from the dorsal hippocampus beneath the area of perfusion (Fig. 2), after a latent period of 15 to 50 min, when K^+ in the perfusing artificial CSF circulates across the hippocampus at a rate of 0.1 to 1.62 μequiv/min. The intensity of discharges is greater and the latent period shorter when the CSF K^+ circulates at the higher rates. Single electrical stimuli delivered to the dorsal hippocampus under the area of the perfusion do not induce convulsive activity when the K^+ in the CSF

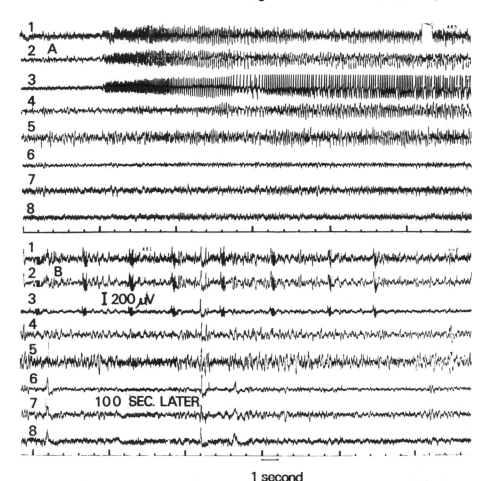

FIG. 2. Paroxysmal discharges appearing from the left dorsal hippocampus after 26 min of perfusion with high K⁺ CSF (16 μequiv/ml) into the left inferior ventricular horn at a rate of 0.05 ml/min. *A:* Onset of seizure with "tonic" (i.e., prolonged) discharges of spikes. *B:* Termination 100 sec later with "clonic" or intermittent bursts of spikes, remaining localized. The stereotaxic locations (Snider and Niemer, 1961) of the electrode placements are: (1) left dorsal hippocampus, Ant. 3.5, Lat. 5.0; (2) left dorsal hippocampus, Ant. 3.5, Lat. 7.0; (3) left dorsal hippocampus, Ant. 0.0, Lat. 10.0; (4) left gyrus lateralis; (5) left gyrus ectosylvius; and (6–8) symmetrical placements in right dorsal hippocampus (corresponding to locations of 1–3). From Zuckermann and Glaser (1968a) with permission of the publisher.

is normal, but do induce such convulsive activity when given during the latent period of a perfusion of high K⁺ CSF (Fig. 3). In most of the experiments, there has been a distinct localization of the discharges from the dorsal hippocampus under the area of perfusion. However, in about 30%

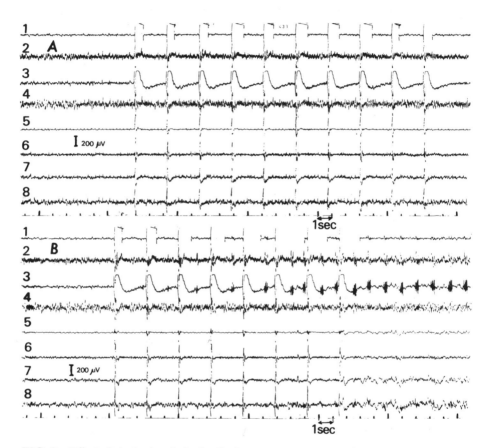

FIG. 3. Effect of single electrical stimuli of square waves (1-msec duration, 15 V) delivered at 2.5-sec. intervals to the left dorsal hippocampus (Ant. 0, Lat. 10). *A:* At 25 min after the start of perfusion with normal artificial CSF at a rate of 0.16 ml/min. No changes are seen after a train of 10 stimuli. *B:* At 26 min after the start of perfusion of the left anterior ventricular horn with high K⁺ CSF (10 μequiv/ml) at a rate of 0.13 ml/min. A gradual build-up of self-sustained paroxysmal bursts of spike discharges is seen. After eight stimuli, the discharges are self-sustained for 15 seconds. Electrode placements: (1) left dorsal hippocampus Ant. 3.5, Lat. 5; (2) left dorsal hippocampus, Ant. 3.5, Lat. 7: (3) left dorsal hippocampus, Ant. 0, Lat. 10; (4) left gyrus lateralis-left caudate nucleus; and (5–8) symmetrical corresponding placements in right hemisphere. From Zuckermann and Glaser (1968*a*) with permission of the publisher.

of the experiments, paroxysmal discharges have appeared from both hippocampi, the contralateral hippocampus showing projected activity, with the same rhythms and patterns as those from the perfused hippocampus, but of lower amplitude. In 17% of the experiments, an independent or mirror focus has developed in the opposite hippocampus, with its own pattern of discharges. In about 17% of instances, also, the activity arising from the perfused hippocampus gradually has spread diffusely to become a major, generalized clinical seizure.

D. Changes in hippocampal evoked responses prior to seizure induced by localized perfusion with high-potassium CSF (Zuckermann and Glaser, 1968b)

The local hippocampal and interhippocampal responses induced by single stimuli (0.5 to 0.25/sec) have been investigated during localized ventricular perfusion with high-K^+ CSF. Typical changes appear soon after the beginning of the perfusion early in the latent period, and reach a peak 10 to 20 min later at the time of the onset of seizure activity (Fig. 4). These responses are recorded from the region of hippocampus just under the area of perfusion, and from the homotopic area in the contralateral hippocampus. Initially, a progressively increasing slow wave is seen, positive in the apical dendritic layer and negative in the basal dendritic layer, together with a depression of the secondary component of the normal response. In a following phase, the slow wave becomes wider as the velocity of its decay decreases, and a later wave of opposite polarity follows it, like an overshoot. Negative spikes of increasing incidence then appear, superimposed. Self-sustained seizure activity is associated, 2 to 4 min after the beginning of the second phase, with a response displaying the wider slower wave and the greatest number of superimposed spikes. The first paroxysmal slow-wave discharge interrupts the late transient, before it reaches its peak, and exhibits an opposite polarity. We assume that development of excitatory postsynaptic potentials in the dorsal layer of hippocampus, the apical dendrites acting as a source, can explain the changes in the first period, and a depression of the inhibitory postsynaptic potential at the same level explain those of the last period. These experiments enabled us to make an analysis of the changes occurring during the latent period of perfusion, prior to the actual induction of seizure activity, clinically and electrographically. Significant modification in excitability of hippocampal neurons occurred early during the perfusion (within 2 to 4 min), since otherwise ineffective single-shock stimuli delivered to dorsal hippocampus during this latent period were able to trigger self-sustained seizure discharges.

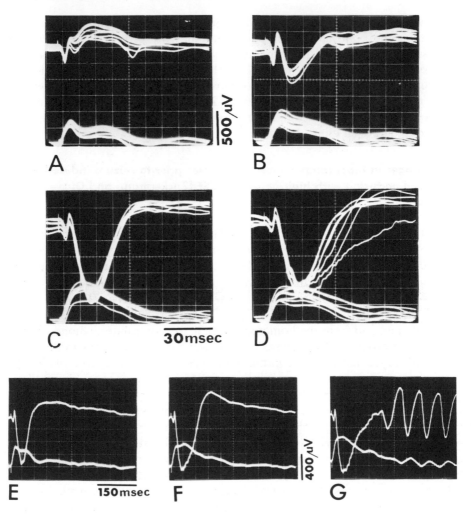

FIG. 4. Changes in local hippocampal response during perfusion of the inferior ventricular horn with high-K$^+$ CSF (12.5 μequiv/ml) at a rate of 0.08 ml/min. Recordings are from the apical dendritic layer (*upper trace*) and the basal dendritic layer (*lower trace*) at 1.5 mm from the point stimulated on the alvear surface. In all frames, negativity is upward, and, unless otherwise indicated, 10 responses to single stimuli at rate of 0.3/sec are recorded superimposed.

A: The normal response, before perfusion. *B:* After 2 min of perfusion; there is general enhancement of all components. *C:* After 7 min the tertiary wave reaches its peak (1.25 mV), and its rising phase is the fastest (125 μV/msec). There is still no induced paroxysmal activity. *D:* After 9 min, the last train of single-stimuli induced responses with a slower decay of the tertiary wave, and spikes become superimposed on the falling phase in the last responses (from apical layer). Self-sustained paroxysmal activity is then triggered, as shown separately in *E, F,* and *G,* second, seventh, and eighth responses, respectively, in the last "triggering" train of such stimuli. From Zuckermann and Glaser (1968*b*) with permission of the publisher.

E. Slow potential shifts in dorsal hippocampus during epileptogenic perfusion of the inferior horn with high-potassium CSF (Zuckermann and Glaser, 1970a)

During the initial experiments of this series, we demonstrated that slow potential shifts do occur associated with seizure discharge activity induced by the localized perfusion with high-K^+ CSF. The paroxysmal activity appears to be generated during the delayed decay of abnormal long-lasting hippocampal responses. We considered it necessary to record and study this type of activity with DC coupled amplifiers to avoid the distortion inherent in an AC coupled system, and such an analysis of slow potential shifts has been performed by utilizing chronically implanted, glass-pipette electrodes prepared specifically for such DC recording. Accordingly, slow potential shifts and responses to ipsi- and contralateral stimulation of dorsal hippocampus have been recorded from basal and apical dendritic layers in awake cats. Perfusion of the inferior horn with increased K^+ concentrations (usually 12 μequiv/ml) in the CSF induces, after 20 to 50 sec, an early DC shift of 1 to 3 mV, only in the basal dendritic layer that reaches a plateau after 2 to 3 min (Fig. 5). During this time, no changes in the pattern of hippocampal-evoked responses have been observed. In the subsequent period, while the DC level is constant, large potentials, negative from basal layer and positive from apical layer, gradually develop in response to single stimuli and reach a peak in 6 to 15 min when a seizure discharge is then triggered. During the last minute preceding the initiation of paroxysmal discharge, the main transient of each response is followed by a long-lasting negative wave from the basal layer at a synchronous positive wave from the apical layer (Fig. 5b). At this moment, another DC shift occurs by the overlapping of these late waves. Paroxysmal discharges are then superimposed on this DC shift.

We have assumed that the early initial DC shift recorded only from the periventricular electrodes is associated with changes in ependymal or glial membranes (Tschirgi and Taylor, 1958; Held et al., 1964), and that the K^+ later increases excitability by another mechanism involving global depolarization of neurons.

F. Epileptogenic effect of localized ventricular perfusion of ouabain over dorsal hippocampus (Pedley et al., 1969)

Concentrations of ouabain greater than 5×10^{-6} M consistently induce focal paroxysmal discharges which spread by projection to the contralateral hippocampus (Fig. 6). Measurements of ionic changes in the perfusion

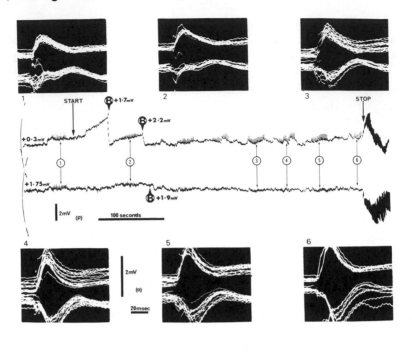

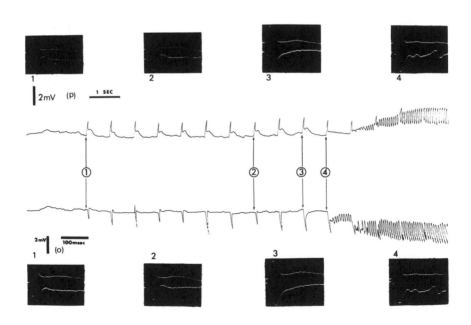

effluent have revealed a rise in the K^+ concentration with no apparent change in the Na^+ concentration during the perfusion. There is a rough correlation between increasing seizure activity and a rise in the K^+ appearing in the effluent. This investigation with ouabain indicates that alterations of active transport enzyme systems, such as the inactivation of Na,K-ATPase by ouabain, are associated with the potential for epileptogenicity (Tower, 1969). The exact mechanism of this effect is not certain, but it is seemingly related to the secondarily induced alterations in ionic activity in the involved area.

G. Activation of experimental epileptogenic foci: action of increased potassium in extracellular spaces of the brain (Zuckermann and Glaser, 1970b)

The reactivity of chronic epileptogenic foci to potassium exhibits a definite trend in relation to the type and age of the focus. The method of production of a subthreshold epileptogenic focus with either cobalt powder or alumina cream has been described above. For the cobalt focus, reactivity is at its peak 3 to 12 days after implantation and then gradually diminishes. For the alumina focus, the peak reactivity is 40 to 60 days after implantation, and afterwards either spontaneous seizures occur or the reactivity decreases. At these respective peaks of reactivity, for both kinds of preparations, the percentage of epileptogenic perfusions is significantly higher for each concentration of K^+ in the artificial CSF than in the control prepara-

←———

FIG. 5.   *Top:* DC recordings from dorsal hippocampus (basal dendritic layer, upper trace; apical, lower trace) under perfusion with high-K^+ CSF (12.5 μequiv/ml at 0.05 ml/min.). The start and stop of perfusion are indicated. Superimposed oscilloscopic records of local hippocampal responses (LHR) to 1/sec stimulation are shown in the inserts. Each number indicates the point in the EEG recording from which each set of responses in the insert was taken. (P) indicates calibration and time base for polygraph-EEG; (0) indicates calibration and time base for oscilloscope. At ⑧, each pen is balanced for the developing DC shift. After the start of the perfusion, the early negative DC shift at the basal layer is not accompanied by any changes in the LHR at ②. Such changes, leading to seizure discharges, begin to appear minutes later, when the DC level already has achieved a constant value. Then, characteristic negative responses gradually develop in the basal dendritic layer along with homologous positive changes in the apical dendritic layer. From Zuckermann and Glaser (1970a) with permission of the publisher.

Bottom: Recordings, both polygraph-EEG (DC coupled amplifier, hfr 3kc) and LHR, to the last train of 1/sec stimulation triggering the seizure discharge (at 6 in top of Fig. 5). The LHR was recorded with AC amplification shown in upper row of inserts, at DC amplification in lower row. Paroxysmal waves are seen becoming superimposed upon a "trailing" negativity from the basal layer, and a "trailing" positivity from the apical layer, which develop as delayed decays of the main transient in each layer. The trend of the slow potential (DC) shift initiated in this way is continued into the first period of self-sustained seizure activity. From Zuckermann and Glaser (1970a) with permission of the publisher.

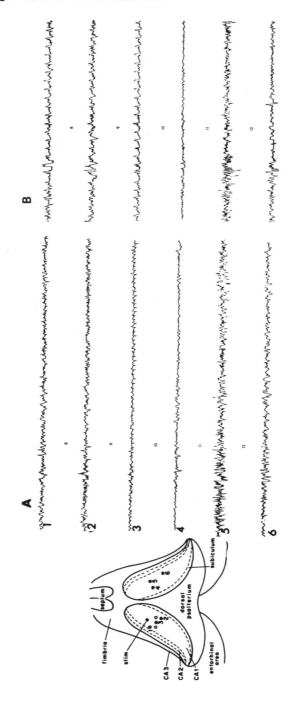

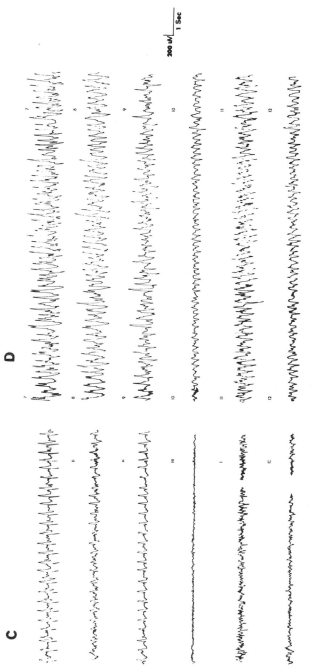

FIG. 6. Localized ventricular perfusion with ouabain (10^{-5} M) over the dorsal hippocampus. *A*: Onset of paroxysmal activity in Channel 3, 18 min after beginning perfusion. *B* and *C*: Subsequent spread of seizure activity, to Channels 1 and 2. *D*: Contralateral spread has occurred, with clinical signs of dilated pupils, blinking, and ear twitches. The positions of the electrodes (solid dots with numbers) and cannulae (open circles without numbers) are shown in the diagram of a dorsal view of the hippocampus and neighboring structures. From Pedley et al. (1969) with permission of the publisher.

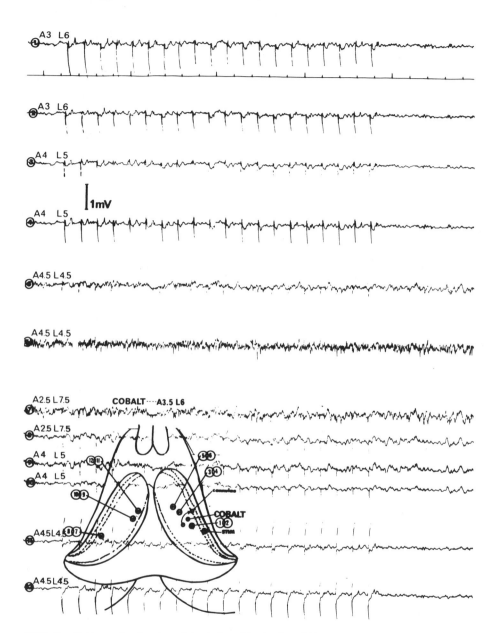

FIG. 7. Pattern of epileptic activity induced in the dorsal hippocampus with a cobalt powder latent focus during perfusion with high-K⁺ CSF (9 μequiv/ml). A train of 20 electrical stimuli at 1/sec initially failed to trigger a seizure discharge, but isolated spikes appeared 10 sec

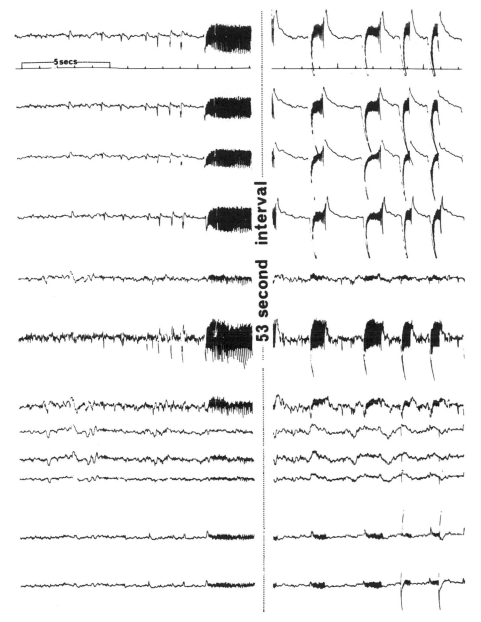

later, followed by prolonged bursts of after-discharge. From Zuckermann and Glaser (1970*b*) with permission of the publisher.

tions. For example, with concentrations of K^+ increased to 7.5 μequiv/ml, the percentage of perfusions inducing epileptogenicity is about 25% with the cobalt or alumina focus, with latent periods in the range of 35 min; in the control preparations, only 10% are reactive, after a latency of about 50 min. At 9 μequiv/ml of K^+, the percentage of perfusions inducing epileptogenicity is 36% in the control preparations, and over 80% in those with foci. The latency of reactivity is reduced to 15 to 20 min as compared to about 45 min in the controls. The combination of 7.5 μequiv/ml of K^+ and Ca^{++}-free CSF doubles the epileptogenic effect of the K^+ increase alone. L-Glutamate added to normal CSF also activates both types of foci, from 5% epileptogenic reactivity at 5 μequiv/ml to 80% at 50 μequiv/ml.

There are also changes among the different variables of the epileptogenic effect. The latent period (with perfusions containing 9 μequiv/ml of K^+) is reduced by more than 50% for the chronic focus preparations; the duration of the induced seizure is increased from 40 ± 16 sec in the controls, to 53 ± 12 sec in the cobalt, to 80 ± 15 sec in the alumina preparations. After the cessation of perfusion, repetitive seizures occur in only 8% of the controls; in the cobalt preparations, there have been repetitive seizures after perfusion in 15% of the cases, and in 32% with alumina. There have been some differences in the pattern of convulsive reactivity. The typical K^+-induced seizure in cobalt preparations is similar to that of the controls, but with more isolated spiking and more prolonged after-discharges (Fig. 7). In alumina preparations, the typical K^+-induced seizure differs from the normally induced seizure, with paroxysmal sharp slow waves (Fig. 8).

IV. COMMENTS AND DISCUSSION

An experimental model for epileptic seizures has been described by which effects of alterations in the extracellular environment of brain can be studied by means of localized perfusion in the inferior horn of the lateral ventricle of an animal. The perfused CSF can be altered by varying the concentrations of its ionic constituents, and by the addition of various pharmacologically active substances. Thus far, extensive studies have been carried out in which perfusions have been performed with increased concentrations of K^+ in the artificial perfusion fluid. Localized hippocampal seizure activity, occasionally spreading to generalization, has been induced and studied by a variety of recording techniques, with and without supplemental electrical stimulation. Characteristic features of epileptogenesis have been confirmed. Since a latent period of 15 to 40 min elapses between the begin-

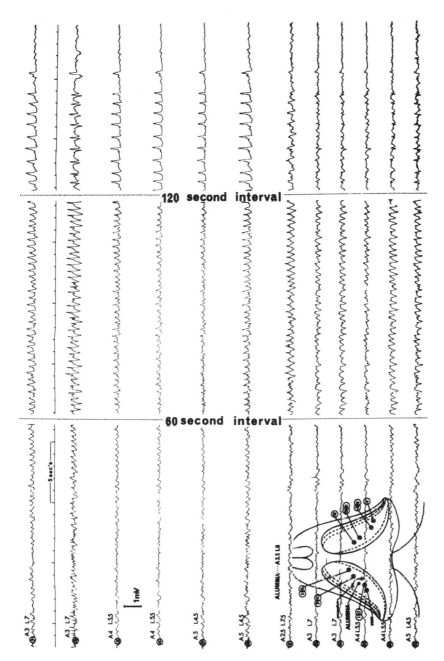

FIG. 8. Pattern of epileptic activity induced in dorsal hippocampus with alumina cream latent focus, during perfusion with high-K⁺ CSF (9 μequiv/ml). The seizure activity consists of paroxysmal slow and often sharp waves gradually spreading from focal derivation. From Zuckermann and Glaser (1970b) with permission of the publisher.

ning of perfusion and the start of seizure activity, there probably are, in normal brain, functional barriers protecting neurons against accumulation of external K^+. We think it is possible that a localized increase of K^+ in extracellular spaces of brain might play a significant role in triggering seizure activity in various physiopathological situations. The critical concentration of K^+ capable of inducing seizure discharges in our hippocampal experiments is 7.5 to 8.5 μequiv/ml in the perfusing CSF (at an average rate of 0.8 μequiv/min). Such concentration could be reached either by cell destruction under pathological circumstances, or by intense neuronal activity, both of which are known to cause a leakage of K^+ from the involved cells (Grafstein, 1963). The experiments with activation of chronic, latent epileptogenic foci tend to support this hypothesis, since most aspects of epileptogenic excitability are increased when latent or subthreshold foci are subjected to high-K^+ perfusion. Under these experimental conditions, the usual rapid clearance of excess K^+ is no longer realized, and K^+ begins to accumulate earlier during the perfusion probably because of derangement of the ordinarily functional barriers which prevent K^+ accumulation at critical neuronal points, bind K^+ or buffer its action, and finally clear the extracellular fluid. At the present time, we have no experimental data to indicate the nature or location of these barriers, whether neuroglia or other extraneuronal structures. At the concentrations of K^+ used, tissue edema was neither expected (Bourke and Tower, 1966a,b) nor found.

Pollen and Trachtenberg (1970) and Trachtenberg and Pollen (1970) have suggested that glial cells adjacent to neurons and presynaptic terminals act to buffer the increases in "external" K^+ that accompany neuronal activity. This concept follows the earlier suggestions by Kuffler and his group (Kuffler and Nicholls, 1966; Orkand et al., 1966). Pollen and Trachtenberg (1970) next postulate that impairment of such neuroglial function could lead to increases in K^+ around neurons and presynaptic terminals and an increase in neuronal excitability. This concept has received support from the experiments described in this chapter and those previously reported (Zuckermann and Glaser, 1968a,b, 1970a,b). The presence of fibrillary gliosis in cerebral lesions (e.g., post-traumatic cicatrices) then assumes more relevant significance as an important factor in epileptogenesis.

Recently, Fertziger and Ranck (1970) have studied the increase in K^+ concentration in "interstitial" cerebral spaces during seizures (induced either by electrical stimulation or pentylenetetrazol), and have related this to a concept of the influence of K^+ in the "regenerative all-or-none" aspect of the initiation of seizures. They used an acute experimental model involving anesthetized animals with exposure of pial surface (cats) and ventricular surface of hippocampus (rats), and perfusion, within a plexiglass chamber, over these surfaces with artificial CSF containing ^{42}K.

In no experiment in our series did we observe any actual "spreading depression" effects induced by perfusions with high K^+ CSF at the concentrations of K^+ utilized. When no seizure is elicited, there is no alteration of background electroencephalographic activity or depression of the DC potential. Epileptic discharges have been induced without any associated sign of depression of electrical activity. Postictally depressed electroencephalographic activity is either absent or brief. These effects differ from those described for K^+ as a powerful and characteristic agent inducing "spreading depression" (Marshall, 1959; Grafstein, 1963). The causes of this apparent contradiction probably are species differences, absence of anesthesia (a predisposing factor in most experiments), and significantly lower K^+ concentrations in the perfusate in present experiments. The last point is the most important factor; in all the studies dealing with K^+-induced spreading depression, very highly concentrated solutions of this ion have been used, usually 1% (w/v) or isotonic (0.15 M) levels. Yet, there may be a relationship between the actual paroxysmal-epileptic phenomena which we have produced with our concentrations of K^+ and some features of spreading depression, since fast, paroxysmal-type discharges, as bursts of spike and random slow waves, have been described (Marshall, 1959) during the development of "spreading depression" (i.e., "spreading activation").

These experimental observations lead us to the assumption that in focal epilepsy latent epileptogenic foci could be activated by a small or moderate increase in extracellular K^+ in the location of the focus. As protective barriers are increasingly disturbed, limited cell destruction, or simply excessive neuronal activity, could induce this relatively small increase in external K^+ concentration. Neurons involved in irritable foci usually display seizure activity before those in normal brain tissue when K^+ is increased, since the latent period for the former is markedly decreased, as we have shown here. Such neurons then become the pacemakers of the epileptic discharge. Oldendorf and Davson (1967) have emphasized that no point in human brain is more than about 2 cm from an ependymal or pial surface, most grey matter being within a few millimeters; however, if various histological abnormalities interfere with the movement of solutes along access pathways to and from CSF, local noxious accumulations can result. Our findings in the series of experiments already described demonstrate that an enforced local accumulation of K^+ exerts a major local effect, with a relatively small tendency to spread to distant areas, except by projection. Most of the effects induced are or can be limited to the perfused hippocampus, often just to the region under perfusion. Thus, there could be limited areas of brain exposed to an altered K^+ environment without appreciable disturbances of the CSF composition or function as a whole. Further, the convulsive effects of single stimuli, delivered during the latent period of high K^+ CSF perfusion, suggest that if abnormal concentrations of K^+ occur in the extracellular spaces of the hippocampus, trivial super-imposed stimuli or, indeed, even additional chemical alterations (such as reduction of Ca^{++} or increase of glutamate), as well as a subthreshold lesion, might be able to trigger a seizure.

V. ACKNOWLEDGMENT

This investigation was supported by U.S. Public Health Service Grant 5–P01–NS–06208 from the National Institute of Neurological Diseases and Stroke.

VI. REFERENCES

Bourke, R. S., and Tower, D. B. (1966a): Fluid compartmentation and electrolytes of cat cerebral cortex *in vitro*. I. Swelling and solute distribution in mature cerebral cortex. *Journal of Neurochemistry*, 13:1071–1097.

Bourke, R. S., and Tower, D. B. (1966b): Fluid compartmentation and electrolytes of cat cerebral cortex *in vitro*. II. Sodium, potassium and chloride of mature cerebral cortex. *Journal of Neurochemistry*, 13:1099–1117.

Bradbury, M. W. B., and Davson, H. (1965): The transport of K^+ between CSF and brain. *Journal of Physiology*, 181:151–174.

Bradbury, M. W. B., and Štulcová, B. (1970): Efflux mechanism contributing to the stability of the potassium concentration in cerebrospinal fluid. *Journal of Physiology*, 208:415–430.

Bronzino, J. D., Morgane, P. J., Stern, W. C., and Bottaro, S. (1972): A new design for an exploring chemode. *Electroencephalography and Clinical Neurophysiology*, 32:195–198.

Cserr, H. (1965): Potassium exchange between CSF plasma and brain. *American Journal of Physiology*, 209:1219–1226.

Feldberg, W. (1963): *A Pharmacologic Approach to the Brain from its Inner and Outer Surface*. E. Arnold, Ltd., London.

Feldberg, W., and Sherwood, S. L. (1957): Effects of Ca^{++} and K^+ injected into the cerebral ventricle of the cat. *Journal of Physiology*, 139:408–416.

Fertziger, A. P., and Ranck, J. B., Jr. (1970): Potassium accumulation in interstitial space during epileptiform seizures. *Experimental Neurology*, 26:571–585.

Glaser, G. H. (1964): Sodium and seizures. *Epilepsia*, 5:97–111.

Glaser, G. H., and Wolf, G. (1963): Seizures induced by intraventricular sodium. *Nature*, 200:44–46.

Glaser, G. H., and Zuckermann, E. C. (1968): Potassium accumulation in extracellular spaces of brain as a possible cause of epileptogenic activity. In: *Brain and Mind Problems*, edited by G. Alema, G. Bollea, W. Floris, B. Guidetti, G. C. Reda, and R. Vizioli. Il Pensiero Scientifico, Rome, pp. 310–329.

Grafstein, B. (1963): Neuronal release of K^+ during spreading depression. In: *Brain Function, Cortical Excitability and Steady Potentials*, edited by M. A. B. Brazier. University of California Press, Berkeley, pp. 87–124.

Held, D., Fencl, V., and Pappenheimer, J. R. (1964): Electrical potential of cerebrospinal fluid. *Journal of Neurophysiology,* 27:942–959.

Hillman, H. (1970): Chemical basis of epilepsy. *Lancet,* 2:23–24.

John, E. R., Tschirgi, R. D., and Wenzel, B. M. (1959): Effects of injections of cations into the cerebral ventricles on conditioned responses in the cat. *Journal of Physiology,* 146:550–562.

Katzman, R., Graziani, L., Kaplan, R., and Escriva, A. (1965): Exchange of CSF K$^+$ with blood and with brain: a study in normal and ouabain perfused cats. *Archives of Neurology,* 13:513–524.

Katzman, R., Weitzman, E. D., Graziani, L., and Escriva, A. (1964): Ventriculo-cisternal perfusion of rhesus. Transport of Ca^{++} and K$^+$ with correlated behavioral changes. *Neurology,* 14:267.

Kuffler, S. W., and Nicholls, J. G. (1966): The physiology of neuroglial cells. *Ergebnisse der Physiologie,* 57:1–90.

Marshall, W. H. (1959): Spreading cortical depression of Leão. *Physiological Reviews,* 39:239–280.

Oldendorf, W. H., and Davson, H. (1967): Brain extracellular space and the sink action of cerebrospinal fluid. *Archives of Neurology,* 17:196–205.

Orkand, R. K., Nicholls, J. G., and Kuffler, S. W. (1966): Effect of nerve impulses on the membrane potential of glial cells in the central nervous system of amphibia. *Journal of Neurophysiology,* 29:788–806.

Pappenheimer, J. R., Heisey, S. R., Jordan, E. F., and Downer, J. D. C. (1962): Perfusion of the cerebral ventricular system in unanesthetized goats. *American Journal of Physiology,* 203:763–774.

Pedley, T. A., Zuckermann, E. C., and Glaser, G. H. (1969): Epileptogenic effects of localized ventricular perfusion of ouabain on dorsal hippocampus. *Experimental Neurology,* 25: 207–219.

Pollen, D. A., and Trachtenberg, M. C. (1970): Neuroglia: Gliosis and focal epilepsy. *Science,* 167:1252–1253.

Snider, R. S., and Niemer, W. T. (1961): *A Stereotaxic Atlas of the Cat Brain.* University of Chicago Press, Chicago.

Tower, D. B. (1960): *Neurochemistry of Epilepsy.* Charles C Thomas, Springfield, Ill.

Tower, D. B. (1969): Neurochemical mechanisms. In: *Basic Mechanisms of the Epilepsies,* edited by H. H. Jasper, A. A. Ward, Jr., and A. Pope. Little, Brown and Co., Boston, pp. 611–638.

Trachtenberg, M. C., and Pollen, D. A. (1970): Neuroglia: Biophysical properties and physiologic function. *Science,* 167:1248–1252.

Tschirgi, R. D., and Taylor, J. L. (1958): Slowly changing bioelectrical potentials associated with the blood-brain barrier. *American Journal of Physiology,* 195:7–22.

Wagner, J. W., and DeGroot, J. (1963): Multipurpose cannula for acute and chronic intracerebral chemical and electrophysiological studies. *Electroencephalography and Clinical Neurophysiology,* 15:125–126.

Zuckermann, E. C., and Glaser, G. H. (1968a): Hippocampal epileptic activity induced by localized ventricular perfusion with high-potassium cerebrospinal fluid. *Experimental Neurology,* 20:87–110.

Zuckermann, E. C., and Glaser, G. H. (1968b): Changes in hippocampal-evoked responses induced by localized perfusion with high-potassium cerebrospinal fluid. *Experimental Neurology,* 22:96–117.

Zuckermann, E. C., and Glaser, G. H. (1970a): Slow potential shifts in dorsal hippocampus during "epileptogenic" perfusion of the inferior horn with high-potassium CSF. *Electroencephalography and Clinical Neurophysiology,* 28:236–246.

Zuckermann, E. C., and Glaser, G. H. (1970b): Activation of experimental epileptogenic foci. Action of increased K$^+$ in extracellular spaces of brain. *Archives of Neurology,* 23:358–364.

14

Audiogenic Seizures

Robert L. Collins

OUTLINE

I. INTRODUCTION

Audiogenic seizures are convulsions triggered by definable sound stimuli. Although uncommon in man (Bickford and Klass, 1969), they can be experimentally induced in housemice (Hall, 1947; Vicari, 1951), deermice

(Dice, 1935; Watson, 1939), rats (Maier and Glaser, 1940a), and rabbits (Nachtsheim, 1937; Nellhaus, 1958).

First described in mice by Studentsov in 1924 (Krushinsky et al., 1970) and in rats by Donaldson (1924), sound-induced convulsions have been rediscovered often and studied extensively from several frames of reference. Accordingly, the literature on audiogenic seizures is vast, international in scope, and occasionally confusing. Important sources of information are found in *Psychophysiologie Neuropharmacologie et Biochimie de la Crise Audiogène* (Colloques Internationaux du Centre National de la Recherche Scientifique, 1963), *Comparative and Cellular Pathophysiology of Epilepsy* (Servít, 1966), and *Physiological Effects of Noise* (Welch and Welch, 1970). Reviews of the early psychological literature are given by Finger (1947) and Bevan (1955), and references to the Soviet literature are provided by Krushinsky et al. (1970).

I believe that audiogenic seizures represent a serviceable experimental model of the epilepsies whose use has yet to be exploited, and I invite the reader to consider the study of sound-induced convulsions from this vantage.

The choice of a laboratory animal is as important a consideration as the choice of an experimental model, and I direct attention to the advantages of using genetically defined mice. Mice are small, inexpensive, and readily available. Experiments calling for testing large numbers of mice are both feasible and economical. The genetic characteristics of mice are the best understood of any laboratory mammal. There exist a number of inbred strains, selectively bred lines, and neurological mutant stocks of mice that are differentially sensitive to convulsion. Relatively efficient techniques for breeding and genetic analysis are available for the isolation of previously undefined hereditary influences as well as for the creation of new stocks possessing specific vulnerabilities. Sensitization-induced convulsibility can be established in otherwise resistant mice by prior auditory exposure to intense sound during a sensitive period of development, and this vulnerability can be restricted unilaterally.

II. DESCRIPTIONS OF AUDIOGENIC SEIZURES

The response pattern of mice and rats undergoing audiogenic seizure consists of pretonic, tonic, and post-tonic phases (Fig. 1). The pretonic phase begins with an initial stun or startle response moments after onset of

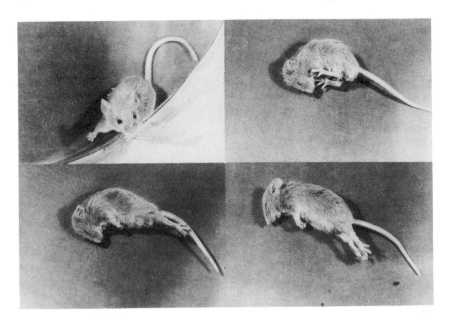

FIG. 1. An audiogenic seizure observed in a 21-day-old mouse of the inherently susceptible DBA/2J inbred strain. *Upper left:* Moments before the onset of bell ringing. *Upper right:* Loss of righting response and clonic spasms of the hindlegs following a burst of rapid running. *Lower left:* Rigid tonic extension of the hindlegs. *Lower right:* Respiratory failure signaled by a relaxation of the pinnae.

sound. A latent period of several seconds is followed by a burst of increasingly rapid running, often punctuated by erratic leaping, until the animal falls over and manifests clonic spasms. The tonic phase begins with an abrupt hindleg flexion followed by an often explosive hindleg extension. Rigid tonic extension may be maintained for 10 to 20 sec. Some mice die during extension. The time of respiratory failure is signaled by a clear-cut relaxation of the pinnae during rigid extension. The post-tonic phase consists of terminal clonus followed by a period of stupor resembling a cataleptic state. The animal may maintain unusual postures (Krushinskii, 1960), and it is generally areflexive to stimuli other than sound (Prokopetz, 1963). The state may be terminated by adventitious sound.

Variations in this basic pattern are seen. The initial running attack may end and the animal appears to resume normal grooming behavior. In mice and rats, this period lasts between 10 and 20 sec, and may be followed by a second episode of running that terminates in convulsion (Fuller and

Smith, 1953; Krushinskii, 1960). The biphasic character of seizure activity during 1 min of sound stimulation is illustrated in Fig. 2. The latencies from the onset of sound to the onset of each episode of running, regardless of whether clonic convulsion ensued, are represented by the gray area, and the latencies to the onset of clonic convulsion are represented by the solid

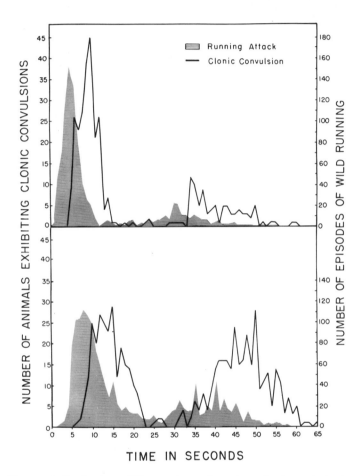

FIG. 2. Temporal distributions of the numbers of running episodes and clonic convulsions observed on tests of mice of 34 different genotypes. Sound stimulation was terminated with the onset of clonus or persisted for a maximum of 60 seconds. All mice were initially tested at 21 days of age. Those that did not display initial clonus on first exposure were retained and tested 48 hr later. *Upper portion:* The distribution of running episodes and clonic convulsions observed on initial tests of 1,720 mice. *Lower portion:* Distributions obtained 48 hr later. The biphasic pattern of seizure activity is seen for both initial and sensitization-dependent convulsions.

line. The bimodal distributions of running episodes and clonic convulsions are clearly visualized for both initial and sensitization-induced audiogenic seizures. The period of relative inhibition of seizure activity in mice occurs between 20 and 30 sec after stimulus onset, and it is during this period that a resumption of grooming behavior is observed.

Minimal convulsions are observed. Animals may exhibit wild running only, or wild running followed by myoclonus. In mice, "standing seizures" are occasionally observed. After a period of motor excitement, a mouse may adopt an immobile upright posture and exhibit a fine tremor. A characteristic of the standing seizure is that the tail becomes slowly raised and rigidly arched over the back. It is held there for several seconds, then slowly lowered horizontally.

Mice and rats may be caused to convulse after occluding one ear. The motor patterns of animals convulsing unilaterally are asymmetrical. In rats, the asymmetry may be signaled by the position adopted at the beginning of the running phase and the initial direction of running (Horák, 1958). These initial signs are not generally observed in mice since they often abruptly change direction during running. However, at the end of running, the forepaw contralateral to the open ear appears to collapse, and the mouse falls to one side with the occluded ear down, and the open ear facing the sound. The forepaw on the side of the open ear may continue to exhibit clonic movements while the opposite forepaw rests on the floor of the chamber. Occasionally, the forepaw ipsilateral to the open ear is extended and displays slow choreiform movements (Ward and Collins, 1971).

Two other types of sound-induced seizure have been reported. Krushinsky et al. (1970) described a "tic-like" myoclonic seizure that may develop in rats that have had typical audiogenic seizures on at least 10 occasions. The myoclonic seizures are first observed in the head region with spasms of the lips, eyelids, and ears. This may later involve the muscles of the neck, forepaws, and hindlegs. The myoclonic seizure differs from normal audiogenic seizures in that it is generally observed to occur during the latent period between two attacks of running. In contrast to normal audiogenic seizures, myoclonic seizures may be eliminated by extirpation of the cortex, or by functional decortication performed by means of spreading depression (Krushinsky et al., 1970).

Multiple seizures resulting from the application of intermittent sound following normal audiogenic seizures are described by Krushinsky et al. (1970). These are obtained during periods of 10-sec sonic bursts following 90 sec of continuous stimulation. These differ from typical audiogenic seizures in that the latency to motor excitation is extremely short (approximately 0.1 sec). Multiple seizures are frequently fatal.

III. AUDIOGENIC SEIZURES AS GENERALIZED CONVULSIONS

The justification for considering audiogenic seizures to be generalized convulsions analagous to those evoked by other means must presently be sought on other than electrographic grounds. It has proved extremely difficult to obtain satisfactory electrographic records of seizure activity in freely running animals. Furthermore, it is generally impossible to provoke audiogenic seizure attacks in restrained mice (Frings and Frings, 1952), rats (Lindsley et al., 1942; Cain et al., 1951; Griffiths, 1953), or rabbits (Nellhaus, 1963). Electrical records of purely derived audiogenic seizure activity are uncommon (Niaussat and Laget, 1963; Krushinsky et al., 1970). Several investigators have recorded electrical activity from animals pretreated with subconvulsive doses of pentylenetetrazol (Bureš, 1953, 1963; Šterc, 1962; Nellhaus, 1963).

The strongest evidence that seizures provoked by acoustic stimuli are analagous to those obtained by other means is obtained by comparing the temporal characteristics of the stages of audiogenic seizure with those obtained following maximal electroshock or pentylenetetrazol-induced seizure. Table 1 summarizes the mean duration in seconds for periods of

TABLE 1. *Patterns and mean durations of components of maximal seizure induced by electroshock, pentylenetetrazol, and sound stimulation in young and adult mice*

Seizure (strain, age)	Mean duration of seizure components (sec)					
				Hindleg tonic		
	Latency	Running	Clonus	Flexion	Extension	Clonus
Audiogenic (Frings, adult)	2.9	2.8	2.7	1.0	12.9	yes
Audiogenic (O'Grady, adult)	3.0	4.0	2.0	1.9	11.1	yes
Electroshock (CF #1, adult)		[a]	[a]	1.8[b]	12.8	yes
Pentylenetetrazol (CF #1, adult)	3.4	[a]	2.5	0.7	12.8	no
Audio-conditioned (CF #1, 20-day)	6.0	3.2	3.0	1.8	15.1	yes
Electroshock (CF #1, 20-day)		[a]	[a]	1.6[b]	17.0	yes
Pentylenetetrazol (CF #1, 20-day)	3.1	[a]	3.0	1.8	20.4	yes

[a] Component absent.
[b] Includes latency.
From Fink and Iturrian (1970) with permission of the publisher.

latency, running, initial clonus, hindleg flexor and extensor components of tonus, and terminal clonus according to the method used to elicit maximal seizure activity in mice (Fink and Iturrian, 1970).

The pretonic component of seizure induced by pentylenetetrazol consists of a period of latency and clonus, while that for electroshock seizure is absent or too short to measure. Mean durations of hindleg flexor and extensor components are remarkably similar for seizures produced by the three methods in adult mice. Although younger mice exhibit longer durations of hindleg extension (Iturrian and Fink, 1969), the durations of this period were similar for the three methods. Terminal clonus, observed following electroshock and audiogenic seizure, is absent following pentylenetetrazol-induced seizure. Although recurrent seizures may be observed in mice treated with pentylenetetrazol, they are not observed following electroshock or audiogenic seizure if the sound is terminated.

The postictal recovery time of maximal electroshock seizure (the time required for 50% of CF #1 mice and Frings' mice to exhibit a second maximal convulsion) was about 90 sec according to studies by Swinyard et al. (1963). Approximately the same recovery time for SJL/J and DBA/2J mice to exhibit a second audiogenic seizure is noted if mice are tested initially with one ear open and then retested with the opposite ear open (Ward, 1971). The recovery time for mice tested bilaterally varies with the strain chosen and may be as long as several hours.

Pharmacological agents possessing known anticonvulsant properties are effective in altering audiogenic seizure. Oral administration of trimethadione (375 mg/kg), phenobarbital (4.6 mg/kg), diphenylhydantoin (5 mg/kg), or meprobamate (29 mg/kg) eliminated the tonic-extensor component of maximal audiogenic seizure in 50% of Frings' mice studied by Swinyard et al. (1963). Higher doses eliminated the running components of seizure.

Chlorpromazine, promazine, triflupromazine, and hydroxyzine have been reported ineffective against the tonic-extensor or running component of maximal audiogenic seizure in doses lower than the neurotoxic level, and reserpine has been shown to increase seizure severity (Fink and Swinyard, 1959).

IV. ONTOGENETIC CONSIDERATIONS

Mouse pups exhibit slow paddling movements of the forelimbs shortly after birth. They pivot sideways by day 3, stand and walk irregularly by days 6 to 7, and are capable of walking a straight line by day 15. Forelimb and hindlimb placing responses are absent at birth and develop from days 3 to 4. The righting reflex is complete by day 7 (Fox, 1965). The development of the Preyer reflex to auditory startle, the initial cochlear potentials, and VIIIth nerve action potentials appear between 9 and 12 days after birth (Alford and Rubin, 1963).

The postnatal development of susceptibility to maximal audiogenic seizure of O'Grady mice studied by Swinyard et al. (1963) is presented in Fig. 3. Spontaneous motor activity was observed in mice aged 1 to 8 days regardless of sonic stimulation. By day 9, hyperkinesia in response to sound was observed; by day 11, the initial startle responses were noted. Running-clonic attacks were observed initially on day 9 and reached a peak by day 15. Tonic flexion was first observed on day 15 and reached maximum incidence on day 18. The tonic-extensor component of maximal audiogenic seizure was first observed on day 17 and reached 100% on day 22.

The age of peak susceptibility to audiogenic seizure in DBA/2J, Frings',

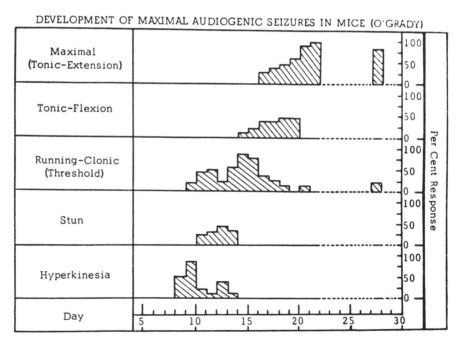

FIG. 3. Postnatal development of maximal audiogenic seizure in mice of O'Grady selected stock. Mice were tested daily except on days indicated by the broken lines. From Swinyard et al. (1963) with permission of the publisher.

and O'Grady mice is between 19 and 24 days; thereafter, susceptibility declines. The pattern of age changes for these three types of mice is similar (Castellion et al., 1965), although the incidence of initial seizures in DBA/2J mice may be quite low by 6 to 8 weeks of age. Since the ability of mice to produce maximal seizures to electrical stimulation is retained throughout adulthood (Castellion et al., 1965), the decline in susceptibility to audiogenic seizures in some mice may be due to a decline in auditory sensitivity. Ralls (1967), measuring auditory evoked potentials from the posterior colliculi, reported marked decreases of auditory sensitivity to high frequencies in DBA/2J mice with increasing age.

In rats selectively bred for susceptibility by Horák (Šterc, 1962), audiogenic seizures were first observed between 3 and 6 weeks of age, reached maximum proportion between 3 and 4 months of age, and decreased thereafter only slightly. The peak susceptibility to audiogenic seizure of rabbits bred by Nellhaus occurred between the 7th and 8th weeks of life and declined to low levels by 18 weeks of age (Nellhaus, 1963: Hohenboken and Nellhaus, 1970).

V. ENHANCING SUSCEPTIBILITY TO AUDIOGENIC SEIZURE

The proportions of convulsible animals observed in genetically heterogeneous populations may be disappointingly low. Occasionally, investigators have had to test large numbers of animals to obtain a sufficient number of sensitive animals for study. The screening of breeds, stocks, or inbred strains may be used to identify groups whose members are sensitive to seizure induction (an example is presented in Section VII). Selective breeding has been practiced to increase the incidence of audiogenic seizures in mice (Frings and Frings, 1953), rats (Maier and Glaser, 1940b; Krushinski, 1963), and rabbits (Nellhaus, 1958; Horák, 1965; Hohenboken and Nellhaus, 1970).

Pretreatment of nonsensitive animals with drugs can elevate susceptibility. Bureš (1963) observed increased sensitivity to audiogenic seizure in rats within 3 to 5 min following administration of subconvulsive doses of pentylenetetrazol (50 mg/kg i.p.). Wada and Ikeda (1966) and Wada and Asakura (1969) produced transient susceptibility to audiogenic seizure in initially nonsensitive rats pretreated with thiosemicarbazide (4.4 mg/kg i.p.) or methionine sulfoximine (300 mg/kg i.p.), and reported that these agents produced a reversible susceptibility to audiogenic seizure in cats and monkeys.

The alumina cream technique of Kopelof et al. (1942) has been adapted for studies of audiogenic seizure. Servít & Šterc (1958) reported that sound-induced seizures could be produced in rats after intracortical injection of aluminum hydroxide (2 to 6 mm³) into motor and cortical areas (Krieg's areas 4 and 41). Seizures were not observed following creation of artificial foci in the cerebellar cortex or in the optic zone. Sound-induced convulsions could be evoked in most rats after a period of about 30 days (Šterc, 1962).

Increases in seizure susceptibility of mice on subsequent exposure to sound have been informally noted by several investigators. Henry (1967), Iturrian and Fink (1968), and Fuller and Collins (1968*a*) formally demonstrated that convulsibility could be induced in otherwise seizure-resistant mice by prior exposure to intense sound. Audiogenic seizures observed on second exposure are called sensitization-dependent, sensitization-induced, or audio-conditioned. Figure 4 presents an example of a sensitization-induced convulsion in an SJL/J mouse.

Sensitization-dependent convulsibility requires a period of development that may vary with the strain of mouse chosen for study and with the age at which it was initially exposed to sound (acoustically primed). Three-week-old SJL/J mice exhibit high risk to convulsion by 36 hr after priming (Fuller

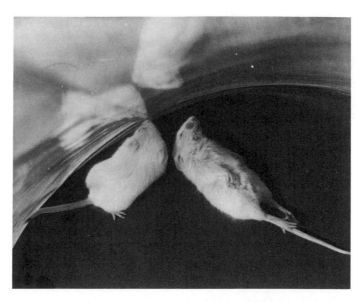

FIG. 4. Example of a sensitization-induced convulsion in a 23-day-old SJL/J mouse. Mice were littermates. The mouse in tonic extension on the right received 30 sec of sound stimulation 48 hr previously.

and Collins, 1968*a*). SJL/J mice tested 21 to 25 weeks following priming have moderate to high convulsive risk, and some mice remain convulsible for as long as 6 months following a 30-sec priming exposure (Fuller and Collins, 1970).

Detectable elevations in convulsive risk have been noted following as little as 1 sec of priming in C57BL/6J mice (Henry and Bowman, 1970), and 5 sec of priming in SJL/J mice (Fuller and Collins, 1968*a*). Sensitization-dependent convulsibility may be obtained in mice primed under sodium pentobarbital or ether anesthesia (Henry, 1967), or in mice primed during bilateral cortical spreading depression (Ward and Sinnett, 1971).

Sensitization-induced convulsibility may be reversibly impaired if mice are repeatedly stimulated with sound at 6- or 12-hr intervals following priming (Fuller and Collins, 1968*a*). The reduction of convulsive risk following repeated exposures behaves as a post-stimulation refractory state possessing a relatively long time constant (Fuller and Collins, 1970).

If the priming stimulus is presented to one ear, unilaterally restricted convulsibility can be obtained. Mice primed after one auditory meatus has been filled with glycerol later convulse only if stimulated through the ear open during priming, and do not convulse when stimulated with the opposite ear open (Fuller and Collins, 1968*b*). Unilateral susceptibility may be achieved by another technique. Intense sound repeatedly presented to one ear at 6- or 12-hr intervals following an initial bilateral priming exposure results in a lateralized inhibition of convulsibility (Collins, 1970*a*). SJL/J mice tested 48 hr post-priming convulse when exposed to sound through the ear that was occluded during intermittent stimulation, and do not convulse when tested with the opposite ear open. Unilateral inhibition does not afford protection against convulsion if mice are tested bilaterally, although the latencies to initial clonus may be lengthened The motor patterns of unilaterally convulsing mice are asymmetrical (Ward and Collins, 1971).

Figure 5 is a flow chart illustrating two methods of preparing mice to become unilaterally susceptible to audiogenic seizure. The proportions of mice displaying clonic convulsion per treatment group are based upon initial experiments using SJL/J mice (Fuller and Collins, 1968*b*; Collins, 1970*a*), and are representative of those consistently obtained in this laboratory.

VI. PRACTICAL ASPECTS

The essential requirements for initiating studies of audiogenic seizures are a source of sound, a sensitive animal, and a method of confining both.

The choice of sound stimuli used to provoke seizure activity has been a

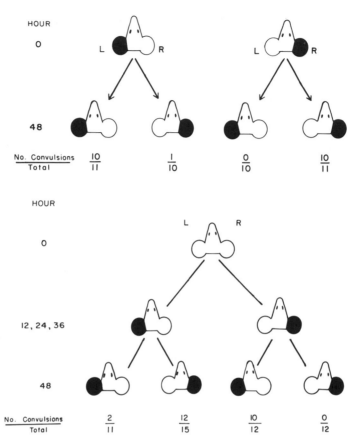

FIG. 5. Flow chart illustrating two procedures used to produce mice unilaterally susceptible to audiogenic seizure. The blackened ear represents the ear occluded with glycerol during sound stimulation. *Upper portion:* Unilateral susceptibility achieved by selective priming. *Lower portion:* Unilateral susceptibility achieved by selective inhibition. Adapted from Fuller and Collins (1968*b*) and Collins (1970*a*).

practical art. A variety of sources has been used; these include jingling keys (Dice, 1935; Maier and Glaser, 1940*a*), jangling metal tubes (Chance and Yaxley, 1949), high-pressure air blasts (Maier and Glaser, 1940*a*), white noise (Antonitis, 1954), and sine-wave tones (Nellhaus, 1963). The ringing of an electric bell has been widely used as a source of high-intensity sound of mixed frequencies.

A sound stimulus must possess an adequate intensity within a delimited bandwidth to provoke seizure activity. Mice exhibit maximum auditory sensitivity to frequencies between 12 and 16 kHz (Berlin and Finck in Fuller and Wimer, 1966; Ralls, 1967). Intense sine-wave stimulation below 8 to 10 kHz is ineffective in producing either audiogenic seizure or sensitization in mice (Morin et al., 1948; Ikeda and Higashi, 1970; Henry et al., 1971). Sound-intensity readings of between 90 and 120 db above 0.0002 dyne/cm^2 at the level of the mouse are sufficient to elicit seizures and initiate sensitization. Since general-purpose sound-level meters are usually calibrated for sine-wave or impulse sounds, their use with sounds of mixed frequencies may provide only indications of relative intensity. All personnel in the testing area and all animals not undergoing actual tests should be afforded protection against the effects of escaping sound.

Whether mice used in experiments are purchased from outside sources (Appendix I) or obtained from an inhouse breeding colony, the investigator should become thoroughly familiar with the recommended methods of care and humane treatment of laboratory mice (Appendix II). In addition, he should be aware of any special requirements of individual strains chosen for study. For example, fumes of chloroform, turpentine, and oxidation products of ethylene oxide are fatal for male mice of DBA/2J and C3H/HeJ strains (Green, 1968). Efforts should be made both to control extraneous variables known to affect susceptibility and to adopt sound practices of the design of experiments. The time of day mice are tested is important. Mice are more susceptible during the onset of the dark cycle (Halberg et al., 1958).

DBA/2J mice have been used extensively for studies of inherent susceptibility to audiogenic seizure. This oldest of inbred strains was developed by C. C. Little in 1909 for experiments on the inheritance of coat color characteristics. The strain name stands for three genes affecting coat color: dilute, brown, and agouti. Nearly 100% of DBA/2J mice tested between 3 and 4 weeks of age exhibit severe, often fatal, audiogenic seizures. DBA/1J mice, another subline formed by Little, are generally nonsusceptible on first exposure. For studies of sensitization-dependent convulsibility, my colleagues and I have relied on the use of SJL/J mice. This strain was inbred by James Lambert in 1955 from Swiss-Webster stocks of three different sources maintained at The Jackson Laboratory. Typically, 1% or so of SJL/J mice convulse on first exposure to sound, while 85% on the average become convulsible within 48 hr after priming. The convulsible state induced by priming may last several months in SJL/J mice, and seizures are seldom fatal. Since male SJL/J mice become vicious fighters, they should not be housed together for long-term experiments.

Mice may be housed singly or in groups in a room adjacent to the testing area. Group-housed mice may be individually identified by banding the tail with ink markings which will persist for a day or so. Permanent identification of mice not subject to auditory tests can be achieved by adopting a system of ear punches (Dickie, 1966).

A mouse can be readied for injection by picking it up by the tail with the right hand and placing it on a piece of $\frac{1}{4}$-inch mesh hardware cloth. The tension exerted by the mouse attempting to move forward against restraint enables the experimenter to place the thumb and forefinger of his left hand safely around the mouse's neck as close to the head as possible. The loose skin is firmly squeezed together to restrict lateral head movements. This position is held while the control of the tail is transferred from the right hand to the palm and little finger of the left hand. The mouse can now be raised from the screen with the left hand, and the right hand is freed for injection.

Glycerol may be introduced into the auditory meatus by means of a small syringe without needle. The pinna is pushed away with the syringe tip, and glycerol is injected until it caps the orifice. Glycerol is sufficiently viscous at room temperature to remain in place for several minutes. It may be removed by swabbing. As a routine control for any possible irritant effects of glycerol, a mouse exposed to sound with one ear blocked should receive an equal amount of glycerol in the other ear after testing.

Audiogenic seizures need not be fatal for mice. Artificial ventilation, performed by means of gentle intermittent blowing into a rubber tube that covers the nose and mouth of the mouse, can be applied until spontaneous respiratory movements reappear.

An adequate test chamber should confine the test animal, provide a measure of attenuation against escaping sound, and permit visual observation. The chamber in use at The Jackson Laboratory resembles a "see-through" file cabinet. It is a double-walled box, insulated with rockwool, with the front face fitted with windows. The interior of the chamber measures 35 cm across, 51 cm deep, and 35 cm high. It is illuminated by two 8-watt fluorescent lamps. Mice are placed into a clear plastic cylindrical container, 30 cm in diameter and 30 cm high, that is fixed to the drawer bed. A 4-inch doorbell, energized by 8 vac, is positioned directly above the container when the front is closed. A battery of stopclocks is started at the same time as the bell, and the latencies of the various components of seizure are recorded to the nearest second.

Information of three types can be obtained from simple experiments. The proportions of mice entering each defined stage of seizure can be calculated and used to evaluate the effects of treatments on empiric risk. Quantitative or qualitative measures obtained from only those animals that entered a defined stage may be used: latencies to each stage, the ratio of the duration of tonic extension to that of tonic flexion, and the side to which an animal falls. A severity score may be obtained on each animal tested. An example of a linearly weighted severity score is: running = 1, clonus = 2, tonus = 3, death = 4. With the exception of reasonable conjecture as to what constitutes a proper severity score, differences between the three types of measures reflect differences in the questions an experimenter asks.

VII. GENETICS AS A TOOL—EXAMPLES

The term "inbred strain" has a specific meaning. A strain may be regarded as inbred if it has been derived by *single pair* brother-by-sister matings for at least 20 consecutive generations, or by parent-by-offspring matings for the same length of time where each mating is made to the younger parent (Staats, 1968). By 20 generations of inbreeding, approximately 99% of all genetic loci are in a homozygous condition. A number of strains of mice have been inbred for more than 150 generations.

The systematic reduction of genetic heterogeneity accomplished by prolonged inbreeding results in a reduction of phenotypic variation associated with hereditary causes. This reduction of biological noise leads to decreased batch-to-batch variability and to practical increases in the precision of detecting treatment differences for a fixed investment of research effort. Since there is no way to predict in advance just which alleles will become fixed during inbreeding, and since different genetic alternatives will become fixed during each inbreeding process, each inbred strain will possess a unique set of heritable characteristics distinguishing it from every other strain. As new research findings accumulate, these become a part of the permanent record of each strain.

Crosses between inbred strains may be made to obtain F_1 hybrids for study. F_1 hybrids are as genetically uniform as their inbred parents, but are genetically heterozygous at many loci. They often possess greater vigor or resistance to stress and thus may be more useful than inbred strains for certain kinds of experiments. In addition, they may be phenotypically less variable than either inbred parent. Strain crossing may be employed to obtain segregating generations, such as backcross or F_2 generations, for preliminary genetic analysis of a trait. F_1 hybrids from differing parents may be crossed to obtain genetically heterogeneous populations that are replicable across space and time.

Nearly 400 mutant genes are known for the mouse, and approximately 200 of these have been assigned positions on one of the 20 linkage groups that comprise the linkage map of the mouse. Approximately 100 of these single gene mutations lead to neurological disorders, and more than a dozen of these have been associated with the production of spontaneous convulsions (Sidman et al., 1965).

Named mutant genes may be used as experimental treatments, whose effects may be difficult or impossible to achieve by other means, or as genetic markers that signal the presence of other genes. Markers may aid in the isolation of carriers of recessive inviable traits, the identification of affected individuals early in development prior to the manifestation of a hereditary anomaly, and in the detection of new, presently unknown, genes that exert major effects upon a character of interest.

Three examples of the use of genetically defined laboratory mice in studies of audiogenic seizure are here presented: the first illustrates the use of multiple, genetically uniform populations to acquire information about the extent to which variation in seizure risk is associated with hereditary causes; the second illustrates the use of segregating generations in a genetic analysis of a particular difference in initial convulsive risk; the third example illustrates a use of a single gene mutation for the test of a hypothesis of a metabolic basis for susceptibility.

Figure 6 presents original data for initial, sensitization-dependent, and cumulative risk to audiogenic seizure obtained from tests of 1,720 mice of 34 genotypes. Mice tested were the progeny of a multiple intercrossing of eight highly inbred strains.

Mice were individually tested at 21 days of age. Those not exhibiting a clonic convulsion were retained and tested again 48 hr later. To estimate the percentage of total variance associated with genetic causes, each of 262 litters was considered to be an experimental unit, and the proportion of convulsing mice per litter was transformed by logits and the data subjected to analyses of variance.

While mice of most groups were resistant to seizure on first exposure to sound, all DBA/2J mice convulsed, and DBA/2J and DBA/1J parents produced hybrids with the highest risks. Genotypic differences accounted for 74% of the total variance for initial audiogenic seizure. The likelihood of sensitization-dependent convulsion was approximately three times that for initial seizure; 29 of 33 groups with defined seizure risks on both tests had numerically higher seizure risk on second exposure. Genotypic differences accounted for 54% of total variance in sensitization-induced convulsibility. Cumulative seizure risk reflected primarily sensitization-dependent convulsibility; 66% of its variance was explained by genotypic differences.

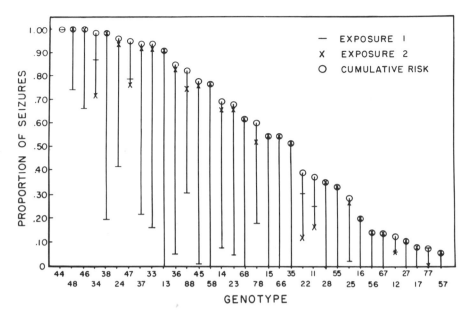

FIG. 6. Summary of data for risk to initial convulsion (bar), sensitization-induced convulsion (X), and cumulative convulsive risk (circle) for mice of 34 different genotypes. Mice (1,720 from 262 litters) were tested for audiogenic seizure at 21 days of age; those not convulsing on initial testing were retained and retested 48 hr later. Mice were obtained from the multiple intercrossing of the following eight highly inbred strains: P/J (11), BDP/J (22), DBA/1J (33), DBA/2J (44), C57BL/6J (55), SJL/J (66), A/J (77), and AKR/J (88). Numbers within parentheses serve to designate the genotype of F_1 hybrids; for example, the hybrid obtained from the mating of P/J and BDP/J is designated "12."

A thoughtful examination of Fig. 6 should lead to an appreciation of the importance of attempting to control, if not indeed exploit, sources of genetic variation. Consider that these data are the test scores of single individuals drawn from a genetically heterogeneous population. An experimenter who randomly chooses individuals and assigns them to experimental treatments will later confront an experimental error term pregnant with hereditary variance.

Figure 7 summarizes the results of a genetic analysis of the difference in risk to convulsion on first exposure to sound between mice of the resistant C57BL/6J strain (P_1) and the sensitive DBA/2J strain (P_2). A total of 940 mice from three genetically uniform generations and six segregating generations were studied (Collins and Fuller, 1968). The segregating generations consisted of the traditional backcross and second filial generations (B_1,

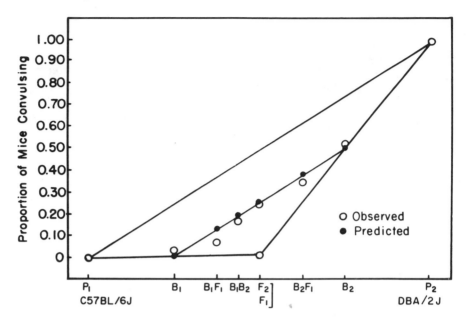

FIG. 7. Geometric representation of the results of a classical crossing experiment conducted to investigate the difference in convulsive risk to initial exposure to intense sound between mice of the sensitive DBA/2J and the resistant C57BL/6J strains. The apices of the triangle are the proportions of convulsing mice observed in the genetically uniform populations. Open circles within the figure are the observed proportions of convulsing mice for each of the six segregating generations, and the solid circles are the values predicted according to a single autosomal model of genetic inheritance. From Collins (1970b) with permission of the publisher.

B_2, and F_2) as well as three additional segregating generations: B_1 by F_1 (B_1F_1), B_2 by F_1 (B_2F_1), and B_1 by B_2 (B_1B_2). All mice were tested at 21 days of age.

Data in Fig. 7 are arranged in the form of a genetic triangle, the apices of which represent the proportions of convulsing mice observed in each of the three genetically uniform generations. The solid circles are the proportions of clonic convulsions per segregating generation expected according to a single-locus model of genetic inheritance (Collins, 1967). The open circles are the proportions observed. Visual inspection and statistical analysis of the data indicate excellent agreement between observed and expected proportions for each of the six segregating generations. The high risk of initial audiogenic seizure of the DBA/2J type is inherited as an autosomal recessive Mendelian character. The genetic locus was designated *asp* (audiogenic seizure prone). Additional studies indicated that the *asp*-locus was loosely linked to three other known genetic loci that reside on Linkage Group VIII of the mouse (Collins, 1970*b*).

These experiments illustrate that new, previously unknown, genetic loci, whose allelic alternatives exert major effect upon convulsive risk, can be identified and genetically mapped in a directed search.

This last example illustrates a use of a named mutant gene in the experimental test of a hypothesis concerning a metabolic defect of genetic origin and seizure susceptibility.

Briefly, Coleman (1960), studying liver phenylalanine hydroxalase activity in dilute and nondilute strains of mice, reported lowered enzyme activities in dilute animals, and he suggested that a deficiency in phenylalanine hydroxalase activity might be responsible for the seizure susceptibility of DBA/2J mice.

This hypothesis is attractive, reasonable, and evergreen for the following reasons: (1) mice homozygous for dilute lethal (d^l/d^l) exhibit spontaneous convulsions; (2) DBA/2J mice, homozygous for dilute (d/d) are highly susceptible to audiogenic seizure; (3) mice of other strains homozygous for dense (D/D) are often resistant to seizure; (4) the incidence of diluted hair color and epilepsies in human phenylketonurics is high (Partington, 1961); and (5) differences in phenylalanine hydroxalase activity have been implicated in all of the above.

A dense mouse appeared in a litter of DBA/2J mice in the Production Department of The Jackson Laboratory. Breeding tests confirmed that a mutation from d/d to D/d occurred. Matings between DBA/2-D/d and DBA/2-d/d were made, and all progeny were tested for audiogenic seizure at 21 days of age. This experiment should be a most sensitive test of the dilute hypothesis since mice were congenic for all genetic loci other than

TABLE 2. *Summary of latencies from onset of bell ringing to onset of stages of seizure for DBA/2-D/d (dense) and DBA/2-d/d (dilute) mice*

Genotype	N	Sex	Average latency (sec) ± SE			
			Run	Clonus	Tonus[a]	Death[b]
DBA/2-D/d	13	female	1.85 ± 0.27	5.69 ± 0.42	9.64 ± 0.59	26.11 ± 0.66
DBA/2-d/d	12	"	1.58 ± 0.23	5.92 ± 0.38	10.91 ± 1.21	26.55 ± 0.95
DBA/2-D/d	16	male	1.63 ± 0.18	5.38 ± 0.26	8.47 ± 0.68	25.31 ± 0.49
DBA/2-d/d	9	"	1.56 ± 0.18	5.78 ± 0.62	9.00 ± 0.54	24.57 ± 0.48

[a] One mouse in each of the four groups failed to exhibit tonic extension.

[b] Latencies to respiratory failure were obtained on 9 dense and 11 dilute female mice, and on 13 dense and 7 dilute male mice. Least squares analyses of variance for all latency differences between dense and dilute mice yielded nonsignificant F ratios ($0.25 < p < 0.50$).

dilute, and mice of both types appeared within each litter. Two replicate experiments were conducted.

All mice convulsed. Table 2 summarizes the data for average latencies to the stages of seizure. Latencies to running, initial clonus, tonic extension, and respiratory failure were statistically indistinguishable for dilute and dense mice of both sexes and both replicates. Therefore, the vulnerability of DBA/2J mice to audiogenic seizure is not predicated on a metabolic defect whose genetic origin resides at the *d*-locus on Linkage Group II of the mouse.

VIII. DISCUSSION

If studies of audiogenic seizure have so far shed little light on problems of the epilepsies (Bickford and Klass, 1969), it is because they have been studied primarily for other reasons. In addition, they have been considered to be, too often, the "audiogenic seizure phenomenon," the curiosity of quadrupeds, rather than (a) seizures, (b) seizures evoked by sound, and (c) seizures evoked by sound in certain sensitive animals.

The most pressing question is not whether audiogenic seizures are a model of a particular human convulsive disorder; they probably are not. Running fits are not terribly common in human beings. The pressing questions concern how the model may be used to provide insights, generate testable extrapolations, and be of general service to those concerned with mechanisms, processes, and treatments of the epilepsies. It is to these questions that each new investigator, who possesses an individual set of research skills and a unique vision, must address himself.

The kinds of research an investigator conducts is in part predicated on his choice of experimental laboratory animal. Mice are genetically sophisticated and neurophysiologically naive. The reverse is true of laboratory primates. The brains of mice weigh less than half a gram and their calvaria are paper-thin, but what mice lack in size is made up by numbers, short intergeneration times, and superb genetic definition. The study of audiogenic seizures in mice is well suited to research problems that demand both the economical testing of large numbers of animals and the stringent experimental control of extraneous variables.

I stress the importance of considering genetical influences one last time. A principle of the conservation of hereditary variance: for a given experiment at a given time, hereditary variance may neither be created nor destroyed, only partitioned. If not treated as an experimental variable, it will appear as part of the experimental error.

In contrast to seizures provoked by other means, audiogenic seizures are somewhat more "natural" convulsions — convulsions precipitated at a distance by an exaggeration of stimuli present in the environment. The running components of audiogenic seizure may well be one of their more useful, rather than disturbing, features. The running bouts, perhaps motor aura, of mice challenged with sound clearly delineate the growth of excitation, inhibition, and excitation, and these may prove to be useful indicators of prodromal seizure activity. The sensitization-induced convulsibility of mice provides one of the more dramatic examples of the creation of a specific vulnerability as an aftermath of a brief, apparently innocent, prior experience. The preparations of mice having convulsible "split personalities" should prove generally useful for studies requiring within-animal control.

The web of interactive influences contributing to seizure risk in mice may be no less complex than that underlying human convulsive disorders, but the opportunities to disentangle and understand these individual processes using laboratory animals appear much greater.

IX. APPENDIX I: SOURCES OF ANIMALS

The Institute of Laboratory Animal Resources, National Research Council of the National Academy of Sciences, periodically publishes a directory of animals useful to research and lists their sources. The current edition is *Animals for Research,* eighth edition-revised (National Academy of Sciences, Washington, D.C., 1971).

Inbred mice are available from a number of suppliers. Inbred strains of mice whose names are suffixed by "J" are available from the Production Department, The Jackson Laboratory, Bar Harbor, Maine 04609. Commercial suppliers of mice include Carworth, Division of Becton, Dickinson and Company, 216 Congers Road, New City, New York 10956; Charles River Breeding Laboratories, Inc., 251 Ballardvale Street, Wilmington, Massachusetts 01887; Cumberland View Farms, Route 3, Clinton, Tennessee 37716; Deblin Farms, Inc., P. O. Box 369, Branchville, New Jersey 07826; Laboratory Supply Company, 5010 Mooresville Road, Indianapolis, Indiana 46241; Simonsen Laboratories, Inc., 5228 Centerville Road, White Bear Minnesota 55110; Sprague-Dawley Company, P. O. Box 4220, Madison, Wisconsin 53711; and Texas Inbred Mice Company, 305 Almeda-Genoa Road, Houston, Texas 77047.

Mice of the O'Grady selected stock are available from Flora O'Grady, 2336 Gunther Avenue, New York City, New York 10469.

Mice originally selected by Frings and Frings for seizure susceptibility do not appear to be available commercially. Lines or inbred strains of Frings' mice are maintained by several individual researchers.

X. APPENDIX II: SOURCES OF INFORMATION ABOUT MICE

The Institute of Laboratory Animal Resources of the National Academy of Sciences has prepared two pamphlets describing recommended standards of care for laboratory animals: *Guide for Laboratory Animals Facilities and Care* (U.S. Public Health Service, Superintendent of Documents, U.S. Government Printing Office, Washington, D.C. 20402), and *Rodents — Standards and Guidelines for the Breeding, Care, and Management of Laboratory Animals* (National Academy of Sciences, Washington, D.C. 20418).

The second edition of *Biology of the Laboratory Mouse*, edited by E. L. Green (McGraw-Hill Book Company, New York, 1966) is a sourcebook of information concerning origins, nomenclature, methods of husbandry, and biological characteristics of inbred and mutant bearing mice. *The Laboratory Mouse — Selection and Management*, by M. L. Simmons and J. O. Brick (Prentice-Hall, Englewood Cliffs, New Jersey, 1970), describes modern methods of animal management and provides details of experimental procedures using mice.

Mouse News Letter (MNL) provides an international exchange of information among those working with mutant mice. It is available from Laboratory Animals Centre, Carshalton, Surrey, England. *Inbred Strains of Mice* is issued twice yearly by The Jackson Laboratory as a companion to MNL. It lists inbred strains of mice actively maintained by contributing laboratories.

Handbook on Genetically Standardized JAX Mice describes biological characteristics of inbred strains, F_1 hybrids, congenic resistant lines, mutant production stocks, and other mutant strains and stocks of mice available from The Jackson Laboratory. It is available on request from The Jackson Laboratory, Bar Harbor, Maine 04609.

XI. ACKNOWLEDGMENTS

I express appreciation to Dr. Roger Ward who aided me in preparing this material. The preparation of the manuscript was supported in part by U.S. Public Health Service research grant MH 11327 from the National Institute of Mental Health, by an allocation from General Research Support Grant RR 05545 to The Jackson Laboratory, and by an allocation from the Richard and Eloise Webber Fund.

XII. REFERENCES

Alford B. R., and Ruben, R. J. (1963): Physiological, behavioral, and anatomical correlates of the development of hearing in the mouse. *Annals of Otology, Rhinology and Laryngology*, 72:237–247.

Antonitis, J. J. (1954): Intensity of white noise and frequency of convulsive reactions in DBA/1 mice. *Science,* 120:139–140.

Bevan, W. (1955): Sound-precipitated convulsions: 1947–1954. *Psychological Bulletin,* 52:473–504.

Bickford, R. G., and Klass, D. W. (1969): Sensory precipitation and reflex mechanisms. In: *Basic Mechanisms of the Epilepsies,* edited by H. H. Jasper, A. A. Ward, Jr., and A. Pope. Little, Brown and Company, Boston, pp. 543–564.

Bureš, J. (1953): Experiments on the electrophysiological analysis of the generalization of an epileptic fit. *Czechoslovak Physiology,* 2:347–356.

Bureš, J. (1963): Electrophysiological and functional analysis of the audiogenic seizure. In: *Colloques Internationaux du Centre National de la Recherche Scientifique No. 112, Psychophysiologie Neuropharmacologie et Biochimie de la Crise Audiogène.* Éditions du Centre National de la Recherche Scientifique, Paris, pp. 165–177.

Cain, J., Mercier, J., and Corriol, J. (1951): Sur l'électroencéphalogramme du rat albinos soumis à la crise audiogène. *Comptes Rendus de Séances de la Société de Biologie,* 145: 915–916.

Castellion, A. W., Swinyard, E. A., and Goodman, L. S. (1965): Effect of maturation on the development and reproducibility of audiogenic and electroshock seizures in mice. *Experimental Neurology,* 13:206–217.

Chance, M. R. A., and Yaxley, D. C. (1949): New aspects of the behavior of *Peromyscus* under audiogenic hyper-excitement. *Behaviour,* 2:96–105.

Coleman, D. L. (1960): Phenylalanine hydroxylase activity in dilute and nondilute strains of mice. *Archives of Biochemistry and Biophysics,* 91:300–306.

Collins, R. L. (1967): A general nonparametric theory of genetic analysis. 1. Application to the classical cross. *Genetics,* 56:551.

Collins, R. L. (1970*a*): Unilateral inhibition of sound-induced convulsions in mice. *Science,* 167:1010–1011.

Collins, R. L. (1970*b*): A new genetic locus mapped from behavioral variation in mice: Audiogenic seizure prone (*asp*). *Behavior Genetics,* 1:99–109.

Collins, R. L., and Fuller, J. L. (1968): Audiogenic seizure prone (*asp*): A gene affecting behavior in linkage group VIII of the mouse. *Science,* 162:1137–1139.

Colloques Internationaux du Centre National de la Recherche Scientifique No. 112 (1963): *Psychophysiologie Neuropharmacologie et Biochimie de la Crise Audiogène.* Éditions du Centre National de la Recherche Scientifique, Paris.

Dice, L. R. (1935): Inheritance of waltzing and of epilepsy in mice of the genus *Peromyscus. Journal of Mammology,* 16:25–35.

Dickie, M. M. (1966): Keeping records. In: *Biology of the Laboratory Mouse,* second edition, edited by E. L. Green. McGraw-Hill, New York, pp. 23–27.

Donaldson, H. H. (1924): *The Rat,* Memoirs of the Wistar Institute of Anatomy and Biology, Philadelphia, No. 6, p. 469.

Finger, F. W. (1947): Convulsive behavior in the rat. *Psychological Bulletin,* 44:201–248.

Fink, G. B., and Iturrian, W. B. (1970): Influence of age, auditory conditioning, and environmental noise on sound-induced seizures and seizure threshold in mice. In: *Physiological Effects of Noise,* edited by B. L. Welch and A. S. Welch. Plenum Press, New York, pp. 211–226.

Fink, G. B., and Swinyard, E. A. (1959): Modification of maximal audiogenic and electroshock seizures in mice by psychopharmacologic drugs. *Journal of Pharmacology and Experimental Therapeutics,* 127:318–324.

Fox, W. M. (1965): Reflex-ontogeny and behavioral development of the mouse. *Animal Behaviour,* 13:234–241.

Frings, H., and Frings, M. (1952): Acoustical determinants of audiogenic seizure in laboratory mice. *Journal of the Acoustical Society of America,* 24:163–169.

Frings, H., and Frings, M. (1953): The production of stocks of albino mice with predictable susceptibilities to audiogenic seizures. *Behaviour,* 5:305–319.

Fuller, J. L., and Collins, R. L. (1968*a*): Temporal parameters of sensitization for audiogenic seizures in SJL/J mice. *Developmental Psychobiology,* 1:185–188.

Fuller, J. L., and Collins, R. L. (1968b): Mice unilaterally sensitized for audiogenic seizures. *Science*, 162:1295.

Fuller, J. L., and Collins, R. L. (1970): Genetic and temporal characteristics of audiogenic seizures in mice. In: *Physiological Effects of Noise*, edited by B. L. Welch and A. S. Welch. Plenum Press, New York, pp. 203–209.

Fuller, J. L., and Smith, M. E. (1953): Kinetics of sound induced convulsions in some inbred mouse strains. *American Journal of Physiology*, 172:661–670.

Fuller, J. L., and Wimer, R. E. (1966): Neural, sensory, and motor functions. In: *Biology of the Laboratory Mouse* (second edition), edited by E. L. Green. McGraw-Hill, New York, pp, 609–628.

Green, E. L. (1968): *Handbook on Genetically Standardized JAX Mice*, second edition. The Jackson Laboratory, Bar Harbor, Maine.

Griffiths, W. J., Jr. (1953): The influence of behavioral factors on the incidence of audiogenic seizures in rats. *Journal of Comparative and Physiological Psychology*, 46:150–152.

Halberg, F., Jacobsen, E., Wadsworth, G., and Bittner, J. J. (1958): Audiogenic abnormality spectra, twenty-four hour periodicity, and lighting. *Science*, 128:657–658.

Hall, C. S. (1947): Genetic differences in fatal audiogenic seizures between two inbred strains of house mice. *Journal of Heredity*, 38:2–6.

Henry, K. R. (1967): Audiogenic seizure susceptibility induced in C57BL/6J mice by prior auditory exposure. *Science*, 158:938–940.

Henry, K. R., and Bowman, R. E. (1970): Acoustic priming of audiogenic seizures in mice. In: *Physiological Effects of Noise*, edited by B. L. Welch and A. S. Welch. Plenum Press, New York, pp. 185–201.

Henry K. R., Thompson, K. A., and Bowman, R. E. (1971): Frequency characteristics of acoustic priming of audiogenic seizures in mice. *Experimental Neurology*, 31:402–407.

Hohenboken, W. D., and Nellhaus, G. (1970): Inheritance of audiogenic seizures in the rabbit. *Journal of Heredity*, 61:107–112.

Horák, F. (1958): A change in seizure susceptibility, the direction of running and type of audiogenic epileptic seizure in rats induced by influencing the auditory receptor. *Physiologia Bohemoslovenica*, 8:306–311.

Horák, F. (1965): Selection of strains of rabbits sensitive to an epileptogenic sound stimulus. *Physiologia Bohemoslovenica*, 14:495–501.

Ikeda, H., and Higashi, T. (1970): The susceptibility of DBA/2 inbred mice to audiogenic seizures (*in Japanese*). *Psychiatria et Neurologia Japonica*, 72:1047–1050.

Iturrian, W. B., and Fink, G. B. (1968): Effect of age and condition-test interval (days) on an audio-conditioned convulsive response in CF #1 mice. *Developmental Psychobiology*, 1:230–235.

Kopeloff, L. M., Barrera, S. E., and Kopeloff, N. (1942): Recurrent convulsive seizures in animals produced by immunologic and chemical means. *American Journal of Psychiatry*, 98:881.

Krushinskii, L. V. (1960): *Animal Behavior—Its Normal and Abnormal Development*. Consultants Bureau, New York.

Krushinski, L. V. (1963): Étude physiologique des differents types de crises convulsives de l'épilepsie audiogène du rat. In: *Colloques Internationaux de Centre National de la Recherche Scientifique No. 112, Psychophysiologie Neuropharmacologie et Biochimie de la Crise Audiogène*. Éditions du Centre National de la Recherche Scientifique, Paris, pp. 71–92.

Krushinsky, L. V., Molodkina, L. N., Fless, D. A., Dobrokhotova, L. P., Steshenko, A. P., Semiokhina, A. F., Zorina, Z. A., and Romanova, L. G. (1970): The functional state of the brain during sonic stimulation. In: *Physiological Effects of Noise*, edited by B. L. Welch and A. S. Welch. Plenum Press, New York, pp. 159–183.

Lehmann, A. G. (1970): Psychopharmacology of the response to noise, with special reference to audiogenic seizure in mice. In: *Physiological Effects of Noise*, edited by B. L. Welch and A. S. Welch. Plenum Press, New York, pp. 227–257.

Lindsley, D. B., Finger, F. W., and Henry, C. E. (1942): Some physiological aspects of audiogenic seizures in rats. *Journal of Neurophysiology*, 5:185–198.

Maier, N. R. F., and Glaser, N. M. (1940a): Studies of abnormal behavior in the rat. II. A comparison of some convulsion producing situations. *Comparative Psychological Monographs*, 16:30.

Maier, N. R. F., and Glaser, N. M. (1940b): Studies of abnormal behavior in the rat. V. The inheritance of the "neurotic pattern." *Journal of Comparative Psychology*, 30:413–418.

Morin, G., Canac, F., Cain, J., and Garveau, V. (1948): Obtention des crises audiogènes du rat par des sons définis. *Comptes Rendus de Séances de la Société de Biologie*, 142:359–360.

Nachtsheim, H. (1937): Erbpathologie des Kaninchens. *Erbatz*, 4:25–30, 50–55.

Nellhaus, G. (1958): Experimental epilepsy in rabbits. *American Journal of Physiology*, 193:567–572.

Nellhaus, G. (1963): Experimental epilepsy in rabbits. In: *Colloques Internationaux du Centre National de la Recherche Scientifique, No. 112, Psychophysiologie Neuropharmacologie et Biochimie de la Crise Audiogène.* Éditions du Centre National de la Recherche Scientifique, Paris, pp. 131–144.

Niaussat, M. M., and Laget, P. (1963): Étude électroencéphalographique de la crise audiogène de la souris. In: *Colloques Internationaux du Centre National de la Recherche Scientifique No. 112, Psychophysiologie Neuropharmacologie et Biochimie de la Crise Audiogène.* Éditions du Centre National de la Recherche Scientifique, Paris, pp. 181–191.

Partington, M. W. (1961): The early symptoms of phenylketonuria. *Pediatrics*, 27:465–473.

Prokopetz, I. M. (1963): Quelques particularités du développement de l'état de catalepsie obtenu chez les animaux à l'aide de l'action des excitants sonores. In: *Colloques Internationaux du Centre National de la Recherche Scientifique No. 112, Psychophysiologie Neuropharmacologie et Biochimie de la Crise Audiogène.* Editions du Centre National de la Recherche Scientifique, Paris, pp. 93–99.

Ralls, K. (1967): Auditory sensitivity in mice: *Peromyscus* and *Mus musculus*. *Animal Behavior*, 15:123–128.

Schlesinger, K., and Griek, B. J. (1970): The genetics and biochemistry of audiogenic seizures. In: *Contributions to Behavior-Genetic Analysis—The Mouse as a Prototype*, edited by G. Lindzey and D. D. Thiessen. Appleton-Century-Crofts, New York, pp. 219–257.

Servít, Z. (1966): *Comparative and Cellular Pathophysiology of Epilepsy.* Proceedings of a symposium held in Liblice, Czechoslovakia. Excerpta Medica Foundation, Amsterdam.

Servít, Z., and Šterc, J. (1958): Audiogenic epileptic seizures evoked in rats by artificial epileptogenic foci. *Nature*, 181:1475.

Sidman, R. L., Green, M. C., and Appel, S. H. (1965): *Catalog of the Neurological Mutants of the Mouse.* Harvard University Press, Cambridge.

Staats, J. (1968): Standardized nomenclature for inbred strains of mice: Fourth listing. *Cancer Research*, 28:391–420.

Šterc, J. (1962): Experimental reflex epilepsy (audiogenic epilepsy). *Epilepsia*, 3:252–273.

Swinyard, E. A. (1963): Some physiological properties of audiogenic seizures in mice and their alteration by drugs. In: *Colloques Internationaux du Centre National de la Recherche Scientifique No. 112, Psychophysiologie Neuropharmacologie et Biochimie de la Crise Audiogène.* Éditions du Centre National de la Recherche Scientifique, Paris, pp. 406–421.

Swinyard, E. A., Castellion, A. W., Fink, G. B., and Goodman, L. S. (1963): Some neurophysiological and neuropharmacological characteristics of audiogenic-seizure-susceptible mice. *Journal of Pharmacology and Experimental Therapeutics*, 140:375–384.

Vicari, E. M. (1951): Fatal convulsive seizures in the DBA mouse strain. *Journal of Psychology*, 32:79–97.

Wada, J. A., and Asakura, T. (1969): Susceptibility to audiogenic seizure induced by thiosemicarbazide. *Experimental Neurology*, 24:19–37.

Wada, J. A., and Ikeda, H. (1966): The susceptibility to auditory stimuli of animals treated with methionine sulfoximine. *Experimental Neurology*, 15:157–165.

Ward, R. (1971): Recovery of susceptibility after audiogenic seizure. *Nature New Biology*, 233:56–57.

Ward, R., and Collins, R. L. (1971): Asymmetric audiogenic seizures in mice: A possible analogue of focal epilepsy. *Brain Research,* 31:207–210.

Ward, R., and Sinnett, E. E. (1971): Spreading cortical depression and audiogenic seizures in mice. *Experimental Neurology,* 31:437–443.

Watson, M. L. (1939): The inheritance of epilepsy and of waltzing in *Peromyscus. Contributions of the Laboratory of Vertebrate Genetics,* University of Michigan, 1939, No. 11, p. 24.

Welch, B. L., and Welch, A. S. (1970): *Physiological Effects of Noise.* Plenum Press, New York.

15

Photogenic Seizures in Baboon

R. Naquet and B. S. Meldrum

OUTLINE

I. INTRODUCTION

For many years, research workers have sought an animal model for use in studying human epilepsy. With the exception of those unusual epileptic manifestations associated with, for example, poisoning and metabolic disturbances which may be identical in man and animals, the similarities were only approximate (Naquet and Lanoir, 1972) between (1) the generalized and/or focal seizures of so-called "essential" epilepsy in man and seizures induced with various convulsant drugs in animals; (2) the generalized and/or focal seizures due to the relatively discrete lesions found in man (lesions following birth anoxia, sequellae of infectious encephalopathies, tumors, vascular lesions); and (3) the seizures caused by irritative lesions created artificially in animals (by tungsten, cobalt, or alumina cream) and transitory focal lesions caused by penicillin or strychnine.

The nature of the afferent events capable of triggering paroxysms preferentially was what differentiated experimental epilepsy from human epilepsy, since in man the most common and accepted form of "reflex" epilepsy was photosensitive epilepsy (Cobb, 1947; Gastaut et al., 1948; Walter and Walter, 1949; Bickford et al., 1952; Gastaut and Tassinari, 1966; Bickford and Klass, 1969), whereas intermittent light stimulation (ILS) was thought until 1966 to be incapable of triggering clinical paroxysms in animals, without induction by any convulsant drugs.

However, Killam et al. (1966a) discovered just such an epilepsy in the Laboratory of Applied Neurophysiology at the Institute of Neurophysiology and Psychophysiology of the CNRS in Marseille. Since then, much work has been carried out in France, Senegal, the United States, and Canada, on elucidating the characteristics of this epilepsy and finding out if it is characteristic of the baboon (*Papio papio*).

We embarked on a systematic study of this type of epilepsy, including its electrical and clinical characteristics as well as the effects of certain cerebral lesions. We have looked for animals of the same genus, group, or species presenting the same symptomatology. Finally, we have investigated applications that can be derived from this work in pharmacology, both in the trial of antiepileptic medication used or usable in man and in improving the understanding of the neurochemical mechanisms of epilepsy.

II. CLINICAL SYMPTOMATOLOGY

The clinical data have been described mainly by Killam et al. (1966b, 1967a), Naquet et al. (1968), Poncet (1968), and Naquet et al. (1969). The clinical symptoms are described below in terms of those which occur during ILS and those which continue after termination of ILS in the form of self-sustained manifestations.

A. Clinical signs occurring during intermittent light stimulation (ILS)

The *Papio papio*, when strapped into a chair which partially immobilizes him, characteristically closes his eyes and falls asleep. With the eyes closed, when ILS is presented either no clinical sign appears or some degree of clonic movements occur.

The first clinical sign of a seizure is "clonus" of the eyelids, which is bilateral, regular, rapid, and of small amplitude. The clonus may stop suddenly after opening the eyes, despite continuation of ILS, or it may increase gradually in amplitude and precede a more diffuse response which involves, in succession, the muscles of the face, the neck, and then the whole body. Polygraphic recordings have shown that the eyelid clonus usually precedes, by between a fraction of a second and several seconds, the clonus of the face, nape, and all the muscles of the neck.

ILS provokes violent clonic jerks affecting the whole body and causes contraction of the facial muscles, sharp flexion of the head onto the trunk, forward projection of both forelimbs, and a retracting movement of both hindlimbs. The jerks occur either in isolation or organized in salvos; they are frequently preceded by a few cloni of the eyelids and face.

ILS provokes at first clonic jerks of the eyelids, then spasm of the facial musculature which tends to spread to the nape of the neck and is suddenly interrupted by a clonic jerk. Tonic contraction then returns, the mouth opens, and the contraction is interrupted by clonic jerks at varying frequency.

The tonic spasm may become generalized to involve the whole body and precedes generalized clonus; the animal utters a cry at the time of certain cloni and may urinate. Here also, polygraphic recordings show that the tonic contraction of the occipital musculature always occurs somewhat after the appearance of the first eye clonus and precedes contraction of the shoulder and trunk musculature.

B. Self-sustained clinical signs persisting after the end of intermittent light stimulation

The self-sustained signs are of three types.

(1) After cessation of ILS, a few clonic jerks of the eyelids and face, and sometimes of the whole body, may persist for several seconds, their frequency declining gradually.

(2) Clonic manifestations may persist for several dozen seconds. The animal has his eyes open and fixed with dilated pupils, and his level of consciousness is certainly lowered; the clonic episodes may be irregular and localized. They may be of small amplitude and predominantly facial, or they may be more violent and accompanied by cries. When the episode is over, the animal remains in a state of confusion for several or many seconds.

(3) After the end of the last generalized clonic jerk provoked by the last flash, the animal has a tonic-clonic attack followed by a period of confusion. It is sometimes possible to see generalized clonic jerks which occur

for several seconds after the end of ILS, and it is only after this that the initial tonic phase of the tonic-clonic seizure occurs.

During the tonic phase, the eyes are open, the pupils dilated, the teeth are bared in a grin, the jaws clenched or half open, the head extended, the arms adducted against the thorax, the forearms flexed on the upper arms, the fists clenched and flexed on the forearms, the thighs in semi-flexion on the abdomen, the legs flexed, the feet in dorsal flexion, and the big toes in plantar flexion.

The clonic phase begins with small-amplitude myoclonic jerks which involve first the muscles of the face, then the whole musculature, while a certain tonic component persists. Gradually the clonic jerks increase and cause saccadic closing of the eyes, opening or increased opening of the jaws, large jerks of the upper limbs which are thrown up and forward, and flexor jerks of the lower limbs. The frequency and amplitude of the clonus diminishes gradually, saliva runs from the corners of the mouth, and then suddenly all motor activity ceases and the animal enters the postictal state of confusion. During this period of confusion, the head is flexed on the thorax, and the limbs are inert and flaccid. A few seconds later, the animal makes a few disorganized jumps, some of which may be very sudden and of large amplitude and resemble true clonic jerks; the animal then seems to "wake up" and his gaze wanders from right to left. Recovery usually takes a few minutes.

A tonic-clonic seizure is variable in duration from one animal to another and in the same animal from one day to another, but usually lasts from 30 to 50 sec.

III. VARIATIONS OF THE DEGREE OF PHOTOSENSITIVITY ACCORDING TO GEOGRAPHICAL DISTRIBUTION, SPECIES, OR GROUP

On all animals for which results are given in this chapter, an initial test was carried out using the same technique: the unanesthetized animal, without implanted electrodes, was restrained in a special chair, and the EEG was recorded using scalp needle electrodes. Only the data reported by Koudry-atzeva (1969) depart from this technique; his animals had implanted electrodes, which may explain the differences in the results.

Killam et al. (1966b), followed by Meldrum et al. (1970b), made a schematic classification of the clinical signs by order of increasing intensity as follows: during ILS, palpebral clonus only (+1); clonus of the eyelids followed by facial clonus and possibly clonus of the facial and head musculature (+2); clonus of the whole body (+3); clonus continuing after the end of ILS (+3+).

Using this classification and considering only those animals with at least (+2) as truly photosensitive, Killam et al. (1966*b*), in an initial study of 100 animals, showed that 60% of the *Papio papio* captured in the Casamance region (the southern part of Senegal) were photosensitive. The degree of photosensitivity was independent of the subject's age, nourishment, habitat, and testing conditions.

Since then, at the Institute of Neurophysiology and Psychophysiology in Marseille, 700 animals from Casamance have been tested and the results give a slightly higher percentage, closer to 67% (Fig. 1). It is lower if we consider the animals presenting self-sustained signs after the end of ILS (+3+), and only about 10% for those presenting generalized seizures. The percentage of photosensitive animals is distinctly smaller when they are captured in other territories of eastern Senegal (Fig. 1) (Serbanescu et al., 1968*a;* Bert and Naquet, 1969; Naquet et al., 1971; Bert et al., 1972, *personal communication*).

At the present time, there is no organization capable of delivering photosensitive *Papio papio*. We are in contact with private organizations from Senegal which sell *Papio papio* captured in the forest. In general, these animals are captured in Casamance, which is the area where the highest percentage of photosensitive baboons can be found; these organizations take care of shipping by air. In general, the animals we receive are not carriers of any germs, but it often happens that they have parasites, and it is preferable to isolate them for a bacteriological analysis of feces and an antiparasite treatment.

Photosensitivity has been investigated in other cercopithecinae: *Papio hamadryas, Papio anubis, Erythrocebus patas, Cercopithecus aethiops sabaeus, Papio cynocephalus* (Killam et al., 1966*b;* Stark et al., 1968; Kitsikis et al., 1970). *Macaca mulatta* (Koudryatzeva, 1969; Rhodes, *personal communication;* Wada et al., 1972*b*). The percentage is generally not more than 10%, although the number of animals tested (a maximum of 100 for the *Papio anubis*) has been smaller. For the *Papio hamadryas*, too few animals have been tested so far to be significant, but their degree of photosensitivity seems to be clear. The *Papio cynocephalus* seems to be less photosensitive than *Papio anubis* (Stark et al., 1968; Kitsikis et al., 1970).

Other species tested in which only rare and not very marked responses to ILS were reported include *Macaca radiata, Macaca irus, Macaca nemestrina, Macaca speciosa, Cerecocebus atys, Hykobates lars,* and *Therpocathecus gelada. Macaca mulata* has usually been reported not to

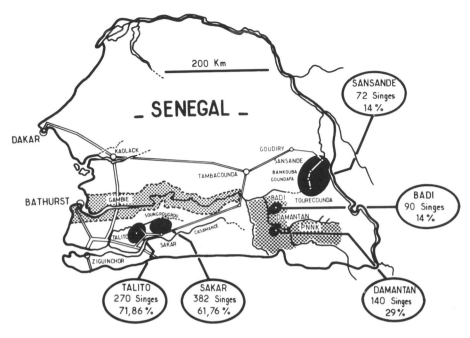

FIG. 1.   Geographical representation of baboons with their corresponding photosensitivity. From Bert et al. (1971, *personal communication*).

be sensitive to the flashing light (Killam et al., *personal communication*) or, at most, to display a +1 response as reported by Wada et al. (1972b), which the authors consider to be insignificant.   However, the percentage was higher in the group tested by Koudryatzcva (1969).   The chimpanzee is not photosensitive (Naquet et al., 1966).   The *Galago senegalensis,* although showing no paroxysmal reaction to ILS when the pupils are myotic, becomes very photosensitive after pupil dilation; this is more marked the younger the animal (Serbanescu et al., 1968b).

Excessive photosensitivity of the Casamance *Papio papio* would therefore seem to be characteristic of a group and not of a species or a genus.

IV. VARIATIONS OF PHOTOSENSITIVITY AT DIFFERENT TIMES

Killam et al. (1967a) reported that "a limited number of animals exhibited a constant high level of sensitivity, others tested at irregular weekly or bi-weekly intervals displayed what appeared to be a cyclic variability in responsiveness to ILS. Sensitivity in a third group of animals appeared partially dependent on the spacing of the test sessions . . . in certain animals, 2, 3, or 4 days rest was necessary for a maximal response to ILS to be elicited."

This finding has recently been confirmed by Wada et al. (1972b): "Longitudinal evaluation of the clinical response to photic stimulation showed a considerable degree of fluctuation in spite of the seemingly standardized testing conditions." These authors even describe the occurrence of spontaneous grand mal attacks in certain animals which were not necessarily the most photosensitive. Killam et al. (1967a), as did Wada et al. (1972b), noticed that an animal who showed low sensitivity in the early tests could later become very photosensitive and, conversely, that an animal very photosensitive at the beginning might be less so in later months, although for the Casamance *Papio* the figure of 67% photosensitive animals is only relative and is certainly less than the actual percentage. These facts led Wada et al. (1972b) to say, "this suggested the presence of a subclinical photosensitive disposition among non-sensitive baboons." However, longterm studies of a colony of 50 to 60 animals from the Casamance area (Killam and Killam, *personal communication*) indicate that reproducible photic stimuli may be used weekly to induce +1 to +3 type responses in *Papio* without loss of responsiveness over a 3- to 4-year period. As in the Killams' earlier studies, some animals appeared stable responders at one of the levels described while others occasionally varied from week to week, but without consistent decrement in seizure sensitivity. In our laboratories, even in the animals showing a stable degree of sensitivity, some of them will show the same type of response to repeated stimulation every half-hour whereas others are only photosensitive once a day.

This phenomenon is even more pronounced when the animal has manifested a +3+ response and particularly after a "generalized" type of seizure occurring after cessation of ILS (Fig. 2). Recovery time is usually 24 hr, but in one animal it was possible to provoke generalized seizures several times during one day, although the length of the seizure become shorter as the photic stimulation occurred at shorter intervals (Fig. 3). The minimal latency for showing a second after-discharge in this animal was 5 hr.

Wada et al. (1972b) also compared the degree of photosensitivity as a function of whether or not the animal performed self-stimulation with an intermittent light. "When the animals were allowed to self-stimulate for a 3-month period, a rather marked and prolonged decrease of the photosensitivity was observed." During the 3 to 5 months following the end of the period of photic stimulation, the photosensitivity of each animal returned to its original level.

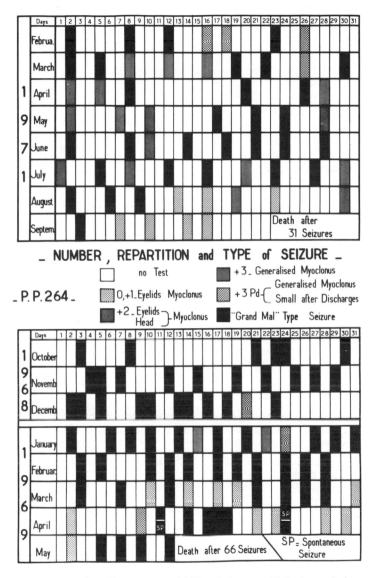

FIG. 2. Examples of long-term variability of photosensitivity in two baboons.

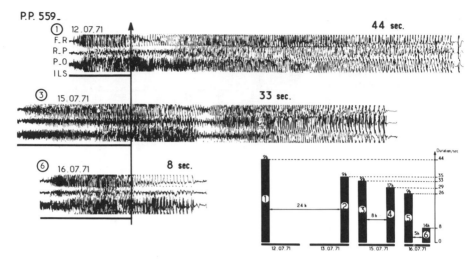

FIG. 3.   Interaction between duration of seizure and interval between presentation of ILS. The figures in the circle correspond between the EEG tracings and the bar graph.

V. ELECTRICAL FINDINGS

Electrical activity data have been reported by Killam et al. (1967*a*), Naquet et al. (1968), Poncet (1968), Naquet et al. (1969), and Naquet and Menini (1972). Wada et al. (1972*b*) have added a few details which modify the descriptions of the above authors.

Electrical activity is described in three parts: without light stimulation, during ILS, and after cessation of ILS, when the latter has triggered a self-sustained seizure discharge.

A. Spontaneous EEG activity

The characteristics of the physiological rhythms recorded during attentive wakefulness, calm wakefulness, and the various sleep states have been described elsewhere (Balzano, 1968; Poncet, 1968; Fischer-Williams et al., 1968; Bert et al., 1970); we concentrate here on the paroxysmal discharges frequently found to occur in the baboon.

Spontaneous paroxysmal discharges of large-amplitude sharp or spike activity have been found in all animals tested but particularly in the most photosensitive animals (Killam et al., 1967*a;* Wada et al., 1972*b*). These discharges occupy mainly the fronto-central regions (Poncet, 1968; Wada et al., 1972*b;* Fischer-Williams et al., 1968; Arfel et al., 1972). They occur only exceptionally in the post-rolandic regions, and, in the rare cases where they do exist, they are always synchronous with those of the pre-rolandic regions. Similar discharges were also found in the basal temporal and orbital regions of *Papio papio* (Wada et al., 1972*b*); however, these authors also found such discharges in their control rhesus monkeys and state that the possible significance of resting paroxysmal electrocortical features remains uncertain.

Bilateral, synchronous, and symmetrical paroxysmal abnormalities occur only when the animal has its eyes closed; they tend to disappear when the animal becomes aroused or attentive (Killam et al., 1967*a;* Poncet, 1968; Fischer-Williams et al., 1968; Wada et al., 1972*b*). They increase during the stages of falling asleep and slow-wave sleep, particularly stages 1 and 2; they disappear during rapid eye movement (REM) sleep (Balzano, 1968; Bert et al., 1970).

Paroxysmal activity of the spike, sharp wave, or spike-and-wave type has never been recorded from deep structures in the absence of such activity in the cortex.[1]

B. EEG activity occurring during intermittent light stimulation

ILS over a wide frequency band produces clear following responses in the occipital regions; for stimulation frequencies close to 25 flashes/sec, paroxysmal discharges occur in the fronto-rolandic regions. These may begin as large-amplitude discharges or they may gradually increase in amplitude. They usually consist of polyspikes, which may be at a frequency close to or independent of ILS, or they may be spike-and-wave. These may occur at about 3/sec; they are bilateral, synchronous, and symmetrical. The discharges may remain localized in the fronto-rolandic regions while the occipital following continues unchanged (Fig. 4). The paroxysmal discharges, like spontaneous discharges, are blocked by sensory stimuli which cause a state of alertness, in which case only the occipital following persists.

In deep structures, several types of response have been recorded. The activity may be unchanged by the appearance of cortical discharges; this is the case for the optic tract and the lateral geniculate body, where following continues unchanged (Fig. 5) (Poncet, 1968; Fischer-Williams et al., 1968;

---

[1] The depth electrodes were implanted using the Horsley-Clarke stereotaxic apparatus and the *Atlas of Papio papio* (Riche et al., 1968). This atlas was constructed from brains of adult females weighing 10 kg.

P.P. 264 _ 07.11.68

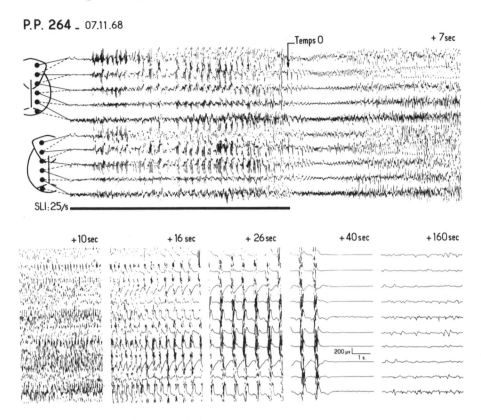

FIG. 4. Paroxysmal discharges during ILS followed by self-sustained paroxysmal activity (grand mal type). From Naquet et al. (1972, *personal communication*).

Naquet et al., 1969; Wada et al., 1972*b*). This may also be the case for other subcortical structures when the changes caused by ILS are not great, according to Poncet (1968) and Fischer-Williams et al. (1968). It was also the case for all the subcortical structures explored by Wada et al. (1972*b*), regardless of the amplitude of the paroxysmal discharge occurring in the cortex: "there was no buildup of electrographic discharges in any localized cortical or deep structures in our study."

The paroxysmal discharges usually spread to certain deep structures when their intensity increases in the cortex and when generalized clonic signs occur. The degree of spread to the subcortical structures varies in the same animal from one time to another and from one structure to another. Poncet (1968) and Fischer-Williams et al. (1968) found paroxysmal activities to occur more often in the thalamus, the internal capsule, the pons,

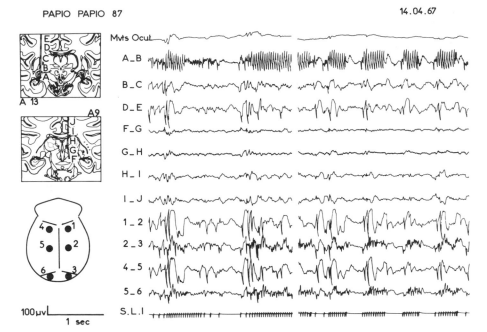

PAPIO PAPIO 87   14.04.67

FIG. 5. A recording of the response to ILS in deep and surface structures of the baboon. Note only following in the geniculate derivation (A–B). At the same time, paroxysmal discharge in the neocortex (1–2; 4–5) and deep cortex (D–E). From Poncet (1968, *personal communication*).

the reticular formation, and certain hypothalamic structures than in the rhinencephalon. Arfel et al. (1972) have recently provided more precise details: the paroxysmal discharges do not invade the white matter, the whole of the thalamus, but only certain nuclei are more affected, in particular, the centrum medianum. The pulvinar is, on the other hand, never involved.

In certain animals, two types of response have been recorded simultaneously. Certain structures are invaded by slow waves occurring simultaneously with the fronto-rolandic paroxysmal discharges, whereas other structures are invaded by rhythmic activity at a frequency close to that of the ILS. This phenomenon suggests that there might be two competitive types of activity: a following response at 25 cps and spike-and-wave discharges related to those which arise in the fronto-rolandic region (Poncet, 1968; Fischer-Williams et al., 1968).

It is worth pointing out in this context that there is no difference between the data of Wada et al. (1972*d*) and those of Poncet (1968), Fischer-Williams et al. (1968), and Arfel et al. (1972). Wada et al. (1972*b*) found no primary paroxysmal discharges in the deep structures and described only a following response to ILS in the visual tracts and reticular formation. The other workers, however, reported that subcortical structures may often be invaded by paroxysmal discharges at the time they are present in the fronto-rolandic regions, although the occurrence of such discharges is not invariable and differs according to the structure.

C. EEG activity occurring after cessation of intermittent light stimulation

In most cases, when ILS stops, all paroxysmal electrical manifestations cease and are not followed by any depression; however, three types of activity may persist after the end of ILS according to Killam et al. (1967*a*), Poncet (1968) and Fischer-Williams et al. (1968).

(1) After ILS is stopped, a few sharp waves or polyspikes persist in strictly localized fronto-central regions, although they may be more diffuse; according to Fischer-Williams et al. (1968) and Poncet (1968), these paroxysmal discharges may spread to certain deep structures.

(2) Generalized polyspike-and-wave discharges may persist over the whole cortex for several dozen seconds; their frequency gradually decreases, and they are followed by a generalized postictal depression.

(3) The cessation of ILS may be followed by complex electrical phenomena, but usually these are identical from one animal to another; only those activities that appear in the first few seconds are not identical according to different authors and for different animals. This may be a consequence of the fact that it is often difficult to identify the beginning of the electrical events which are going to be responsible for the self-sustained ictal activity. However, Wada et al. (1972*b*) insist that the onset of clinical seizure was coincident with the abrupt alteration of the pre-existing pattern in all the structures, with diffuse 4 to 5 cps activity followed by a rhythmic 14 cps synchronized sharp activity prior to the commencement of an organized cortical discharge. Killam et al. (1967*a*), Poncet (1968) and Wada et al. (1972*b*) are in almost complete agreement that the ictal discharge starts throughout the cortex as a rapid, small-amplitude activity, followed in the anterior region by "organized and sustained repetitive spike, multiple spike-and-sharp-wave discharges" spreading gradually to the whole cortex (Fig. 4). At first, there is no spread to the deep structures; then they gradually become involved more or less intensely, depending on the structure. Some structures may not be invaded, notably the rhinencephalic structures (Fischer-Williams et al., 1968; Naquet, 1969). Synchrony between the anterior and posterior regions and involvement of all the deep structures (always excluding the rhinencephalon) only occurs gradually, and specifi-

cally at the stage when the rhythmic polyspike discharges are occurring at a rate of 1 to 2/sec.

The last burst of polyspike-and-wave is followed by a depression of activity which is predominant in the neocortical structures but also involves the deep structures. The depression lasts for a variable time depending on the length of the seizure, and the original physiological activity reappears only very gradually. These electrical phenomena are sometimes preceded by a few generalized synchronous and symmetrical polyspike-and-wave discharges which persist after the cessation of ILS.

VI. ELECTROCLINICAL CORRELATIONS

It is rare for animals without implanted depth electrodes to have spontaneous seizures. Wada et al. (1972b) report that two animals of eight they studied were found to have recurrent spontaneous convulsive seizures prior to the cerebral electrode implantation. Riche et al. (1970, 1971) have also reported the spontaneous occurrence of seizures identical to those elicited by ILS in one of their most photosensitive animals which had no implanted electrodes.

The spontaneous paroxysmal discharges recorded in all animals in the fronto-central regions have never been accompanied by clinical signs (Killam et al., 1967b; Fischer-Williams et al., 1968; Poncet, 1968; Wada et al., 1972b).

A. Correlations between clinical and EEG signs during intermittent light stimulation

Close correlations between clonus and paroxysmal electrical activity are thought to exist according to Killam et al. (1967a), Naquet et al. (1969), and Fischer-Williams et al. (1968). Wada et al. (1972b) report that "isolated photomyoclonic responses did not always have paroxysmal electrographic concomitants." Poncet (1968) stated that each cortical discharge of polyspikes, spike-and-wave, or polyspike-and-wave has a clonus corresponding to it; he also reported that he had never observed clonus without paroxysmal electrical phenomena in the motor cortex, but that it is not rare for paroxysmal discharges provoked by ILS to be unaccompanied by motor phenomena. Wada et al. (1972b) found that "there were often, but not always, polyspike-and-wave patterns in the cortex anteriorly at the time of an isolated photomyoclonic jerk."

When the clonic activity involves only the eyelids and face, the paroxysmal discharge is usually restricted to the superficial frontal regions. When the clonus is generalized, the electrical discharge spreads slightly to the whole cortex, excluding the visual cortex; recordings from the deep structures usually show that a great number give rise to paroxysmal activity (Poncet, 1968; Fischer-Williams et al., 1968). When there is a tonic component at the same time as the clonic manifestations, the paroxysmal activities involve the whole cortex and the deep structures. Wada et al. (1972b) confirm some of these results, but report that "this was not time-locked to the clinical responses . . . there was no buildup of electrographic discharge in any localized cortical or deep structures in our study;" this is, again, in disagreement with the data published by Killam et al. (1967b), Poncet (1968), and Fischer-Williams et al. (1968).

B. Correlations between clinical and electrical signs which persist after the end of intermittent light stimulation

When the clinical signs consist only of a few myoclonic jerks limited to the eyelids and face, the topography of the paroxysmal EEG activities is comparable to that of the discharges which accompany clonus occurring during ILS. The morphology of this activity is, however, somewhat modified by the disappearance of the light stimuli.

When the self-sustained phenomena take the form of a generalized clonic seizure, a paroxysmal discharge is associated with each clonus. When the self-sustained signs consist of a grand mal seizure, the descriptions given by Killam et al. (1967a), Poncet (1968), Fischer-Williams et al. (1968), and Wada et al. (1972b) are, on the whole, similar.

During the tonic phase, there is no specific type of EEG activity. The ictal discharges are either limited to the frontal regions or more diffuse, involving other cortical and sub-cortical regions. There is not necessarily any synchrony between the activity recorded from the cortex and from the deep structures.

During the clonic phase, the ictal discharges are better organized, with polyspike-and-wave involving the whole cortex and gradually the deep structures. However, only in the "latter stages of the seizure did the deep structure appear to participate more actively" (Wada et al., 1972b).

All these authors are in agreement that during the postictal phase there is a widespread depression of electrical activity which is predominant in the cortex. When a few cloni reappear preceding the return of coordinated movements, it is not rare to see a few cortical paroxysmal elements occurring.

C. Factors facilitating or inhibiting the appearance of clinical and EEG paroxysmal signs induced by intermittent light stimulation

The age factor has never appeared to be significant between adolescence and adulthood. However, with a few exceptions, very young animals are not photosensitive [the first signs of excessive photosensitivity have been found in animals aged 7 to 8 months from the group captured in eastern Senegal (Balzano, 1971, *personal communication*)]. Highly photosensitive *Papio* are found in groups captured in Africa or born in a primate center and raised with extensive care.

As stated previously, the frequency most likely to elicit paroxysmal discharges is about 25 cps, and discharges are most likely to appear with the eyes closed.

Serbanescu (1970) and Serbanescu et al. (1972) have shown that EEG discharges and clinical signs are more likely to appear when the pupils are dilated and less likely to occur under the effect of pilocarpine. These differences apply not only to the intensity and percentage of appearance of these discharges in a given animal, but also to the latency of their appearance. The same authors have also shown that the wavelength of the light used may affect the triggering of these paroxysms. The least efficient wavelengths in animals correspond to red light (lambda 676 nm) and green light (lambda 548.8 nm), whereas in man green, blue, and white lights are less effective in triggering paroxysmal discharges than is red light.

Rhythmic, painless periocular stimulation, combined with ILS, is likely to cause appearance of ocular clonus and spread of clonus to the face and whole body. On the other hand, curarization of the animal reduces the size of the paroxysmal EEG discharges triggered by ILS. These discharges may, however, persist, even though less intense, in the very photosensitive animals. Curarization may produce this effect either by suppressing the possibility of clonic signs appearing or because of the consequent emotional stress which accompanies it. Killam et al. (1967a) have demonstrated that "all disturbing influences in the laboratory during the test session markedly attenuated the response or blocked it entirely. These included excessive noise, light and general traffic."

Periocular anesthesia with 0.5% procaine blocks the clonic jerks elicited by ILS; the paroxysmal EEG discharges persist. Saline injected in the same region has no effect on the clinical or EEG signs elicited by ILS. More concentrated doses of procaine block the electrical discharges as well, but it is impossible to be certain that the decrease in photosensitivity is not a consequence of a general effect of this product (Naquet et al., 1971a; Naquet and Menini, 1972).

Bilateral section of the facial nerve, which prevents spontaneous closing of the eyelids and destroys the motor reflex to light, alters the clinical signs provoked by ILS; in the absence of eyelid clonus, certain very photosensitive animals show clonus of the lower jaw, the head, and the whole body, while the eyes remain half open. In other animals, the usual organization of the seizure disappears and a few isolated cloni of the body may occur with a latency usually rather long in relation to the paroxysmal EEG discharges.

These results suggest that although the eyelid clonus may be an important link in the chain or organization of the clinical seizure, probably through a "feed-back" mechanism similar to that suggested for certain photosensitive epilepsies in man (Naquet et al., 1971a), it is not, however, vital to the appearance of clinical ictal manifestations.

D. Correlations between paroxysmal EEG discharges and unit recordings

Because it is difficult to obtain paroxysmal manifestations after curarization, very few convulsive episodes have been recorded with microelectrodes. In a few special cases, extracellular unit recordings have been possible using tungsten microelectrodes.

When there are no paroxysmal cortical discharges, the neuronal behavior is normal in all cortical regions in all *Papio papio* whether or not they are photosensitive and whether or not there is ILS.

When electrical paroxysmal discharges occur, certain neurons in the fronto-rolandic cortex show activation of a nature very similar to that seen in man and animals after a scar lesion or local application of a convulsant agent (Fig. 6).

The close correlations seen between activation of fronto-rolandic neurons and the paroxysmal EEG discharges have not been demonstrated either following stimulation of other sensory modalities or in other cortical zones following ILS. Also, although a cortical paroxysmal discharge is always in synchrony with a unit burst in the fronto-rolandic cortex, it is possible to see cellular activation without the paroxysmal EEG discharges. These findings led Menini et al. (1968a) and Morrell et al. (1969) to conclude that these discharges had a local origin, this cortical area behaving like a true epileptogenic focus even if no lesion or other abnormality could be demonstrated in that area (Riche et al., 1970, 1971). Jami (1972) showed that correlations of the same type exist in the cat, not only in the pre-cruciate gyrus but also in other cortical regions after intravenous injection of pen-

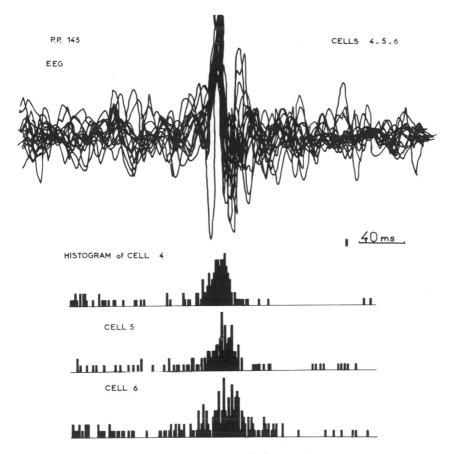

FIG. 6.   Patterns of firing in three cells in area 6 of a photosensitive baboon when paroxysmal activity appeared. *Upper tracing:* The superimposition of all wave complexes analyzed below. The histogram indicates the distribution of firing around the paroxysmal complexes. From Morrell et al. (1969, *personal communication*).

tylenetetrazol.   These facts do not rule out the possibility of a local origin for the paroxysmal EEG signs with concomitant activation of the cortical neurons in the baboon; but they do tend to indicate that this mode of reactivity does not necessarily imply that a local epileptogenic focus exists. Instead, the pattern of negativity with associated spikes may simply be the specific mode of reactivity of the cortex under the effect of particular afferents and convergence patterns.

VII. STUDY OF EVOKED POTENTIALS

A. Visual evoked potentials

Killam et al. (1967*b*), Menini et al. (1968*b,c,* 1970), and Wada et al. (1972*b*) all consider that the largest-amplitude responses are obtained from the visual tract and the occipital part of the cortex. In the pre-rolandic region, an evoked response of small amplitude and short latency (50 msec) is found in all animals. This response is particularly clear from the inferior frontal sulcus and the caudal branch of the cingulate gyrus (Fig. 7).

For Wada et al. (1972*b*) in all animals of their group, and for Menini et al. (1970), especially for the most photosensitive animals, a late rhythmic after-discharge is seen, localized to area 6 for Menini et al. (1970), more or less diffuse but predominantly fronto-central for Wada et al. (1972*b*). This only occurs when the animal has closed eyes, and is most likely to be elicited by double flashes 40 msec apart. It may involve a facilitation of as much as 600 to 700% for the most photosensitive animals (Dimov et al., 1969; Menini et al., 1970). For the latter group this after-discharge occurs only for the visual modality, whereas for Wada et al. (1972*b*) it may also be found for auditory stimulation. Wada et al. reported (1972*b*) that this type of late response elicited by either isolated flashes or sounds is characteristic of the baboon and does not exist in the rhesus.

Menini and Rostain (1969, 1970) have demonstrated visual afferents recorded from cell units in the same fronto-rolandic area. The shortest latencies to single flashes (20 msec) were found in the deep cortical layers. Under the effect of ILS, certain fronto-rolandic units are activated in a tonic manner by the very first flashes; others, without undergoing any noticeable activation, show a following at the same frequency as the stimulation or at a harmonic frequency.

B. Somesthetic evoked potentials

This study of somesthetic evoked potentials, which is only in an early stage, concerns the effect of stimulating the fore- and hindpaws and particularly the effects of stimulating the periocular skin (Catier et al., 1971). Apart from the early response localized to the post-rolandic cortex, evoked responses occur in the premotor cortex for all the areas stimulated. In the premotor cortex, a convergence of somatic afferents is found which presents no precise somatotopy. However, the response evoked by stimulation of the eyebrows exceeds those from the forelimbs.

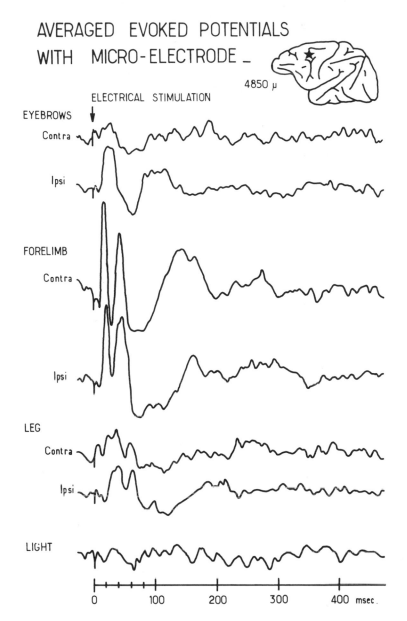

FIG. 7. Recording from a single unit in the fronto-rolandic cortex. In each section can be seen: *above,* the artifact from photic stimulation; *then,* a frontal derivation, an occipital derivation, and below the single unit record. Spontaneous activity shows few bursts of unit discharges (*left, above*). The cell responds to each flash of light (*left, below*). *On the right:* frontal spikes triggered by photic stimulation. A spike is always synchronous with a burst of unit discharges but there are bursts seen in the absence of spikes. From Naquet et al. (1972, *personal communication*).

The shortest latencies (14 msec for the forepaw) and the most complete convergence are localized for the frontal lobe in the region of the superior frontal sulcus. For stimulation of the eyebrows, the ipsilateral frontal responses are of greater amplitude (200 to 300%) than the contralateral responses. This has not been found elsewhere, either in other explored cortical regions or for other stimulations used (Menini et al., 1971).

The existence of somesthetic afferents going to the frontal cortex has been verified at a unitary level; many cortical units are activated with brief latencies for the various stimulations carried out, tactile as well as electrical (Fig. 7).

Although no precise somatotopy has been clarified, early results tend to imply that certain units possess specificity. Some are activated only by stimulation of the forelimbs and others by stimulation of the face. The receptor fields are very extensive and bilateral. Certain units show heterotopic convergence, and, for stimulation of the eyebrows, the homolateral unit responses are often longer with a greater frequency of discharge than the responses to contralateral stimulation (Menini et al., 1971).

VIII. EFFECTS OF CEREBRAL LESIONS

Various types of experimental lesions have been performed in an attempt to determine the role of different cortical regions in generating seizures. These experiments have been done only recently, and certain results (e.g., for frontal lobe ablations) still need confirmation.

A. Chronic occipital and frontal epileptogenic lesions

Irritative occipital lesions were created by injecting an epileptogenic agent, made of a mixture of alumina cream and pure cobalt powder, under the pia matter (Dimov and Lanoir, 1969). We shall not say much about the characteristics of this occipital focus, but it is interesting to note that the lesion did not lower the threshold of appearance of fronto-rolandic paroxysmal discharges in response to ILS in any animal; it almost seems as if the chronic occipital epileptogenic focus, during its period of development, clearly raised the threshold of photosensitivity in all the animals, since ILS was ineffective even in the most photosensitive. In a single case, ILS triggered a seizure which originated occipitally, but this involved the cortex contralateral to the lesion and the seizure remained localized to the posterior region.

A progressive lesion of one occipital cortex, whether irritative or not, is therefore capable of blocking photosensitivity temporarily; this finding, like certain data recorded from cell units, suggests the possibility that the occipital cortex plays a role of triggering paroxysmal discharges by light stimulation. In contrast, when the animal has an irritative lesion of the same type in the fronto-rolandic cortex of one hemisphere, the paroxysmal discharges elicited by ILS are facilitated during the progressive phase of the focus (Dimov and Lanoir, *in preparation*).

B. Lesion of the superior colliculus

Wada et al. (1972*b*) created lesions of the superior colliculus under direct vision in some very photosensitive *Papio papio*. These lesions had only a transitory effect on photosensitivity.

C. Bilateral ablations of various cortical regions

Complete bilateral ablations of the occipital, temporal, or frontal lobes (excluding area 4) were carried out on several photosensitive baboons; frontal lobe ablation was carried out only in one animal; its survival time of 3 weeks after the operation was inadequate to validate completely the corresponding results. After each operation, the degree of photosensitivity of each animal was tested (Wada et al., 1972*b*). Some of these experiments are not yet complete, but it is already possible to conclude the following. (1) The animal deprived of occipital lobes will show an immediate and persistent loss of photosensitivity lasting for 6 to 9 months after the operation. Since a transient reduction in photosensitivity following any neurosurgical procedure does not usually last more than 2 weeks, such a loss in the occipital group appears highly significant. (2) Animals who undergo ablation of frontal or temporal lobes will show no change in photosensitivity, although the limitations mentioned above must be remembered in these cases.

D. Section of the corpus callosum in the photosensitive *Papio papio*

Recordings were carried out over a long period of time (up to 15 months) in *Papio papio* after complete section of the corpus callosum. The EEG activity, apart from any paroxysmal discharge, was generally bilateral, synchronous, and symmetrical, and the power spectra established for homologous derivations were superimposable; these data are confirmed by Batini et al. (1967). However, the spontaneous paroxysmal abnormalities recorded in the fronto-rolandic region generally occurred asynchronously.

When they were provoked by ILS, the abnormalities occurred either asynchronously or synchronously, and could be predominant on the homo- or contralateral side to that on which the surgical approach was made. Also, the discharges that persisted after the end of ILS could start asymmetrically and predominate in one hemisphere; for example, in the same animal they may have remained localized to one hemisphere during one recording and then spread temporarily to the other hemisphere during another recording. Clinically, the seizure no longer assumed the form of tonic-clonic manifestations of generalized appearance but rather of a seizure which was either unilateral or bilateral but always predominant in one half of the body, the side corresponding to the opposite hemi-cortex from which the maximal ictal discharge was recorded.

When the section of the corpus callosum involved an extensive lesion of the fronto-rolandic cortex of one hemisphere, the asynchrony between the two hemispheres became even more exaggerated; electrically the seizure triggered by ILS occupied only the "healthy" hemisphere, and clinically it remained localized to the opposite side of the body. The seizure is followed by an electrical depression involving only the hemisphere which had discharged and also by a transient paralysis (Catier et al., 1970; Naquet et al., 1972).

This series of experiments demonstrates, first, that section of the corpus callosum decreases the synchrony of paroxysmal discharges, both spontaneous and those elicited by ILS, and, second, that it transforms seizures which were previously generalized into focal, or rather hemispheric, seizures. Also, these experiments seem to confirm that the fronto-rolandic cortex may play a part in the genesis of seizures, since when this region was destroyed in association with section of the corpus callosum, the animal subsequently had only unilateral seizures on the side opposite that of the lesion. The lesion or ablation experiments involving the occipital cortex indicate that it also plays an important role.

IX. PHARMACOLOGICAL STUDIES

The syndrome of photosensitive epilepsy in the baboon may well be of great value in future pharmacological studies of epilepsy. There are two reasons for this. Firstly, it resembles the "idiopathic epilepsy" of man more closely than any other "experimental" epilepsy. It thus provides an appropriate animal model for studying the effects of drug treatments, either those already in use or those undergoing preclinical evaluation. Accurate comparative assessments of the antiepileptic potency of drugs can be made. Their mode of action and their influence on the acute and chronic evolution of epileptic processes can be studied. This approach is being successfully pursued by the Killam's and their group (University of California), and some detailed results are given below. Secondly, pharmacological agents, with relatively well-established actions on synaptic transmission, can be employed to study the biochemical and synaptic mechanisms involved in the onset and development of epileptic seizures. This approach is aided by the growing body of data about neurophysiological mechanisms involved in this syndrome, but it is limited insofar as no drug has a mode of action that is entirely specific. However, the judicious selection of a number of drugs whose principal modes of action are known permits certain conclusions. Some of those that have been reached on the basis of this approach are outlined below.

A. Antiepileptic drugs

Because of day-to-day variations in the responsiveness of experimental animals, it is necessary to test each animal over a long period of time to establish his mean responsiveness and his variability. The antiepileptic drug must be tested in both acute and chronic doses in animals of high and low photosensitivity.

The syndrome of photosensitive epilepsy resembles myoclonus "petit mal" or non-focal "grand mal" in that barbiturates have a high therapeutic effectiveness (e.g., phenobarbital, 15.0 mg/kg i.m., suppresses all motor epileptic responses for 2 to 3 days), whereas hydantoins, which act in focal epilepsy and particularly temporal lobe epilepsy in man, are much less effective in single doses. However, as in man, cumulative doses of hydantoins are more effective. Diphenylhydantoin, for example, does not block seizures at single doses up to 50 mg/kg, but 15 mg/kg will prevent seizure responses to ILS in 75% of animals if given in three successive daily doses; the most highly photosensitive animals show only modifications of pattern and severity of response at this dose (Stark et al., 1970).

Trimethadione modifies seizure patterns at doses up to 100 mg/kg, but usually fails to block abnormal activity completely in the *Papio* (Killam et al., 1972), although it acts with success in human "petit mal." Benzodiazepines have been found to be very effective in blocking the syndrome. Diazepam blocks seizure responses in some animals in single doses as low as 0.013 mg/kg and is fully effective in single or long-term chronic dosage at 0.5 mg/kg. The 7-chloro (RO 5807) and 7-nitro derivatives (RO 4023) also block seizures at doses which do not cause muscle relaxation (Stark et al., 1970). The 7-nitro compound has been shown to have an ED_{50} for seizure control of 0.005 mg/kg in single doses (Killam et al., 1972). The relative effectiveness of RO 4023 to diazepam in *Papio papio* is closely similar to recent results in human patients with petit mal attacks (Gastaut, 1970). With either diazepam or RO 4023, animals maintained on doses initially just sufficient to control seizure responses tend to escape from therapeutic control, but an increased dose restores the antiepileptic effect (Killam et al., 1972).

Table 1 summarizes data about the effective doses of some established antiepileptic drugs and the approximate time course of their action. For comparison, data relating to drugs acting on synaptic transmission (discussed below) are also given.

TABLE 1. *Drugs diminishing or abolishing myoclonic responses to photo stimulation*

Drug	Dose (mg/kg)	Latency of effect (min)	Duration of effect (hr)
Diazepam	0.02–0.5	<5	>2 <24
RO 4023	0.005–0.05	<5	>2 <24
Phenobarbital	5–15	<5	24– 48
Diphenylhydantoin	15–50	(repetitive dosage required)	
LSD 25	0.04–0.1	<5	0.5–1.5
Psilocybin	1–4	<5	1–2
Dimethyltryptamine	2–4	<5	0.5
Methysergide	2–5	5	1–2
Methylergometrine	0.05–2	5	2–3
L-5-Hydroxytryptophan	10–30	30	2–3
Tranylcypromine	15–30	60–240	8–24
Amino-oxyacetic	10–15	30–40	6–24
Di-N-Propylacetic acid	25–150	5–15	1–3

B. CNS pathways and synaptic mechanisms

A wide variety of techniques (including microiontophoresis, enzyme histochemistry, histofluorescent staining for amines, lesions combined with biochemical measurements, subcellular fractionation techniques, and studies with isotopically labeled precursors) have increased our knowledge of CNS transmitter substances, synaptic mechanisms and the neuronal pathways concerned in certain physiological functions. Considerably more data are available for the rat than for the primate; very little work has been done on synaptic mechanisms in *Papio papio*. However, pharmacological experiments performed so far do permit some conclusions about the synaptic mechanisms involved in the epileptic responses. These are conveniently considered in relation to the different putative neurotransmitters found in the brain.

1. Acetylcholine

There is histochemical and physiological evidence for two cholinergic pathways within the cerebral cortex. One is part of the ascending reticular formation and contributes to EEG activation following arousing stimuli. Excessive activity in this system may explain the seizures seen in rats after toxic doses of eserine or diisopropylfluorophosphate (DFP). There is also evidence for an intracortical cholinergic inhibitory system that may contribute to cortical spikes produced by the local application of anticholinergic agents (Bhargava and Meldrum, 1969). However, in *Papio papio,* intravenous doses of atropine or eserine sufficient to modify the ascending activating system (as shown by changes in background EEG rhythms) do not modify photosensitivity (Meldrum et al., 1970*b*). It is, therefore, unlikely that cholinergic pathways play a critical role in the initiation or evolution of the epileptic responses in the baboon.

2. Gamma-aminobutyric acid (GABA)

There is good evidence that GABA is an inhibitory transmitter within the cerebral cortex, cerebellum, hippocampus, and thalamus. Many drugs that impair the synthesis of GABA by inhibiting the enzyme glutamic acid decarboxylase produce generalized seizures in a wide range of animals, e.g., in the baboon, isoniazid at a dose of 100 to 160 mg/kg, or 4-deoxypyridoxine at a dose of 100 to 160 mg/kg. Seizures induced by these drugs in *Papio papio* differ from those induced by photic stimulation in that they characteristically originate in one occipital lobe. These drugs in subconvulsive doses (e.g., isoniazid 40 to 80 mg/kg, 4-deoxypyridoxine 40 to 80 mg/kg) produce a marked enhancement of photosensitivity, beginning after 15 to 45 min and lasting 1 to 4 hr (Meldrum et al., 1970*a;* Meldrum and Horton, 1971). Pentylenetetrazol, a convulsant which does not block the synthesis of GABA, also enhances photosensitivity but with a very short latency from the injection.

Amino-oxyacetic acid increases the cerebral content of GABA by blocking its further metabolism by the enzyme GABA-transaminase. In the baboon at a dose of 10 to 15 mg/kg, it blocks the photically induced myoclonic responses for several hours (Meldrum et al., 1970*a*). However, higher doses provoke spontaneous seizures by an unknown mechanism.

Bicuculline, an alkaloid that blocks the postsynaptic inhibitory action of GABA on cortical neurons, produces convulsions in cats, monkeys and baboons at intravenous doses of 0.2 to 0.4 mg/kg. Subconvulsive doses do not produce any marked enhancement of sustained myoclonic responses to photic stimulation (Meldrum and Horton, 1971).

Table 2 shows the contrast between the delayed and prolonged action of the pyridoxine antagonists (that inhibit glutamic acid decarboxylase) and the rapid onset of action of bicuculline and two other drugs (pentamethylenetetrazol and picrotoxin) which produce similar but briefer seizures.

TABLE 2. *Drugs enhancing photosensitivity and/or inducing seizures in the absence of photic stimulation*

Drug	Dose enhancing photosensitivity (mg/kg)	Dose provoking seizures (mg/kg)	Latency of effect (min)	Duration of effect (hr)
Isoniazid	65–100	100–150	7–40	1–2
Thiosemicarbazide	4–7	4–10	60–240	1–3
4-Deoxypyridoxine	40–100	105–150	15–45	1–4
Pentamethylenetetrazol	5–15	15	<1–5	0.1–0.4
Bicuculline	–	0.2–0.4	<1	0.1–5.0
Picrotoxin	0.5–0.8	1	1–5	1–1.5

GABA undoubtedly plays an important role in many forms of seizure, including photically induced epilepsy. There is however no evidence for any specific abnormality in the GABA inhibitory system in *Papio papio*.

3. Serotonin

A serotonergic system ascending from the nuclei of the median raphé to the hypothalamus and cerebral cortex has been identified morphologically and shown by pharmacological experiments and by lesion studies to be involved in the initiation and maintenance of slow-wave sleep, and probably also in other behavioral mechanisms such as habituation. Drugs which have been shown to modify activity in this system have pronounced effects on photically induced responses in *Papio papio*.

LSD 25 (40 to 100 μg/kg i.v.) completely abolishes the myoclonic and EEG paroxysmal responses to intermittent photic stimulation (Walter et al., 1971) (Fig. 8). A similar effect is produced by some hallucinogenic derivatives of tryptamine (e.g., psilocybin 1 to 4 mg/kg, or dimethyltrypta-

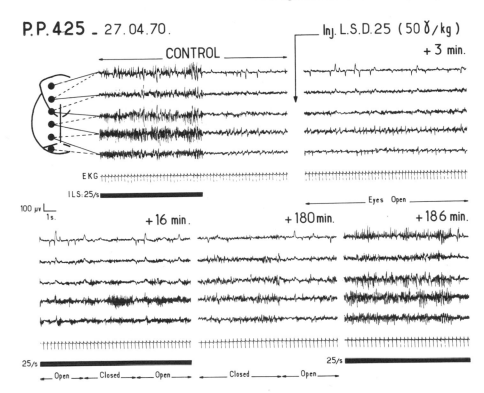

FIG. 8. The effects of LSD 25 on paroxysmal discharge in a baboon. From Meldrum and Naquet (1971, *personal communication*).

mine 2 to 4 mg/kg) and by some relatively non hallucinogenic derivatives of lysergic acid (e.g., methysergide 2 to 5 mg/kg, or methylergometrine 0.5 to 2 mg/kg) (Meldrum and Naquet, 1971; Vuillon-Cacciuttolo and Balzano, 1972). All these compounds block the smooth-muscle-contracting action of serotonin. Their action on central synapses is less well understood. LSD 25 and most of the other drugs that block photically induced responses modify electrical activity within the visual pathway. They reduce both postsynaptic responses at the lateral geniculate nucleus and photically evoked responses at the cortex. These drugs may reduce photosensitivity by an action on the afferent pathway, but an additional action at a cortical or subcortical site cannot be excluded.

The synthesis of serotonin (5-HT) in the brain can be impaired by the administration of an inhibitor of tryptophan hydroxylase, *para*-chloro-phenylalanine (PCPA). This drug in appropriate doses produces insomnia in rats, cats, and monkeys. At the time of the greatest reduction in brain 5-HT (48 hr), baboons show some enhancement of photosensitivity, but subsequently (4 to 7 days) they cease to show any myoclonic responses (Wada et al., 1972a, 1972c).

The immediate precursor of 5-HT, *l*-5 hydroxytryptophan (5-HTP), when given i.v. or i.p. at 15 to 50 mg/kg, abolishes the photically induced myoclonus (Wada et al., 1972a). It is not yet clear whether this is due to enhancement of brain 5-HT content, or to some pharmacological action of 5-HTP, which is known, for example, to reduce postsynaptic responses at the lateral geniculate.

Thus, although drugs known to modify activity in serotoninergic systems have powerful effects on photosensitive epilepsy, further studies are required before the physiological mechanisms involved can be precisely defined.

4. Catecholamines

Neuronal systems containing noradrenaline and dopamine have been identified in various subcortical areas. A dopaminergic system plays an important role in the control of movement, and the noradrenaline-containing system is apparently concerned with appetitive behavior, various homeostatic mechanisms, and the paradoxical phase of sleep. Studies are in progress in Marseille, Carshalton, Davis, and Vancouver to elucidate the possible role of catecholamines in epileptic responses, but it is too early to attempt to draw definite conclusions.

X. CONCLUSION

Since photosensitive epilepsy in the *Papio papio* was first discovered in 1966, additional studies have supported the 1967 opinion of Killam and co-workers that here was an animal model of great importance in the study of epilepsy. Also, because the model is found in a primate, it is closer to man than any other model commonly used in the laboratory. It is a natural model triggered by external physical stimuli very similar to physiological stimuli and, moreover, analogous to those effective in man. This animal model provides a means of investigating genetic, neurochemical, neuropharmacological, neuroanatomical, and neurophysiological aspects which no artificially produced animal model can provide.

Experimentation is at a stage where the clinical data are no longer in doubt; with regard to the EEG data, certain points such as the exact origin and mechanism of photosensitivity still require clarification. The neuro-anatomical investigation is just beginning, and this model will allow the study of neuropathologic events secondary to epileptic seizures (Riche et al., 1971). The entire field is still open for neurophysiological study, both of cell units and of preparations involving destruction of various cortical and subcortical regions; the possibility of a metabolic or neurochemical explanation is still only tentative. Breeding of animals with excessive and stable photosensitivity, which has already been done for audiogenic epilepsy, may well provide answers to these various problems. It will also permit genetic studies such as those done with domestic fowl (Crawford, 1970) and those newly in progress with *Papio papio* at the Centre d'Hémotypologie in Toulouse (Gourdin et al., 1972).

Leaving aside the idea of breeding, it is still a fact that this animal model exists and is already being used by many laboratories. The agreement of results from the various teams working on this problem suggests that we can confidently expect within a few years to have acquired a much more extensive understanding of photosensitive epilepsy in the *Papio papio* and, by extrapolation, of certain human epilepsies.

XI. REFERENCES

Arfel, G., Walter, S., and Christolomme, A. (1972): Extension thalamique des décharges paroxystiques chez un babouin *Papio papio* photosensible. *Rev. EEG Neurophysiol.* (*in press*).

Balzano, E. (1968): Etude polygraphique du sommeil nocturne du *Papio papio* babouin du Sénégal. Thèse de 3ème cycle Neurophysiologie, Marseille, 135 pp.

Batini, C., Radulovacki, M., Kado, R. T., and Adey, W. R. (1967): Effect of interhemispheric transection on the EEG pattern in sleep and wakefulness in monkeys. *Electroencephalography and Clinical Neurophysiology*, 22:101–112.

Bert, J., and Naquet, R. (1969): Variations géographiques de la photosensibilité chez le babouin *Papio papio*. *Revue Neurologique*, 121:364–365.

Bert, J., Pegram, V., Rhodes, J. M., Balzano, E., and Naquet, R. (1970): A comparative sleep study of two cercopithecinae. *Electroencephalography and Clinical Neurophysiology*, 28:32–40.

Bhargava, V. K., and Meldrum, B. S. (1969): The strychnine-like action of curare and related compounds on the somatosensory evoked response of the rat cortex. *British Journal of Pharmacology*, 37:112–122.

Bickford, R. G., and Klass, D. W. (1969): Sensory precipitation and reflex mechanisms. In: *Basic Mechanisms of the Epilepsies*, edited by H. H. Jasper, A. A. Ward, Jr., and A. Pope. Little, Brown and Co., Boston, pp. 543–564.

Bickford, R. G., Sem-Jacobsen, C. W., White, P. T., and Daly, D. (1952): Some observations on the mechanisms of photic and photo-metrazol activation. *Electroencephalography and Clinical Neurophysiology*, 4:275.

Catier, J., Choux, M., Cordeau, J. P., Dimov, S., Riche, D., Eberhard, A., and Naquet, R.

(1970): Résultats préliminaires des effets électrographiques de la section du corps calleux chez le *Papio papio* photosensible. *Revue Neurologique,* 122:521–522.

Catier, J., Menini, C., Charmasson, G., and Carlier, E. (1971): Evidence for somatosensory cortical projections to frontal lobe in the baboon. *Journal of Physiology* (Paris), 63:121*A*–122*A*.

Cobb, S. (1947): Photic driving as a cause of clinical seizures in epileptic patients. *Archives of Neurology and Psychiatry* (Chicago), 58:70–71.

Dimov, S., and Lanoir, J. (1969): Effets de lésions épileptogènes chroniques occipitales (cobalt-alumine) chez le *Papio papio. Revue Neurologique,* 120:480.

Dimov, S., Menini, C., and Naquet, R. Cortical recovery cycles to light stimulation in *Papio papio* and their relation to the photomyoclonic manifestations. Communication at symposium "Visual information processing and control of motor activity," Sofia, July 1969 (*in press*).

Fischer-Williams, M., Poncet, M., Riche, D., and Naquet, R. (1968): Light-induced epilepsy in the baboon *Papio papio:* Cortical and depth recordings. *Electroencephalography and Clinical Neurophysiology,* 25:557–569.

Gastaut, H. (1970): Exceptional anticonvulsive properties of a new benzodiazepine. In: *Modern Problems of Pharmacopsychiatry,* Vol. IV: Epilepsy. Edited by E. Niedermeyer. S. Karger, Basel, pp. 261–269.

Gastaut, H., Roger, J., and Gastaut, Y. (1948): Les formes expérimentales de l'épilepsie humaine: l'épilepsie induite par la stimulation lumineuse intermittente rythmée ou "épilepsie photogénique." *Revue Neurologique,* 80:161–183.

Gastaut, H., and Tassinari, A. (1966): Triggering mechanisms in epilepsy. The electroclinical point of view. *Epilepsia,* 7:85.

Gourdin, D., Vergnes, H., Bouloux, C., and Gherardi, M. (1972): Polymorphism of erythrocyte G6PD in the baboon. *American Journal of Medical Anthropology* (*in press*).

Jami, L. (1972): Pattern of cortical population discharge. *Electroencephalography and Clinical Neurophysiology,* 32:641–654.

Killam, K. F., Killam, E. K., and Naquet, R. (1966*a*): Mise en évidence chez certains singes d-un syndrome photomyoclonique. *Comptes Rendus de l'Académie des Séances* (Paris), 262:1010–1012.

Killam, K. F., Killam, E. K., and Naquet, R. (1967*a*): An animal model of light sensitive epilepsy. *Electroencephalography and Clinical Neurophysiology,* 22:497–513.

Killam, K. F., Killam, E. K., and Naquet, R. (1967*b*): Evoked potential studies in response to light in the baboon (*Papio papio*). *Electroencephalography and Clinical Neurophysiology,* Suppl. 26:108–113.

Killam, E. K., Matsuzaki, M., and Killam, K. F. Studies of anticonvulsant compounds in the *Papio papio* model of epilepsy. In: *Advances in Biochemical Psychopharmacology,* Vol. 7. Raven Press, New York (*in press*).

Killam, K. F., Naquet, R., and Bert, J. (1966*b*): Paroxysmal responses to intermittent light stimulation in a population of baboons (*Papio papio*). *Epilepsia,* 7:215–219.

Kitsikis, A., Dimov, S., Dubouch, P., Pons, C., and Naquet, R. (1970): Etude de la photosensibilité du *Papio anubis,* du *Papio cynocephalus* et de *Papio nés* de leur croisement. *Revue Neurologique,* 121:366–367.

Koudryatzeva, N. N. (1969): Response to rhythmic photostimulation in lower monkeys. *Sechenov Physiological Journal of the USSR,* 55:132–137.

Meldrum, B. S., Balzano, E., Gadea, M., and Naquet; R. (1970*a*): Photic and drug-induced epilepsy in the baboon (*Papio papio*); the effects of isoniazid, thiosemicarbazide, pyridoxine and amino-oxyacetic acid. *Electroencephalography and Clinical Neurophysiology,* 29: 333–347.

Meldrum, B. S., and Horton, R. W. (1971): Convulsive effects of 4-deoxypyridoxine and of bicuculline in photosensitive baboons (*Papio papio*) and in rhesus monkeys (*Macaca mulatta*). *Brain Research,* 35:419–436.

Meldrum, B. S., and Naquet, R. (1971): Effects of psilocybin, dimethyltryptamine, mescaline and various lysergic acid derivatives on the EEG and on photically induced epilepsy in the baboon, *Papio papio. Electroencephalography and Clinical Neurophysiology,* 31:563–572.

Meldrum, B. S., Naquet, R., and Balzano, E. (1970*b*): Effects of atropine and eserine on the electroencephalogram, on behaviour and on light-induced epilepsy in the adolescent baboon *Papio papio. Electroencephalography and Clinical Neurophysiology,* 28:449–458.

Menini, C., Catier, J., Charmasson, G., and Carlier, E. (1971): Projections corticales des afférences péri-oculaires chez le *Papio papio. Rev. EEG Neurophysiol,* 4:432–433.

Menini, C., Dimov S., Vuillon-Cacciuttolo, G., and Naquet, R. (1970): Réponses corticales évoquées par la stimulation lumineuse chez le *Papio papio. Electroencephalography and Clinical Neurophysiology,* 29:233–245.

Menini, C., Morrell, F., and Naquet, R. (1968*a*): Enregistrements corticaux au moyen de microélectrodes chez le *Papio papio* photosensible. *Journal de Physiologie,* 60:498–499.

Menini, C., and Rostain, J. C. (1969): Enregistrements unitaires dans le cortex fronto-rolandique *du Papio papio* photosensible. *Journal de Physiologie, 61,* suppl. 2:352.

Menini, C., and Rostain, J. C. (1970): Activités unitaires évoquées par la stimulation lumineuse dans différents territoires corticaux chez le *Papio papio. Journal de Physiologie, 62,* suppl. 3:414–415.

Menini, C., Vuillon-Cacciuttolo, G., and Lesevre, N. (1968*b*): Chronologie et topographie des réponses corticales évoquées par différents types de stimulations chez le *Papio papio. Journal de Physiologie,* 60:277–278.

Menini, C., Vuillon-Cacciuttolo, G., and Naquet, R. (1968*c*): Etude morphologique, chronologique et topographique des potentiels évoqués visuels d'un cercopithecinae. *Revue Neurologique,* 118:474–475.

Morrell, F., Naquet, R., and Menini, C. (1969): Microphysiology of cortical neurons in *Papio papio. Electroencephalography and Clinical Neurophysiology,* 27:708–709.

Naquet, R. (1969): Discussion. *Photogenic seizures in baboon.* In: *Basic Mechanisms of the Epilepsies,* H. H. Jasper, A. A. Ward, Jr., and A. Pope, editors. Little, Brown and Co., Boston, pp. 566–573.

Naquet, R., Ames, F., Carlier, E., Charmasson, G., Catier, J., and Menini, C. (1971*a*): Afférences périoculaires et photosensibilité du *Papio papio.* Etude clinique et électroencéphalographique. *Rev. EEG Neurophysiol.,* 4:430–431.

Naquet, R., Bert, J., and Guillon, R. (1971): Répartition de la photosensibilité dans plusieurs populations de babouins (*Papio papio*). Proceedings of the Third International Congress of Primatology, Zurich, Vol. 8, pp. 45–48, Karger, Basel.

Naquet, R., Killam, K. F., and Killam, E. K. (1969): Photomyoclonic epilepsy of *Papio papio.* In: *The Physiopathogenesis of the Epilepsies,* H. Gastaut, H. Jasper, J. Bancaud, and A. Waltregny, editors. Charles C Thomas, Springfield, Ill., pp. 268–272.

Naquet, R., Killam, K. F., Killam, E. K., Bimar, J., and Poncet, M. (1968): Un nouveau "modèle animal" pour l'étude de l'épilepsie: Le *Papio papio.* In: *Actualités Neurophysiologiques,* 8ème série. Masson & Cie Ed., Paris, pp. 213–230.

Naquet, R., Killam, K. F., Rhodes, J. M. (1966): Flicker stimulation with chimpanzees. *Life Sciences,* 6:1575–1578.

Naquet, R., and Lanoir, J. (1972): Détermination de l'activité anti-épileptique expérimentale. Tests spéciaux. In: *The International Encyclopedia of Pharmacology and Therapeutics.* Pergamon Press, Oxford (*in press*).

Naquet, R., and Menini, C. (1972): La photosensibilité excessive du *Papio papio.* Approches neurophysiologiques et pharmacologiques de ses mécanismes. Communication au Colloque International en Sciences Neurologiques en Hommage à H. H. Jasper, Montréal, September 1970. *Electroencephalography and Clinical Neurophysiology (in press).*

Naquet, R., Menini, C., and Catier, J. (1972): Photically-induced epilepsy in *Papio papio.* The initiation of discharges and the role of the frontal cortex of the corpus callosum. Symposium on "Mechanisms of synchronization in epileptic seizures," Vienna, September 1971 (*in press*).

Poncet, M. (1968): L'épilepsie photosensible du singe *Papio papio.* Etude clinique et électroencéphalographique. Structures corticales et profondes. Thèse de Médecine, Marseille, p. 138.

Riche, D., Christolomme, A., Bert, J., and Naquet, R. (1968): *Atlas Stéréotaxique du Cerveau de Babouin* (*Papio papio*). C.N.R.S., Paris, p. 207.

Riche, D., Gambarelli-Dubois, D., Dam, M., and Naquet, R. (1971): Repeated seizures and cerebral lesions in photosensitive baboons (*Papio papio*). A preliminary report. In: *Brain Hypoxia*, J. B. Brierley and B. S. Meldrum, editors. Spastics International Medical Publishers, London, pp. 297–301.

Riche, D., Gambarelli-Dubois, D., and Naquet, R. (1970): Crises fréquentes et lésions anatomiques chez le *Papio papio* photosensible. *Revue Neurologique*, 123:257–258.

Serbanescu, F. T. (1970): Epilepsia fotosensibilă a Babuinului *Papio papio* (Studiu comparativ intre om şi animal). Teza de Doctorat, Bucarest.

Serbanescu, T., Bert, J., Guillon, R., and Naquet, R. (1968a): Etude de la photosensibilité du *Papio papio* du Sénégal oriental. *Journal de Physiologie*, 60:399–403.

Serbanescu, T., Godet, R., Orsini, J. C., and Naquet, R. (1968b): La stimulation lumineuse intermittente chez le Galago senegalensis. *Journal de Physiologie*, 60:391–398.

Serbanescu, T., Naquet, R., and Menini, C. (1972): Various physical parameters which influence photosensitive epilepsy in the *Papio papio*. *Brain Research* (*in preparation*).

Stark, L. G., Joy, R. M., Hance, A. J., and Killam, K. F. (1968): Further studies of photic stimulation in subhuman primates (*unpublished data*).

Stark, L. G., Killam, K. F., and Killam, E. K. (1970): The anticonvulsivant effects of phenobarbital, diphenylhydantoin and two benzodiazepines in the baboon, *Papio papio*. *Journal of Pharmacology and Experimental Therapeutics*, 173:125–132.

Vuillon-Cacciuttolo, G., and Balzano, E. (1972): Action de quatre dérivés de l'ergot sur la photosensibilité et l'EEG du *Papio papio*. *Journal de Pharmacologie*, 3:31–45.

Wada, J. A., Balzano, E., Meldrum, B. S., and Naquet, R. (1972a): Effects of L-5-hydroxytryptophan and D-L-parachlorophenylalanine on the photomyoclonic syndrome in the Senegalese baboon, *Papio papio*. *Electroencephalography and Clinical Neurophysiology*.

Wada, J. A., Terao, A., and Booker, H. E. (1972b): Longitudinal correlative analysis of epileptic baboon, *Papio papio*. (*in preparation*).

Wada, J. A., Meldrum, B. S., and Balzano, E. (1972c): Modified level of brain serotonin in *Papio papio*; study of parachloro-phenylalanine. *Journal de Pharmacologie* (*in press*).

Wada, J. A., Catier, J., Charmasson, G., Menini, C., and Naquet, R. (1972d): Elimination of photogenic seizure susceptibility by bilateral occipital lobectomy in photosensitive epileptic baboon, *Papio papio*. *Science* (*in press*).

Walter, S., Balzano, E., Vuillon-Cacciuttolo, G., and Naquet, R. (1971): Effets comportementaux et électrographiques du diéthylamide de l'acide D-lysergique (LSD 25) sur le *Papio papio* photosensible. *Electroencephalography and Clinical Neurophysiology*, 30:294–305.

Walter, V. J., and Walter, W. G. (1949): The central effects of rhythmic sensory stimulation. *Electroencephalography and Clinical Neurophysiology*, 1:57–86.

16

Systemic Chemical Convulsants and Metabolic Derangements

William E. Stone

Outline

I. INTRODUCTION

The scientific study of convulsing agents and their effects on experimental animals began more than a century ago. Wiedemann (1877) described epileptiform seizures induced in animals by administration of camphor, and referred to earlier experiments with this drug. Marcé (1864) induced convulsions in dogs and rabbits by administration of absinth. The effects of picrotoxin were described in detail by J. Crichton Browne (1875). At that time the actions of strychnine were known and had been studied rather extensively; however, the convulsions induced by strychnine cannot be considered epileptiform in the light of modern investigations to be discussed. Thujone, an isomer of camphor, is the active ingredient of absinth and is obtainable from the oils of wormwood, thuja, tansy, and sage. Purified preparations were in use by the beginning of this century, when Hildebrandt (1902) found that thujone was a more potent convulsant than camphor. Wortis et al. (1931) introduced camphor monobromide. Pentylenetetrazol was synthesized by Schmidt (1924), and its convulsive action was observed by Hildebrandt (1926). It soon became the most widely used chemical convulsant. Agents of the camphor group fell into disuse, while many new convulsants were introduced and have been utilized to some extent.

The use of systemically administered convulsants has the advantage that the excitatory agent is distributed to all parts of the brain, a consideration that is particularly important in neurochemical studies. The relevance to human epileptogenic processes is difficult to evaluate, and must be considered in relation to the type of convulsant employed since different types undoubtedly act by different mechanisms. However, some convulsants are antagonized by drugs that are of therapeutic value in human epilepsy, and epileptogenic foci in patients can be activated by small doses of agents such as pentylenetetrazol. These facts can be taken to indicate the relevance to the epilepsy problem of studies employing convulsant drugs.

Metabolic derangements that tend to precipitate seizures include severe hypoglycemia, vitamin B_6 deficiency, and parathyroid hypofunction. Alterations in steroid levels also may play a role, at least by influencing the convulsive threshold.

II. METHODS

A. General procedures

It is assumed that the investigator will have acquired a degree of familiarity with procedures commonly used in animal experimentation. Excellent technical guides are available containing basic information on laboratory equipment, procedures for the care and handling of animals, injection of drugs, local and general anesthesia, pre-anesthetic medication, common surgical procedures, and physiological monitoring (Lumb, 1963; Graham-Jones, 1964; Miller et al., 1969). Electrophysiological methods are described in detail by Bureš et al. (1960). Longo (1962) gives procedures for studying drug actions in rabbits. Barnes and Eltherington (1964) give, for various animals, tabulated dosages of anesthetics, convulsants, and many other drugs.

B. Experiments on intact animals

1. Drug administration and monitoring of seizures

The simplest method of producing a model of epilepsy with a systemic chemical convulsant is to administer an adequate dose to an intact animal. Since the sensorium is disrupted to the point of complete unconsciousness during a generalized seizure, the use of analgesia or anesthesia usually is not required. This model is often used to test the effects of pharmacologic agents, brain lesions, or other factors on the convulsive threshold and has played an important role in the evaluation of new anticonvulsants. Testing procedures have been developed in which standard doses of pentylenetetrazol are given subcutaneously or intravenously in rats or mice (Swinyard et al., 1952; Goodman et al., 1953; Swinyard, 1969). Others who have used various convulsants and species in this way include Everett and Richards (1944), Chen and Portman (1952), Banziger and Hane (1967), and Chusid and Kopeloff (1969).

A variant of these methods is the timed infusion procedure, in which the convulsant is given slowly by vein at a standard rate and the time required for the initiation of a seizure is recorded (Jenny and Pfeiffer, 1956; Kopeloff and Chusid, 1967; Adler, 1969). A newer and very practical method employs flurothyl, a volatile convulsant that can be administered by inhalation. The animal is placed in a closed chamber and flurothyl is introduced at a fixed rate, the time required for the induction of convulsive activity being observed (Truitt et al., 1960; Adler, 1969; Prichard et al., 1969).

These and other techniques for the evaluation of anticonvulsants have been reviewed by Domer (1971). They are dependent upon observation of overt convulsive symptoms; however, a refinement permitting electrographic recording of cerebral activity can be attained by prior implantation of electrodes (Delgado, 1955; McLean, 1957; Bureš et al., 1960; Spehlmann and Colley, 1968; Milstein, 1969; Record et al., 1969).

2. *Quick-freezing of small animals and sampling procedures*

When the objective is to study neurochemical changes associated with the convulsive state, a suitable method of sampling is required. McIlwain and Rodnight (1962) have described procedures for obtaining, fixing, and extracting neural tissues. For the measurement of relatively stable constituents it suffices to decapitate the animal and obtain the desired samples by dissection. The study of intermediary metabolites, however, requires a technique that will eliminate rapid postmortem changes as far as possible. Some workers have frozen the head in liquid N_2 immediately after decapitation, but this procedure allows anoxic changes in some intermediates (e.g., energy-rich phosphate compounds, lactate, gamma-aminobutyric acid). The usual method is to submerge the head or the whole animal suddenly into liquid N_2 at the chosen time. Animals no larger than the rat can be dropped into liquid N_2, and it is advantageous to restrain the animal in a small wire cage for this purpose. Takahashi and Aprison (1964), using this procedure, submerged adult rats for measured periods of time and recorded temperature changes in the brain from implanted thermistors. After a delay of about 10 sec, the temperature of the cortex dropped rapidly, reaching 0°C at 20 to 40 sec. The thalamic region began to cool after 30 sec and reached 0°C at 70–85 sec. By keeping the animals immersed only for carefully measured short-time intervals, with subsequent decapitation, it was possible to cool the brain quickly to 0°C without freezing; this "near-freezing" technique facilitated dissection at 0°C and gave satisfactory values for acetylcholine content.

Dissection of frozen brain at very low temperatures to obtain specific regions is very difficult because of the brittleness of the tissue. However, if the temperature is brought to between -15 and $-20°C$, enough softening occurs to make dissection feasible. The samples can then be stored for weeks in liquid N_2 or for shorter periods with solid CO_2.

Lowry et al. (1964) froze mice in Freon-12 cooled to $-150°C$ with liquid N_2. Although this coolant freezes very small tissue samples more rapidly than does liquid N_2 (Cain and Davies, 1964), it has been found to be less effective than liquid N_2 for adult rats. Bazán et al. (1971) compared the two methods, using a thermocouple in the hypothalamic region, and found that the time required to reach $0°C$ was 58 to 71 sec in liquid N_2 and 91 to 108 sec in Freon-12. In smaller animals, less time was required in liquid N_2, but no comparison was made with Freon-12.

According to Granholm et al. (1968), freezing by submersion in liquid N_2 is not fast enough to prevent completely anoxic changes in the levels of certain intermediary metabolites. This was shown by comparing data on anesthetized rats frozen in liquid N_2 with findings on rats given the same anesthetic and artificially ventilated while the brain was being frozen *in situ*. Presumably the differences were due to the absence of respiration in the submerged animals while freezing was in progress.

An alternative to the freezing method is to kill the animal quickly by microwave irradiation, which destroys enzymes by heat inactivation and may be applicable when heat-stable intermediates are to be measured (Schmidt et al., 1971). This is a new method that has not yet been thoroughly tested.

3. Processing frozen samples

The removal of the brain from the frozen head is described by McIlwain and Rodnight (1962). A block of solid CO_2 makes a convenient platform for this operation. The tissue is frequently replaced in liquid N_2 for cooling during the procedure. A cartilage knife or a large scalpel and large forceps are useful instruments. Various types of chisels and a motor-driven routing tool or saw also may be used. The instruments are chilled intermittently in liquid N_2. Frozen tissues as well as cold instruments may be handled with pigskin gloves. The procedure is often carried out in a cold room, but this is not essential.

A small wire basket on a long handle is convenient for retrieving tissue specimens from liquid N_2 in a Dewar flask. A mortar and pestle cooled with liquid N_2 may be used to grind the frozen sample to a powder. A small amount of liquid N_2 should be added and allowed to evaporate just before the grinding. However, the tissue should first be crushed in a stainless steel percussion mortar (Stone, 1938; Cain and Davies, 1964) since large pieces of the very brittle frozen material are not easily ground in an ordinary mortar without losses. A small aluminum spoon attached to a wooden handle is useful for handling the powdered tissue. The sample may be weighed in a cold room on a chilled piece of thick sheet aluminum (bent into a shape suitable for pouring), or the vessel may be tared and weighed again after addition of the sample, being dried with a towel before each weighing if necessary. In some instances it is most convenient to weigh the small tube or bottle containing the powdered tissue before and after removal of the sample.

The extractant to be used must be selected with regard to the constituents to be measured. Extraction in aqueous media at 0°C allows changes in some constituents at the moment of thawing (Granholm et al., 1968); hence, extraction in organic solvents at temperatures well below 0°C is preferable when consistent with the analytical methods to be used (Minard and Davis, 1962; King et al., 1967; Minsker et al., 1970). The extractant is best contained in a small glass-stoppered Erlenmeyer flask. The powdered sample is introduced through a chilled aluminum funnel, the stopper replaced, and the flask immediately shaken. Dispersion is more rapid in such a flask than in a test tube. However, a homogenizer tube can be used when the sample is to be homogenized immediately.

C. Acute experiments requiring surgical preparation

Surgical procedures are often required for neurophysiological, neurochemical, or other studies. The brain may have to be exposed for the placing of various types of electrodes, excision of samples, or freezing *in situ*. Cannulation of blood vessels is often desirable for sampling of arterial or venous blood, for intravenous injections, and for monitoring arterial blood pressure, pH, or gas tensions. The monitoring of arterial blood pressure and oxygenation, and the use of a respiration pump when necessary, are of particular importance when it is essential to rule out the complicating effects that would arise from arterial or ischemic anoxia.

1. Problems of anesthesia

The surgical approach is fraught with problems related to the use of anesthetics and the restraint or immobilization of the animal. Most anesthetics are interdicted because of their antagonism to convulsants. A few workers have avoided anesthetics entirely by using curarizing agents to immobilize the animal and a pump to provide artificial respiration. However, it must be remembered that curarization does nothing to diminish the sensory inputs or the perception of pain (Smith et al., 1947). It is necessary that effective means be employed to eliminate pain.

Some workers have used chloralose or chloralose with urethan for anesthesia in cats and dogs (Nadler and Berger, 1938; Gellhorn et al., 1939; Ajmone Marsan and Marossero, 1950). These agents apparently exhibited little anticonvulsive activity in the experiments reported, but their suitability has been questioned (R. Naquet, *personal communication*). In dogs, Gurdjian et al. (1946) used large doses of morphine sulfate (20 mg/kg s.c.) supplemented with local infiltration of procaine hydrochloride where necessary. Pscheidt et al. (1954) modified this procedure, using morphine sulfate at 5 mg/kg s.c. supplemented with thiopental sodium (12 mg/kg i.v., with additional doses as needed) until the surgical procedures were completed. This dose of the briefly acting barbiturate is about one-half of that which would be required in the absence of morphine, and, after its effects disappear, the actions of morphine continue for at least 4 hr. A curarizing agent can be used in this preparation to suppress the peripheral manifestations of the convulsive discharge. Since morphine does not antagonize convulsants, and since control animals receive the same dose of morphine as do those given convulsants, this procedure can be used for studies of seizures in dogs and in some other animals. A detailed description is given in the Appendix. However, morphine cannot be used in cats (Miller et al., 1969). Beresford et al. (1969), working with dogs, used nitrous oxide rather than morphine. Venes et al. (1971) studied the use of nitrous oxide in cats and recommended it for neurophysiological experiments.

Numerous workers have used transient anesthesia (ether, vinyl ether, thiopental, or thiamylal) during surgical procedures, followed by an agent to block neuromuscular transmission (artificial respiration being provided), but in this type of preparation great care must be taken to infiltrate all operative sites and pressure points with a local anesthetic (Meyer et al., 1962; Sutton and Oldstone, 1969). The paralyzing agents chosen have included d-tubocurarine (Crescitelli and Gilman, 1946; Preston, 1955), β-erythroidine (Starzl et al., 1953), dihydro-β-erythroidine (Klein and Olsen, 1947; Wang and Sonnenschein, 1955), gallamine triethiodide (Vanasupa et al., 1959; Harris, 1964; Beresford et al., 1969), and succinylcholine (Amato et al., 1969). d-Tubocurarine has the disadvantage that it often induces severe hypotension. At dose levels sufficient for paralysis, these agents do not appear to influence the cerebral electrographic patterns, probably because of failure to pass the blood-brain barrier. They do not inhibit convulsive activity. At much higher doses, however, gallamine triethiodide induces a pattern resembling the arousal reaction (Whisler et al., 1968), and *d*-turbocurarine blocks dendritic potentials (Purpura and Grundfest, 1956).

When artificial respiration must be maintained for a considerable period of time, it is important to monitor the end-expiratory CO_2 tension with an infrared gas analyzer and to regulate the pump so that the CO_2 tension is kept within the normal range. Without this precaution, it is almost impossible to avoid a respiratory acidosis or alkalosis.

A suitable head holder is essential for experiments of this type. When depth electrodes are to be used, a Horsley-Clarke stereotaxic instrument is commonly employed (Bureš et al., 1960). Lim et al. (1960) described a modification suitable for the dog. When only cortical leads are required, a simple inexpensive head holder can be constructed. Thompson et al. (1951) described a very suitable model, adaptable to various animals.

2. *Freezing in situ and sampling procedures*

Several procedures have been described for obtaining samples of cerebral tissue frozen *in situ* (McIlwain and Rodnight, 1962). Kerr (1935) introduced the method of freezing with liquid air. In young cats, rabbits, and smaller animals, the brain can be frozen through the calvarium; in larger animals, the dura mater must be exposed and may also be opened and reflected. For obtaining small serial samples from the cortex, Dobkin (1970) used a metal container filled with a mixture of solid CO_2 and acetone, applying the bottom to the exposed cortex for a few seconds and excising the frozen area. A similar procedure described by Schmahl et al. (1965) appears to be more advantageous; they used an aluminum suction device chilled in liquid N_2. Minsker et al. (1970), in a study on the isolated, perfused brain of the dog, used a cryoprobe cooled by evaporation of Freon-22 within the tip and equipped with a rotating knife blade. The probe is inserted into the cortex, and the blade is rotated to cut around the plug of frozen tissue. Several small serial samples can be obtained with this device. Cooper (1962) described a probe cooled by liquid N_2, designed for neurosurgical use but applicable in neurochemical studies.

III. CHEMICAL CONVULSANTS

Convulsing agents are far too numerous to be cataloged here. Representative data for a few selected agents are given in Table 1. Major convulsants or groups will be considered very briefly. Except as noted, the

TABLE 1. *Chemical convulsants*

Drug	Animal	Convulsant dose (mg/kg)	Latent period	Reference	Remarks
Pentylenetetrazol	Mouse	85 s.c.	—	Swinyard et al. (1952)	Seizures in 97%
	"	50–75 i.p.	1–3 min	Stone (1970)	
	Rat	70 s.c.	—	Swinyard et al. (1952)	Seizures in 97%
	"	40–70 i.p.	—	Blum and Zacks (1958)	
	Guinea pig	60–70 i.p.	4–15 min	Watterson (1939)	
	Rabbit	15–25 i.v.	9 sec	Longo (1962)	
	Cat	20–40 i.v.	—	Wang and Sonnenschein (1955)	
	Dog	25–30 i.v.	8–20 sec	Gurdjian et al. (1946)	Animal under morphine
	Monkey	8.5–29 i.v.	—	Chusid and Kopeloff (1969)	Threshold
Bemegride	Rat	21 i.p.	—	Hahn and Oberdorf (1962)	Seizures in 50%
	Rabbit	5.6 i.v.	—	Hahn and Oberdorf (1962)	Seizures in 50%
	Dog	8–15 i.v.	10–20 sec	Stone (*unpublished*)	Animal under morphine
	Monkey	5–9 i.v.	>1 min	Chusid and Kopeloff (1969)	
Picrotoxin	Mouse	5.9 s.c.	—	Hahn and Oberdorf (1962)	Seizures in 50%
	Rabbit	0.8 i.v.	15 min	Werner and Tatum (1939)	Minimum convulsant dose
	Dog	2 i.v.	2–15 min	Bircher et al. (1962)	
	Monkey	0.45–0.9 i.v.	15–25 min	Chusid and Kopeloff (1969)	Threshold
Thujone	Cat, rabbit	5–7 i.v.	a few sec	Opper (1939)	20% in propylene glycol
Methyl fluoroacetate	Dog	1 i.v.	51–88 min	Tews and Stone (1965)	Animal under morphine
DL-Methionine-DL-sulfoximine	"	10 i.v.	16–18 hr	Tews and Stone (1964)	
	"	700–800 i.v.	1–2 hr	Harris (1964)	
Thiosemicarbazide	Dog	20 i.v.	43–87 min	Tews and Stone (1965)	Animal under morphine
1,1-Dimethylhydrazine	Mouse	150 i.p.	76±19 min	Furst and Gustavson (1967)	
4-Deoxypyridoxine hydrochloride	Monkey	100–150 i.v.	29–104 min	Meldrum and Horton (1971)	
Methylpyridoxine	Cat	50 i.v.	35–40 min	Purpura and Gonzales-Monteagudo (1960)	
Bicuculline	Monkey	0.1–0.4 i.v.	A few sec	Meldrum and Horton (1971)	Threshold
Tetraethyl pyrophosphate	Dog	2 i.v.	3–15 min	Stone (1957)	Animal under morphine, atropine, artificial respiration

discussion will be limited to agents known to induce epileptiform cortical electrographic patterns. Further information may be found in an extensive review by Hahn (1960) and a handbook by Barnes and Eltherington (1964).

A. Tetrazoles

The only commonly used agent of the tetrazole group is pentylenetetrazol (pentamethylenetetrazol, Metrazol®, Cardiazol®, Leptazol®). Although a number of others are more potent convulsants (Hahn, 1960; Stone, 1970), the uniquely high solubility of pentylenetetrazol is an advantage. At high enough doses, this agent acts on all parts of the central nervous system, but the most sensitive region is the cerebral cortex (Bircher et al., 1962).

Purpura and Gonzalez-Monteagudo (1960) referred to pentylenetetrazol as a "synaptically acting convulsant," with the implication that it directly activates excitatory synapses (in contrast to the blocking action of strychnine on inhibitory synapses). The activating mechanism remains unexplained. Pentylenetetrazol does not directly activate muscle or nerve fibers, but Eyzaguirre and Lilienthal (1949) reported that it has veratrine-like effects; i.e., it increases the tension and duration of the twitch on direct or indirect stimulation, this effect being associated with a train of spikes following the normal diphasic action potential. The nerve also showed a train of spikes in response to a single shock. Anguiano and McIlwain (1951) suggested a similar action in the cortex, on the basis of chemical studies showing that in isolated cortex there were chemical changes in response to electrical stimulation but no comparable changes on treatment with pentylenetetrazol. Thus the action of pentylenetetrazol might be to potentiate the response to a stimulus rather than to initiate activity. However, Dripps and Larrabee (1940) found that pentylenetetrazol stimulated autonomic ganglia even when all preganglionic impulses had been eliminated by nerve section. Esplin and Zablocka-Esplin (1969) described microelectrode studies bearing on the mechanism of action of pentylenetetrazol.

B. Glutarimides

Bemegride (Megimide®) causes general stimulation of the central nervous system. Its actions are quite comparable to those of pentylenetetrazol (Hahn, 1960). Bemegride has found clinical use as an analeptic and as an activator in the diagnosis of focal epilepsy. A related. compound, β-methyl-β-isopropyl glutarimide, has actions like those of bemegride but is a more potent convulsant (MacFarlane and McKenzie, 1960).

C. Picrotoxin

The actions of picrotoxin are very similar to those of pentylenetetrazol, except that the effects develop more slowly after injection (Hahn, 1960). In dogs given 2 mg/kg i.v., there is a slow "build-up" in the cortical electrical activity starting in 1 to 5 min. Spikes and slow waves appear and increase gradually in size and frequency. Muscular twitching is not noticeable at first, but appears early during the build-up and gradually increases, merging into a severe clonic convulsion. In some instances the developing clonic pattern is interrupted by the onset of a severe tonic-clonic seizure (Stone et al., 1960).

D. Compounds of the camphor group

Camphor compounds have been used very little since the introduction of electroencephalography, and few recordings of their electrographic effects are available. Lennox et al. (1936) found that camphor induced epileptiform cortical activity in a patient. Dusser de Barenne et al. (1938) recorded seizure patterns from a dog and a monkey after administration of camphor monobromide. Klein and Olsen (1947) apparently observed the same type of activity in cats given thujone, but published no record or detailed description. Opper (1939), who carried out histological studies on the brain after injection of thujone or camphor monobromide, reviewed some of the early literature on these agents.

E. Monofluoroacetates and related compounds

Monofluoroacetates are metabolic poisons. Through enzymatic processes they are converted to fluorocitric acid, which partially blocks the tricarboxylic acid cycle by inhibiting the enzyme aconitase (Peters, 1957; Goldberg et al., 1966). In addition, fluoroacetates have a blocking action on the synthesis of glutamine (Lahiri and Quastel, 1963). The relation of the metabolic effects to the initiation of seizures has not been clarified; possible mechanisms have been discussed by Patel and Koenig (1971).

The effects of these agents and the required dosages vary considerably from one species to another (Chenoweth, 1949). In dogs and guinea pigs, the brain is primarily affected, with the development of severe tonic-clonic seizures after a latent period that varies inversely with the dosage. In some animals (e.g., rabbit, goat), the heart is primarily affected, whereas in others (e.g., cat, pig, monkey), both brain and heart are involved. Rats, mice, and guinea pigs sometimes respond with seizures, but not consistently.

F. Methionine sulfoximine

Seizures induced by methionine sulfoximine have a relatively long latent period that varies inversely with the dosage (Table 1). A massive dose may induce convulsions in less than 2 hr, whereas a low convulsant dose induces a semi-epileptoid condition with intermittent seizures that begin many hours after injection and continue for a day or two. Gradual recovery may follow, or death in status epilepticus may occur. The syndrome was described by Tower (1958) as it occurs in dogs, and by Proler and Kellaway (1962) as seen in cats. There are wide species differences in sensitivity to this agent (Gershoff and Elvehjem, 1951). Proler and Kellaway (1965) recorded the gradually developing electrical patterns in the cat over a period of many hours. Hřebíček and Koloušek (1968), in a similar study, found alterations in visual-evoked potentials that differed from those seen with convulsants such as pentylenetetrazol.

Methionine sulfoximine inhibits glutamine synthetase and alanine transferase in the brain, and induces alterations in cerebral levels of ammonia and several amino acids. It is antagonized by methionine. These biochemical effects have been reviewed (Stone, 1969; Van den Berg, 1970). Peters and Tower (1959) studied the altered metabolism of glutamate and glutamine in slices of cortical tissue obtained from animals that had been treated with methionine sulfoximine. Van den Berg and Van den Velden (1970) observed that the drug reduces the rate of incorporation of carbon from glucose into cerebral amino acids related to the tricarboxylic acid cycle, while increasing the incorporation from acetate and phenylalanine. It also decreases the uptake of labeled methionine by brain structures, presumably by blocking its incorporation into proteins (Hřebíček et al., 1971). The significance of the biochemical effects in relation to the convulsive phenomena remains obscure.

G. Convulsants affecting pyridoxal-5-phosphate-dependent enzyme systems

There is a large group of agents that bring about what has been described as a drug-induced vitamin B_6 deficiency. Although pyridoxal phosphate acts as a coenzyme in a number of metabolic processes involving amino acids, the reactions by which γ-aminobutyric acid (GABA) is formed and removed seem to be the ones most affected by convulsants of this group. Glutamic acid decarboxylase (GAD), the enzyme that forms GABA, is particularly sensitive to a deficiency of pyridoxal phosphate (Tapia et al., 1969; Tower, 1969).

Three types of drug action are to be considered. Antimetabolites such as 4-deoxypyridoxine and its phosphorylated analog are believed to compete with B_6 vitamers for enzymic binding sites, whereas carbonyl-trapping agents such as the hydrazides inactivate pyridoxal phosphate by combining with the aldehydic 4-CHO group to form hydrazones (Holtz and Palm, 1964; Nishie et al., 1966). In addition, some hydrazones have a potent convulsing action (Furst and Gustavson, 1967). This is attributed to inhibition of pyridoxal kinase, the enzyme that phosphorylates B_6 vitamers; thus, the supply of the active coenzyme is cut off, and a deficiency quickly develops (Tapia et al., 1969).

All of these convulsants reduce the formation of GABA by GAD. Some of them also inhibit GABA transaminase, the enzyme that removes GABA, while others do not. Hence, there are variable effects on the level of GABA in the brain. However, Tapia et al. (1969) have suggested that inhibition of GAD may be the critical factor in the development of seizures. This enzyme is found mainly in the axoplasm of nerve endings. If GABA is an inhibitory transmitter released at certain nerve endings, excitation could develop owing to failure of its synthesis and release. GABA transferase is a mitochondrial enzyme, and its inhibition might have little or no effect at nerve endings. Wood and Abrahams (1971) have further elaborated this hypothesis, suggesting that the concentration of GABA attained in the synaptic cleft may be influenced not only by the GAD activity but also by a membrane transport process involved in removal of GABA from the cleft.

There are some convulsants that inhibit GAD in ways other than through action on pyridoxal phosphate. These include allylglycine (Alberici et al., 1969) and mercaptopropionic acid (Lamar, 1970). Apparently the electrographic effects of these agents have not yet been reported. Thiosemicarbazide seems to have two modes of action, one resembling that of other hydrazides and another appearing at lower dose levels (Wood and Abrahams, 1971).

Large doses of pyridoxine counteract the convulsive and other effects of agents that inactivate pyridoxal phosphate, but do not antagonize other convulsants (Holtz and Palm, 1964).

H. Bicuculline

The convulsant alkaloid bicuculline is a phthalide isoquinoline derivative isolated from fumaraceous plants. Intravenous injection induces epileptiform seizures immediately. Baboons given adequate doses develop a status epilepticus in which seizures may be sustained for 150 to 300 min without interruption by isoelectric periods (Meldrum and Horton, 1971; Brierley et al., 1972). Bicuculline is a GABA antagonist, and its mode of action is believed to be to block inhibitory systems employing GABA as the inhibitory transmitter (Curtis, et al., 1971a; Curtis and Felix, 1971). It is possible to classify inhibitory amino acids as "GABA-like" (antagonized by bicuculline) and "glycine-like" (antagonized by strychnine), although in some instances tests on supraspinal neurons yield results that differ from those obtained on spinal neurons.

I. Strychnine

Strychnine is one of the longest known and most extensively studied convulsants. Ajmone Marsan (1969) has tabulated many central and peripheral actions described in the literature. Esplin and Zablocka-Esplin (1969) recently reviewed studies on the mode of action of strychnine and pharmacologically similar agents, a subject which remains controversial. Bradley et al. (1953) introduced the concept that strychnine blocks direct inhibition by competing with an inhibitory transmitter for postsynaptic receptor sites. The resulting disinhibition might account for the excitatory effects. Further studies have shown that at low concentrations strychnine specifically antagonizes the inhibitory effects of glycine, the probable transmitter (Curtis et al., 1971b). It remains an open question whether this is due to competition for the same steric configurations on the postsynaptic membrane or to a direct action on the membrane altering its capacity to undergo changes in ionic conductance in the presence of the transmitter (Pollen and Ajmone Marsan, 1965; Stefanis and Jasper, 1965). The latter effect may occur only at higher concentrations of strychnine, as may a direct excitatory effect (Curtis et al., 1971b).

It is important to note that the convulsions induced by systemic administration of strychnine are not epileptiform. They consist only of tonic extension and extensor jerks which may be triggered by any sensory stimuli (Esplin and Zablocka-Esplin, 1969). Electrographic studies have shown that the drug acts principally in the spinal cord, brainstem, and cerebellum, inducing waves of very high frequency and amplitude (Markham et al., 1952; Longo and Chiavarelli, 1962). The cortex usually shows only an arousal pattern, although Amato *et al.* (1969) noted cortical spiking in cats paralyzed with succinylcholine and given strychnine systemically. (For further discussion, see Chapter X.)

J. Inhibitors of cholinesterase

There are many compounds that exhibit anticholinesterase activity, including agents such as physostigmine and a large group of organophosphorus compounds (Heath, 1961). The blood-brain barrier is not permeable to all of these, but a number of them do enter the brain and induce convulsive phenomena when introduced into the blood stream. Tower (1969) has discussed this model and reviewed the occurrence of seizures and other symptoms of toxicity in persons accidentally exposed to these compounds.

Systemic administration of anticholinesterases has found only limited use in attempts to induce experimental epilepsy. To study the central actions, it is necessary to protect the animal from peripheral muscarinic effects with a small dose of atropine or preferably methyl atropine (Meldrum et al., 1970) and to provide adequate ventilation with a respiration pump. The convulsive action of tetraethyl pyrophosphate in the dog has been studied in this way (Stone, 1957). The cerebral level of acetylcholine increases, presumably because it is being synthesized and released as in normal activity but is not being destroyed. The initial electrographic effect is an intense arousal reaction, a sudden increase in frequency followed by increasing amplitude for a few minutes and then gradually decreasing amplitude. In some dogs the high frequency pattern continues indefinitely, but more often epileptiform convulsive activity supervenes.

This type of seizure is distinguished by the fact that it can be prevented or quickly suppressed by a massive dose of atropine or scopolamine (5 to 10 mg/kg i.v.), drugs that do not inhibit seizures of other types. (Scopolamine is preferable since it has no hypotensive effect.) There seems to be little doubt that seizures induced by anticholinesterases are brought about by the action of accumulated acetylcholine on cholinoceptive neurons.

K. Miscellaneous convulsants

Flurothyl (Indoklon®) is hexafluorodiethyl ether. It can be given either by inhalation or intravenously (Krantz, 1963). The effects resemble those of pentylenetetrazol. There are also convulsant barbiturates, which are of special interest in that they are specifically antagonized by the closely related depressant barbiturates (Esplin and Zablocka-Esplin, 1969; Downes et al., 1970). Diethylbutanediol is a convulsant homolog of the depressant diethylpropanediol (Slater et al., 1954).

Eidelberg et al. (1963) studied the convulsive action of cocaine. In cats, the seizures begin in the amygdala, spreading to become generalized. A similarity to temporal lobe epilepsy has been suggested. Local anesthetics such as lidocaine and butacaine also act as convulsants when given in large doses (Munson and Wagman, 1969; Tuttle and Elliott, 1969).

Chusid et al. (1956) described convulsive effects of high doses of two antihistamines, tripelennamine (Pyribenzamine®) and diphenhydramine

(Benadryl®). Similar studies by Wallach et al. (1969) dealt with antidepressive drugs (amitriptyline, imipramine, and desmethylimipramine). Winters et al. (1969) described seizures induced by a hallucinogen, phencyclidine. Sutton and Oldstone (1969) showed that massive doses of penicillin given systematically induce epileptiform seizures.

Convulsant acridones have the property of fluorescence, which makes possible the application of fluorescence microscopy (Mayer and Bain, 1956). Pollock and Bain (1950) investigated a series of β-chlorinated amines (nitrogen mustards). Wang and Sonnenschein (1955) studied one of these further, and Pradhan and Ajmone Marsan (1963) tested a related compound, chlorambucil. Several chlorinated insecticides are known to have convulsive actions (Crescitelli and Gilman, 1946; McNamara and Krop, 1948; Pollock and Wang, 1953; St. Omer, 1971). Acrylamide, another industrial chemical, also induces seizures (Kuperman, 1958).

Nicotine, which has long been of interest to physiologists because of its ganglionic and other peripheral effects, has been shown to induce epileptiform cerebral activity under favorable experimental conditions. These studies have been reviewed by Silvette et al. (1962).

IV. METABOLIC DERANGEMENTS

A. Hypoglycemia

Insulin hypoglycemia has been studied extensively. McQuarrie et al. (1940) used dogs treated with large doses of insulin as a model of the epileptic. Seizures usually occurred in intact animals not subjected to additional experimental procedures. However, when the dog is prepared surgically under morphine with transient thiopental anesthesia, seizures occur much less regularly even when hexamethonium is used to block release of epinephrine (Stone, 1969). Electrographic recordings have been taken during hypoglycemic convulsions in several laboratories (reviewed by Stone, 1969). More recent observations have been made on cats by Waltregny (1969) and on baboons by Naquet et al. (1970). Poiré (1969) recorded hypoglycemic convulsive activity in human patients, and reviewed the relevant clinical literature.

Gastaut et al. (1968) found, in cats with epileptogenic foci produced by local application of penicillin or tungsten paste, that moderate hypoglycemia decreased the cerebral excitability, whereas marked hypoglycemia increased excitability and lowered the convulsive threshold. In baboons susceptible to seizures induced by intermittent light stimulation, however, hypoglycemia did not increase the sensitivity to photic stimulation (Naquet et al., 1970). Insulin has not been found to precipitate seizures in epileptic patients (Ziskind and Bolton, 1936; Zolliker, 1938).

B. Vitamin B₆ deficiency

Convulsions develop in association with vitamin B_6 deficiency in most of the common species. The seizures are comparable to those induced by antimetabolites of pyridoxine, discussed previously. Vitamin B_6 deficiency has been thoroughly reviewed by Tower (1969), including its effects in human patients and the occurrence of vitamin B_6 dependency.

C. Parathyroid hypofunction

In parathyroid deficiency, the resulting hypocalcemia brings about an increase in excitability at all levels of the neuromuscular system. Recent observations by Corriol et al. (1969) make it clear that in dogs the symptoms include seizures of the grand mal type, with epileptiform cortical activity.

D. Adrenal steroid imbalance

After reviewing the relationships between adrenal cortical activity and the convulsive state, Glaser (1953) concluded that "there is a strong suggestion that a heightened susceptibility to seizures or an increase in cerebral excitability" may be correlated with increased activity of glucocorticoids, whereas the reverse may occur with mineralocorticoids. A few years later, Heuser and Eidelberg (1961) found that large doses of Reichstein's substance S (cortexolone, 17α-hydroxy-11-deoxycorticosterone) induced seizures in cats and rats. Epileptiform electrographic patterns were recorded from the cortex and other regions of the cat brain. The seizures began in the hippocampus, and resembled those of temporal lobe epilepsy. Cortexolone, a precursor of cortisol, was initially classified as a mineralocorticoid but was later shown to have glucocorticoid properties as well (Applesweig, 1962).

V. APPENDIX: DETAILED PROCEDURE FOR AN EXPERIMENT ON A DOG

The purpose of this Appendix is to describe fully details not previously published regarding experiments on the dog to study convulsive agents. It will be apparent that the procedure could be altered in many ways and adapted to other species.

The dog is allowed water but no food for 18 hr before the experiment. Morphine sulfate is given subcutaneously (5 to 6 mg/kg), and after 45 min thiopental sodium (12 mg/kg) is given intravenously. Should respiratory arrest occur at this point, as often happens, artificial respiration is given manually until breathing is resumed. Polyethylene cannulae are placed in a femoral artery and a femoral vein. The arterial cannula is filled with heparinized saline, and is later connected to a pressure transducer for recording. The venous catheter, to be used for all injections, is connected to a bottle of normal saline (0.15 M NaCl) and a very slow infusion is given to keep the cannula open.

The head is fastened firmly in a head holder, and an endotracheal tube with an inflatable cuff is inserted. Should the animal show any signs of awakening before surgical procedures are completed, additional thiopental is given in doses of about 4 mg/kg as often as needed.

A long midline incision is made in the scalp, the skin is retracted, and the temporal muscles are detached and reflected, exposing the calvarium. A large part of each temporal muscle is carefully excised; cut vessels are clamped with hemostats and subsequently tied. The calvarium is opened with a large trephine, and a rongeur is used to remove most of the calvarium. Bleeding from the bone is controlled with bone wax. It is not necessary to leave a bridge of bone over the sagittal sinus. Emissary veins over the anterior part of the sinus are usually ruptured, but the bleeding can be stopped by pressing a pledget of Gelfoam (absorbable gelatin sponge) or a piece of muscle over the opening and applying a moderate pressure until clotting occurs. The dura mater may be opened if desired.

For electrographic recording, disposable electrodes are made from short lengths of No. 18 copper wire. These are thrust through tight holes in a 10×50 mm strip of polyethylene cut from a thick sheet. One end of the strip is fastened to the bone over the frontal sinus with a sheet metal screw, and the electrodes (with U-shaped ends) are bent so as to make firm but gentle contact with the dural or cortical surface. Short flexible wires clipped to the electrodes lead to larger clips attached to the head holder. The EEG leads are connected here. For monopolar recording, the indifferent lead is connected to a screw in the bone over the frontal sinus region. This electrode assembly is not easily dislodged by convulsive movements. Electrocardiographic leads are also attached and connected to one EEG channel.

To prepare for freezing the brain, a "crown" made from a strip of cardboard (the ends being fastened with skin clips) is set in place surrounding the exposed brain. The retracted skin is pulled up and fastened with skin clips to the "crown," all around. If the head is at the correct angle and the cardboard has been trimmed to fit properly, the brain will now lie at the bottom of a cup-like container for the liquid N_2.

Recordings are made intermittently until the effects of thiopental have subsided (about 30 min). The dog remains heavily sedated, but responds to a strong pinch of toe or tail. At this point, the infrared CO_2 analyzer intake is connected to the endotracheal tube and an end-expiratory reading is taken. The respiratory pump is started and connected, gallamine triethiodide (4 mg/kg) is injected, and the pump is adjusted to maintain the end-expiratory CO_2 at the normal level. The reading must be watched continually and the pump adjusted as required.

Within a few minutes, the convulsant is injected, while recording continues. At the time chosen for freezing, liquid N_2 is poured on the brain, forming a pool which is maintained by frequent additions for a period of 4 min. About 1 liter of liquid N_2 is required. The EEG channels are turned off when freezing begins. A sample of arterial blood may be drawn at this time, and the adequacy of oxygenation checked either visually or by analysis. After 2 min of freezing, the heart is stopped by injection of 10 ml of saturated KCl.

The "crown," frozen skin, and electrodes are quickly broken away with a large rongeur or other instrument, the samples to be removed are circumscribed with a motor-driven routing tool or saw, and a chilled cartilage knife is used to separate the pieces of tissue. An assistant uses chilled forceps to remove the pieces and place them in liquid N_2. Later they are carefully trimmed before processing. The operators' hands are protected by pigskin gloves during these procedures.

In control or other experiments in which the animal may retain some consciousness, the KCl injection is preceded by a dose of thiopental (given when the region to be sampled has been frozen). Stopping the heart serves to avoid bleeding from deep, unfrozen regions while the frozen samples are being removed.

VI. REFERENCES

Adler, M. W. (1969): Laboratory evaluation of antiepileptic drugs. *Epilepsia (Fourth Series)*, 10:263–280.

Ajmone Marsan, C. (1969): Acute effects of epileptogenic agents. In: *Basic Mechanisms of the Epilepsies*, edited by H. H. Jasper, A. A. Ward, Jr., and A. Pope. Little, Brown & Co., Boston, pp. 299–319.

Ajmone Marsan, C., and Marossero, F. (1950): Electrocorticographic and electrochordographic study of the convulsions induced by cardiazol. *Electroencephalography and Clinical Neurophysiology*, 2:133–142.

Alberici, M., Rodrigues de Lores Arnaiz, G., and De Robertis, E. (1969): Glutamic acid decarboxylase inhibition and ultrastructural changes by the convulsant drug allylglycine. *Biochemical Pharmacology*, 18:137–143.

Amato, G., La Grutta, V., Militello, L., and Enia, F. (1969): The function of the caudate nucleus in the control of some paroxystic activities in the neuraxis. *Archives Internationales de Physiologie et de Biochimie*, 77:465–484.

Anguiano, G., and McIlwain, H. (1951): Convulsive agents and the phosphates of brain examined *in vitro*. *British Journal of Pharmacology and Chemotherapy*, 6:448–453.

Applezweig, N. (1962): *Steroid Drugs*. McGraw-Hill, New York.

Banziger, R., and Hane, D. (1967): Evaluation of a new convulsant for anticonvulsant screening. *Archives Internationales de Pharmacodynamie et de Thérapie*, 167:245–249.

Barnes, C. D., and Eltherington, L. G. (1964): *Drug Dosage in Laboratory Animals: A Handbook*. University of California Press, Berkeley.

Bazán, N. G., Jr., de Bazán, H. E. P., Kennedy, W. G., and Joel, C. D. (1971): Regional distribution and rate of production of free fatty acids in rat brain. *Journal of Neurochemistry*, 18:1387–1393.

Beresford, H. R., Posner, J. B., and Plum, F. (1969): Changes in brain lactate during induced cerebral seizures. *Archives of Neurology*, 20:243–248.

Bircher, R. P., Kanai, T., and Wang, S. C. (1962): Intravenous, cortical and intraventricular dose-effect relationship of pentylenetetrazol, picrotoxin and deslanoside in dogs. *Electroencephalography and Clinical Neurophysiology*, 14:256–267.

Blum, B., and Zacks, S. (1958): Analysis of the relationship between drug-induced convulsions and mortality in rats. *Journal of Pharmacology and Experimental Therapeutics*, 124:350–356.

Bradley, K., Easton, D. M., and Eccles, J. C. (1953): An investigation of primary or direct inhibition. *Journal of Physiology*, 122:474–488.

Brierley, J. B., Horton, R. W., and Meldrum, B. S. (1972): Physiological observations during prolonged epileptic seizures in primates and their relation to subsequent brain damage. *Proceedings of the Physiological Society*, 74 P, December, 1971; *Journal of Physiology* (*in press*).

Browne, J. C. (1875): On the actions of picrotoxine, and the antagonism between picrotoxine and chloral hydrate. *British Medical Journal*, 1:409–411.

Bureš, J., Petráň, M., and Zochar, J. (1960): *Electrophysiological Methods in Biological Research* (translated by P. Hahn). Publishing House of the Czechoslovak Academy of Sciences, Praha.

Cain, D., and Davies, R. E. (1964): Rapid arrest of metabolism with melting Freon. In: *Rapid Mixing and Sampling Techniques in Biochemistry*, edited by B. Chance, R. H. Eisenhardt, Q. H. Gibson, and K. K. Lonberg-Holm. Academic Press, New York, pp. 229–237.

Chen, G., and Portman, R. (1952): Titration of central nervous system depression. *A.M.A. Archives of Neurology and Psychiatry*, 68:498–505.

Chenoweth, M. B. (1949): Monofluoroacetic acid and related compounds. *Pharmacological Reviews*, 1:383–424.

Chusid, J. G., and Kopeloff, L. M. (1969): Use of chronic irritative foci in laboratory evaluation of anti-epileptic drugs. *Epilepsia*, 10:239–262.

Chusid, J. G., Kopeloff, L. M., and Kopeloff, N. (1956): Convulsant action of antihistamines in monkeys. *Journal of Applied Physiology*, 9:271–274.

Cooper, I. S. (1962): A cryogenic method for physiologic inhibition and production of lesions in the brain. *Journal of Neurosurgery*, 19:853–858.

Corriol, J., Papy, J. J., Rohner, J. J., and Joanny, P. (1969): Electroclinical correlations established during tetanic manifestations induced by parathyroid removal in the dog. In: *The Physiopathogenesis of the Epilepsies*, edited by H. Gastaut, H. Jasper, J. Bancaud, and A. Waltregny, Charles C Thomas, Springfield, Ill., pp. 128–140.

Crescitelli, F., and Gilman, A. (1946): Electrical manifestations of the cerebellum and cerebral cortex following DDT administration in cats and monkeys. *American Journal of Physiology*, 147:127–137.

Curtis, D. R., Duggan, A. W., Felix, D., Johnston, G. A. R., and McLennan, H. (1971a): Antagonism between bicuculline and GABA in the cat brain. *Brain Research*, 33:57–73.

Curtis, D. R., Duggan, A. W., and Johnston, G. A. R. (1971b): The specificity of strychnine as a glycine antagonist in the mammalian spinal cord. *Experimental Brain Research*, 12:547–565.

Curtis, D. R., and Felix, D. (1971): The effect of bicuculline upon synaptic inhibition in the cerebral and cerebellar cortices of the cat. *Brain Research*, 34:301–321.

Delgado, J. M. R. (1955): Evaluation of permanent implantation of electrodes within the brain. *Electroencephalography and Clinical Neurophysiology*, 7:637–644.

Dobkin, J. (1970): Reversible changes in glutamine levels in the cat cerebral cortex evoked by afferent electrical stimulation and by administration of pentamethylenetetrazol. *Journal of Neurochemistry*, 17:237–246.

Domer, F. R. (1971): *Animal Experiments in Pharmacological Analysis*. Charles C Thomas, Springfield, Ill., pp. 319–349.

Downes, H., Perry, R. S., Ostlund, R. E., and Karler, R. (1970): A study of the excitatory effects of barbiturates. *Journal of Pharmacology and Experimental Therapeutics*, 175:692–699.

Dripps, R. D., and Larrabee, M. (1940): Electrical activity of the cortex and changes in cortical blood flow induced by Metrazol© and other exciting agents. *Archives of Neurology and Psychiatry*, 44:684–687.

Dusser de Barenne, J. G., Marshall, C. S., McCulloch, W. S., and Nims, L. F. (1938): Observations on the pH of the arterial blood, the pH and electrical activity of the cerebral cortex. *American Journal of Physiology*, 124:631–636.

Eidelberg, E., Lesse, H., and Gault, F. P. (1963): An experimental model of temporal lobe epilepsy: Studies of the convulsant properties of cocaine. In: *EEG and Behavior*, edited by G. H. Glaser. Basic Books, New York, pp. 272–283.

Esplin, D. W., and Zablocka-Esplin, B. (1969): Mechanisms of actions of convulsants. In: *Basic Mechanisms of the Epilepsies*, edited by H. H. Jasper, A. A. Ward, Jr., and A. Pope. Little, Brown & Co., Boston, pp. 167–183.

Everett, G. M., and Richards, R. K. (1944): Comparative anticonvulsive action of 3,5,5-trimethyloxazolidine-2,4-dione (Tridione®), Dilantin® and phenobarbital. *Journal of Pharmacology and Experimental Therapeutics*, 81:402–407.

Eyzaguirre, C., and Lilienthal, J. L., Jr. (1949): Veratrinic effects of pentamethylenetetrazol (Metrazol®) and 2,2-bis(p-chlorophenyl) 1,1,1 trichloroethane (DDT) on mammalian neuromuscular function. *Proceedings of the Society for Experimental Biology and Medicine*, 70:272–275.

Furst, A., and Gustavson, W. R. (1967): A comparison of alkylhydrazines and their B_6-hydrazones as convulsing agents. *Proceedings of the Society for Experimental Biology and Medicine*, 124:172–175.

Gastaut, H., Lyagoubi, S., Mesdjian, E., Saier, J., and Ouahchi, S. (1968): Generalized epileptic seizures, induced by "non-convulsant" substances. *Epilepsia*, 9:311–316.

Gellhorn, E., Darrow, C. W., and Yesinick, L. (1939): Effect of epinephrine on convulsions. *Archives of Neurology and Psychiatry*, 42:826–836.

Gershoff, S. N., and Elvehjem, C. A. (1951): The relative effect of methionine sulfoximine on different animal species. *Journal of Nutrition*, 45:451–458.

Glaser, G. H. (1953): On the relationship between adrenal cortical activity and the convulsive state. *Epilepsia*, 2:7–14.

Goldberg, N. D., Passonneau, J. V., and Lowry, O. H. (1966): Effects of changes in brain metabolism on the levels of citric acid cycle intermediates. *Journal of Biological Chemistry*, 241:3997–4003.

Goodman, L. S., Grewal, M. S., Brown, W. C., and Swinyard, E. A. (1953): Comparison of maximal seizures evoked by pentylenetetrazol (Metrazol®) and electroshock in mice, and their modification by anticonvulsants. *Journal of Pharmacology and Experimental Therapeutics*, 108:168–176.

Graham-Jones, O. (1964): *Small Animal Anesthesia*. MacMillan, New York.

Granholm, L., Kaasik, A. E., Nilsson, L., and Siesjö, B. K. (1968): The lactate/pyruvate ratios of cerebrospinal fluid of rats and cats related to the lactate/pyruvate, the ATP/ADP, and the phosphocreatine/creatine ratios of brain tissue. *Acta Physiologica Scandinavica*, 74:398–409.

Gurdjian, E. S., Webster, J. E., and Stone, W. E. (1946): Cerebral metabolism in Metrazol® convulsions in the dog. *Proceedings of the Association for Research in Nervous and Mental Disease*, 26:184–204.

Hahn, F. (1960): Analeptics. *Pharmacological Reviews*, 12:447–530.

Hahn, F., and Oberdorf, A. (1962): Vergleichende Untersuchungen über die Krampfwirkung von Bemegrid, Pentetrazol und Pikrotoxin. *Archives Internationales de Pharmacodynamie et de Therapie*, 135:9–30.

Harris, B. (1964): Cortical alterations due to methionine sulfoximine. *Archives of Neurology*, 11:388–407.

Heath, D. F. (1961): *Organophosphorus Poisons*. Pergamon Press, Oxford.

Heuser, G., and Eidelberg, E. (1961): Steroid-induced convulsions in experimental animals. *Endocrinology*, 69:915–924.

Hildebrandt, F. (1926): Pentamethylenetetrazol (Cardiazol®). *Archiv für experimentelle Pathologie und Pharmacologie*, 116:100–109.

Hildebrandt, H. (1902): Zur Pharmacologie der Kamphergruppe. *Archiv für experimentelle Pathologie und Pharmacologie*, 48:451–456.

Holtz, P., and Palm, D. (1964): Pharmacological aspects of vitamin B₆. *Pharmacological Reviews*, 16:113–178.

Hřebíček, J., and Koloušek, J. (1968): Preparoxysmal changes of spontaneous and evoked electrical activity of the brain after administration of methionine sulphoximine. *Epilepsia*, 9:145–162.

Hřebíček, J., Koloušek, J., Wiederman, M., and Charamza, O. (1971): Changes of the incorporation of [⁷⁵Se]methionine and of the electrical activity in various brain structures of the cat after administration of methionine sulphoximine. *Brain Research*, 28:109–117.

Jenney, E. H., and Pfeiffer, C. C. (1956): The predictable value of anticonvulsant indices. *Annals of the New York Academy of Sciences*, 64:679–689.

Kerr, S. E. (1935): Studies on the phosphorus compounds of brain. I. Phosphocreatine. *Journal of Biological Chemistry*, 110:625–635.

King, L. J., Lowry, O. H., Passonneau, J. V., and Venson, V. (1967): Effects of convulsants on energy reserves in the cerebral cortex. *Journal of Neurochemistry*, 14:599–611.

Klein, J. R., and Olsen, N. S. (1947): Effect of convulsive activity upon the concentration of brain glucose, glycogen, lactate and phosphates. *Journal of Biological Chemistry*, 167:747–756.

Kopeloff, L. M., and Chusid, J. G. (1967): Indoklon® and Metrazol® convulsions in epileptic and control monkeys. *International Journal of Neuropsychiatry*, 3:174–178.

Krantz, J. C. (1963): Volatile anesthetics and Indoklon®. *Journal of Neuropsychiatry*, 4:157–161.

Kuperman, A. S. (1958): Effects of acrylamide on the central nervous system of the cat. *Journal of Pharmacology and Experimental Therapeutics*, 123:180–192.

Lahiri, S., and Quastel, J. H. (1963): Fluoroacetate and the metabolism of ammonia in the brain. *Biochemical Journal*, 89:157–163.

Lamar, C., Jr. (1970): Mercaptopropionic acid: A convulsant that inhibits glutamate decarboxylase. *Journal of Neurochemistry*, 17:165–170.

Lennox, W. G., Gibbs, F. A., and Gibbs, E. L. (1936): Effect on the electroencephalogram of drugs and conditions which influence seizures. *Archives of Neurology and Psychiatry*, 36:1236–1245.

Lim, R. K. S., Liu, C.-N., and Moffitt, R. L. (1960): *A Stereotaxic Atlas of the Dog's Brain*. Charles C Thomas, Springfield, Ill.

Longo, V. G. (1962): *Electroencephalographic Atlas for Pharmacological Research. Effects of Drugs on the Electrical Activity of the Rabbit Brain.* Elsevier, Amsterdam.

Longo, V. G., and Chiavarelli, S. (1962): Neuropharmacological analysis of strychnine-like drugs. In: *Proceedings of the First International Pharmacological Meeting, Vol. 8, Pharmacological Analysis of Central Nervous Action*, edited by W. D. M. Paton. Pergamon Press, Oxford, pp. 189–198.

Lowry, O. H., Passonneau, J. V., Hasselberger, F. X., and Schulz, D. W. (1964): Effect of ischemia on known substrates and cofactors of the glycolytic pathway in brain. *Journal of Biological Chemistry*, 239:18–30.

Lumb, W. V. (1963): *Small Animal Anesthesia*. Lea and Febiger, Philadelphia.

MacFarlane, A. W., and McKenzie, J. S. (1960): The pharmacology of a new central nervous system stimulant, ββ-methyl isopropyl glutarimide. *Archives Internationales de Pharmacodynamie et de Thérapie*, 127:379–401.

Marcé, M. (1864): Sur l'action toxique de l'essence d'absinthe. *Comptes Rendus Hebdomadaires Des Séances de l'Académie des Sciences*, 58:628–629.

Markham, J. W., Browne, K. M., Johnson, H. C., and Walker, A. E. (1952): Convulsive patterns in cerebellum and brain stem. *Proceedings of the Association for Research in Nervous and Mental Disease*, 30:282–298.

Mayer, S. E., and Bain, J. A. (1956): The intracellular localization of fluorescent convulsants. *Journal of Pharmacology and Experimental Therapeutics*, 118:1–16.

McIlwain, H., and Rodnight, R. (1962): *Practical Neurochemistry*. Little, Brown & Co., Boston.

McLean, P. D. (1957): Chemical and electrical stimulation of hippocampus in unrestrained animals. *A.M.A. Archives of Neurology and Psychiatry*, 78:113–127.

McNamara, B. P., and Krop, S. (1948): Observations on the pharmacology of the isomers of hexachlorocyclohexane. *Journal of Pharmacology and Experimental Therapeutics*, 92:140–146.

McQuarrie, I., Ziegler, M. R., and Stone, W. E. (1940): Studies on the mechanism of insulin convulsions. *Chinese Medical Journal*, 58:1–25.

Meldrum, B. S., and Horton, R. W. (1971): Convulsive effects of 4-deoxypyridoxine and of bicuculline in photosensitive baboons (*Papio papio*) and in rhesus monkeys (*Macaca mulatta*). *Brain Research*, 35:419–436.

Meldrum, B. S., Naquet, R., and Balzano, E. (1970): Effects of atropine and eserine on the electroencephalogram, on behavior and light-induced epilepsy in the adolescent baboon (*Papio papio*). *Electroencephalography and Clinical Neurophysiology*, 28:449–458.

Meyer, J. S., Gotoh, F., Tazaki, Y., Hamaguchi, K., Nouailhat, F., and Symon, L. (1962): Regional cerebral blood flow and metabolism in vivo. *Archives of Neurology*, 7:560–581.

Miller, E., Ben, M., and Cass, J. S., editors (1969): Comparative anesthesia in laboratory animals. *Federation Proceedings*, 28:1369–1586.

Milstein, V. (1969): Implantation of sterile electrodes in chronic animals. *Electroencephalography and Clinical Neurophysiology*, 27:442–443.

Minard, F. N., and Davis, R. V. (1962): The effects of electroshock on the acid-soluble phosphates of rat brain. *Journal of Biological Chemistry*, 237:1283–1289.

Minsker, D. H., Gilboe, D. D., and Stone, W. E. (1970): Effects of shock and anoxia on nucleotides and creatine phosphate in the isolated brain of the dog. *Journal of Neurochemistry*, 17:253–259.

Munson, E. S., and Wagman, I. H. (1969): Acid-base changes during lidocaine induced seizures in *Macaca mulatta*. *Archives of Neurology*, 20:406–412.

Nadler, J. E., and Berger, A. R. (1938): Action of pentamethylenetetrazol (Metrazol®) on splanchnic circulation of the dog. *Proceedings of the Society for Experimental Biology and Medicine*, 38:381–383.

Naquet, R., Meldrum, B. S., Balzano, E., and Charrier, J. P. (1970): Photically induced epilepsy and glucose metabolism in the adolescent baboon (*Papio papio*). *Brain Research*, 18:503–512.

Nishie, K., Weary, M., and Berger, R. (1966): Anticonvulsant and convulsant effects of chemically related thiosemicarbazide, thiourea and urea derivatives. *Journal of Pharmacology and Experimental Therapeutics*, 153:387–395.

Opper, L. (1939): Pathologic picture of thujone and monobromated camphor convulsions. *Archives of Neurology and Psychiatry*, 41:460–470.

Patel, A., and Koenig, H. (1971): Some neurochemical aspects of fluorocitrate intoxication. *Journal of Neurochemistry*, 18:621–628.

Peters, E. L., and Tower, D. B. (1959): Glutamic acid and glutamine metabolism in cerebral cortex after seizures induced by methionine sulphoximine. *Journal of Neurochemistry*, 5:80–90.

Peters, R. A. (1957): Mechanism of the toxicity of the active constituent of *Dichapetalum cymosum* and related compounds. *Advances in Enzymology and Related Subjects of Biochemistry*, 18:113–159.

Poiré, R. (1969): Hypoglycemic epilepsy: Clinical, electrographic and biological study during induced hypoglycemia in man. In: *The Physiopathogenesis of the Epilepsies*, edited by H. Gastaut, H. Jasper, J. Bancaud, and A. Waltregny. Charles C Thomas, Springfield, Ill., pp. 75–110.

Pollen, D. A., and Ajmone Marsan, C. (1965): Cortical inhibitory post-synaptic potentials and strychninization. *Journal of Neurophysiology*, 28:342–358.

Pollock, G. H., and Bain, J. A. (1950): Convulsions in cerebellum and cerebrum induced by β-chlorinated amines. *American Journal of Physiology*, 160:195–202.

Pollock, G. H., and Wang, R. I. H. (1953): Synergistic actions of carbon dioxide with DDT in the central nervous system. *Science*, 117:596–597.

Pradhan, S. N., and Ajmone Marsan, C. (1963): Chlorambucil toxicity and EEG "centrencephalic" patterns. *Epilepsia*, 4:1–14.

Preston, J. B. (1955): Pentylenetetrazole and thiosemicarbazide: A study of convulsant activity in the isolated cerebral cortex preparation. *Journal of Pharmacology and Experimental Therapeutics,* 115:28–38.

Prichard, J. W., Gallagher, B. B., and Glaser, G. H. (1969): Experimental seizure-threshold testing with flurothyl. *Journal of Pharmacology and Experimental Therapeutics,* 166:170–178.

Proler, M., and Kellaway, P. (1962): The methionine sulfoximine syndrome in the cat. *Epilepsia,* 3:117–130.

Proler, M. L., and Kellaway, P. (1965): Behavioral and convulsive phenomena induced in the cat by methionine sulfoximine. *Neurology,* 15:931–940.

Pscheidt, G. R., Benitez, D., Kirschner, L. B., and Stone, W. E. (1954): Effects of fluoroacetate poisoning on citrate, lactate and energy-rich phosphates in the cerebrum. *American Journal of Physiology,* 176:483–487.

Purpura, D. P., and Gonzalez-Monteagudo, O. (1960): Acute effects of methoxypyridine on hippocampal end-blade neurons: An experimental study of "special pathoclisis" in the cerebral cortex. *Journal of Neuropathology and Experimental Neurology,* 19:421–432.

Purpura, D. P., and Grundfest, H. (1956): Nature of dendritic potentials and synaptic mechanisms in cerebral cortex of cat. *Journal of Neurophysiology,* 19:573–595.

Record, N. B., Prichard, J. W., Gallagher, B. B., and Seligson, D. (1969): Phenolic acids in experimental uremia. *Archives of Neurology,* 21:387–394.

Schmahl, F. W., Betz, E., Talke, E., and Hohorst, H. J. (1965): Energieriche Phosphate und Metabolite des Energiestoffwechsels in der Grosshirnrinde der Katze. *Biochemische Zeitschrift,* 342:518–531.

Schmidt, K. F. (1924): Uber den Imin-Rest. *Berichte der Deutsche Chemischen Gesellschaft,* 57:704–706.

Schmidt, M. J., Schmidt, D. E., and Robison, G. A. (1971): Cyclic adenosine monophosphate in brain areas: Microwave irradiation as a means of tissue fixation. *Science,* 173:1142–1143.

Silvette, H., Hoff, E. C., Larson, P. S., and Haag, H. B. (1962): The actions of nicotine on central nervous system functions. *Pharmacological Reviews,* 14:137–173.

Slater, I. H., Leary, D. E., and Dresel, P. E. (1954): Diethylbutanediol, a convulsant homologue of the depressant, diethylpropyldiol. *Journal of Pharmacology and Experimental Therapeutics,* 111:182–196.

Smith, S. M., Brown, H. O., Toman, J. E. P., and Goodman, L. S. (1947): The lack of cerebral effects of *d*-tubocurarine. *Anesthesiology,* 8:1–14.

Spehlmann, R., and Colley, B. (1968): Effect of diazepam (Valium) on experimental seizures in unanesthetized cat. *Neurology,* 18:52–60.

Starzl, T. E., Niemer, W. T., Dell, M., and Forgrave, P. R. (1953): Cortical and subcortical electrical activity in experimental seizures induced by Metrazol. *Journal of Neuropathology and Experimental Neurology,* 12:262–276.

Stefanis, C., and Jasper, H. (1965): Strychnine reversal of inhibitory potentials in pyramidal tract neurons. *International Journal of Neuropharmacology,* 4:125–138.

St. Omer, V. (1971): Investigations into mechanisms responsible for seizures induced by chlorinated hydrocarbon insecticides: The role of brain ammonia and glutamine in convulsions in the rat and cockerel. *Journal of Neurochemistry,* 18:365–374.

Stone, W. E. (1938): The effects of anesthetics and of convulsants on the lactic acid content of the brain. *Biochemical Journal,* 32:1908–1918.

Stone, W. E. (1957): The role of acetylcholine in brain metabolism and function. *American Journal of Physical Medicine,* 36:222–255.

Stone, W. E. (1969): Action of convulsants: Neurochemical aspects. In: *Basic Mechanisms of the Epilepsies,* edited by H. H. Jasper, A. A. Ward, Jr., and A. Pope, Little, Brown & Co., Boston, pp. 184–193.

Stone, W. E. (1970): Convulsant actions of tetrazole derivatives. *Pharmacology,* 3:367–370.

Stone, W. E., Tews, J. K., and Mitchell, E. N. (1960): Chemical concomitants of convulsive activity in the cerebrum. *Neurology,* 10:241–248.

Sutton, G. G., and Oldstone, M. B. A. (1969): Evidence against pyridoxine deficiency as the mechanism in penicillin seizures. *Neurology*, 19:859–864.

Swinyard, E. A. (1969): Laboratory evaluation of antiepileptic drugs. *Epilepsia*, 10:107–119.

Swinyard, E. A., Brown, W. C., and Goodman, L. S. (1952): Comparative assays of antiepileptic drugs in mice and rats. *Journal of Pharmacology and Experimental Therapeutics*, 106:319–330.

Takahashi, R., and Aprison, M. H. (1964): Acetylcholine content of discrete areas of the brain obtained by a near-freezing method. *Journal of Neurochemistry*, 11:887–898.

Tapia, R., Pérez de la Mora, M., and Massieu, G. H. (1969): Correlative changes of pyridoxal kinase, pyridoxal-5'-phosphate and glutamate decarboxylase in brain, during drug-induced convulsions. *Annals of the New York Academy of Sciences*, 166:257–266.

Tews, J. K., and Stone, W. E. (1964): Effects of methionine sulfoximine on levels of free amino acids and related substances in the brain. *Biochemical Pharmacology*, 13:543–545.

Tews, J. K., and Stone, W. E. (1965): Free amino acids and related compounds in brain and other tissues: Effects of convulsant drugs. *Progress in Brain Research*, 16:135–163.

Thompson, R. K., Smith, G. W., and Crosby, R. M. N. (1951): Head rest for experimental cranial surgery. *Journal of Neuropathology and Experimental Neurology*, 10:338–340.

Tower, D. B. (1958): Discussion. In: *Temporal Lobe Epilepsy*, edited by M. Baldwin and P. Bailey. Charles C Thomas, Springfield, Ill., pp. 288–295.

Tower, D. B. (1969): Neurochemical mechanisms. In: *Basic Mechanisms of the Epilepsies*, edited by H. H. Jasper, A. A. Ward, Jr., and A. Pope. Little, Brown & Co., Boston, pp. 611–638.

Truitt, E. B., Jr., Ebersberger, E. M., and Ling, A. S. C. (1960): Measurement of brain excitability by use of hexafluorodiethyl ether (Indoklon®). *Journal of Pharmacology and Experimental Therapeutics*, 129:445–453.

Tuttle, W. W., and Elliott, H. W. (1969): Electrographic and behavioral study of convulsants in the cat. *Anesthesiology*, 30:48–64.

Vanasupa, P., Goldring, S. and O'Leary, J. I. (1959): Seizure discharges effected by intravenously administered convulsant drugs. *Electroencephalography and Clinical Neurophysiology*, 11:93–106.

Van den Berg, C. J. (1970): Glutamate and glutamine. In: *Handbook of Neurochemistry*, Vol. 3, edited by A. Lajtha. Plenum Press, New York, pp. 355–379.

Van den Berg, C. J., and Van den Velden, J. (1970): The effect of methionine sulphoximine on the incorporation of labelled glucose, acetate, phenylalanine and proline into glutamate and related amino acids in the brains of mice. *Journal of Neurochemistry*, 17:985–991.

Vencs, J. L., Collins, W. F., and Taub, A. (1971): Nitrous oxide: An anesthetic for experiments in cats. *American Journal of Physiology*, 220:2028–2031.

Wallach, M. B., Winters, W. D., Mandell, A. J., and Spooner, C. E. (1969): A correlation of EEG, reticular multiple unit activity and gross behavior following various antidepressant agents in the cat. *Electroencephalography and Clinical Neurophysiology*, 27:563–573.

Waltregny, A. (1969): Epilepsy and insulinic hypoglycemia: An experimental study. In: *The Physiopathogenesis of the Epilepsies*, edited by H. Gastaut, H. Jasper, J. Bancaud, and A. Waltregny. Charles C Thomas, Springfield, Ill., pp. 111–124.

Wang, R. I. H., and Sonnenschein, R. R. (1955): pH of cerebral cortex during induced convulsions. *Journal of Neurophysiology*, 18:130–137.

Watterson, D. J. (1939): On the mechanisms of convulsive phenomena, with reference to the effects of vasodilator drugs. *Journal of Mental Science*, 85:904–924.

Werner, H. W., and Tatum, A. L. (1939): A comparative study of the stimulant analeptics picrotoxin, Metrazol® and Coramine®. *Journal of Pharmacology and Experimental Therapeutics*, 66:260–278.

Whistler, K. E., Tews, J. K., and Stone, W. E. (1968): Cerebral amino acids and lipids in drug-induced status epilepticus. *Journal of Neurochemistry*, 15:215–220.

Wiedeman, C. (1877): Beiträge zur Pharmakologie des Camphers. *Archiv für experimentelle Pathologie und Pharmakologie*, 6:216–232.

Winters, W. D., Mori, K., Wallach, M. B., Marcus, R. J., and Spooner, C. E. (1969): Reticular multiple unit activity during a progression of states induced by CNS excitants. *Electroencephalography and Clinical Neurophysiology*, 27:514–522.

Wood, J. D., and Abrahams, D. E. (1971): The comparative effects of various hydrazides on γ-aminobutyric acid and its metabolism. *Journal of Neurochemistry*, 18:1017–1025.

Wortis, S. B., Coombs, H. C., and Pike, F. H. (1931): Monobromated camphor, a standard convulsant. *Archives of Neurology and Psychiatry*, 26:156–161.

Ziskind, E., and Bolton, R. (1936): Insulin hypoglycemia in epilepsy. *Archives of Neurology and Psychiatry*, 36:331–341.

Zolliker, A. (1938): The insulin tolerance in epilepsy. *American Journal of Psychiatry*, 94:Suppl., 198–207.

17

Electrically Induced Convulsions

Ewart A. Swinyard

OUTLINE

I. INTRODUCTION

Although Fritsch and Hitzig (1870) first demonstrated electroshock seizures in animals in 1870, and Albertoni (1882) studied the effect of faradic stimulation of the cerebral cortex through the trephined skull in 1882, little was done with these procedures during the next 50 years. In 1922, Schilf adopted Jellinek's (1920) method of stimulation through corneal electrodes and measured seizure threshold for alternating current applied for 0.5 sec. In 1937, Spiegel also employed corneal electrodes but measured threshold in terms of both time and intensity, expressing threshold in ampere-seconds. Also in 1937, Putnam and Merritt applied rectangular pulses of direct current for 10 sec through skull and mouth electrodes in cats, as did Knoefel and Lehmann (1942). Kozelka and Hine (1940, 1943) employed alternating current of fixed strength; shock duration rather than current was varied in determination of seizure threshold. Bárány and Stein-Jensen (1946a,b) passed alternating current through electrodes placed in the auditory meatus and, in contrast to previous workers, observed the effects of drugs on seizure pattern as well as on seizure threshold.

These achievements stimulated a search for more sophisticated ways of inducing electroshock seizures in laboratory animals and resulted in the development of a number of novel laboratory models of epilepsy. In 1946, Goodman and co-workers initiated an intensive study of the "physiology and therapy of experimental convulsive disorders." These studies led not only to the development of four classical electrical models of experimental epilepsy (Toman et al., 1946; Swinyard, 1949a; Swinyard et al., 1952) but also to the design of an apparatus for the induction of electroshock seizures (Woodbury and Davenport, 1952). These studies also directed attention to the characteristics of maximal seizure pattern evoked by supramaximal electroshock stimulation (Toman et al., 1946). Since electroshock therapy for psychiatric patients had previously been introduced by Cerletti and Bini (1938) and other workers (Hemphill and Walter, 1941; Kalinowsky and Kennedy, 1943) had studied the effect of antiepileptic drugs on the *threshold* for such seizures, it was only logical to extend this work to include the characteristics and modification of *seizure pattern* in nonepileptic human patients undergoing electroshock therapy for psychiatric disorders (Toman et al., 1947). Subsequently, these basic electrical procedures, as shown in Table 1, were adapted to virtually every laboratory animal and man.

Numerous minor modifications in the parameters employed in these electrical procedures have been reported. These include the type of stimulator, stimulus frequency and duration, electrode implacement, and others.

TABLE 1. *Models for electrically induced convulsions*

Species	Seizure type	Major manifestations	Reference
Salamander	?	stiffening and quivering[a]	Peters and Vonderahe, 1956
Frog	?	stiffening and quivering[b]	Servit, 1959
Mouse	threshold	stun[c]	Swinyard et al., 1962
Mouse	threshold	clonus[d]	Swinyard et al., 1952
Mouse	threshold	tonic extension[d]	Swinyard et al., 1963
Mouse	maximal	tonic flexion and extension, clonus[d]	Swinyard et al., 1952
Rat	threshold	clonus[d]	Swinyard, 1949a
Rat	threshold	tonic extension[d]	Swinyard, 1971
Rat	maximal	tonic flexion and extension, clonus[d]	Toman et al., 1946
Hamster	threshold	clonus[c]	Orcutt and Prytherch, 1956
Rabbit	maximal	tonic flexion and extension, clonus[d]	Toman et al., 1946
Cat	maximal	tonic flexion and extension, clonus[d]	Toman et al., 1946
Sloth	maximal	tonic *extension* and *flexion*, clonus[d]	Esplin and Woodbury, 1961
Monkey	maximal	tonic flexion and extension, clonus[d]	Goodman et al., 1946
Man	maximal	tonic flexion and extension, clonus[f]	Toman et al., 1947

[a] Grass Stimulator: 300 Hz, 0.3 sec, needle electrodes.
[b] Stimulation: 50 Hz, 0.2 sec, mouth and head electrodes.
[c] Grass Stimulator: 6 Hz, 3 sec, ear-clip electrodes.
[d] Woodbury & Davenport Stimulator: 60 Hz, 0.2 sec, corneal electrodes.
[e] Variable-Voltage Trans: 60 Hz, buccal electrodes.
[f] Offner Stimulator: 60 Hz, 0.2 sec, corneal electrodes.

For the most part, such technical changes have contributed little either to improving the basic procedures or to the ultimate usefulness of the model. However, two modifications (Bogue and Carrington, 1953; Paalzow, 1969) have certain inherent advantages and will be described herein.

II. CHARACTERISTICS OF ELECTROSHOCK CONVULSIONS

A. Classification of seizures

It may be seen from Table 1 that electroshock seizures in laboratory animals may be classified on the basis of either seizure type or overt motor manifestations. In general, experimental electroshock seizures are either threshold or maximal. Threshold seizures may be induced in mice or rats by low-frequency electroshock stimulation (6 Hz-ES; unidirectional rectangular pulses 0.2 msec, 6 pulses/sec, applied through corneal electrodes for 3 sec), in mice, rats, and other laboratory animals by conventional 60-cycle alternating current (60 Hz-ES, applied through corneal electrodes for 0.2 sec), or in mice by high-frequency electroshock stimulation (800 Hz-ES,

0.6-msec pulse width, 400-msec stimulus duration). It should be noted that the latter two procedures can also be used to measure the *threshold* for tonic flexor and extensor (maximal) seizures. Maximal seizures are evoked in laboratory animals by supramaximal electroshock stimulation (60 Hz-ES, applied through corneal electrodes for 0.2 sec). The details of these procedures are provided in the Appendix.

Threshold seizures, irrespective of the exciting stimulus, are characterized by a stun reaction (catatonia) or by localized clonic movements of the vibrissae, face, ears, and, more commonly, forelimbs. Maximal seizures, irrespective of the exciting stimulus, are characterized by tonic flexion and extension followed by terminal clonus. It should be noted from Table 1 that the sloth contrasts markedly with this generalization. Maximal seizures in this species, as shown by Esplin and Woodbury (1961), are characterized by tonic *extension* and *flexion* followed by terminal clonus. The reverse sequence in the sloth validates the predictions that the terminal tonic phase represents the most powerful limb muscles; in the sloth the flexors, which serve an antigravity function, are more powerful than the extensor limb muscles — hence, the reverse tonic pattern. Thus, the principal overt motor manifestations of electroshock seizures are stun (catatonia), clonic movements, and various intensities and combinations of tonic flexion and extension.

B. Profile of electroshock seizures

The overt manifestations of electrically induced seizures in rats as a function of a stimulus intensity are shown in Fig. 1. This figure (a modification of the unpublished observations of D. W. Esplin and D. M. Woodbury; see Woodbury and Vernadakis, 1967) relates the degree of motor activity to the current intensity in milliamperes (mA). The solid thick line in the figure represents the overt manifestations at the different current strengths. The variously labeled thin lines represent the underlying neurological and physiological processes which take place in the brain as a result of stimulation. At low current values, the motor responses result from discharge of sensory pain receptors in the region of the stimulating electrodes. As the current is increased, hyperkinesia occurs as a result of a combination of maximal sensory discharge and low-intensity stimulation of the collection of neurons involved in minimal seizure discharge. (The latter has been defined by Toman and Taylor [1952] and others as the "oscillator.") At current intensities around 18 mA, a rage reaction is seen as a result of intense sensory discharge, increased discharge of neurons involved in minimal seizures, and involvement of other subcortical areas responsible for

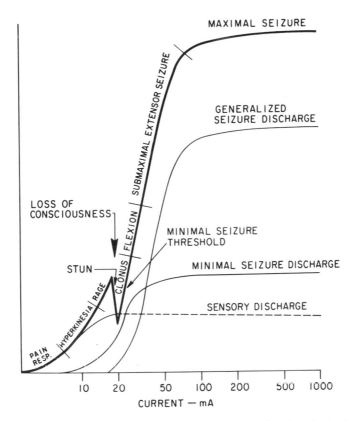

FIG. 1. Profile of experimentally induced seizures in rats as a function of stimulus intensity. See text for explanation. Modified from Woodbury and Vernadakis (1967) with permission of the publisher.

rage-type reactions. When the stimulating current is increased further, consciousness is lost and, although sensory discharge continues, sensation is lost, a stun reaction (catatonia) occurs, and motor activity is reduced. Stimulation with current values only slightly above this level evokes minimal seizure discharge which is characterized by clonic activity. Clonic activity which persists for a period of 5 sec is arbitrarily defined as the minimal electroshock seizure threshold (EST). The EST is a definite endpoint characterized by clonic activity of the vibrissae, face, and ears; it is easily identified, since a stun reaction appears only slightly below the threshold, and clonic activity of the forelimbs appears slightly above the stimulus intensity required to evoke this response. With stimulus intensities higher than threshold, the animal loses its balance, flexion of the hind limbs followed by clonus occurs as a result of intense stimulation of the collection of neurons responsible for seizure discharge, and there is generalized spread of the seizure activity to involve other networks and parts of the brain (as illustrated in Fig. 1 on the curve labeled "Generalized Seizure Discharge").

At still higher current intensities, maximal seizures occur; these are characterized by maximal tonic flexion and extension, followed by clonic activity. The maximal seizure represents maximal discharge of the entire cerebrospinal axis.

C. Spinal cord convulsions

The studies of Esplin and co-workers (Esplin and Laffan, 1957; Esplin and Freston, 1960; Vernadakis, 1962) on the direct stimulation of the cervical spinal cord have contributed greatly to the understanding of seizure mechanisms and of the relative role of the spinal cord and supraspinal sites in this phenomenon. As shown in Fig. 2, these workers studied the effect

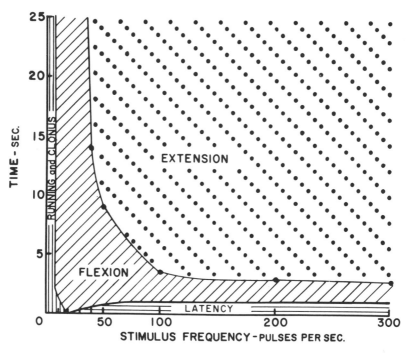

FIG. 2. Hindlimb motor responses to cervical spinal cord stimulation in the cat. Square-wave stimuli, 1 msec in width and 30 V intensity. Ordinate indicates the time in seconds from the beginning of stimulation. Stimulation is continuous at the indicated frequency. From Esplin (1959) with permission of the publisher.

of stimulus frequency on the profile of experimental seizures in cats. It can be seen from this figure that at low frequencies (less than about 10/sec) only running movements and clonus are produced. At intermediate frequencies (10 to 50/sec), the hindlimbs are maintained in tonic flexion. At still higher frequencies (above 50/sec), the pattern in the hindlimbs has all the components seen in a maximal electroshock, or grand mal, convulsion, namely, a latent period, tonic flexion, and tonic extension. This and other evidence suggests that the spinal cord serves as a conduction pathway for impulses generated at the supraspinal level and that seizure type is determined largely by the extent of brain discharge and the frequency of the impulses coming from supraspinal levels.

D. Stimulus intensity (6 Hz-ES and 60 Hz-ES) and seizure type

Seizures evoked by low-frequency electroshock stimulation (6 Hz-ES) or by conventional 60-cycle alternating current (60 Hz-ES) are remarkably similar qualitatively, but differ markedly in the stimulus intensity required to evoke a particular type of seizure. The relation between stimulus intensity and seizure type induced by 6 Hz-ES and 60 Hz-ES in mice is shown in Table 2. It may be seen that 7.2 mA is required to elicit a stun response

Table 2. *The relation of stimulus intensity and seizure type by the 6 Hz-EST and 60 Hz-EST in mice*

Endpoint	CV50 6 Hz-EST (V)	CC50 60 Hz-EST (mA)
Stun	23.0 (21.3–24.8)	7.2 (6.9–7.6)
Clonus	136 (128–144)	7.7 (7.3–8.1)
Hindleg tonic-ext.	>150	10.4 (9.7–10.8)

with 60 Hz-ES and that 23 V is required to elicit the same response with 6 Hz-ES. A 60 Hz-ES stimulus intensity 10 and 45% above that required for a stun response results in a threshold clonic seizure and a hindlimb tonic extensor seizure, respectively. In marked contrast, it requires a 6 Hz-ES stimulus intensity 5.9 times and greater than 7.0 times that required to evoke a stun response to produce a threshold clonic seizure and a tonic ex-

tensor seizure, respectively. Thus, 6 Hz-ES is preferred for definitive threshold studies, whereas 60 Hz-ES is preferred for studies on maximal seizure pattern.

E. Seizure threshold and extent of neuronal discharges

In view of the above, it is interesting to correlate the seizure threshold, as determined by the 6 Hz-ES, 60 Hz-ES, and 60 Hz-MES techniques, with the extent of neuronal discharge. In minimal seizures evoked by 6 Hz-ES, the collection of neurons responsible for minimal seizure discharge is excited with maximum efficiency, but the discharge spreads very little to adjacent areas and maximal spread is never obtained. Indeed, the current intensity employed in this technique may be increased several-fold without change in seizure pattern (Toman, 1951; Tedeschi et al., 1956). Minimal seizures evoked by 60 Hz-ES are the result not only of a more intense discharge of neurons associated with minimal seizures, but also of some spread of the discharge to other areas of the brain. That seizure spread does occur is indicated by the rather limited range over which the current intensity may be increased and still evoke only a minimal clonic seizure and by the generalized seizure which occurs with only slightly higher stimulus intensities (see Table 2). With 60 Hz-MES, on the other hand, the collection of neurons responsible for minimal seizures discharges maximally, and the discharge spreads over the entire brain. The overt motor manifestations of such a generalized discharge of the brain is a maximal tonic-clonic seizure.

F. Postictal recovery

Laffan et al. (1957) have shown in rats that recovery time (RT_{50}) for rats shocked with 600 mA was 12.5 min, whereas for those shocked with 37.5 mA, the RT_{50} was 6.8 min. These workers also observed a linear decrease in the mean duration of hindleg tonic flexion and an increase in the mean duration of hindleg tonic extension as stimulus intensity was increased. Thus, flexor/extensor (F/E) ratio progressively decreased as the stimulus intensity increased. These observations indicate that in rats maximal seizure severity increases with increased stimulus intensity.

Tedeschi et al. (1956) determined the RT_{50} in mice for a "second" maximal seizure given after a "first" maximal. The RT_{50} and 95% confidence limits were 75 (65 to 86) sec. The order in which the durations of the various components of the "second" seizure returned to control values was as follows: total seizure duration, terminal clonus, tonic extension, and tonic flexion.

III. MATURATION OF THE CNS AND DEVELOPMENT OF ELECTROSHOCK SEIZURES

Since seizure disorders frequently have their onset in early childhood, it is important to have some insight into the maturation of the central nervous system and the development of electroshock seizures in laboratory animals. Such studies are also a prelude to the search for appropriate models for inducing abnormalities in structure and function associated with exquisite convulsant activity in immature and mature animals.

A. Development of threshold seizures

Several studies have contributed to an understanding of the developmental properties of seizure activity assessed by responses of the developing central nervous system to brain electroshock stimulation (Millichap, 1957; Castellion, 1964; Vernadakis and Woodbury, 1969) and to direct stimulation of the spinal cord (Vernadakis, 1962). The changes in threshold for 6 Hz-ES and 60 Hz-ES in mice as a function of increasing age, as reported by Vernadakis and Woodbury (1965), are shown in Fig. 3. The

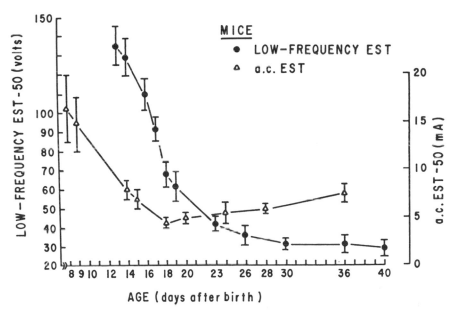

FIG. 3. Change in 6 Hz-ES threshold (low-frequency EST) and 60 Hz-ES threshold (a.c. EST) in mice during maturation. From Vernadakis and Woodbury (1965) with permission of the publisher.

threshold for 60 Hz-ES progressively and markedly decreased up to 18 days of age and slowly increased somewhat thereafter. The threshold for 6 Hz-ES decreased markedly up to 30 days and remained relatively constant thereafter. The progressive decrease in thresholds for both 6 Hz-ES and 60 Hz-ES has been interpreted by Vernadakis and Woodbury (1965) to indicate the development of those neurons responsible for minimal seizures and the discharge of more excitatory neuronal elements. At early postnatal periods, the 6 Hz-ES is high, probably because the neuronal elements responsible for minimal seizures have not fully matured and a self-sustained discharge cannot occur. With 60 Hz-ES stimulation, both the neuronal elements essential to a sustained minimal discharge and other developing excitatory and inhibitory systems are stimulated; hence, minimal seizures appear somewhat earlier. As maturation progresses, the discharge elicited by 60 Hz-ES stimulation spreads to other developing areas of the brain, and the 60 Hz-ES threshold decreases. Vernadakis and Woodbury (1965) suggest that the progressive decrease in the 60 Hz-ES threshold might represent a measure of the extent to which neuronal elements other than those associated with minimal seizures participate in the seizure discharge.

B. Development of maximal electroshock seizures

The effect of maturation on the development and reproducibility of electroshock seizure *pattern* in mice is shown in Fig. 4. These unpublished observations of Castellion (1964) indicate that on day 8 some symmetrical movements resembling clonic activity appeared; peak incidence (100%) occurred on day 12 and could no longer be elicited with supramaximal electroshock stimulation on day 20. All animals exhibited some type of seizure activity by day 15. Maximal seizures were first elicited on day 16 (63%) and reached peak incidence (100%) on day 20. Mice continued to respond to supramaximal electroshock stimulation with a maximal seizure throughout life.

These observations in intact animals contrast markedly with those reported by Vernadakis (1962) for spinal cord convulsions in developing rats. In these studies, tonic flexor-extensor seizures characteristic of adult animals were observed in rats as young as 1 day old. It would appear that the inability of intact rats and mice to exhibit a flexor-extensor convulsion before 16 to 21 days of age is due to lack of maturation of the brain rather than the spinal cord.

The development of excitatory and inhibitory pathways involves many factors, such as myelination and development of synaptic transmission.

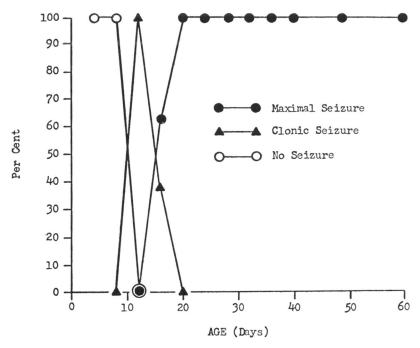

FIG. 4. The effect of maturation on the development of maximal electroshock seizures (60 Hz-MES) in mice (Castellion, 1964).

Since both seizure threshold and maximal seizure pattern first appear in normal intact mice 16 to 18 days after birth, these studies suggest brain maturation is virtually complete at this time. This is of particular interest since other reports indicate that brain cortex thickness (Sugita, 1918), packing density of the brain neurons (Haddara, 1956), and brain weight/body weight ratio (Kobayashi, 1963) are indistinguishable in 15- to 17-day-old mice and mature animals.

IV. CHOICE OF LABORATORY ANIMALS

Available data do not establish one laboratory animal species as superior to another for use as an electrical model of epilepsy. Nevertheless, each species has certain inherent advantages which will be mentioned at this point. Mice present certain advantages for the routine study of antiepileptic drugs. The cost of mice is considerably less than that of rats, as is also the cost of feeding and housing. Mice are preferred for use in the 6 Hz-ES threshold model, since the various endpoints, stun, and clonic activity, are easier to elicit in this species. Mice are also preferred for experimental procedures based on maximal electroshock seizure (60 Hz-MES) pattern. Mice invariably exhibit the full maximal seizure pattern when stimulated with a supramaximal electroshock, whereas about 10% of young rats and a higher percent of older rats may fail to do so. If the supply of a drug is limited, more data can be obtained in mice than rats. There is also a greater cumulation of postictal refractoriness in rats than in mice after repeated maximal electroshock stimulation. On the other hand, the rat is probably preferred for such studies as EEG recording and problems of fate and excretion. Also, rats are more suitable for critical electroshock threshold studies and long-range chronic studies. In addition, it is easier to detect discrete neurological changes or alterations in electrolyte distribution in the larger animal.

The specialized use of hamsters, rabbits, cats, sloths, and monkeys are more difficult to justify. The hamster offers no particular advantages, except it is possible to use buccal electrodes in this species. Rabbits and cats have been used extensively for studies involving EEG recordings simultaneously with electroshock convulsions. The former species is rather fragile; many animals exhibit fractured vertebrae after stimulation with supramaximal electroshock. For obvious reasons related to the safety of the investigator, cats and monkeys are usually employed for studies based only on maximal electroshock seizure pattern. The sloth, as mentioned previously, is unique in that its flexor muscles are most powerful, since it hangs upside-down from trees.

In general, the choice of animal depends on the kind of study contemplated and on the electrical model to be used.

V. APPLICATION OF ELECTROSHOCK SEIZURES TO RESEARCH

A. Factors which alter seizure susceptibility

There are a number of factors which affect the susceptibility and response of laboratory animals to experimentally induced seizures. If these variables are not rigidly controlled, they can compromise the results obtained with the laboratory models of epilepsy described herein. These factors have been summarized by Woodbury (1969) and are listed in Table 3. The various factors are shown in the column on the left, specific substances or procedures which increase seizure susceptibility in the middle column, and those which decrease seizure susceptibility in the column on the right. It can be seen that a variety of endocrine, gaseous, water, electrolyte, acid-base, nutritional, and temperature changes can alter susceptibility to seizures.

TABLE 3. *Factors that alter susceptibility to experimental seizures*

Factors	Increase	Decrease
Endocrine changes	cortisol thyroxine triiodothyronine estradiol insulin adrenalectomy pancreatectomy	deoxycorticosterone aldosterone progesterone testosterone growth hormone thyroidectomy hypophysectomy
Gases	hypoxia carbon dioxide (2nd phase) decreased pCO_2	hyperoxia carbon dioxide (1st and 3rd phase)
Water, electrolyte, and acid-base changes	hydration hypocalcemia hyperkalemia hyponatremia hypermagnesemia bicarbonate increase	dehydration hypercalcemia hypernatremia bicarbonate decrease
Nutritional changes	starvation pyridoxine deficiency	
Temperature	hypothermia	hyperthermia

Data from Woodbury (1969).

Factors other than those listed in Table 3 are known to alter the susceptibility of laboratory animals to seizures. For example, age and circadian and other types of rhythms alter seizure susceptibility. The ES threshold for electroshock seizures in rats normally varies as a result of daily (circadian) and hormonally induced rhythms. Woolley and Timiras (1962) have shown that ES threshold is significantly lower in the late evening and during estrus. These observations emphasize the importance of evoking seizures at the same time each day and using male animals when experimental conditions permit.

B. Application to research

The numerous factors which modify seizure susceptibility (see Table 3) provide adequate documentation of the useful application of these procedures to research. Laboratory models, such as the 6 Hz-ES and 60

Hz-ES threshold procedures, make it possible to determine the effect of virtually any biochemical, pharmacological, or physiological procedure on brain sensitivity. Indeed, their application to research is limited largely by the ingenuity of the investigator.

VI. SUMMARY

Electrical models of epilepsy have been adapted to virtually every laboratory animal and man. These evoked seizures may be classified on the basis of either seizure type or overt motor manifestations. Thus, seizures may be classified as threshold or maximal seizures. The profile of threshold seizures includes stun (catatonia) and/or minimal clonic activity. The profile of maximal seizures includes tonic flexion and extension followed by terminal clonus. The relation between these overt seizure manifestations and stimulus intensity has been reviewed. Attention has also been directed to spinal cord convulsions and the relative role of stimulus frequency on the profile of such seizures. These studies suggest that seizure type is largely determined by the extent of brain discharge and the frequency of impulses originating at supraspinal levels. Threshold convulsions are commonly evoked either by low-frequency electroshock (6 Hz-ES) or by 60-cycle electroshock (60 Hz-ES) stimulation. Seizures elicited by these techniques are qualitatively similar, but differ markedly with regard to stimulus intensity and the type of seizure evoked. Thus, 6 Hz-ES is preferred for precise mimimal threshold studies, whereas 60 Hz-ES is preferred for maximal seizure threshold and maximal seizure pattern studies.

Available evidence indicates that *6 Hz-ES threshold* correlates well with minimal neuronal discharge and with minimal spread to adjacent areas of the brain; *60 Hz-ES threshold* seizures result not only from minimal neuronal discharge but also from some spread of discharge to other areas of the brain; *supramaximal stimulation* with 60 Hz-ES current discharges the collection of neurons responsible for minimal seizures maximally, and the discharge spreads over the entire brain. Indeed, all neuronal circuits are nearly maximally active following this type of stimulation, which results in a maximal tonic-clonic seizure.

Postictal recovery (RT_{50}) was observed to be 12.5 min in rats and 75 sec in mice. Flexor/extensor (F/E) ratio was observed to provide a useful measure of maximal seizure severity.

Studies on the maturation of the CNS and the development of seizures indicate *threshold* for *60 Hz-ES* markedly decreased from birth to 18 days postnatally and slowly increased thereafter; the *threshold* for *6 Hz-ES* decreased markedly up to 30 days and then remained relatively constant. The marked initial decrease in 6 Hz-ES and 60 Hz-ES correlates with the development of neuronal elements necessary to sustain a minimal seizure discharge; the subsequent increase in 60 Hz-ES threshold probably represents maturation of other neuronal elements. Maturation and development studies in mice indicate that *maximal* seizures first appeared on day 16 and reached peak incidence at day 20. Since spinal cord convulsions can be elicited in 1-day-old animals, it would appear that the inability of the intact animal to sustain a seizure during the first 8 days of life is due to a lack of maturation of the brain elements rather than of the spinal cord.

Although available data do not indicate one laboratory animal to be superior to another as a model, data are presented which suggest that advantages and disadvantages attend the use of certain animals for specific electrical models. Attention was also directed to the numerous factors which modify electroshock seizure threshold and to the importance of controlling these factors insofar as possible. Finally, reference was made to the extensive application of electrical models to research on experimental epilepsy.

VII. APPENDIX

General methods

Adult male albino rats and adult male albino mice are usually employed as experimental animals, although the tests to be described may also be conducted in hamsters, guinea pigs, rabbits, cats, and monkeys. All animals are maintained on an adequate diet and allowed free access to food and water, except during the short time they are subjected to the experimental procedure. Spiegel (1937) corneal electrodes are used and the electrical stimulus delivered either by means of an apparatus similar to that designed by L. A. Woodbury (Woodbury and Davenport, 1952) or by means of a Grass Stimulator (Model S4B). The former apparatus is used for models in which 60-cycle alternating current (60 Hz-ES) is utilized. (The current delivered by this apparatus is independent of the external resistance.) The latter apparatus is used for models based on low-frequency (6 Hz-ES) and high-frequency (800 Hz-ES) electrical stimulation. In all electrically induced convulsions, the animal is restrained only by hand and released at the moment of stimulation in order to permit observation of the seizure throughout its entire course.

Special considerations

Starvation modifies maximal electroshock seizure pattern (shortens tonic flexion and prolongs tonic extension) and reduces the threshold for minimal electroshock seizures (Davenport and Davenport, 1948). Therefore, all animals are allowed free access to food and water except during the actual procedure. Animals newly received in the laboratory are allowed several days to correct for possible food and water restriction incurred during transit. Male CF #1 mice and male Holtzman or Sprague-Dawley rats are preferred for electrically induced seizures, since these strains are easier to handle. Furthermore, the electroshock procedure is rarely lethal in CF #1 mice (Torchiana and Stone, 1959). For accurate evaluations, all laboratory animals used in these tests should be of the same sex and be approximately the same age and weight (Woolley et al., 1961). Approximately 10% of young rats fail to give a full maximal seizure; this incidence is higher in older rats and in animals which struggle during electrode placement. Rats exhibiting excessive struggle are discarded. New rats are not used as laboratory models of epilepsy until they have had a series of three or four control supramaximal electroshocks at 24-hr intervals to establish seizure pattern. A drop of 0.9% sodium chloride solution is applied routinely to the eyes of each mouse prior to the application of the corneal electrodes; a drop of local anesthetic solution is applied to the eyes of all other laboratory animals. This not only assures adequate electrode contact, but in mice it reduces almost to zero the incidence of fatalities resulting from electroshock seizures. If this precaution is not taken, a majority of mice will fail to resume breathing after termination of the maximal seizure, the reason probably being that, in the absence of electrolyte solution, current spread to the medulla is such that severe postictal and often lethal respiratory depression occurs. Nevertheless, some animals may require artificial respiration in order to survive.

In the determination of *threshold* for minimal or maximal electroshock seizures, mice and rats are given single shocks at intervals of not less than 24 hr until the threshold is stabilized and does not vary more than 3% (0.25 mA in mice; 0.5 mA in rats) for three successive determinations; more frequent shocks may elevate threshold and thus render subsequent test data impossible to interpret (Woodbury and Davenport, 1952; Brown et al., 1953). Repetitive electroshock stimulation in cats also induces a tolerance-like increase in electroshock seizure threshold (Essig, 1969). For definitive threshold studies, long, flexible electrodes are recommended so that the animal can be returned to its home environment for approximately 30 sec prior to stimulation, since restraint itself significantly lowers minimal seizure threshold (Swinyard et al., 1962).

Electroshock procedures

The usual laboratory models employed may be divided into two categories: seizure threshold models and maximal seizure pattern models.

Seizure threshold models

Minimal electroshock seizure threshold (60 Hz-EST) model

The details of inducing these seizures, as performed with electroshock apparatus designed by Woodbury and Davenport (1952), have been described (Swinyard, 1949a; Swinyard et al., 1952; Brown et al., 1953). Initial (control) electroshock threshold is determined by giving individual animals shocks of 0.2-sec stimulus duration at intervals of 24 hr, with small increments or decrements in current intensity until the minimal seizure threshold has been established. A minimal seizure consists of 7 to 12 sec of clonic activity of the vibrissae, lower jaw, or forelimbs, without loss of posture. With this criterion, the current required to elicit these seizures varies from 6 to 9 mA in adult mice (Swinyard et al., 1952; Brown et al., 1953) and 20 to 26 mA in rats (Swinyard, 1949a). The threshold current is quite constant for each individual animal. For group studies, the minimal current required to elicit seizures in 50% of animals (convulsive-current fifty; CC_{50}) may be determined by use of the "staircase" procedure described by Finney (1952), in which the stimulus intensity for the next animal is determined by the response of the animal just tested. Thus, stimulus intensity is increased to the next higher increment if the previous animal failed to exhibit a seizure and to the next lower increment if the animal exhibits a seizure. With this procedure, the CC_{50} can either be estimated for a single group of animals on one day and the experimental procedures initiated 24 hr later, or, by using two groups of animals (test group and control group), the entire procedure can be completed the same day. The individual threshold of the treated animals is redetermined and the percentage increase or decrease in threshold induced by a given procedure is calculated. When groups of animals are employed, the CC_{50} of the control group and that of the experimental group are determined and the percent increase or decrease in the CC_{50} calculated. Although the elapsed time necessary before a second threshold seizure can be evoked at the same current intensity in 50% of mice is relatively short (7.5 min with 95% fiducial limits of 6.5 to 8.6 min), for precise studies the electroshock stimulus should not be repeated more frequently than every 24 hr.

Minimal electroshock seizure threshold (6 Hz-EST) model

6 Hz-EST seizures, originally described as psychomotor seizures (Toman, 1951; Toman et al., 1952) and as low frequency electroshock seizures (Swinyard et al., 1962), are induced in mice with unidirectional rectangular pulses of 0.2-msec duration delivered through corneal electrodes for 3 sec at a frequency of 6 pulses per sec. The Grass Stimulator (Model S4B) is commonly utilized for this test (Swinyard et al., 1957, 1962). The resulting seizure is characterized by the following overt manifestations: the mouse is stunned; the posture is awkward but upright; the forelimbs are crossed and the hindlimbs spread apart; the tail is vertical; and the

movements of the face and forelimbs resemble automatisms. Seizure duration varies from 10 to 75 sec and, at the end of the seizure, the animal rather suddenly resumes normal locomotion and normal exploratory activity. The minimal stimulus required to elicit such a seizure is 23 V (21.3 to 24.8). When the 6 Hz-EST model is used to measure a biological phenomenon, the minimal voltage required to elicit the above-described seizure in individual animals or groups of mice is first determined as described above. The mice are allowed 24 hr for full recovery, and then subjected to the specific procedure and the threshold redetermined. The percentage increase or decrease in individual or group seizure threshold can then be calculated.

Hyponatremic electroshock seizure threshold (60 Hz-HEST) model

The phenomenon of water intoxication has received considerable attention since the studies by Rowntree (1926) on the effects in mammals of the administration of excessive quantities of water. In particular, the role of water and electrolyte metabolism in clinical epilepsy has been extensively investigated. Stimulated by these investigations, Swinyard and co-workers (1946) reported on a systematic study of the influence of alterations in the internal environment (induced by the oral administration of water and by the intraperitoneal injection of isosmolar glucose) on the threshold for convulsive seizures in laboratory animals. These workers reported that depletion of 40% of the extracellular electrolyte by the intraperitoneal injection of isosmolar glucose lowered electroshock 60 Hz-ES seizure threshold by 56%. A similar reduction in the concentration of extracellular electrolyte by orally administered water lowered threshold to an equal extent. Combination of these two methods resulted in an even greater reduction in 60 Hz-EST, and spontaneous seizures were observed in some animals. Since some clinically effective antiepileptic drugs, such as diphenylhydantoin, cannot raise the electroshock seizure threshold in normal animals but can significantly elevate the threshold lowered by the removal of extracellular electrolyte, Swinyard et al. (1946) recommended that this model be used for the evaluation of anticonvulsant drugs. Subsequently, the *hyponatremic electroshock seizure threshold (60 Hz-HEST) model* was included in the battery of tests employed by these workers (Swinyard, 1949a; Swinyard et al., 1952).

This procedure may be performed in either mice or rats. The control minimal electroshock seizure threshold for *individual* animals is first determined as previously described. Each animal is then injected intraperitoneally with a 5.5% glucose solution (10 ml/100 g body weight). The maximal hyponatremic state is reached in mice and rats 2 and 4 hr, respectively, after glucose administration, at which time extracellular electrolyte concentration is reduced approximately 20% (Swinyard, 1949b) and electroshock seizure threshold reduced approximately 55% (Swinyard, 1949b; Brown et al., 1953). To determine the effectiveness of various procedures in elevating this experimentally lowered threshold the minimal electroshock seizure threshold is redetermined, and the percentage change in threshold is calculated. Other details are the same as those described for the minimal seizure model.

Maximal seizure threshold (60 Hz-MEST) model

The threshold for maximal seizure threshold is determined in precisely the same way as the threshold for minimal seizures, except that either hindleg tonic flexion or hindleg tonic extension is used as the endpoint. This model is of particular value for studying the effect of biological procedures on the spread of seizure discharge.

Maximal seizure pattern model

Maximal electroshock seizure pattern (60Hz-MES) model

Maximal electroshock seizures are elicited with a current intensity five to seven times that necessary for minimal electroshock seizures: 50 mA, mice; 150 mA, rats; 300 mA, rabbits; 400 mA, cats (Toman et al., 1946). Corneal electrodes are usually employed and the current delivered for 0.2 sec. It should be remembered, however, that approximately 10% of rats (Swinyard et al., 1952) and 30% of cats (Toman et al., 1946) fail to exhibit a tonic hindlimb extensor component with this procedure. In mice the maximal seizure consists of 1.6 sec of latency and initial tonic flexion, 13.2 sec of hindleg tonic extension, and 7.6 sec of terminal clonus. The total duration of the seizure is 22.3 sec (Swinyard et al., 1963). The patterns of maximal seizures, irrespective of how they are induced, are remarkably similar, except for time scales. The average elapsed time from stimulation to the end of the tonic phase is 14 sec in rats, 19 sec in rabbits, and 15 sec in cats (Toman et al., 1946), and 36 sec in man (Toman et al., 1947). This model is useful for evaluating the effect of biological procedures either on seizure spread or on seizure severity. For the former, alterations in the pattern of the seizure are noted and compared with control values. For the latter, the F/E ratio provides a reliable measure.

Maximal electroshock seizures can also be induced by the technique of continuous brain stimulation with low current intensity, as originally described by Bogue and Carrington (1953). Current intensities of 7.5 to 30 mA, depending on the animal employed, are usually sufficient. A timing switch is inserted in the circuit of the stimulator employed and the time in seconds to the onset of a maximal seizure measured. The results obtained may then be expressed in seconds or in milliampere seconds (millicoulombs). Zablocka and Esplin (1964) have shown that rats which respond to the conventional 60 Hz-MES test with only a tonic hindlimb *flexor* component invariably exhibit a tonic hindlimb *extensor* component with this procedure. Thus, this technique eliminates the necessity for pretesting rats and cats for the ability to exhibit a maximal tonic hindlimb extensor seizure in response to electrical stimulation.

Combined maximal seizure pattern and threshold (800 Hz-MES) model

Paalzow (1969) recommends a high-frequency electrical model in mice which involves both pattern and threshold. Electrical stimulation is induced with two Grass Stimulators (S4), coupled in train to deliver electrical square waves of 800 pulses/

sec, pulse width of 0.6 msec, and delivered for 400 msec via temporal needle electrodes. Tonic extension of the hindlimbs is taken as the endpoint. After determination of the individual 800 Hz-MES threshold for a tonic extensor seizure in two preliminary tests, the animals are given repeated shocks at 15- or 30-min intervals at a voltage 20% above that of the control threshold; abolition of the tonic hindleg extensor component is taken as the endpoint. Paalzow reports this technique can be repeated every 15 min and can be used to follow the duration of action of anticonvulsant drugs in individual animals.

Spinal cord convulsions. Direct stimulation of the spinal cord duplicates all the motor patterns seen during generalized motor seizure activity in the intact animal (Esplin and Laffan, 1957). The technique of direct spinal cord stimulation was first described by Esplin and Freston (1960) and modified for younger animals by Vernadakis (1962). The stimulating electrode is a stainless steel wire or 26-gauge needle insulated except for the portion in contact with the spinal cord. Animals are decapitated at the cervical region, and the noninsulated portion is inserted into the cord from C_1 to C_4. The cord electrode is the cathode; the anode is attached to surrounding tissues. Square-wave stimuli are delivered by a Grass Stimulator. Maximal stimulus parameters, in terms of the intensity, are 1 to 2 msec and 30 to 50 V. With maximal parameters, the entire cord is stimulated and both hindlimbs move in synchrony even if the electrode is placed along one side of the cord. Simple motor sequences, such as flexor-extensor convulsions, are timed. With supramaximal stimulation of the spinal cord, various responses, namely, phasic movements, flexion, and flexion followed by extension, are observed as a function of stimulus frequency. This model is of particular value for studies intended to determine the relative contribution of supraspinal and spinal functions in laboratory models.

Statistical analysis

The electrical models described are either based on electroshock seizure pattern or electroshock seizure threshold. Examples will be given herein for the statistical analysis of data obtained by use of representative models of each type.

When the *maximal electroshock seizure pattern (60 Hz-MES) model* is used to evaluate candidate antiepileptic drugs, groups of 8 to 10 animals are given various doses of the drug to be tested and stimulated with a supramaximal electroshock at the previously determined time of peak drug effect and the presence or absence of a full hindleg tonic extensor component noted for each animal. Some investigators (Toman et al., 1952) have used abolition of the entire tonic phase as the endpoint. This procedure is repeated with different groups of animals and various doses of the drug until at least three points are established between the dose which abolishes the hindlimb tonic extensor component in all the animals and that which does not abolish the tonic extensor component in any of the animals. The data obtained are then plotted on logarithmic probability paper (No. 3228, Codex Book Co., Inc., Norwood, Mass.) and a straight line visually fitted to the plotted points. The dose of drug required to abolish the hindleg tonic extensor component in 50% of animals

(ED_{50}) and 95% fiducial limits are then calculated by the method of Litchfield and Wilcoxon (1949).

The effect of drugs and other procedures on seizure severity may also be determined by the 60 Hz-MES model. Sixteen to 20 animals are randomly divided into two groups: one group is subjected to the experimental procedure and the other group serves as a control. Both groups are then given a supramaximal electroshock and the durations of the hindleg tonic flexor and extensor components recorded for each group. The average duration for the flexor and for the extensor components are calculated and the extensor flexor ratio (E/F ratio) determined for each group. An E/F ratio of the test group smaller than that of the control group indicates the seizures of the test group are less severe. Conversely, an E/F ratio larger than that for the control group indicates the seizures in the test group are more severe.

When the 60 Hz-MES model is elicited by the Bogue and Carrington (1953) technique, body weight and the stimulus time to induce a maximal seizure are recorded for each animal, and the data obtained for experimental and control groups are evaluated by the analysis of co-variance (Finney, 1952).

When *threshold* models are employed, the effect of drugs and other procedures on threshold may be determined either in individual animals or in groups of animals. For definitive studies, the individual threshold of each animal is determined over a period of several days, during which time the animal is stimulated with various current intensities until the threshold can be accurately estimated. Twenty-four hours later, the animals are subjected to the experimental procedure and the threshold redetermined. The average increase or decrease in threshold and standard error can then be calculated. Alternatively, each animal can be stimulated with a current intensity a fixed percent above or below the determined threshold and the presence or absence of a seizure recorded. The data are then analyzed as described under the 60 Hz-MES model. For group studies, 24 to 30 animals are tested by the "staircase" procedure (see Finney, 1952) and the data are plotted on logarithmic probability paper, a line fitted to the plotted points, and the convulsive current fifty (CC_{50}) or convulsive voltage fifty (CV_{50}) calculated (see example, Table 4 and Fig. 5). Twenty-four hours later, the animals are subjected to the experimental procedure and the group threshold (CC_{50} or CV_{50}), and the 95% fiducial limits are calculated. Alternatively, the above procedure can be completed in one day by using two groups of 24 to 30 animals (one control and one experimental) and calculating the CC_{50} or CV_{50} for each group as described above. The data obtained can then either be expressed as a percent change in threshold, or the procedure can be repeated daily to follow changes in threshold over a period of time.

Presented below is an example of the application of *the graphic method of Litchfield and Wilcoxon* (1949) to the estimation of the CV_{50} and the calculation of the 95% fiducial limits. Preliminary experiments indicated the CV_{50} and 95% fiducial limits for the group of 42 mice as determined by the 6 Hz-EST test were 17.4 V (16.1–18.8). Twenty-four hours later, all animals were given 200 mg/kg of phenaglycodol orally, and the CV_{50} for the group determined 60 min later by means of the 6 Hz-EST and the "staircase" procedure. The data obtained are shown in Table 4 and plotted in Fig. 5.

TABLE 4. *Protocol: Effect of phenaglycodol[a] on 6 Hz-ES threshold*

Volts	No. animals tested	No. seizures	Observed seizures (%)	Expected seizures[b] (%)	Observed Minus expected (absolute value)	Contributions to (Chi)^2 (obtained from nomograph 1)[c]
40	10	3	30	29	1	0.001
45	12	6	50	50	0	0.000
50	10	7	70	69	1	0.001
55	10	8	80	82.5	2.5	0.003
					Total	0.005

[a] 200 mg/kg orally.
[b] Determined from Fig. 5.
[c] Litchfield and Wilcoxon, 1949.

Calculation of CV$_{50}$ and 95% fiducial limits

Total number of animals = 42 (see Table 4)
Total number of groups (K) = 4
Total contributions to (Chi)^2 (A) = 0.005
Degrees of freedom (K-2) = 2
Animals/dose (B) = 10.5
(A×B) = 0.005×10.5 = 0.0525
Chi^2 for 2 degrees of freedom is 5.99 (Table II, Litchfield and Wilcoxon, 1949)
∴ Heterogeneity *is not* significant.
Number of animals whose *expected* effects are between 16 and 84%: (N) = 42
CV$_{84}$ = 55.5 (Determined from Fig. 5)
CV$_{50}$ = 45.0 (Determined from Fig. 5)
CV$_{16}$ = 36.5 (Determined from Fig. 5)

$$\text{Slope function} = \frac{CV_{84}/CV_{50} + CV_{50}/CV_{16}}{2} = \frac{55.5/45.0 + 45.0/36.5}{2} = 1.23$$

fCV$_{50}$ = 1.23$^{(2.77/\sqrt{N})}$, where N is the number of animals whose *expected* effects are between 16 and 84%
$$= 1.23^{(2.77/\sqrt{42})} = 1.23^{(0.43)} = 1.10$$

Fiducial limits: lower, 45.0 ÷ 1.10 = 40.9
                   upper, 45.0 × 1.10 = 49.5
CV$_{50}$ = 45.0 (40.9–49.5)

Calculation of EST ratio (threshold drug group/threshold control group)

(1) CV$_{50}$ of control group = 17.4 V
(2) fCV$_{50}$ of control group = 1.08

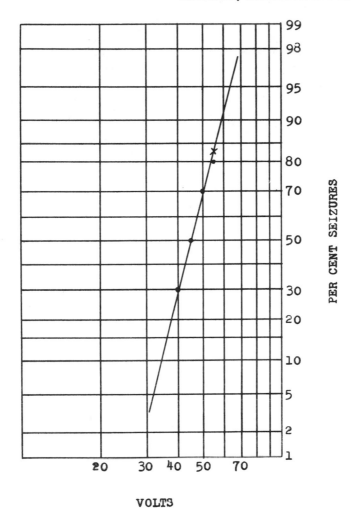

FIG. 5. Observed percent of animals which exhibited seizures plotted on logarithmic probability paper (only one-half sheet shown) against the voltage employed. The "x" indicates the expected percent for 55 V. See text for explanation.

(3) CV_{50} of drug treated group = 45.0 V

(4) fCV_{50} of drug treated group = 1.10

(5) EST ratio = CV_{50} drug group/CV_{50} control group = 45.0/17.4 = 2.59

(6) fEST ratio = 1.16 (obtained from nomograph No. 4, Litchfield and Wilcoxon, 1949) with the use of (2) and (3) above

(7) The 95% fiducial limits for the EST ratio are obtained by first dividing and then by multiplying the ratio by the fEST as follows:

Lower limit = EST ratio/fEST ratio = 2.59/1.16 = 2.23
Upper limit = EST ratio × fEST ratio = 2.59 × 1.16 = 3.00
Thus, the EST ratio and 95% fiducial limits = 2.59 (2.23–3.00).

Interpretation. The above calculations indicate that the CV_{50} and 95% fiducial limits for the control group and the phenaglycodol group are 17.4 (16.1 to 18.8) and 45.0 (40.9 to 49.5) V, respectively, and that phenaglycodol increased the EST 2.59 (2.23 to 3.00) times. Since the EST ratio (2.59) exceeds the factor of the ratio (1.16), the increase in threshold induced by phenaglycodol is significant.

VIII. REFERENCES

Albertoni, P. (1882): Untersuchung über die Wirkung einiger Arzneimittel auf die Erregbarkeit des Grosshirns nebst Beiträgen zur Therapie der Epilepsie. *Archiv für experimentelle Pathologie und Pharmacologie*, 15:248–288.

Bárány, E. H., and Stein-Jensen, Erna. (1946*a*): The mode of action of anticonvulsant drugs on electrically induced convulsions in the rabbit. *Archives Internationales de Pharmacodynamie et de Thérapie*, 73:1–47.

Bárány, E. H., and Stein-Jensen, Erna. (1946*b*): The action of di-allyl-barbituric acid on the electrically induced epileptic fit. *Acta Pharmacologica et Toxicologica*, 2:264–267.

Bogue, J. Y., and Carrington, H. C. (1953): The evaluation of Mysoline – A new anticonvulsant drug. *British Journal of Pharmacology and Chemotherapy*, 8:230–236.

Brown, W. C., Schiffman, D. O., Swinyard, E. A., and Goodman, L. S. (1953): Comparative assay of antiepileptic drugs by "psychomotor" seizure test and minimal electroshock threshold test. *Journal of Pharmacology and Experimental Therapeutics*, 107:273–283.

Castellion, A. W. (1964): Some neurophysiological and neurochemical characteristics of audiogenic-seizure-susceptible mice. Ph.D. Thesis, University of Utah.

Cerletti, U., and Bini, L. (1938): L'elettroshock. *Archivio di Psicologia, Neurologia e Psichiatria*, 19:266–268.

Davenport, V. D., and Davenport, H. W. (1948): The relation between starvation, metabolic acidosis and convulsive seizures in rats. *Journal of Nutrition*, 36:139–151.

Esplin, D. W., and Freston, J. W. (1960): Physiological and pharmacological analysis of spinal cord convulsions. *Journal of Pharmacology and Experimental Therapeutics*, 130:68–80.

Esplin, D. W., and Laffan, R. J. (1957): Determinants of flexor and extensor components of maximal seizures in cats. *Archives Internationales de Pharmacodynamie et de Thérapie*, 113:189–202.

Esplin, D. W., and Woodbury, D. M. (1961): Spinal reflexes and seizure patterns in the two-toed sloth. *Science*, 133:1426–1427.

Essig, C. F. (1969): Frequency of repeated electroconvulsions and the acquisition rate of a tolerance-like response. *Experimental Neurology*, 25:571–574.

Finney, D. J. (1952): *Probit Analysis*. Cambridge University Press, Cambridge.

Fritsch, G., and Hitzig, E. (1870): Ueber die elecktrische Erregbarkeit des Grosshirns. *Archiv für Anatomie und Physiologie wissenschaftlichen Medizin*, 37:300.

Goodman, L. S., Swinyard, E. A., and Toman, J. E. P. (1946): Studies on the anticonvulsant properties of diphenylhydantoin. *Federation Proceedings*, 5:180.

Haddara, M. (1956): A quantitative study of the postnatal changes in the packing density of the neurons in the visual cortex of the mouse. *Journal of Anatomy*, 90:494–501.

Hemphill, R. E., and Walter, W. G. (1941): Epanutin and electric convulsion therapy. *Lancet*, 240:446–448.

Jellinek, S. (1920): Electropathologic studies on direct current and alternating current; inference from type of excitation in experimental animal as to kind of current used; contribution to experimental epilepsy. *Medizinische Klinik*, 16:1128.

Kalinowsky, L. B., and Kennedy, F. (1943): Observations in electric shock therapy applied to problems of epilepsy. *Journal of Nervous and Mental Disease*, 98:56–67.

Knoefel, P. K., and Lehmann, G. (1942): The anticonvulsant action of diphenylhydantoin and some related compounds. *Journal of Pharmacology and Experimental Therapeutics*, 76:194–201.

Kobayashi, T. (1963): Brain-to-body ratios and time of maturation of the mouse brain. *American Journal of Physiology*, 204:343–346.

Kozelka, F. L., and Hine, C. H. (1940): Distribution, rate of disappearance, and excretion of Dilantin® (sodium salt of 5,5-diphenyl-hydantoin). *Journal of Pharmacology and Experimental Therapeutics*, 69:292.

Kozelka, F. L., and Hine, C. H. (1943): Degradation products of Dilantin®. *Journal of Pharmacology and Experimental Therapeutics*, 77:175–179.

Laffan, R. L., Swinyard, E. A., and Goodman, L. S. (1957): Stimulus intensity, maximal electroshock seizures, and potency of anticonvulsants in rats. *Archives Internationales de Pharmacodynamie et de Thérapie*, 111:60–69.

Litchfield, J. T., Jr., and Wilcoxon, F. (1949): A simplified method of evaluating dose-effect experiments. *Journal of Pharmacology and Experimental Therapeutics*, 96:99–113.

Millichap, J. G. (1957): Development of seizure patterns in newborn animals. Significance of brain carbonic anhydrase. *Proceedings of the Society for Experimental Biology and Medicine*, 96:125–129.

Orcutt, J. A., and Prytherch, J. P. (1956): Anticonvulsant assays utilizing electroshock induced via buccal electrodes in hamsters. *Archives Internationales de Pharmacodynamie et de Thérapie*, 106:60–67.

Paalzow, L. (1969): An electrical method for estimation of anticonvulsant in mice. Part I. Methodological investigations. *Acta Pharmaceutica Suecica*, 6:163–176. Part II. Application of the method in investigations of some anticonvulsant drugs. *Acta Pharmaceutica Suecica*, 6:177–192.

Peters, J. J., and Vonderahe, A. R. (1956): Localization and threshold studies of electrically induced seizures in the salamander. *Journal of Comparative Neurology*, 104:273–283.

Putnam, T. J., and Merritt, H. H. (1937): Experimental determination of the anticonvulsant properties of some phenyl derivatives. *Science*, 85:525–526.

Rowntree, L. G. (1926): Effects on mammals of administration of excessive quantities of water. *Journal of Pharmacology*, 29:135–159.

Schilf, E. (1922): Ueber experimentelle Erzeugung epileptischer Anfaelle durch dosierte starkstomenergie. Einfluss von Massnahmen pharmakologischer, chirurgischer und serologischer Art auf die kuenstliche erzeugte Epilepsie. *Zeitschrift fur die Gesamte experimentelle Medizin einschliesslich experimentelle Chirurgie*, 28:127.

Servit, Z. (1959): Contribution to the comparative pharmacology of antiepileptic drugs. Analysis of the action of some antiepileptic drugs on the seizures evoked by localized electroshock in the frog. *Ceskoslovenska Fysiologie*, 8:458–459.

Spiegel, E. A. (1937): Quantitative determination of the convulsive reactivity by electrical stimulation of the brain with the skull intact. *Journal of Laboratory and Clinical Medicine*, 22:1274–1276.

Sugita, N. (1918): Comparative studies on the growth of the cerebral cortex. VIII. General review of data for the thickness of the cerebral cortex and the size of the cortical cells in several mammals, together with some postnatal growth changes in these structures. *Journal of Comparative Neurology*, 29:241–278.

Swinyard, E. A. (1949a): Laboratory assay of clinically effective antiepileptic drugs. *Journal of the American Pharmaceutical Association*, 38:201–204.

Swinyard, E. A. (1949b): Effect of extracellular electrolyte depletion on brain electrolyte pattern and electroshock seizure threshold. *American Journal of Physiology*, 156:163–169.

Swinyard, E. A., Brown, W. C., and Goodman, L. S. (1952): Comparative assays of antiepileptic drugs in mice and rats. *Journal of Pharmacology and Experimental Therapeutics,* 106:319–330.

Swinyard, E. A., Castellion, A. W., Fink, G. B., and Goodman, L. S. (1963): Some neurophysiological and neuropharmacological characteristics of audiogenic-seizure-susceptible mice. *Journal of Pharmacology and Experimental Therapeutics,* 140:375–384.

Swinyard, E. A., Chin, L., Cole, F. R., and Goodman, L. S. (1957): Anticonvulsant properties of L-glutamine and L-asparagine in mice and rats. *Proceedings of the Society for Experimental Biology and Medicine,* 94:12–15.

Swinyard, E. A., Radhakrishnan, N., and Goodman, L. S. (1962): Effect of brief restraint on the convulsive threshold of mice. *Journal of Pharmacology and Experimental Therapeutics,* 138:337–342.

Swinyard, E. A., Toman, J. E. P., and Goodman, L. S. (1946): The effect of cellular hydration on experimental electroshock convulsions. *Journal of Neurophysiology,* 9:47–54.

Tedeschi, D. H., Swinyard, E. A., and Goodman, L. S. (1956): Effects of variations in stimulus intensity on maximal electroshock seizure pattern, recovery time, and anticonvulsant potency of phenobarbital in mice. *Journal of Pharmacology and Experimental Therapeutics,* 116:107–113.

Toman, J. E. P. (1951): Neuropharmacologic considerations in psychic seizures. *Neurology,* 1:444–460.

Toman, J. E. P., Everett, G. M., and Richards, R. K. (1952): The search for new drugs against epilepsy. *Texas Reports on Biology and Medicine,* 10:96–104.

Toman, J. E. P., Loewe, S., and Goodman, L. S. (1947): Physiology and therapy of convulsive disorders. I. Effect of anticonvulsant drugs on electroshock seizures in man. *Archives of Neurology and Psychiatry,* 58:312–324.

Toman, J. E. P., Swinyard, E. A., and Goodman, L. S. (1946): Properties of maximal seizures and their alteration by anticonvulsant drugs and other agents. *Journal of Neurophysiology,* 9:231–240.

Toman, J. E. P., and Taylor, J. D. (1952): Mechanism of action and metabolism of anticonvulsants. *Epilepsia,* 1:31–48.

Torchiana, M. L., and Stone, C. A. (1959): Post-seizure mortality following electroshock convulsions in certain strains of mice. *Proceedings of the Society for Experimental Biology and Medicine,* 100:290–293.

Woodbury, D. M. (1969): Role of pharmacological factors in the evaluation of anticonvulsant drugs. *Epilepsia,* 10:121–144.

Woodbury, D. M., and Vernadakis, A. (1967): Influence of hormones on brain activity. *Neuroendocrinology,* 2:335–375.

Woodbury, L. A., and Davenport, V. D. (1952): Design and use of a new electroshock seizure apparatus, and analysis of factors altering seizure threshold and pattern. *Archives Internationales de Pharmacodynamie et de Thérapie,* 92:97–107.

Woolley, D. E., and Timiras, P. S. (1962): Estrous and circadian periodicity and electroshock convulsions in rats. *American Journal of Physiology,* 202:379–382.

Woolley, D. E., Timiris, P. S., Rosenzweig, M. R., Krech, D., and Bennett, E. L. (1961): Sex and strain differences in electroshock convulsions of the rat. *Nature,* 190:515–516.

Vernadakis, A. (1962): Spinal cord convulsions in developing rats. *Science,* 137:532.

Vernadakis, A., and Woodbury, D. M. (1965): Effects of diphenylhydantoin on electroshock seizure thresholds in developing rats. *Journal of Pharmacology and Experimental Therapeutics,* 148:144–150.

Vernadakis, A., and Woodbury, D. M. (1969): Maturational factors in development of seizures. In: *Basic Mechanisms of the Epilepsies,* edited by H. H. Jasper, A. A. Ward, and L. A. Pope. Little, Brown and Co., Boston, pp. 535–541.

Zablocka, B., and Esplin, D. W. (1964): Role of seizure spread in determining maximal convulsion pattern in rats. *Archives Internationales de Pharmacodynamie et de Thérapie,* 147:525–542.

18

Systemic Oxygen Derangements

J. D. Wood

OUTLINE

I. INTRODUCTION

Seizures can occur in various species, including man, when the environmental pO_2 levels are abnormally high (hyperoxia) or abnormally low (hypoxia, anoxia). The hypoxia- or anoxia-induced convulsions are associated with events closely preceding coma and death and are not always observed. Since this phenomenon therefore provides an unsuitable model for the study of seizures, it is dealt with here in a rather cursory manner. The emphasis of the chapter is placed on a description of the more controllable hyperbaric oxygen-induced seizures, together with a discussion of their suitability as a model for epilepsy.

II. HYPOXIA

For the sake of conciseness, the term hypoxia is used here to describe conditions with low oxygen levels including those where oxygen is absent. In view of the hazard to life associated with hypoxia-induced convulsions, studies on this phenomenon must be limited to animal experiments. Hypoxic conditions are established by placing the experimental animal in a decompression chamber and lowering the pressure (simulated altitude) or by exposing the animal at ambient pressure to pure nitrogen or to gas mixtures low in oxygen content. The former procedure, although requiring more elaborate equipment, is the method of choice since the intensity and duration of the hypoxic episode can be more precisely controlled (Luft and Noell, 1956).

The sensitivity of animals to hypoxia varies with age and species (Wood et al., 1968; Wood and Peesker, 1971). Although susceptibility to seizures was not included as a parameter in the above studies, it would seem wise to standardize the two variables — age and species — during any studies on hypoxia-induced seizures. Hypoxia-induced convulsions were first reported by Robert Boyle (1660), who observed seizures in a sparrow, a lark, a cat, and mice which had been exposed to abnormally low pressures of air in a decompression chamber. The simulated altitude required to induce seizures has not been well documented, but Russian workers are reported as having observed seizures in rats exposed to altitudes of 25,000 to 140,000 meters (Tower, 1969). In view of the results described below for gas mixtures of low oxygen content, the onset of seizures might be expected to occur at lesser simulated altitudes than those employed by the Russians, possibly as low as 10,000 meters. Passouant et al. (1967a,b) exposed cats to 4% oxygen at ambient pressure and observed hippocampal spike-and-wave discharges within a few minutes of the initiation of the hypoxic conditions. If pure nitrogen is used as the breathing mixture, the onset of seizures is extremely rapid. For example, adult mice convulse within 9.5 ± 0.5 sec (mean $\pm$ SE) after they are placed in a nitrogen atmosphere (Nelson and Mantz, 1971). The seizures consist of bursts of clonic movement which last for 11.0 ± 0.9 sec. Respiratory failure follows 8 sec later.

Excitation of the nervous system is also observed in animals recovering from an hypoxic episode (Gellhorn and Heymans, 1948; Passouant et al., 1967a,b). The latter workers exposed cats to 4% oxygen until the animals were in coma and all electrical activity in the brain had ceased. The cats were then revived by returning them to an air environment in conjunction with chest massage. During the recovery period, organized discharges arising in the hippocampus were observed.

Although severe hypoxia induces seizures, less drastic conditions may have an anticonvulsant action. Hypoxia prevents or delays seizures induced by pentylenetetrazol (Metrazol®) (Jasper and Erickson, 1941), semicarbazide (Baumel et al., 1969a), methionine sulfoximine (Baumel et al., 1969b), and isonicotinic acid hydrazide (Wood and Peesker, 1971).

The mechanisms responsible for the convulsant and anticonvulsant actions of hypoxia are poorly understood. Interference with oxidative metabolism and associated production of high-energy compounds necessary for the normal functioning of the nervous system has been reported (Gurdjian et al., 1949) and is an obvious candidate for consideration as a potential cause of the actions of hypoxia. On the other hand, hypoxia produces striking increases in brain levels of gamma-aminobutyric acid (GABA) (Lovell and Elliott, 1963; Wood et al., 1968), and the high concentrations of this putative inhibitory transmitter substance may be the source of the anticonvulsant action.

In conclusion, hypoxia-induced convulsions are difficult to reproduce in a precise manner except under the most severe conditions and therefore provide a rather poor model for the study of epilepsy. Nevertheless, the potentially interesting etiology of the seizures may elicit a more determined effort in the future to elucidate the mechanisms involved.

III. HYPERBARIC OXYGEN

The occurrence of seizures in animals breathing oxygen at high pressure (OHP) was first described by Bert (1878). The onset of OHP-induced seizures in man is also well established (Bornstein and Stroink, 1912; Thomson, 1935; Behnke et al., 1934–5; Behnke, 1940). Up to the early 1940's, investigations concerning OHP-induced seizures and the physiological effects of OHP are well documented in the reviews of Stadie et al., (1944) and Bean (1945). More recent investigations, including biochemical studies, are covered in the reviews by Lambertsen (1966), Haugaard (1968), and Wood (1969).

A. Experimental procedures

1. Chamber design. Hyperbaric oxygen experiments can be divided into two categories: animal experiments using relatively simple equipment and human studies where sophisticated, expensive chambers are required and where personnel highly trained in diving procedures and hyperbaric medicine are essential. The latter category falls outside the scope of this chapter which will be devoted to animal studies using appropriately sized chambers.

Elaborate chambers are sometimes used for animal experiments but more simply designed ones are, in most cases, satisfactory. They may be procured directly from firms specializing in such items (e.g., Bethlehem Corporation, Bethlehem, Pa.), but small, simply designed chambers can usually be manufactured locally. However, it must always be borne in mind that a chamber at pressure is a potentially lethal piece of equipment and the specifications for its construction should be drawn up accordingly.

The size of the chamber required depends on the species to be studied. Large dogs, for example, require chambers 4 ft or more in length, whereas small table-top chambers suffice for the smaller species such as mice and rats. Small chambers can be constructed of transparent plastic as illustrated in Fig. 1 which shows a series of these units connected to a source of high pressure oxygen. This type of chamber design has the advantage that the animal can be readily viewed from various angles. If, however, the chamber is constructed of nontransparent material, such as steel, a window must be provided which gives a clear view of the entire interior of the chamber. In this respect, a window in the end of a cylindrical chamber is superior to a port midway along the cylinder axis since the latter design leads to significant blind areas in the chamber.

The advantages of closed-circuit television viewing of animals during their exposure in the window type of chamber is readily apparent to any investigator who has had to make continual observations over a protracted period. In direct viewing through a port, the observer is severely limited in his movements since his eyes must be fairly close to the window. On the other hand, the use of a television camera close to the window with projection of the picture on a monitor allows considerable movement of the observer about the room. This procedure, of course, adds considerably to the cost of the equipment required for the hyperbaric studies but may be considered worthwhile if a large number of lengthy exposures is planned and if a window-type chamber is already available in the laboratory. Otherwise, direct viewing using simple plastic chambers would seem to be the procedure of choice for those persons setting up *de novo* an installation primarily for the purpose of using OHP-induced seizures as a model for epilepsy.

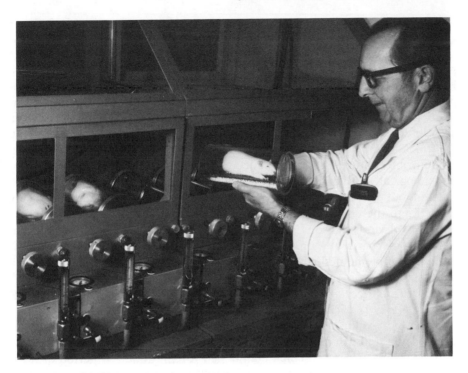

FIG. 1. Small chambers of simple design used for hyperbaric studies. Published with permission of Dr. M. W. Radomski, Defense and Civil Institute of Environmental Medicine.

The chamber should be equipped with a means of removing respired CO_2. The simplest procedure is to combine CO_2 absorption with venting of the chamber at pressure. A tray of soda-lime absorbent is placed in the bottom of the chamber, and the outflow valve is adjusted so that a controlled leak exists. A flow rate of 2 liters/min for a unit of 7-liter capacity has been found satisfactory. Although this procedure introduces a noise factor, this has not, in the writer's experience, significantly affected the sensitivity of the animals to OHP seizures. Chambers should be designed to handle at least 6 atmospheres absolute (ATA), i.e., approximately 75 p.s.i. gauge pressure, and preferably somewhat more. An accurate pressure gauge is an obvious requirement on all chambers.

If more than one animal is being exposed at the same time, they may be placed in individual chambers (as shown in Fig. 1) or they may be placed in individual transparent compartments within the same chamber. Lucite boxes containing large (1-cm diameter) perforations in all surfaces to allow adequate circulation of the experimental gas mixture are suitable for such a purpose.

2. Safety measures. Small animal chambers are simple to operate but strict attention must be paid to certain fundamental safety precautions. First, there are those precautions normally taken when using any high-pressure gas cylinders, such as ensuring that the cylinders are strapped or fixed to some rigid support such as a bench, and that the cylinder valves are closed at the end of each experiment. With oxygen studies, there is the additional hazard of fire. Care must therefore be taken that material of an inflammable nature is not introduced into the chamber. Where electro-physiological studies are to be carried out, the EEG equipment must be located outside the pressure chamber and only normal screened leads passed into the chamber. The potential hazards which have been stressed here for obvious reasons may cause some apprehension to the potential user of hyperbaric oxygen techniques. However, if the basic safety measures are implemented, the experimental technique may be considered a safe laboratory procedure.

3. Pressurization and decompression. A typical exposure to OHP (e.g., 6 ATA) is carried out as follows. Initial flushing of the chamber is effected by a vigorous flow of oxygen for 2 min. The pressure is then increased at a uniform rate over a 2-min period until the experimental pressure is reached, this pressure being maintained for the required period of time. Decompression from 6 ATA or less is carried out over a 5-min period, a rate which is tolerable to the animals.

It is customary to designate zero time for an exposure as that time when the desired experimental pressure is reached rather than when pressurization is commenced. This is an arbitrary procedure, however, since the animals will be exposed to a certain degree of high pressure during the compression period. In any event, the exact procedure followed should be clearly designated in any reports on hyperbaric oxygen studies.

4. Quantitative measure of susceptibility to OHP seizures. It is essential that the sensitivity of experimental animals to OHP seizures be placed on a quantitative basis if biochemical data are to be related to the convulsive activity. This is best done by using the CT_{50} values, where this value, expressed in minutes, denotes the length of exposure required to produce seizures in 50% of the animals. The CT_{50} value is a more accurate expression of susceptibility than is the mean convulsion time since the latter value is often unduly influenced by one or two animals from the experimental group that appear to be exceedingly resistant to OHP-induced seizures.

The CT_{50} values may be determined from the plot of the cumulative percent convulsed as a function of exposure time. This type of graphical presentation gives the reader a ready appreciation of the overall seizure picture, but deviations in the curve around the 50% point can lead to significant errors in the determined CT_{50} value. A more accurate estimate of the CT_{50} value is obtained, particularly when only a limited amount of data are available, by plotting the same results on logarithmic probability paper as described by Miller and Tainter (1944). This procedure provides a linear relationship which facilitates estimation of the CT_{50} value.

B. Variables requiring control during hyperbaric oxygen studies

1. Pressure. The pressure in the chamber must be closely controlled during the exposure if the results are to be meaningful and reproducible. Hyperbaric oxygen-induced convulsions seldom occur at pressures less than 3 ATA (Lambertsen, 1955), although pulmonary pathology develops at these pressures. This holds true for both humans and animals. Even pressures slightly greater than this, e.g., 3.8 ATA, are unsuitable for seizure studies, since at this pressure the aforementioned pulmonary damage is still a significant factor. At greater pressures, the onset of convulsions is rapid and overshadows the pulmonary damage which takes longer to become manifest. However, extremely high oxygen pressures are to be avoided because seizures occur so rapidly, within a few minutes, that a relatively large experimental error may be introduced into the calculations of the CT_{50} value and into the determination of biochemical events brought about by the hyperbaric oxygen. Although the optimum pressure varies somewhat depending upon the species being investigated, 5 to 6 ATA (60 to 75 p.s.i. gauge pressure) would appear to be the optimum range of pressure for most studies. The CT_{50} values at various pressures for mice are shown in Fig. 2.

2. Carbon dioxide. The removal of respired CO_2 in the chamber has already been mentioned. This precaution is necessary since the presence of CO_2 in the breathing mixture reduces considerably the time to the onset of OHP seizures (Table 1), presumably due to CO_2-induced vasodilation which in turn increases the supply of oxygen to the cerebral tissues (Lambertsen et al., 1955–56).

3. Environmental temperature. Although no studies appear to have been carried out on the effect of temperature on the sensitivity of animals to seizures, it would seem wise to control this factor within certain fairly close limits. In the experience of the author, variation in chamber temperature between 20 and 25°C did not produce a demonstrable alteration in seizure susceptibility.

4. Species. A considerable species variation exists with respect to

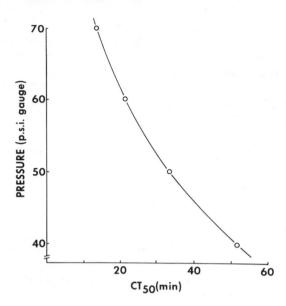

FIG. 2. Susceptibility of mice to hyperbaric oxygen as a function of pressure. The CT_{50} value is the length of exposure required to bring about seizures in 50% of the mice.

susceptibility to OHP seizures (Fig. 3). Avian species are extremely susceptible to seizures, as are mice and hamsters. The rat and rabbit are somewhat more resistant and guinea pigs even more so. Cats are relatively sensitive to OHP seizures (Shilling and Adams, 1933). Cold-blooded species such as the alligator are extremely resistant to OHP-induced sei-

TABLE 1. *Factors influencing susceptibility of animals to OHP-induced seizures*

Species and age	Special conditions	CT_{50} (min)	Reference
Mouse, adult	–	21.3	Wood et al. (1969)
	0.5% CO_2 in breathing mixture	14.0	
	1.0% CO_2 in breathing mixture	5.7	
Chick, 2 days	–	22.5	Wood (1970)
1 week	–	12.0	
2 weeks	–	9.9	
3 weeks	–	8.4	
Chick, 2 weeks	–	9.9	Wood (*un-published*)
	fasted 24 hr prior to exposure	15.0	
	fasted 48 hr prior to exposure	14.0	

Animals exposed to 60 p.s.i. (gauge pressure) oxygen.
CT_{50} = length of exposure required to induce seizures in 50% of the animals.

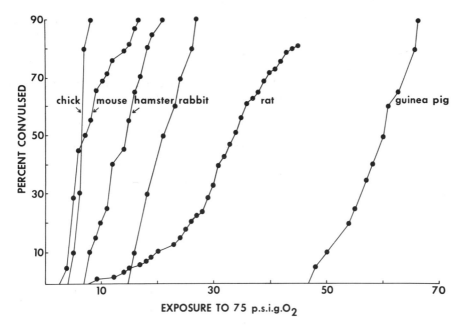

FIG. 3. Susceptibility of various species to hyperbaric oxygen-induced seizures. The values for the exposure to 75 p.s.i. (gauge pressure) O$_2$ are given in minutes.

zures (Thompson, 1889). The recommended species for biochemical studies on hyperbaric oxygen are the mouse, rat, and chick because of their ready availability and because of their suitable sensitivity to OHP-induced seizures. Rabbits are a suitable species if a somewhat larger animal is required.

5. *Sex.* Differences in the susceptibility to OHP-induced seizures of the male and female have been reported (Wood, 1966). The reason is uncertain but hormonal effects are possibly involved. The sex of the animals used in hyperbaric oxygen studies should therefore be stated clearly in any publication ensuing from the investigation. Since most previous studies on the subject have been conducted on male animals, experiments using this sex allow more widespread comparison with the work of other research groups. On the other hand, comparison between results obtained with males and females of the same species might well provide a useful tool in relating biochemical events to susceptibility to seizures.

6. *Nutritional status.* The susceptibility of a given species to OHP-induced seizures is governed by the nutritional status of the animal at the time of exposure (Table 1). Fasting for 24 hr produces a small but signifi-

cant increase in CT_{50} value (i.e., there is a decrease in susceptibility) over that for fed animals. Extension of the fasting period to 48 hr does not cause any further change in the CT_{50} value. Although fed animals have been used predominantly in past studies with good reproducibility of results, maximum reproducibility would seem to warrant 24-hr fasted animals. In any case, the nutritional status of the animals should be clearly stated in any publication.

7. *Age.* The susceptibility of animals to OHP seizures varies with age, mature animals being more susceptible than immature ones. The effect of age is most noticeable during the neonatal period. Day-old chicks are twice as susceptible as are 3-week-old chicks, most of the change occurring during the first week post-hatch (Table 1). The young mature adult is therefore the animal of choice in hyperbaric oxygen experiments.

8. *Time of sampling.* The convulsant action of OHP is rapidly reversible (Lambertsen, 1955), and consequently the biochemical derangement responsible for the seizures must also of necessity be of a rapidly reversible nature. Indeed, Abrahams and Wood (1970) have shown in rats that the brain levels of GABA decreased by OHP return to normal very rapidly (0.07 μmoles/g/min) after removal of the animals from the hyperbaric oxygen environment. Hence when OHP is used as a model to study the mechanisms involved in seizures, the following procedures should be adhered to: (i) the time between commencement of the decompression and the killing of the animals should be constant from experiment to experiment and should be as short as possible bearing in mind that too rapid a decompression may introduce other stress factors, and (ii) the rate of reversibility of any OHP-induced changes should be determined experimentally.

In addition to the specific reversibility of OHP changes, there is also to be overcome the more general problem of post-mortem changes in brain metabolite level. Hence, as in many other neurochemical studies, it is mandatory that these changes be kept to a minimum by either dropping the whole animal into liquid nitrogen or by decapitating the animal so that the head falls directly into the liquid nitrogen.

C. Rationale for using hyperbaric oxygen as a model for human epilepsy

1. Similarity between hyperbaric oxygen-induced convulsions and epileptic seizures. Hyperbaric oxygen-induced seizures appear to be a suitable model for the study of epilepsy since both the outward appearances and EEG patterns of the two types of seizures are similar. Moreover, the OHP-induced seizures in man and in animals are of a similar nature, thereby indicating the suitability of animal studies as a model for the situation in the human.

In animals, the seizures take the form of generalized tonic-clonic convulsions which are frequently, but not always, preceded by minor twitching of the head and fore-limbs. The progressive symptoms of oxygen poisoning in man are most aptly expressed by Lambertsen (1965) who describes the course of events as follows: "The convulsions are usually, but not always, preceded by the occurrence of localized muscular twitching especially about the eyes, mouth and forehead. Small muscles of the hand may be involved and incoordination of diaphragm activity in respiration may occur. These phenomena increase in severity over a period which may vary from a few minutes to nearly an hour with essentially clear consciousness being retained. Eventually an abrupt spread of excitation occurs and the rigid tonic phase of the convulsion begins. The tonic phase lasts for about 30 seconds and is accompanied by an abrupt loss of consciousness. Vigorous clonic contractions of the muscular groups of head and neck, trunk and limbs then occur becoming progressively less violent over about one minute."

The electrical activity of the brain during the fully developed OHP-induced seizure is similar to the pattern observed in grand mal epilepsy (Cohn and Gersh, 1945; Sonnenschein and Stein, 1953). The EEG pattern in OHP-induced seizures has been described in detail by various workers (Cohn and Gersh, 1945; Batini et al., 1954a,b; Sonnenschein and Stein, 1953; Stein, 1955; Rucci et al., 1967, 1968), and a typical effect of OHP on cortical and subcortical electrical activities is shown in Fig. 4. Rucci et al. (1967), using unrestrained, unanesthetized rats, showed that seizures are usually preceded by preseizure activity which is most evident in the subcortical centers. This activity consists of increases in voltage and discharge rate and in spindle-like waves. The onset of the seizure is simultaneous in all cortical records, and the subcortical leads fire at the same time as those in the cortex. The cerebral cortex is not necessary for initiating and developing seizures since convulsions are observed in decorticate rats. The cerebellum does not show preseizure activity and fires later than the extracerebellar formations (Rucci et al., 1968). Total cerebellectomy increases both the preseizure activity and the duration of the first seizure which led Rucci and co-workers to suggest that the cerebellum may play an inhibitory role in the development of the hyperoxic seizure.

2. Comparison of the etiologies of epileptic seizures and OHP-induced convulsions. The major consideration with regard to the choice of a particular model for epilepsy is, of course, an assessment of the possibility that the basic biochemical mechanisms involved in the etiologies of the two types

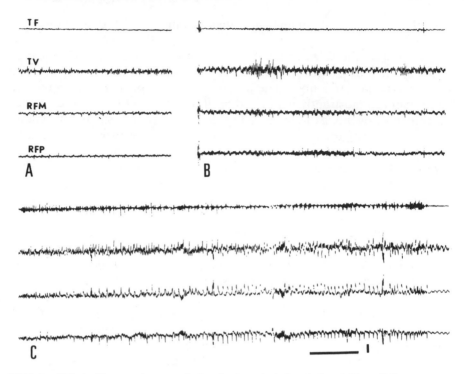

FIG. 4.   Effect of hyperoxia on cortical and subcortical electrical activities.   T.F., transverse frontal lead; T.V., unipolar record from right ventral nucleus of thalamus; R.F.M., unipolar record from left mesencephalic reticular formation; R.F.P., unipolar record from pontine reticular formation.   A: Before hyperoxia; B: 20 min after beginning of hyperoxia (4 ATA); C: 23 min after beginning of hyperoxia; generalized seizure.   Note spindle-like waves in the subcortical leads, particularly evident in T.V. before the onset of the first seizure.   Calibrations: 6 sec and 150 μV.   From Rucci et al. (1967) with permission of the publisher.

of seizures are similar, at least in part.   The merits of hyperbaric oxygen will now be assessed in this regard.

The primary event in the mechanism of OHP-induced seizures is almost certainly the oxidation of cellular constituents in the nervous tissue.   The oxidation of sulfhydryl groups is likely to be of particular importance in this respect since these groups are necessary for the proper functioning of enzymes and cellular membranes.   The oxidation of unsaturated lipids may likewise affect cellular function.   Regardless of the exact nature of this primary action, it is unlikely that it will duplicate events leading to epileptic seizures; however, the rather remote possibility that one type of epilepsy is due to a lack of available antioxidant material in the tissue cannot be rejected out of hand.

The secondary effects caused by the above oxidation are probably varied since, for example, many enzymes require sulfhydryl groups for activity and their oxidation could therefore result in changes in the levels and availability of various metabolites. However, Wood et al. (1966) have shown that the enzyme glutamic acid decarboxylase is particularly susceptible to oxidation by OHP and that inhibition of this enzyme *in vivo* results in decreased concentrations of cerebral GABA, the product of the reaction. Since GABA is believed to be an inhibitory transmitter substance in the central nervous system (Krnjević and Schwartz, 1966), Wood (1971) has suggested that low levels of the amino acid brought about by OHP may be the direct cause of the seizures. Indeed, a good correlation between susceptibility to seizures and decrease of brain GABA was found (Fig. 5), and administration of GABA ameliorated the seizures (Wood et al., 1963).

The question must now be asked whether a deranged GABA metabolism is involved at some stage of the epileptogenic process. Evidence to date, although indirect, suggests that this possibility must be given serious consideration. Most apropos is the report by Tower (1960) that orally administered GABA had an anticonvulsant action in some epileptic patients. Most dramatic was the effect of GABA on a 14-year-old girl with petit mal seizures where an oral dose of 2 mmoles/kg four times daily reduced the incidence of seizures from 402 per month to zero. Lesser but still significant protection by GABA against petit mal and/or generalized seizures was reported in three other patients. On the other hand, these results must be tempered by others where no response to GABA was obtained in several patients. The efficacy of GABA treatment in certain patients could be attributed to various mechanisms: (i) the patients were afflicted with a rather uncommon type of epilepsy which was caused by a deranged GABA metabolism and which could be counteracted by the exogenously supplied GABA; (ii) the patients suffered from a reasonably common form of the disease involving a deranged GABA metabolism, but in addition, and rather unusually, they possessed a defective blood-brain barrier which allowed the exogenous GABA to reach the tissue of the central nervous system [normally GABA does not readily penetrate the blood brain barrier, at least in animals (Van Gelder and Elliott, 1958)]; or (iii) a defective blood-brain barrier in the patients allowed exogenous GABA to penetrate into the central nervous system where, by its general depressant action, it counteracted the seizures which were caused by a mechanism not involving GABA. It is clear from the above that although the evidence for a role for GABA in epileptic seizures is indirect and rather tenuous, the possibility nevertheless exists and the employment of a model involving a deranged GABA metabolism (i.e., hyperbaric oxygen-induced seizures) seems valid and potentially useful.

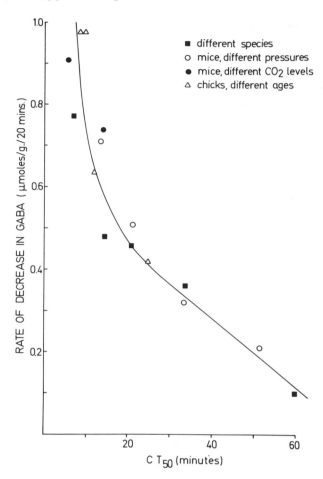

FIG. 5. Correlation between susceptibility to hyperbaric oxygen-induced seizures and the rate of decrease in cerebral GABA levels. CT_{50} indicates the time required for 50% of the animals to convulse. $\bigcirc$, mice at 40, 50, 60 and 70 p.s.i.g. oxygen; $\bullet$, mice at 60 p.s.i.g. oxygen + 0.5% or 1.0% carbon dioxide; $\blacksquare$, mice, hamsters, rats, and guinea pigs at 75 p.s.i.g. oxygen; $\triangle$, chicks ages 2 days, 1 week, 2 weeks and 3 weeks at 60 p.s.i.g. oxygen. From Wood (1970) with permission of the publisher.

3. Application of the OHP model to drug evaluation studies. How suitable is OHP as a model for evaluating drugs as antiepileptic agents? Examination of various agents protecting animals against oxygen toxicity (Wood, 1969) indicates that the compounds may be divided into two broad classifications. First, there are those compounds which can be considered antioxidants, e.g., vitamin E and 2,5-bis (1,1-dimethylpropyl) hydroquinone. Their ability to afford protection against the toxic effects of OHP is not surprising since the primary effect of hyperbaric oxygen is the oxidation of cellular constituents. However, as pointed out above, this effect is unlikely to be involved in the etiology of epileptic seizures. OHP is therefore an unsuitable model for evaluating the antiepileptic action of drugs whose prophylactic effect with respect to OHP-induced seizures is dependent on their antioxidant properties.

In the second classification are the agents which protect against OHP-induced seizures but which do not rely on an antioxidant action to do so; e.g., compounds such as GABA, tris(hydroxymethyl)aminomethane, and the barbiturates. These compounds probably exert their prophylactic action by influencing or counteracting secondary events triggered by the initial oxidation. Since similar events may occur during the epileptogenic processes, OHP could serve as a suitable model for evaluating the antiepileptic efficacy of this rather diverse group of compounds.

4. Specific advantages of the OHP model. In any discussion of the suitability of hyperbaric oxygen as a model for studying the mechanisms of seizures, mention must be made of certain powerful tools which this model provides to the investigator. As mentioned previously, there are striking species differences in susceptibility to OHP-induced seizures (Fig. 3). In order for a particular biochemical derangement to be considered the cause of the seizures, an exacting criterion must therefore be met; i.e., the biochemical derangement and the susceptibility of the animals to seizures must vary in a similar quantitative manner between species. Age differences in susceptibility to OHP-induced seizures allow a similar type of critical analysis to be made. In addition, the rapidly reversible nature of oxygen poisoning (see Section III, B, 8) provides another criterion to be satisfied if a biochemical defect is to be considered the cause of the seizures; i.e., the defect must disappear rapidly on the return of the animals from the hyperbaric oxygen environment to normal conditions. Altogether, the above criteria form a very precise test of the involvement of a biochemical defect in the seizure process.

D. Conclusions

Hyperbaric oxygen may be a suitable model for simulating certain types of epilepsy, particularly if a deranged GABA metabolism is suspected of being involved in the epileptogenic processes. The hyperbaric oxygen model is also suitable for evaluating the anticonvulsant effect of drugs whose mode of action does not depend on antioxidant properties. Conversely, compounds which protect against OHP-induced seizures by virtue of an antioxidant effect are unlikely to be generally efficacious in the prevention of epileptic seizures.

IV. REFERENCES

Abrahams, D. E., and Wood, J. D. (1970): Hydrazide-induced seizures and cerebral levels of γ-aminobutyric acid. *Journal of Neurochemistry,* 17:1197–1204.

Batini, C., Parma, M., Ricci, G. F., and Zanchetti, A. (1954*a*): Aspetti electroencefolografici della syndrome convulsive iperossica. *Archivio di Fisiologia,* 53:346–353.

Batini, C., Parma, M., Ricci, G. F., and Zanchetti, A. (1954*b*): Meccanismi piramidali ed extra-piramidali delle convulsioni iperossiche. *Archivio di Fisiologia,* 53:362–369.

Baumel, I., Schatz, R., DeFeo, J., and Lal, H. (1969*a*): Protection against semicarbazide-induced convulsions in mice at a hypobaric pressure. *Journal of Pharmacy and Pharmacology,* 21:119–120.

Baumel, I., Schatz, R., DeFeo, J., and Lal, H. (1969*b*): Hypoxia and methionine sulphoximine seizures in mice. *Journal of Pharmacy and Pharmacology,* 21:703–704.

Bean, J. W. (1945): Effects of oxygen at increased pressure. *Physiological Reviews,* 25:1–147.

Behnke, A. R. (1940): High atmospheric pressures; physiological effects of increased and decreased pressure; application of these findings to clinical medicine. *Annals of Internal Medicine,* 13:2217–2228.

Behnke, A. R., Johnson, F. S., Poppen, J. R., and Motley, E. P. (1934–5): The effect of oxygen on man at pressures from 1 to 4 atmospheres. *American Journal of Physiology,* 110:565–572.

Bert, P. (1878): *La Pression Barométrique.* English Translation by M. A. Hitchcock and F. A. Hitchcock. College Book Company, Columbus, Ohio. 1943.

Bornstein, A., and Stroink, M. (1912): Ueber Sauerstoffvergiftung. *Deutsche medizinische Wochenschrift,* 38:1495–1497.

Boyle, R. (1660): *New Experiments Physico-mechanical, Touching the Spring of Air, and Its Effects.* H. Hall, Oxford.

Cohn, R., and Gersh, I. (1945): Changes in brain potentials during convulsions induced by oxygen under pressure. *Journal of Neurophysiology,* 8:155–160.

Gellhorn, E., and Heymans, C. (1948): Differential action of anoxia, asphyxia and carbon dioxide on normal and convulsive potentials. *Journal of Neurophysiology,* 11:261–273.

Gurdjian, E. S., Webster, J. E., and Stone, W. E. (1949): Cerebral constituents in relation to blood gases. *American Journal of Physiology,* 156:149–157.

Haugaard, N. (1968): Cellular mechanisms of oxygen toxicity. *Physiological Reviews,* 48:312–373.

Jasper, H., and Erickson, T. C. (1941): Cerebral blood flow and pH in excessive cortical discharge induced by Metrazol® and electrical stimulation. *Journal of Neurophysiology,* 4:333–347.

Krnjević, K., and Schwartz, S. (1966): Is γ-aminobutyric acid an inhibitory transmitter? *Nature,* 211:1372–1374.

Lambertsen, C. J. (1955): Respiratory and circulatory actions of high oxygen pressure. In: *Proceedings of the Underwater Physiology Symposium,* edited by L. G. Goff. National Academy of Sciences–National Research Council, Washington, pp. 25–38.

Lambertsen, C. J. (1965): Effects of oxygen at high partial pressure. In: *Handbook of Phys-*

iology, Vol. 2., Section 3, edited by W. O. Fenn and H. Rahn. American Physiological Society, Washington, pp. 1027–1046.

Lambertsen, C. J. (1966): Physiological effects of oxygen inhalation at high partial pressures. In: *Fundamentals of Hyperbaric Medicine,* prepared by Committee on Hyperbaric Oxygenation. National Academy of Sciences–National Research Council, Washington, pp. 12–20.

Lambertsen, C. J., Ewing, J. H., Kough, R. H., Gould, R., and Stroud, M. W. (1955–6): Oxygen toxicity. Arterial and internal jugular blood gas composition in man during inhalation of air. 100% O_2 and 2% CO_2 in O_2 in O_2 at 3.5 atmospheres ambient pressure. *Journal of Applied Physiology,* 8:255–263.

Lovell, R. A., and Elliott, K. A. C. (1963): The γ-aminobutyric acid and factor I content of brain. *Journal of Neurochemistry,* 10:479–488.

Luft, V. C., and Noell, W. K. (1956): Manifestations of brief instantaneous anoxia in man. *Journal of Applied Physiology,* 8:444–454.

Miller, L. C., and Tainter, M. L. (1944): Estimation of the ED_{50} and its error by means of logarithmic-probit graph paper. *Proceedings of the Society for Experimental Biology and Medicine,* 57:261–264.

Nelson, S. R., and Mantz, M. L. (1971): Brain energy reserve levels at the onset of convulsions in hypoxic mice. *Life Sciences,* 10:901–907.

Passouant, P., Cadilhac, J., Pternitis, C., and Baldy-Moulinier, M. (1967a): Épilepsie temporale et decharges ammoniques provoquées par l'anoxie exprive. *Revue Neurologique,* 117:65–70.

Passouant, P., Cadilhac, J., Pternitis, C., and Baldy-Moulinier, M. (1967b): Temporal epilepsy and hippocampal discharges induced by oxyprivic anoxia. *Electroencephalography and Clinical Neurophysiology,* 23:379.

Rucci, F. S., Giretti, M. L., and La Rocca, M. (1967): Changes in electrical activity of the cerebral cortex and of some subcortical centers in hyperbaric oxygen. *Electroencephalography and Clinical Neurophysiology,* 22:231–238.

Rucci, F. S., Giretti, M. L., and La Rocca, M. (1968): Cerebellum and hyperbaric oxygen. *Electroencephalography and Clinical Neurophysiology,* 25:359–371.

Shilling, C. W., and Adams, B. H. (1933): A study of the convulsive seizures caused by breathing oxygen at high pressures. *U.S. Naval Medical Bulletin,* 31:112–121.

Sonnenschein, R. R., and Stein, S. N. (1953): Electrical activity of the brain in actue oxygen poisioning. *Electroencephalography and Clinical Neurophysiology,* 5:521–524.

Stadie, W. C., Riggs, B. C., and Haugaard, N. (1944): Oxygen poisoning. *American Journal of Medical Science,* 207:84–114.

Stein, S. N. (1955): Neurophysiological effects of oxygen at high partial pressure. In: *Proceedings of the Underwater Physiology Symposium,* edited by L. G. Goff. National Academy of Sciences–National Research Council, Washington, pp. 20–24.

Thompson, W. G. (1889): The therapeutic value of oxygen inhalation with exhibition of animals under high pressure of oxygen. *Medical Records,* 36:1–7.

Thomson, W. A. R. (1935): The physiology of deep-sea diving. *British Medical Journal,* 2:208–210.

Tower, D. B. (1960): The administration of gamma-aminobutyric acid to man: Systemic effects and anticonvulsant action. In: *Inhibition in the Nervous System and Gamma-Aminobutyric Acid,* edited by E. Roberts. Pergamon Press, Oxford, pp. 562–578.

Tower, D. B. (1969): Reports on visits to scientific institutions and laboratories. In: *Neurochemistry in the Soviet Union,* p. 44. The National Institute of Neurological Diseases and Stroke, National Institutes of Health, Bethesda, Md.

Van Gelder, N. M., and Elliott, K. A. C. (1958): Disposition of γ-aminobutyric acid administered to mammals. *Journal of Neurochemistry,* 3:139–143.

Wood, J. D. (1966): Development of a strain of rats with greater than normal susceptibility to oxygen poisoning. *Canadian Journal of Physiology and Pharmacology,* 44:259–265.

Wood, J. D. (1969): Oxygen toxicity. In: *The Physiology and Medicine of Diving and Com-*

pressed Air Work, edited by P. B. Bennett and D. H. Elliott. Bailliere, Tindall and Cassell, London, pp. 113–143.

Wood, J. D. (1970): Seizures induced by hyperbaric oxygen and cerebral γ-aminobutyric acid in chicks during development. *Journal of Neurochemistry,* 17:573–579.

Wood, J. D. (1971): Toxicity in neuronal elements. In: *Proceedings of the Fourth Symposium on Underwater Physiology,* edited by C. J. Lambertsen. Academic Press, New York, pp. 9–17.

Wood, J. D., and Peesker, S. J. (1971): The effect of hypoxia on isonicotinic acid hydrazide-induced seizures in chicks during ontogenesis. *Journal of Pharmacy and Pharmacology,* 23:637–638.

Wood, J. D., Watson, W. J., and Clydesdale, F. M. (1963): Gamma-aminobutyric acid and oxygen poisoning. *Journal of Neurochemistry,* 10:625–633.

Wood, J. D., Watson, W. J., and Ducker, A. J. (1968): The effect of hypoxia on brain γ-aminobutyric acid levels. *Journal of Neurochemistry,* 15:603–608.

Wood, J. D., Watson, W. J., and Murray, G. W. (1969): Correlation between decreases in γ-aminobutyric acid levels and susceptibility to convulsions induced by hyperbaric oxygen. *Journal of Neurochemistry,* 16:281–287.

Wood, J. D., Watson, W. J., and Stacey, N. E. (1966): A comparative study of hyperbaric oxygen-induced and drug-induced convulsions with particular reference to γ-aminobutyric acid metabolism. *Journal of Neurochemistry,* 13:361–370.

19

Systemic Carbon Dioxide Derangements

C. D. Withrow

OUTLINE

I. INTRODUCTION

The major purpose of this chapter is to give the prospective investigator in experimental epilepsy a grasp of the use of systemic carbon dioxide (CO_2) derangements as a model for the study of seizures and of anticonvulsant drugs.   Background material, experimental details and current theories about interpretation of results have been given in some detail. Thus, a person not familiar with these types of investigations can, hopefully, use this chapter without much additional reading to decide whether CO_2 derangements are useful to him, and begin experimental work if the decision is favorable.   The chapter is not intended to be either a comprehensive review of the effects of CO_2 on the central nervous system (CNS) or a complete summary of acid-base metabolism.   Rather, these subjects have been included only to the extent that they serve the primary purpose of the chapter.

II. CARBON DIOXIDE EFFECTS ON THE CENTRAL NERVOUS SYSTEM

A. Introduction

The effects of CO_2 on the CNS will be considered only insofar as the changes produced by CO_2 are related to experimental models for the study of seizure processes and of drugs which have anticonvulsant effects.   Emphasis will be placed on CO_2-induced responses in the electroencephalograph (EEG) and in motor movements because these effects have been most widely used for experimentation with antiseizure agents.   Finally, for the sake of convenience, hypocarbia and hypercarbia will be considered separately because, as will become obvious below, CO_2 effects on the CNS are not a simple continuum of a single CO_2 action.

B. Hypocarbia

It has been known for many years (see Brown, 1953, and Wyke, 1963, for early references) that hyperventilation can precipitate seizures in epileptic patients.   Although patients suffering from petit mal are more susceptible to a decrease in blood CO_2 tensions, grand mal EEG patterns can also be induced by hyperventilation (Toman and Davis, 1949).   It is not possible, however, to produce true seizures of any kind in a person not prone to epilepsy.

Extensive use of the EEG by clinicians and by laboratory investigators has shown that hyperventilation causes an increase in high-voltage, slow waves in the EEG patterns of both epileptic and some normal persons. These slow waves qualitatively resemble those EEG variations observed in classic petit mal epilepsy to the extent that both are high voltage and slow.   In epileptic patients with petit mal, the hypernea-induced slow waves are followed by paroxysmyal bursts of the 3/sec, spike-dome EEG waves so characteristic of this disorder. Motor manifestations of the changes in brain electrical patterns may or may not be present. In contrast, in normal persons the EEG slow waves caused by hyperventilation do not change into classic petit mal patterns (Toman and Davis, 1949), and no motor movements attributable to CNS activity are observable.

Whether hypocapnea is a suitable model for experimentation with anticonvulsant drugs is a moot point. Although the abnormal EEG waves recorded in petit mal patients and those observed in hyperventilated normal persons are both high voltage and slow, the two wave types are not identical. The spike-dome waves of petit mal are not necessarily activated only by changes in respiration and can be elicited by several other methods that probably have effects different from CO_2 changes (Cobb, 1963). With regard to drugs, it is known that abnormal EEG patterns in petit mal patients can be dramatically suppressed by oxazolidinediones, and that this effect is associated with complete control of petit mal seizures. The oxazolidinediones, however, do not have any consistent effects on the EEG patterns of normal persons unless sedative doses are given. In contrast, it is frequently found that drugs of the hydantoin-type give good clinical control of seizures without affecting the disappearance of abnormal activity in the EEG (Toman and Davis, 1949). Schwab et al. (1941) observed that diphenylhydantoin and phenobarbital decreased the incidence of hyperventilation-induced slow waves in epileptic patients. However, a systematic study of anti-petit mal drugs, or any other types of anticonvulsant drugs for that matter, on the EEG of hyperventilated normal animals or patients has not been made. Thus, it is possible, but not likely, that a potential experimental model has been overlooked. Experimental problems, discussed below, would limit the usefulness of this type of model even if drug effects can be studied in this way. The use of hyperventilation is nevertheless a very valuable and commonly used aid for the diagnosis of epilepsy.

C. Hypercarbia

Increases of CO_2 concentration in inspired air can cause profound effects on the CNS. Since these have been extensively reviewed and discussed elsewhere (Woodbury et al., 1958; Woodbury and Karler, 1960; Wyke, 1963), only a brief summary will be given here.

The first CNS effect observed when CO_2 levels in inspired air are increased is a depression of cortical excitability as measured by elevations of the electroshock seizure threshold, protection against convulsions induced by maximal electroshock, and prevention of seizures induced by a variety of chemical agents (see Woodbury and Karler, 1960, for pertinent references). Low concentrations of CO_2 enhance high-pressure O_2 seizures, but this effect is more likely due to changes in brain blood flow rather than to a specific effect of CO_2 on neuronal activity (Marshall and Lambertsen, 1961). As CO_2 concentrations are further increased to between 20 and 30%, a phase of cortical excitability is observed in which experimental animals and man exhibit the minimal type seizures described in section III, B (see Woodbury et al., 1958, and Wyke, 1963, for additional information). Supporting evidence for the cortical excitatory effects of CO_2 is found in the experiments of Pollock and Bain (1950) in which they observed that seizures caused by β-chlorinated amines were potentiated by 15 to 30% CO_2. Although they attributed these potentiations to differences in the effects of the chemicals on the cortex and cerebellum, later work (Pollock and Wang, 1954) showed that convulsant nitrogen mustards topically applied to the cortex and cerebellum act similarly. It should be pointed out that inhalation of CO_2 in this range—which includes the low anesthetic range—results in the rather unusual situation in which anesthetized animals or patients exhibit seizures (Leake and Waters, 1929; Seevers, 1944; Gyarfas et al., 1949; Meduna and Gyarfas, 1949; Cassels et al., 1940; Woodbury et al., 1958). Finally, when concentrations of CO_2 are greater than approximately 40% in the inspired air, complete narcosis and anesthesia is attained (Leake and Waters, 1929; Seevers, 1944; Poulsen, 1952).

Rapid withdrawal from very high concentrations of CO_2 also affects CNS function; CNS excitation is most commonly seen in experimental animals (Pollock and Bain, 1950; Woodbury et al., 1958; Brown, 1971a; Petty and Sulkowski, 1971) and in man (Gibbs et al., 1938; Clowes et al., 1955). Thus, a rapid decrease in blood CO_2 levels causes a clonic seizure of the type recorded in section III, B.

The effects of CO_2 on the CNS have also been extensively studied by use of the EEG (see Wyke, 1963, for a detailed discussion). The triphasic effects of CO_2 described above have been confirmed by systematic EEG studies in rats and dogs (Woodbury et al., 1958; Wyke, 1963). Numerous studies in animals and man indicate that CO_2 concentrations in the inspired air of 5 to 10% cause the appearance of fast, low-voltage waves in the EEG. An increase in CO_2 levels to the 30 to 35% range results in slow, high-voltage activity in the EEG (Pollock, 1949; Clowes et al., 1955; Morrice, 1956; Swanson et al., 1958; Meyer et al., 1961). Thus, as pointed out by Morrice (1956), the interesting situation exists that both hypo- and hypercarbia cause high-voltage, slow waves in the EEG. They differ, however, in that CO_2-induced slow waves are not affected by blood glucose levels (Morrice, 1956). A more important difference insofar as seizure studies are concerned is the fact that slow waves caused by hyperventilation only are associated with motor movements in epileptic patients, whereas motor movements have been correlated with EEG slow-wave activity in normal humans (Meduna and Gyarfas, 1949) and normal rats (Woodbury et al., 1958) exposed to elevated CO_2 concentrations. Also of interest are the observations of Woodbury and co-workers (1958) that the EEG patterns of rats exposed to 30% CO_2 are similar to those recorded when rats were suddenly withdrawn from 50% CO_2.

Anticonvulsant drugs have been shown to have effects on both the in-chamber and CO_2 withdrawal seizures. Woodbury et al. (1958) showed that phenobarbital, trimethadione, and acetazolamide changed the incidence of seizures in both types of challenges, whereas diphenylhydantoin exacerbated seizures in both exposure and withdrawal experiments. Withrow et al. (1968) showed that dimethadione (DMO) changed the peak effect concentration of CO_2 in exposure experiments. Since all of the drugs affecting CO_2 seizures are anti-petit mal agents, it appears that CO_2 seizures are suitable models for the study of antiepileptic drugs of this type. This is not surprising since the CO_2 seizures are nonfocal, generalized seizures and probably of subcortical origin. CO_2 seizures do not appear to be useful as models for the study of drugs that affect seizure spread such as the hydantoins.

Another application of CO_2 seizures was to study maturation of CNS in rats (Withrow et al., 1967).

D. Summary

Systemic CO_2 derangements produce dramatic changes in CNS electrical activity that can be, in the case of hypercarbia, manifested in observable clonic movements in normal animals. These seizures, and those precipated by withdrawal from high CO_2 concentrations, are useful for the study of anticonvulsant drugs and are considered in some detail below. It has been pointed out that hyperventilation does not appear to be a useful laboratory tool for the study of anticonvulsant drugs. However, some of the experimental difficulties of hyperventilation experiments are briefly discussed in the experimental section.

III. EXPERIMENTAL DETAILS

A. Hyperventilation

Hyperventilation at present is useful for the study of anticonvulsant drugs only in patients prone to seizures. Even then, however, it is not a simple procedure. Hyperventilation requires effort and cooperation, neither of which may be forthcoming in a young child, a balky teenager, or a senile adult. The classic study of Blinn and Noell (1949), confirmed later by Meyer and Waltz (1960a), showed that even in healthy, cooperative adults, a standard 3-min hyperventilation test produced hypocapnia of a range from 10 to 28 mm Hg. Therefore, even in ideal patients, it is not possible to conclude that all persons have had the same hypocapnic challenge unless blood or alveolar gas measurements are made. An even more important finding in their experiments was the fact that the first appearance of slow waves in the EEG occurred at a wide range (10 to 38 mm Hg) of alveolar CO_2 tensions. Later experiments by Meyer and Waltz (1960a,b) showed that this range of activation of CO_2 tensions was found in both normal and epileptic subjects. Thus, there appear to be wide differences in neuronal "stability" (Morrice, 1956) in different normal and diseased populations. These differences in sensitivity to CO_2 complicate drug testing in humans by hyperventilation even if all the ethical and logistical problems were solved.

Common laboratory animals do not have spontaneous seizures of any type. Gibbs et al. (1936) mention EEG work by Kornmüller on rabbits having spontaneous seizures but only scant details were given. Therefore, activation of seizures by hyperventilation, and the effect of drugs on this activation, are not able to be studied in the laboratory. Even if a readily available species is found that has seizure foci that can be activated by overbreathing, the technical difficulties of hyperventilating animals are numerous. Animals must be anesthetized, tracheotomized or intubated, and, ideally, paralyzed. Also, body temperature must be maintained. All these procedures are somewhat tedious, but perhaps the most serious objection is that anesthesia would seriously complicate the interpretation of drug effects on the EEG. It might perhaps be possible to stimulate respiration in unanesthetized animals with drugs (Lambertsen, 1966), but, once again, interpretation of other drug effects would be confused.

B. CO_2 seizures

1. General. CO_2 seizures are produced by exposure to and/or withdrawal from high concentrations of the gas. A typical experiment is performed as follows.

A few animals are placed in a chamber filled with a gas mixture containing CO_2, N_2, and O_2. CO_2 concentrations usually range from 5 to 50%, O_2 is usually constant at 20%, and the remainder of the gas mixture is N_2. The animals are kept in the box for 6 to 10 min and observed for seizure activity. If an animal exhibits either jaw or forelimb clonus or both while being exposed to CO_2, this animal is said to have had an in-chamber or exposure seizure. The highest incidence of exposure seizures is usually seen in 35% CO_2 (Woodbury et al., 1958).

At the end of the 6- to 10-min time period, all animals are taken from the box and allowed to breathe room air. In seconds, susceptible animals then manifest so-called withdrawal seizures characterized by rapid jaw and forelimb clonus, marked salivation, piloerection, and a rearing-up movement. Withdrawal from 50% CO_2 is usually employed to induce withdrawal seizures.

2. Equipment. The equipment required for CO_2 seizure studies usually consists of a CO_2 chamber and a supply of several gas mixtures containing different CO_2 concentrations. In our laboratory, most studies have been done with mice and rats. Therefore, the exposure chamber is a small box made from plastic to allow easy observation of animals in the chamber. The different gas mixtures used are made in the laboratory immediately prior to use by mixing gases from commercial tanks of CO_2, N_2, and O_2 in a Collins 120L spirometer. Details of the construction of the box and of mixing the gases have been given by Woodbury et al. (1958). Obviously, more elaborate equipment may be assembled to work with larger animals, to prepare gas mixtures, and to measure and monitor gas concentrations.

3. Animals. All systematic studies of CO_2 seizures have used either rats or mice as experimental animals. The obvious advantages of small rodents are the ease with which large numbers of animals can be handled and the lack of necessity for large CO_2 chambers that require large amounts of gas mixtures to fill and flush. Another advantage of the use of rats is that an enormous amount of information is available concerning CO_2-induced changes in brain electrolyte and acid base metabolism. Thus, interpretation of results is aided by this knowledge. Withdrawal studies in larger mammals, however, may be limited by the fact that rapid withdrawal from CO_2 concentrations can cause fatal ventricular fibrillation (Brown and Miller, 1952), although there is considerable difference between breathing CO_2 for a few minutes in withdrawal experiments and for 4 hr in fibrillation studies.

4. Suggestions and possible errors

a. Care must be taken to insure that the gas tensions in the chamber are not altered by CO_2 production or O_2 consumption of animals placed there for study. Therefore, the chamber must either be large or be continuously flushed with the gas mixture. In our laboratory, a Collins spirometer full of a gas mixture contains sufficient gas to allow a slow flushing of the chamber for 6 to 12 min. Another advantage of a chamber which is kept under positive pressure during flushing is that the addition of animals to the chamber does not cause dilution of the enclosed gas mixture with room air.

b. In most papers dealing with CO_2 seizures, CO_2 concentrations are given as percent CO_2. It would be more exact to report CO_2 levels in pressure units since 35% CO_2 in Salt Lake City (normal barometric pressure = 640 mm Hg) has a much lower Pco_2 than does 35% CO_2 compounded at sea level. Caution must therefore be exercised when comparisons of data from different laboratories are made to ensure that CO_2 tensions in the gas mixtures are comparable.

c. Seizure observations must be made carefully. In-chamber seizures are particularly difficult to detect. Crowding in the chamber should therefore be avoided, and practice and concentration are rewarded by more reproducible results. Great care must be exercised when immature animals are studied to separate seizure activity from random exploratory and feeding-type movements.

Withdrawal seizures are easily detected and are often dramatic. In

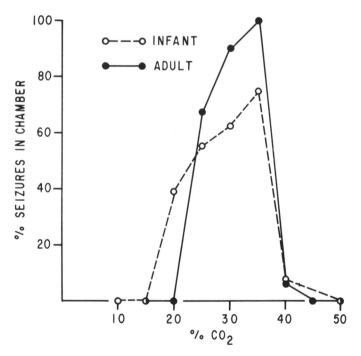

FIG. 1. Percent seizures in infant and adult rats exposed to various concentrations of CO_2. From Withrow et al. (1967) with permission of the publisher.

fact, rats have been observed sitting like trained dogs while exhibiting jaw and forelimb clonus, and often toppling straight back over their tails rather than to one side or the other. Woodbury et al. (1958) should be studied for more details of the seizures.

5. *Presentation of data.* The incidence of seizures in the CO_2 chamber is usually presented either in tabular form or in graphic form as shown in Fig. 1. The graphic presentation allows ready comparison of the position of curves along the abscissa. Two kinds of changes have been observed when data are plotted this way. In the experiments depicted, the highest incidence of seizures in both the young and adult groups was observed in animals being exposed to 35% CO_2. The frequency of seizures, however, was less in the younger animals. In other experiments, the frequency of seizures is the same in two experimental groups, but the percent CO_2 causing the maximum incidence of seizures is changed by drug treatment. This type of response is shown in Fig. 2. Interpretation of these results is discussed below.

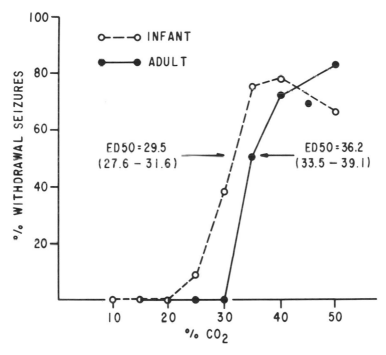

FIG. 2. Percent seizures in infant and adult rats after withdrawal to room air from various CO_2 concentrations. From Withrow et al. (1967) with permission of the publisher.

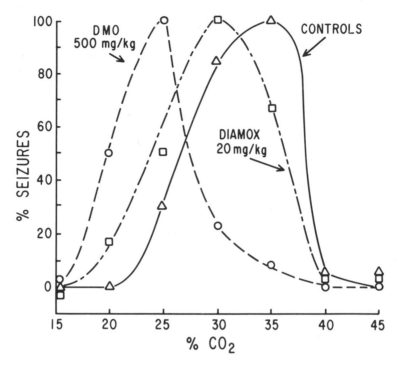

FIG. 3. Effect of DMO and acetazolamide on seizures induced by exposure to high CO_2 concentrations. From Withrow et al. (1968) with permission of the publisher.

Typical results from a withdrawal seizure experiment are shown in Fig. 3. Curves of this type are very similar in shape to dose-effect curves and amenable to probit analysis by the method of Litchfield and Wilcoxon (1949). Interpretations of typical data are discussed in the Appendix.

6. *Advantages and disadvantages.* CO_2 seizures of either type as experimental tools have several advantages. The equipment and gases used are cheap, readily available, and can be used by nonexperts. Although many animals are needed for a single experiment, the animals can be used repeatedly and thus keep down the cost. Anesthesia and surgery are unnecessary. The method gives fast results and is thereby useful for screening purposes.

A major disadvantage of the CO_2-seizures method for studying drugs is that it is a kinetic experiment in which rapid changes are taking place in both intracellular and extracellular fluids. It is therefore extremely difficult to do appropriate electrolyte and acid-base analyses.

A possible problem with CO_2 experiments is that CO_2 excess and deficit can affect the entry of drugs into the CNS (Goldberg et al., 1961). Any major effects of CO_2 on brain concentration of drugs are unlikely, however, because of the very short duration of CO_2 distortions in CO_2 seizure studies.

IV. APPENDIX

Acid-base distortions

1. Introduction. A discussion of acid-base changes in hyperventilation or CO_2 seizure experiments is, in a sense, easy. The experiments are so acute that intra-cellular-extracellular shifts of ions (Brown, 1971b), except in the red blood cell (RBC), can be ignored. The contribution of intracellular active processes to cell pH regulation (Siesjö and Messeter, 1971) is probably also insignificant. Finally, renal compensation is so slow that this effect on acid-base balance is not important (Woodbury, 1965; Brown, 1971b).

On the other hand, there are very little data available defining acid-base changes that occur in a few minutes. Tissue data are particularly scarce because of the technical problem of getting samples rapidly. Withdrawal seizures in which changes occur in seconds present extreme technical difficulties. The summary that follows, then, must necessarily be brief and incomplete.

2. Blood and extracellular fluid. In the acute experiments being considered, a decrease or increase in the CO_2 tension of alveolar air results in a rapid decrease or increase, respectively, of the partial pressure of CO_2 in blood. The change in blood P_{CO_2} rapidly changes blood pH. HCO_3^- levels in plasma are also varied because of the buffer reactions with plasma proteins and with hemoglobin in the RBC. The protein and hemoglobin buffer reactions are somewhat different even though they both mitigate blood pH changes. Their functions can be illustrated by consideration of what happens when blood P_{CO_2} is elevated.

When P_{CO_2} in blood is increased, some of the CO_2 is hydrated by plasma water to form carbonic acid (H_2CO_3) which rapidly dissociates into H and HCO_3 ions. Some of the H ions combine then with anionic sites on plasma proteins to form a weaker acid than H_2CO_3. Hence, some of H^+ added to plasma as a result of an increased P_{CO_2} is neutralized. It is important to note that the neutralization of one mole of H_2CO_3 results in the addition of one mole of HCO_3^- to the plasma.

Some of the CO_2 added to blood rapidly diffuses into the RBC. In the RBC, the hydration of CO_2 to H_2CO_3 by cell H_2O is accelerated by carbonic anhydrase (CA), an enzyme present in the RBC but not in plasma. The H_2CO_3 ionizes inside the RBC and some of the H^+ is buffered by hemoglobin. Once again, the neutralization of a mole of H^+ results in the appearance of one mole of HCO_3^-. Consequently, HCO_3^- concentration in the RBC rises above that of plasma. Since the RBC membrane is permeable to HCO_3^-, the HCO_3^- begins to diffuse out of the

RBC. Electrical neutrality in the RBC is preserved by a movement of Cl ions from the plasma into the RBC. This exchange of intracellular HCO_3^- for extracellular Cl^-, called the chloride shift, increases plasma HCO_3^- and decreases plasma Cl^- when blood CO_2 tensions are elevated. The buffering effect of the RBC is much more important than that of plasma proteins because (i) the quantities of hemoglobin in the RBC are greater than the quantities of plasma protein in normal plasma, and (ii) the uncatalyzed rate of hydration of CO_2 in plasma is much slower than the CA-catalyzed hydration in the RBC.

A decrease in blood P_{CO_2} essentially reverses the changes described above. Plasma HCO_3^- levels fall and plasma Cl^- concentrations rise. In extreme hyperventilation, the appearance of large amounts of lactate from cells titrates plasma HCO_3^- and diminishes blood pH elevations secondary to a CO_2 loss. Small amounts of lactate disappear from plasma in hypercarbia, but this effect is quantitatively minor in buffering a carbonic acid acidosis (Pitts, 1963).

A confusing point often is the apparent change in blood buffering shortly after a rapid increase in CO_2 tensions in blood. That is, plasma HCO_3^- concentrations are greatest within a few minutes after CO_2 levels are elevated. During the next 5 to 30 min, plasma bicarbonate decreases. This lowering of plasma HCO_3^- is due to the redistribution of HCO_3^- formed only in blood into the rest of the extracellular fluids which contain little buffer substances. Therefore, *in vivo* buffering of CO_2, as measured by plasma HCO_3^- levels, appears to be much less than the buffering of CO_2 by blood *in vitro*. It is worth emphasizing again that blood buffering *in vivo* is time dependent in that it is apparently higher very soon after P_{CO_2} is elevated.

In summary, it can be stated that the RBC is the keystone of extracellular H_2CO_3 buffering. Thus, changes in blood pH and blood HCO_3^- levels when blood CO_2 tensions are varied will depend strongly upon the amount of RBCs, or more specifically, hemoglobin, present. Although plasma proteins are relatively minor buffers, their absence will also affect blood acid-base balance. Finally, buffering *in vivo* appears to be less than buffering *in vitro* because the large amounts of non-buffer-containing fluids *in vivo* dilute HCO_3^- generated by the blood buffers. It must be emphasized, however, that the actual buffering by blood protein and hemoglobin is the same in either case.

3. Brain and CSF. CO_2 is rapidly transported to the brain where it penetrates into brain cells and into CSF. The time constant for this rate is 2.7 min (Farhi and Rahn, 1960).

When CO_2 penetrates brain cells, it is coped with in three ways: (i) physicochemical buffering; (ii) active transport of H^+ out of cells; and (iii) consumption of organic acids (Siesjö and Messeter, 1971). The reaction with physicochemical buffers and with various organic acids begins to take place immediately and is clearly evident 15 min after hypercarbia is produced. The effects of transmembrane fluxes of HCO_3^- and H^+, active transport, are measurable in 45 min and return cell pH to approximately normal in 48 hr. Thus, in acute experiments changes in intracellular HCO_3^- levels are due to passive reactions of H_2CO_3 with buffers and organic acids present in the cell.

In severe, acute hyperventilation, the production of lactate becomes more significant for buffering brain tissue and CSF (Plum et al., 1968). Otherwise, acute hyperventilation is the reverse of acute hypoventilation, and active transport processes are of minor importance in maintaining normal values of cell pH (Siesjö and Messeter, 1971).

Entry of CO_2 into CSF causes a rapid decrease in CSF pH. CSF HCO_3^- concentrations in the very acute experiments considered here do not change immediately because CSF contains little buffer substances. Continued elevation of CO_2 in blood, however, results in a rise of HCO_3^- levels in CSF (Merwarth and Sieker, 1961; Lee et al., 1969) for a number of reasons.

First, the buffering of CO_2 in blood increases the concentration gradient from plasma into CSF. Brain cell HCO_3^- also increases because of CO_2 buffering there (see above). Even though it has been speculated that CSF HCO_3^- comes from brain cells when CO_2 levels are increased (Swanson and Rosengren, 1962), brain cell HCO_3^- concentrations are much less than CSF HCO_3^- levels so the normal concentration gradient is from CSF into brain cells. Second, the normal positive potential difference between CSF and blood (+4 mV) is made more positive by CO_2 inhalation. Hence, the electrical gradient for HCO_3^- from blood to CSF is increased. Third, Maren (1971) has found that respiratory acidosis increased the formation of HCO_3^- in CSF by choroid plexus cells. Finally, the active process that maintains HCO_3^- against an electrochemical gradient between CSF and blood in normal animals may help regulate CSF pH when CO_2 tensions in blood are changed (see various discussions in Siesjö and Sørensen, 1971, for details). Whatever the reason, the increase in HCO_3^- in CSF nevertheless increases CSF pH toward normal values in hypercarbia.

Hyperventilation of normal animals essentially reverses the above processes described for hypercarbia. Extreme hyperventilation, however, results in acute rises of lactate concentrations in CSF which keep pH values close to normal. The lactate comes from brain tissue since increased blood lactate concentrations do not elevate CSF lactate levels (see Posner and Plum, 1967, for some experiments and pertinent references), and it has been shown that hyperventilation elevates brain lactate values rapidly (Messeter and Siesjö, 1971). Granholm et al. (1968) reported some data which indicated that lactate is passively distributed between brain and CSF. However, later experiments (Granholm and Siesjö, 1969) showed that other factors, e.g., active transport, may be important. This issue is not settled at present.

Acid base distortions in the CNS by hypocarbia and hypercarbia are mitigated primarily by brain tissue. In acute changes in CO_2 tensions, active processes regulating intracellular pH are probably not of quantitative importance in brain. CSF pH (HCO_3^-) is also defended when CO_2 distortions are produced in blood. It is clear that part of the regulation depends strongly on exchanges between brain and CSF and perhaps between CSF and blood. In very acute experiments, e.g., CO_2 withdrawal seizure studies, the very rapid diffusion of CO_2 between blood and CSF becomes the most important determinant of CSF pH because CSF has no buffer capacity (the interested reader is referred to the volume edited by Siesjö and Sørensen, 1971, for very complete discussions of the complexities of ion regulation in brain and CSF). Additional acid-base information can be obtained from Woodbury (1965) and Masoro and Siegel (1971).

Mechanisms of CNS effects and of seizures in hypo- and hypercarbia

1. Hypocarbia. There is much evidence, both direct and indirect, to indicate the EEG slowing caused by hyperventilation is due to cerebral hypoxia: hypoxia and syncope produce similar effects (Gibbs et al., 1935; Meyer and Waltz, 1960*a,b*); hyperbaric O_2 eliminates or decreases the effect (Reivich et al., 1966); hyperoxic hyperventilation prevents much of the rise in CSF and brain lactate levels (Plum et al., 1968); and jugular Po_2 was the only factor measured (others were jugular Pco_2, pH, Na^+, and K^+) that correlated statistically with EEG slowing (Gotoh et al., 1965). Most investigators that favor the hypoxia theory believe that the hypoxia is due to the well-described cerebral vasoconstriction (Sokoloff, 1960) caused by a decrease in blood CO_2 tensions.

The argument, however, is not settled. The recent findings of Granholm and Siesjö (1971) in which they reported that hyperventilation did not result in a decrease in brain high-energy phosphates are difficult to reconcile with tissue hypoxia. Older experiments, summarized by Dawson and Greville (1963), bring into the discussion compensatory vasoconstriction and a reduction in cholinergic supply to the blood vessels as being important. The common thread of vasoconstriction, nevertheless, appear often. Whatever the mechanism of slow-wave production, it seems clear that hypocapnia rather than blood pH changes *per se* is of primary importance (Swanson et al., 1958).

2. Hypercarbia

a. In-chamber seizures. The localized clonic seizures observed while animals are being exposed to moderate (15 to 30%) CO_2 concentrations have been attributed by Woodbury and co-workers (Woodbury et al., 1958; Woodbury and Karler, 1960) to activation of subcortical centers by CO_2. The subcortical centers, in turn, overcome any cortical depression by CO_2 and seizures occur. The hyperexcitability of this phase of CO_2 effects is enhanced by the release of epinephrine and adrenal cortical hormones of the cortisol-type, both of which increase cortex excitability (see Woodbury and Karler, 1960, and Tenny and Lamb, 1965, for details).

Why subcortical neurons are excited more than cortical nerves is not known. Even cortical neurons are affected differently by CO_2, although the prominent effect is depression, or more correctly stabilization, secondary to hyperpolarization (Krnjević et al., 1965). Walker and Brown (1970) have shown that CO_2 can either hyperpolarize or depolarize *Aplysia* ganglion cells, depending on whether the membrane potential is more or less positive than the chloride equilibrium potential. No effect such as this has been shown in mammalian CNS. Even if some difference is found in the response to CO_2 of various CNS neurons, the complexities of the interconnected pathways in brain make simple interpretations almost impossible at present.

b. Withdrawal seizures. The clonic seizure caused by sudden withdrawal from high CO_2 concentrations has been explained as follows (Woodbury et al., 1958; Woodbury and Karler, 1960). When rats are exposed to 40 to 50% CO_2 for a few minutes, a rapid rise in Pco_2 of the cell occurs. Intracellular H^+ and HCO_3^- concentrations increase as a result of the change in cellular Pco_2 (Brodie and Woodbury, 1958). At the same time, brain intracellular Na^+ levels decreases and the ratio of Na^+ extracellular to Na^+ intracellular increases. Upon withdrawal, the Pco_2 of the cell rapidly declines but cell HCO_3^- levels remain elevated. Hence, brain cells become alkaline. Concurrently, Na^+ rapidly enters cells and decreases the elevated Na^+ ratio caused by the inhalation of high CO_2 concentrations. The influx of Na^+ into cells depolarizes the membrane and generates an action potential which, in turn, results in seizures. It is likely that a decrease of H^+ concentration in the cell decreases ionizable Ca^{++} in the cell. Since such a decrease is known to enhance the permeability of cells to Na^+, the seizures most probably are a consequence of cell pH changes.

The reader interested in more complex and sophisticated discussions of the biochemical and neurophysiological effects of CO_2 on the CNS is referred to the very complete book by Wyke (1963).

c. *Summary.* The discussion of the in-chamber seizures was empirical and essentially correlated neurophysiological observations made on brain electrical activity. It was suggested that different parts of the brain were affected differently by CO_2. The summary of withdrawal seizures mechanisms was based upon electrolyte and acid-base data obtained only from cerebral cortex. It is obvious that both biochemical and neurophysiological studies must be done together in all parts of the brain, or more exactly the entire CNS, before the biochemical and physiological events underlying seizures are understood completely.

V. ACKNOWLEDGMENTS

This investigation was supported by U.S. Public Health Service Program-Project Grant 5 PO1–NS–04533 from the National Institute of Neurological Diseases and Stroke.

The expert typing and library assistance of Mrs. Jill Jones is gratefully acknowledged.

VI. REFERENCES

Blinn, K. A., and Noell, W. K. (1949): Continuous measurement of alveolar CO_2 tension during the hyperventilation test in routine electroencephalography. *Electroencephalography and Clinical Neurophysiology,* 1:333–342.

Brodie, D. A., and Woodbury, D. M. (1958): Acid-base changes in brain and blood of rats exposed to high concentrations of carbon dioxide. *American Journal of Physiology*, 192:91–94.

Brown, E. B., Jr. (1953): Physiological effects of hyperventilation. *Physiological Reviews*, 33:445–471.

Brown, E. B., Jr. (1971a): Drugs and respiratory control. *Annual Review of Pharmacology*, 11:271–284.

Brown, E. B., Jr. (1971b): Whole body buffer capacity. In: *Ion Homeostasis of the Brain*, edited, by B. K. Siesjö and S. C. Sørensen. Munksgaard, Copenhagen, pp. 317–333.

Brown, E. B., Jr., and Miller, F. (1952): Ventricular fibrillation following a rapid fall in alveolar carbon dioxide concentration. *American Journal of Physiology*, 169:56–60.

Cassels, W. H., Becker, T. J., and Seevers, M. H. (1940): Convulsions during anesthesia, an experimental analysis of the role of hyperthermia and respiratory acidosis. *Anesthesiology*, 1:56–68.

Clowes, G. H. A., Jr., Hopkins, A. L., and Simeone, F. A. (1955): A comparison of the physiological effects of hypercapnia and hypoxia in the production of cardiac arrest. *Annals of Surgery*, 142:446–460.

Cobb, W. A. (1963): The normal adult EEG. In: *Electroencephalography*, edited by D. Hill and G. Parr. Macmillan Company, New York, pp. 232–249.

Dawson, M. E., and Greville, G. D. (1963): Biochemistry. In: *Electroencephalography*, edited by D. Hill and G. Parr. Macmillan Company, New York, pp. 147–192.

Farhi, L. E., and Rahn, H. (1960): Dynamics of changes in carbon dioxide stores. *Anesthesiology*, 21:604–614.

Gibbs, F. A., Davis, H., and Lennox, W. G. (1935): The electroencephalogram in epilepsy and in conditions of impaired consciousness. *Archives of Neurology and Psychiatry*, 34:1133–1148.

Gibbs, F. A., Gibbs, E. L., and Lennox, W. G. (1938): Cerebral dysrhythmias of epilepsy. *Archives of Neurology and Psychiatry*, 39:298–314.

Gibbs, F. A., Lennox, W. G., and Gibbs, E. L. (1936): The electroencephalogram in diagnosis and in localization of epileptic seizures. *Archives of Neurology and Psychiatry*, 36:1225–1235.

Goldberg, M. A., Barlow, C. F., and Roth, L. J. (1961): The effects of carbon dioxide on the entry and accumulation of drugs in the central nervous system. *Journal of Pharmacology and Experimental Therapeutics*, 131:308–318.

Gotoh, F., Meyer, J. S., and Takagi, Y. (1965): Cerebral effects of hyperventilation in man. *Archives of Neurology*, 12:410–423.

Granholm, L., Kaasik, A. E., Nilsson, L., and Siesjö, B. K. (1968): The lactate/pyruvate ratios of cerebrospinal fluid of rats and cats related to the lactate/pyruvate, the ATP/ADP, and the phosphocreatine/creatine ratios of brain tissue. *Acta Physiologica Scandinavica*, 74:398–409.

Granholm, L., and Siesjö, B. K. (1969): The effects of hypercapnia and hypocapnia upon the cerebrospinal fluid lactate and pyruvate concentrations and upon the lactate, pyruvate, ATP, ADP, phosphocreatine and creatine concentrations of cat brain tissue. *Acta Physiologica Scandinavica*, 75:257–266.

Granholm, L., and Siesjö, B. K. (1971): The effect of combined respiratory and nonrespiratory alkalosis on energy metabolites and acid-base parameters in the rat brain. *Acta Physiologica Scandinavica* 81:307–314.

Gyarfas, K., Pollock, G. H., and Stein, S. N. (1949): Central inhibitory effects of carbon dioxide. IV Convulsive phenomena. *Proceedings of the Society for Experimental Biology and Medicine*, 70:292–293.

Krnjević, K., Randić, M., and Siesjö, B. K. (1965): Cortical CO_2 tension and neuronal excitability. *Journal of Physiology*, 176:105–122.

Lambertsen, C. J. (1966): Drugs and respiration. *Annual Review of Pharmacology*, 6:327–378.

Leake, C. D., and Waters, R. M. (1929): The anesthetic properties of carbon dioxid. *Anesthesia and Analgesia*, 8:17–19.

Lee, J. E., Chu, F., Posner, J. B., and Plum, F. (1969): Buffering capacity of cerebrospinal fluid in acute respiratory acidosis in dogs. *American Journal of Physiology*, 217:1035–1038.

Litchfield, J. T., Jr., and Wilcoxon, F. (1949): A simplified method of evaluating dose-effect experiments. *Journal of Pharmacology and Experimental Therapeutics*, 96:99–113.

Maren, T. H. (1971): The effect of acetazolamide on HCO_3^- and Cl^- uptake into cerebrospinal fluid of cat and dogfish. In: *Ion Homeostasis of the Brain*, edited by B. K. Siesjö and S. C. Sørensen. Munksgaard, Copenhagen, pp. 290–311.

Marshall, J. R., and Lambertsen, C. J. (1961): Interactions of increased P_{O_2} and P_{CO_2} effects in producing convulsions and death in mice. *Journal of Applied Physiology*, 16:1–7.

Masoro, E. J., and Siegel, P. D. (1971): *Acid-Base Regulation: Its Physiology and Pathophysiology.* W. B. Saunders Company, Philadelphia.

Meduna, L. J., and Gyarfas, K. (1949): Motor and sensory phenomena during therapeutical CO_2 inhalations. *Diseases of the Nervous System*, 10:3–7.

Merwarth, C. R., and Sieker, H. O. (1961): Acid-base changes in blood and cerebrospinal fluid during altered ventilation. *Journal of Applied Physiology.* 16:1016–1018.

Meyer, J. S., Gotoh, F., and Tazaki, Y. (1961): CO_2 narcosis, an experimental study. *Neurology*, 11:524–537.

Meyer, J. S., and Waltz, A. G. (1960a): Arterial oxygen saturation and alveolar carbon dioxide during electroencephalography. *A.M.A. Archives of Neurology*, 2:631–643.

Meyer, J. S., and Waltz, A. G. (1960b): Arterial oxygen saturation and alveolar carbon dioxide during electroencephalography. *A.M.A. Archives of Neurology*, 2:644–656.

Morrice, J. K. W. (1956): Slow wave production in the EEG, with reference to hypernoea, carbon dioxide and autonomic balance. *Electroencephalography and Clinical Neurophysiology*, 8:49–72.

Petty, W. C., and Sulkowski, T. S. (1971): CO_2 narcosis in the rat: 1. Effects on respiration and blood parameters. *Aerospace Medicine*, 42:547–552.

Pitts, R. F. (1963): *Physiology of the Kidney and Body Fluids.* Year Book Medical Publishers, Inc., Chicago.

Plum, F., Posner, J. B., and Smith, W. W. (1968): Effect of hyperbarichyperoxic hyperventilation on blood, brain, and CSF lactate. *American Journal of Physiology*, 215:1240–1244.

Pollock, G. H. (1949): Central inhibitory effects of carbon dioxide. *Journal of Neurophysiology*, 12:315–324.

Pollock, G. H., and Bain, J. A. (1950): Convulsions in cerebellum and cerebrum induced by β-chlorinated amines. *American Journal of Physiology*, 160:195–202.

Pollock, G. H., and Wang, R. I. H. (1954): Synergistic convulsive activity of topical nitrogen mustard and carbon dioxide inhalation. *Archives Internationales de Pharmacodynamie et de Therapie*, 98:490–492.

Posner, J. B., and Plum, F. (1967): Independence of blood and cerebrospinal fluid lactate. *Archives of Neurology*, 16:492–496.

Poulsen, T. (1952): Investigations into the anesthetic properties of carbon dioxide. *Acta Pharmacologica et Toxicologica*, 8:30–46.

Reivich, M., Cohen, P. J., and Greenbaum, L. (1966): Alterations in the electroencephalogram of awake man produced by hyperventilation: Effects of 100% oxygen at 3 atmospheres (absolute) pressure. *Neurology*, 13:304.

Schwab, R. S., Grunwald, A., and Sargant, W. M. (1941): Regulation of the treatment of epilepsy by synchronized recording of respiration and brain waves. *Archives of Neurology and Psychiatry*, 46:1017–1034.

Seevers, M. H. (1944): The narcotic properties of carbon dioxide. *New York State Journal of Medicine*, 44:597 602.

Siesjö, B. K., and Messeter, K. (1971): Factors determining intracellular pH. In: *Ion Homeostasis of the Brain*, edited by B. K. Siesjö and S. C. Sørensen. Munksgaard, Copenhagen, pp. 244–262.

Siesjö, B. K., and Sørensen, S. C., Editors, (1971): *Ion Homeostasis of the Brain.* Munksgaard, Copenhagen.

Sokoloff, L. (1960): The effects of carbon dioxide on the cerebral circulation. *Anesthesiology,* 21:664–673.

Swanson, A. G., and Rosengren, H. (1962): Cerebrospinal fluid buffering during acute experimental respiratory acidosis. *Journal of Applied Physiology,* 17:812–814.

Swanson, A. G., Stavney, L. S., and Plum, F. (1958): Effects of blood pH and carbon dioxide on cerebral electrical activity. *Neurology,* 8:787–792.

Tenny, S. M., and Lamb, T. W. (1965): Physiological consequences of hypoventilation and hyperventilation. In: *Respiration,* Vol. 2, edited by W. O. Fenn and H. Rahn. American Physiological Society, Washington, D.C., pp. 979–1010.

Toman, J. E. P., and Davis, J. P. (1949): The effects of drugs upon the electrical activity of the brain. *Journal of Pharmacology and Experimental Therapeutics,* Part 2, 97:425–491.

Walker, J. L., Jr., and Brown, A. M. (1970): Unified account of the variable effects of carbon dioxide on nerve cells. *Science,* 167:1502–1504.

Withrow, C. D., Nord, N. M., Turner, L. M., Jr., and Woodbury, D. M. (1967): Carbon dioxide seizures in immature rats. *Proceedings of the Society for Experimental Biology and Medicine,* 125:288–291.

Withrow, C. D., Stout, R. J., Barton, L. J., Beacham, W. S., and Woodbury, D. M. (1968): Anticonvulsant effects of 5,5-dimethyl-2,4-oxazolidinedione (DMO). *Journal of Pharmacology and Experimental Therapeutics,* 161:335–341.

Woodbury, D. M., and Karler, R. (1960): The role of carbon dioxide in the nervous system. *Anesthesiology,* 21:686–703.

Woodbury, D. M., Rollins, L. T., Gardner, M. D., Hirschi, W. L., Hogan, J. R., Rallison, M. L., Tanner, G. S., and Brodie, D. A. (1958): Effects of carbon dioxide on brain excitability and electrolytes. *American Journal of Physiology,* 192:79–90.

Woodbury, J. W. (1965): Regulation of pH. In: *Physiology and Biophysics,* edited by T. C. Ruch and H. D. Patton. W. B. Saunders Company, Philadelphia, pp. 899–934.

Wyke, B. (1963): *Brain Function and Metabolic Disorders.* Butterworths, London.

20

Drug Withdrawal Convulsions in Animals

Carl F. Essig

OUTLINE

I. INTRODUCTION

It is well established that both man and several species of animals are liable to develop abstinence convulsions as a result of physical dependence on drugs of the alcohol-barbiturate type (Isbell et al., 1950, 1955; Essig, 1967; Essig and Lam, 1968; Victor, 1968). Physical dependence is described as an altered biological state induced by the repeated consumption of a drug, so that its use must be continued in order to prevent the emergence of a stereotyped illness known as an abstinence syndrome. In the parlance of drug abuse, sedative-hypnotic agents, minor tranquilizers, central relaxants, psychotropic agents, and others, that can induce physical dependence like that of alcohol or the barbiturates, are classified as drugs of the alcohol-barbiturate type. Such dependence can result in an abstinence syndrome marked by generalized convulsions, a delirium or both (Isbell et al., 1950, 1955; Essig, 1966a, 1967). In addition to these major features, the syndrome includes many so-called minor abstinence manifestations, but in this discussion the latter will not be emphasized.

Abstinence convulsions related to drugs of the alcohol-barbiturate type have been reported in five species of animals (mouse, rat, cat, dog, and monkey). In contrast, it is doubtful that there is a reliable animal model of opiate or opioid (synthetic opiate-like compounds) abstinence convulsions. Thus, in a tabular reference to morphine abstinence convulsions in man, monkey, dog, and rat, the term "rare" is appended (Seevers and Deneau, 1963).

The following discussion is limited to the practical aspects of reproducing seizure phenomena caused by the withdrawal of drugs of the alcohol-barbiturate type. Several reviews dealing with other experimental work in this area have been presented elsewhere (Essig, 1967; Wikler and Essig, 1970).

II. RATIONALE FOR THE USE OF ANIMAL MODELS OF DRUG WITHDRAWAL CONVULSIONS

There is a need for more information about the mechanisms underlying convulsions of various etiologies that occur in man. A better understanding of the mode of action of depressant drugs and physical dependence might be derived from basic studies of abstinence convulsions. Since many experiments on these phenomena cannot be done in man, it is useful to reproduce the condition in animals. Abstinence seizures are of theoretical interest with regard to their basic pathophysiological and possible neuro-chemical mechanisms of origin. More information about such mechanisms might be applicable in part to seizure states of other etiologies. Also, it is possible that an improved understanding of the pharmacological aspects of the problem could be important in the development of sedative drugs that would not induce physical dependence. Similarly, some new anticonvulsant drugs might be devised.

From a more practical viewpoint, abstinence convulsions in animals have been used to study various drug treatments of this condition in man (Essig and Carter, 1962; Essig et al., 1969). Such testing can be used to screen different pharmacotherapeutic agents for trial in patients or to do more controlled or basic studies of various treatments than could be done in man (Essig et al., 1969). Another applied use of studying abstinence con-vulsions in animals is that of testing depressant drugs in order to predict or confirm if they can induce physical dependence in man (Essig, 1958, 1963). Even though convulsions are not the only feature of the abstinence syn-drome, they are such an important aspect of the syndrome that they can be highly useful in such tests.

III. GENERAL METHOD OF INDUCING PHYSICAL DEPENDENCE AND DRUG WITHDRAWAL CONVULSIONS

Seevers and Tatum (1931) observed that dogs physically dependent on sodium barbital were liable to have convulsions if the drug was discontinued. Later it was reported (Fraser and Isbell, 1954) that some dogs developed bizarre behavior ("canine delirium") as well as convulsions following sodium barbital withdrawal. Subsequent to these observations, other species and different drugs have been used to induce abstinence convulsions. The gen-eral principles described here have been derived empirically. They are presented for use with drugs that have not yet been tested for their effective-ness in producing physical dependence and abstinence convulsions. More specific information about methods that already have been used for this purpose is presented in Table 1.

A. Establishing the early dosage regimen for untested drugs

Drugs of the alcohol-barbiturate type usually can induce ataxia and sleep. In estimating a dose effect, ataxia can be a helpful behavioral index.

TABLE 1. *Dosage regimens of drugs given orally to induce physical dependence and abstinence convulsions*

Species	Drug	Final dose range before abstinence (mg/kg/day)	Total days of Intoxication	Percent of animals that convulse	Reference
Dog	Sodium barbital	148–158	165–170	75%	Essig (*unpublished*)
Dog	Meproba-mate	656 to 814 divided into 3 doses daily	124–188	100%	Essig (1958)
Dog	Gluteth-imide	114–424	113–168	20%	Essig (1963)
Cat	Sodium barbital	173–279	23–217	91%	Essig and Flanary (1959)
Rat	Sodium barbital	396±53	111	100%	Essig (1966a)

Swaying or unsteadiness of the head and trunk, high steppage and/or a broad-based staggering gait are useful signs of intoxication. Such behavior is sometimes followed by sleep. At the beginning of an experiment, it is best to find a dose of the drug to be used that will cause minimal signs of ataxia or only a short interval of sleep. Such doses are repeated often enough during each 24-hr cycle to maintain some degree of drug effect throughout most of the day and night. After variable periods of drug administration, enough physical dependence develops to be useful—if necessary—in revising the daily dosage schedule. Thus, if signs of abstinence develop, the interval between doses is probably too long. An animal that is trembling, hyperactive, and sensitive to external stimuli is probably exhibiting early abstinence signs. Under these conditions, it is best to shorten the interval between doses. For example, it has been found (Essig, 1958) that meprobamate must be administered at 8-hr intervals every day, whereas sodium barbital can be given once daily.

B. Increasing the daily dosage of drug during chronic intoxication

Since the drug must be given every day, arrangements have to be made to administer it during the night (if necessary) and over weekends. The daily dose of drug is increased within the limits of maintaining the animals in good physical condition. Increasing the dose too rapidly might result in the animal's refusal to eat or drink, and prolonged periods of drug-induced sleep increase susceptibility to pneumonia. The duration of chronic intoxication varies with the drug. As a rough guide, the original dose is increased 2.5-

to 3.5-fold in 4 to 6 months. During chronic intoxication, records of dosage increases should be maintained. Body weights should be measured periodically to detect any significant weight loss which might indicate that the dose is being increased too rapidly or that the drug is toxic.

C. Preparation for withdrawal and discontinuance of the drug

Arrangements for discontinuing the drug depend on the purpose of the study. It is best to make observations that might be required prior to withdrawal, after the final dose increase has been made. Such observations include food and fluid consumption, and body weight and temperature. If indicated, blood and urine samples can be obtained to determine blood levels of drug, hemograms, and urinalyses. The animals are placed in individual cages that permit adequate observation of behavior. Well-lighted cages fitted with clear plastic fronts are useful for this purpose.

The drug must be completely and abruptly discontinued.

If the purpose of the study requires recording the occurrence of convulsions or other abnormal behavior, continuous observation should be made for the first 7 days of withdrawal. If the drug is known to be eliminated slowly, it might be necessary to extend the period of continuous observation to 10 or 12 days.

In addition to convulsions, the animals can be observed for bizarre or hallucinatory behavior, tremulousness, increased startle response, weight loss, decreased food consumption, variation in water intake, and changes in body temperature. If necessary, blood samples can be obtained to measure declining levels of the drug in relation to the occurrence of convulsions. Proper care of the animals is critical at these stages since they will not groom themselves during the withdrawal period.

IV. METHODS FOR INDUCING ABSTINENCE CONVULSIONS IN ANIMALS TO STUDY UNDERLYING MECHANISMS

Workers interested in the mechanisms underlying abstinence seizures can do basic studies in various categories such as behavioral, neurophysiological (ablation, stimulation, recording), neuroendocrinological, neurochemical, histochemical, and histological. Some of these techniques can be applied in a sequential manner during various stages of the development of physical dependence, withdrawal, and recovery. Certain animal species are more feasible for particular experimental methods. Neurochemical investigations often require quick-freezing techniques which can be done in mice and rats. Both species develop abstinence convulsions, and comparatively short periods of intoxication have been used (Crossland and Leonard, 1963; Freund, 1969).

Cats have been utilized in EEG studies of sodium barbital intoxication and withdrawal (Essig and Flanary, 1961). The cat also offers an opportunity to study petit mal-like behavior during sodium barbital withdrawal (Essig and Flanary, 1959, 1961). It is notable that evidence for physical dependence on pentobarbital has been demonstrated in cats after only 26 hr of exposure to the drug (Jaffe and Sharpless, 1965). Barbiturate abstinence convulsions have been observed in this species after such drugs have been administered for about 3 weeks (Essig and Flanary, 1959; Jaffe and Sharpless, 1965). An apparatus has been used for monitoring the occurrence of abstinence convulsions in cats (Essig and Flanary, 1957), and is probably adaptable for use in rats, but it has not proven feasible in dogs.

Dogs are probably the best species to use for experiments requiring surgical ablations. They seem better able to survive the stresses of surgery and chronic intoxication than are smaller animals. Decorticate and decerebellate dogs have been used in experimental studies of barbiturate abstinence convulsions (Essig, 1962b, 1964). Both dogs and rats are useful in testing drugs for their effectiveness in preventing barbiturate abstinence convulsions (Essig and Carter, 1962; Essig, 1968). Such experiments have been used to gain information about possible biochemical mechanisms underlying the withdrawal seizures (Essig, 1967). Rats have been utilized to study the effects of hypophysectomy or adrenalectomy on the occurrence of abstinence convulsions (Essig, *unpublished data*).

A. Methods of administering drugs to animals

Most dogs are tractable enough to receive pills or capsules orally. The drug can be incorporated in a small amount of ground meat, and the bolus is placed in the pharynx. Massaging the anterior neck seems to aid the swallowing process. If the dog tries to bite the laboratory aid when he inserts the bolus, the dog's cheeks are pressed inward posteriorly so that the dog tends to bite the inside of his cheek rather than the aid's hand. The oral administration of drugs to cats usually requires two people. One helps to hold the cat while the other places the tablet or capsule in the posterior pharynx by means of a forceps.

It has been demonstrated that laboratory rats become physically dependent on sodium barbital if it is dissolved in their drinking water (Crossland and Leonard, 1963). Fluid intake is limited to solutions containing increasing concentrations of the drug. Abstinence convulsions have been observed in rats that were exposed to this drug for 4 to 5 weeks before it was discontinued. A dietary method has been used to make mice ingest alcohol, phenobarbital, and potassium bromide (Freund, 1969, *in press*). Body weight is reduced by means of caloric deprivation, and then the drug is offered in a Metrecal ® liquid diet. It has been reported that rats maintained at 80% of their free-feeding weights will drink pentobarbital by means of schedule-induced polydipsia (Meisch, 1969). It is not known to the writer if this method can be used to induce physical dependence on drugs of the alcohol-barbiturate type.

Alcohol has been administered to dogs via surgically implanted gastric cannulae (Essig and Lam, 1968). This drug has been given to monkeys by gastric intubation (Ellis and Pick, 1969). Both methods were used to induce physical dependence and abstinence convulsions. A self-administration system has been used to give drugs to monkeys. A lever pressed by the monkey activates an injection device which delivers a measured amount of the drug intravenously. Physical dependence on drugs of the alcohol-barbiturate type has been self-induced by monkeys (Deneau et al., 1965; Woods and Schuster, 1970).

A summary of various methods of drug administration is given in Table 2.

B. Some aspects of testing drugs for their abuse liability

It has been suggested that developers of new drugs of certain chemical classes be asked to test such agents in dogs and one other animal species (Isbell, 1959). Dogs have proven most reliable for this purpose since they become physically dependent on the same drugs that man does. Moreover, the abstinence syndromes — including convulsions — also parallel those seen in man. Dogs become dependent on alcohol, sodium barbital, pentobarbital, meprobamate, and glutethimide (Seever and Tatum, 1931; Frazer and Isbell, 1954; Essig, 1958, 1963; Essig and Lam, 1968).

In such tests, groups of 10 to 12 dogs are given the drug orally in increasing doses for long periods as already outlined. A sincere and concerted attempt is made to induce physical dependence. This might mean giving the drug up to 6 months in final daily amounts which are quite large. Such high dosages can be justified because some patients also increase their daily doses to exhorbitant levels. After the drug is discontinued, continuous observations for abstinence signs must be carried out for at least a week. Failure to detect abstinence signs or convulsions sometimes reflects sporadic or random rather than continuous observation. One limita-

TABLE 2. *Methods of inducing abstinence convulsions for their investigation in animals*

Species	Drug used	Duration of intoxication	Final dose range of drug	Special methods of administering drug	Abstinence convulsions	Reference
Mouse (ICR-DUB)	Ethanol	4 days	Alcohol blood levels of 400–650 mg/100 ml	Weight-reduced mice consumed liquid diet with 35% of calories derived from ethanol	In 60–95%	Freund (1969)
Mouse	Phenobarbital	4 days	218 mg/kg (mean)	0.30 mg phenobarbital per ml of liquid diet (½ Metrecal® ½ water)	In 87%	Freund (*in press*)
Mouse	Potassium bromide	4–6 days	1,930–2,710 mg/kg/day	4–5 mg KBr/ml of undiluted Metrecal® (liquid)	In 83–100%	Freund (*in press*)
Rat	Sodium barbital	4–5 weeks	280–400 mg/kg/day	Drug dissolved in drinking water as only source of fluid	Yes (%?)	Crossland and Leonard (1963)
Cat	Pentobarbital	2–3 weeks	86–110 mg/kg (?)	Intravenous injection 3–4 × daily to induce surgical anesthesia	Yes (%?)	Jaffe and Sharpless (1965)
Dog (mongrel beagle)	Ethanol	57 days	7.6–11.1 ml/kg of 95% alcohol divided in 4 doses daily	Alcohol (20% v/v) injected into stomach via surgically implanted cannula	In 83%	Essig and Lam (1968)
Monkey	Ethanol	10–18 days	4–8 g/kg/day mean daily dose	Gastric intubation of 25% (w/v) alcohol in 2 or 3 daily doses	In 80%	Ellis and Pick (1970)
Monkey	Pentobarbital	15 days	550–700 mg/kg/day	Self administration by animal pressing a lever to deliver 5 mg/kg doses intravenously	Yes (%?)	Woods and Schuster (1970)

tion of this method is the inability of dogs to survive chronic intoxication as the dose is increased. In the case of glutethimide, 5 of 10 dogs died during the course of chronic intoxication (Essig, 1963). Such a high death rate did not occur during chronic meprobamate or sodium barbital intoxication (Essig, 1963).

The rat might be used to supplement the dog in such studies. It seems feasible to use the method of limiting water intake to increasingly concentrated solutions of the drug (Crossland and Leonard, 1963). This method might require less time than chronic intoxication studies in dogs (Essig, 1966a). However, such an approach is limited to drugs that are soluble enough in water to supply increasing amounts of drug within the limits of daily fluid requirements.

Drug self-administration by monkeys might become an important technique in testing drugs for their abuse liability in man. In general, monkeys will press a lever to inject themselves repeatedly with some drugs but not others. Thus far, drugs selected for self-injection correspond to those abused by man. Such drugs are termed "reinforcers," and the importance of psychic rather than physical dependence is emphasized (Yanagita et al., 1965; Deneau et al., 1965; Woods and Schuster, 1970).

C. Episodic and seizure behaviors other than generalized convulsions during drug withdrawal

Focal clonic seizures as well as generalized convulsions occur following barbiturate withdrawal in small dogs. Aluminum hydroxide had been injected into a focal area of one cerebral cortex prior to chronic intoxication and withdrawal (Essig, 1962a). Partial as well as major seizures occurred in some Wistar rats following withdrawal of sodium barbital. During such partial seizures, the rat's forelegs are off the floor, and its head, face and forelegs undergo twitching movements (Essig, 1966a). Episodic behavior reminiscent of "running fits" has been observed in rats following sodium barbital withdrawal. In some cases, an auditory stimulus results in violent running activity (Crossland and Leonard, 1963).

Petit mal-like movements have been described in cats following withdrawal of sodium barbital. Such behavior occurs during periods of inactivity when the cats appear drowsy but unable to sleep. Under these conditions, repetitive eyelid blinking is associated with slight head jerking or facial twitching. Some cats develop a single myoclonic jerk after their eyelids had been closed momentarily (Essig and Flanary, 1959). Episodic, sham rage behavior has been observed in dogs that had both cerebral

TABLE 3. *Episodic and seizure-like behavior (plus convulsions) following sodium barbital withdrawal*

Species	Description of behaviors	Special treatment	Period intoxicated	Final dose range of sodium barbital (mg/kg/day)	Reference
Small dogs	Focal myoclonic jerks of extremities opposite cortical lesion (epilepsia-partialis continuans)	Aluminum hydroxide lesion of cerebral cortex	125 days	177–186	Essig (1962a)
Cats	Petit mal-like behavior especially when drowsy: 1) Rhythmic blinks of eyelids and slight jerks of head or facial twitches. 2) Single generalized myoclonic jerk.	None	23–217 days	173–278	Essig and Flanary (1959, 1961)
Albino rats	Wild running—especially in response to auditory stimulation	None	4–5 weeks	280–400	Crossland and Leonard (1963)
Wistar rats	Twitching movements of head, face, forelegs while sitting on hind legs	None	111 days	396±53	Essig (1966a)
Dog	Episodes of violent non-convulsive motor activity or "sham rage" behavior	Bilateral cerebral decortication	262–372 days	190–248	Essig (1962b)

cortices removed prior to chronic sodium barbital intoxication and withdrawal (Essig, 1962*a*).

Methods used to obtain the various abstinence behavioral phenomena described here are summarized in Table 3.

V. SOME LIMITATIONS OF THE RESEARCH METHOD ON THE CONVULSIVE PROCESS

It is unfortunate that more quantitative data are not available on the relative importance of the variables involved in the development of physical dependence and the occurrence of abstinence convulsions. Instead, the method has evolved in an empirical way without controlled experiments on the relative importance of such variables as duration of intoxication, rate of dosage increase, and final dosage. There is some indication in cats that the final dosage range of sodium barbital is an important factor in the subsequent development of abstinence convulsions. Thus, at the end of intoxication, over 95% of cats that had received daily 173 mg/kg or larger doses of sodium barbital had one or more convulsions when the drug was discontinued (Essig and Flanary, 1959). There is also some clinical evidence that the occurrence of abstinence convulsions is related to the dose of barbiturate that was being taken when the drug was discontinued (Fraser et al., 1958). It seems likely that the final daily dosage attained is more directly related to the occurrence of abstinence convulsions than is the total time of exposure to the drug.

Swinyard et al. (1957) and Chin and Swinyard (1958) have developed a useful graphical method of presenting quantitative correlations between withdrawal hyperexcitability (expressed as a ratio of the electroshock seizure thresholds in the drug group to those in the control group of animals) and the temporal course of drug administration and withdrawal.

The objection that prolonged periods of intoxication are required can no longer be sustained. It has been reported that the threshold for pentylenetetrazol (Metrazol®) seizures was decreased when pentobarbital was discontinued after 26 hr of administration (Jaffe and Sharpless, 1965). Abstinence convulsions have been observed after 4 days to several weeks of intoxication in mice, rats, and cats (Crossland and Leonard, 1963; Jaffe and Sharpless, 1965; Freund, 1969). If a continuous supply of animals ready for withdrawal is needed, it is possible to start one or more of them on the drug at appropriate intervals.

Some animals die during the period of chronic intoxication. The death rate in cats during chronic sodium barbital intoxication can be excessive. Wistar rats that drink increasing concentrations of sodium barbital have a modest death rate. Dogs that receive sodium barbital on a chronic basis seldom die.

Those interested in basic studies of abstinence seizures should be aware of variations that occur under these conditions. All of the animals do not have convulsions, and even those that do vary considerably in the number of seizures they develop. Perhaps such variations have potential advantages in that finding methods of counteracting them might help reveal some of the mechanisms underlying the seizure process.

Experimental animals sometimes die during withdrawal. This seems to be more prevalent in animals that develop status epilepticus. Depending on the experimental design, it might be well to make several preparations if electrodes are to be implanted or if other special techniques are required. In experiments related to mechanisms of seizure onset, the occurrence of status epilepticus might be advantageous if repeated convulsions occurred before death. Thus, animals that develop the usual number of abstinence convulsions do so randomly or unpredictably. This can be a handicap in experiments designed to study the onset of such seizures. Again, the development of methods designed to trigger abstinence convulsions might help reveal their mode of onset.

VI. REFERENCES

Chin, L., and Swinyard, E. A. (1958): Tolerance and withdrawal hyperexcitability induced in mice by chronic administration of Phenaglycodol®. *Proceedings of the Society for Experimental Biology and Medicine,* 97:251–254.

Crossland, J., and Leonard, B. E. (1963): Barbiturate withdrawal convulsions in the rat. *Biochemical Pharmacology,* Suppl. 12:103.

Deneau, G. A., Yanagita, T., and Seevers, M. H. (1965): Psychic dependence studies in self-administration techniques in the rhesus monkey. *Committee on Problems of Drug Dependence,* NAS-NRC appendix 21:4267–4269.

Ellis, F. W., and Pick, J. R. (1970): Experimentally induced ethanol dependence in rhesus monkeys. *Journal of Pharmacology and Experimental Therapeutics,* 175:88–93.

Essig, C. F. (1958): Withdrawal convulsions in dogs following chronic meprobamate intoxication. *Archives of Neurology,* 80:414–417.

Essig, C. F. (1962a): Focal convulsions during barbiturate abstinence in dogs with cerebrocortical lesions. *Psychopharmacologia,* 3:432–437.

Essig, C. F. (1962b): Convulsive and sham rage behaviors in decorticate dogs during barbiturate withdrawal. *A.M.A. Archives of Neurology,* 7:471–475.

Essig, C. F. (1963): Addictive and possible toxic properties of glutethimide. *American Journal of Psychiatry,* 119:993.

Essig, C. F. (1964): Barbiturate withdrawal convulsions in decerebellate dogs. *International Journal of Pharmacology,* 3:453–456.

Essig, C. F. (1966*a*): Barbiturate withdrawal in white rats. *International Journal of Pharmacology*, 5:103–107.

Essig, C. F. (1966*b*): Newer sedative drugs that can cause states of intoxication and dependence of barbiturate type. *Journal of the American Medical Association*, 196:714–717.

Essig, C. F. (1967): Clinical and experimental aspects of barbiturate withdrawal convulsions. *Epilepsia*, 8:21–30.

Essig, C. F. (1968): Possible relation of brain gamma-aminobutyric acid (GABA) to barbiturate abstinence convulsions. *Archives Internationales de Pharmacodynamie et de Thérapie*, 176:97–103.

Essig, C. F., and Carter, W. W. (1962): Failure of diphenylhydantoin in preventing barbiturate withdrawal convulsions in the dog. *Neurology*, 12:481–484.

Essig, C. F., and Flanary, H. G. (1957): An activity method of recording generalized convulsions in experimental animals. *Electroencephalography and Clinical Neurophysiology*, 9:348.

Essig, C. F., and Flanary, H. G. (1959): Convulsions in cats following withdrawal of sodium barbital. *Experimental Neurology*, 1:529–533.

Essig, C. F., and Flanary, H. G. (1961): Convulsive aspects of barbital sodium withdrawal in the cat. *Experimental Neurology*, 3:149–159.

Essig, C. F., Jones, B. E., and Lam, R. C. (1969): The effect of pentobarbital on alcohol withdrawal in dogs. *Archives of Neurology*, 20:554–558.

Essig, C. F., and Lam, R. C. (1968): Convulsions and hallucinatory behavior following alcohol withdrawal in the dog. *Archives of Neurology*, 18:626–632.

Fraser, H. F., and Isbell, H. (1954): Abstinence syndrome in dogs after chronic barbiturate medication. *Journal of Pharmacology and Experimental Therapeutics*, 112:261–267.

Fraser, H. F., Wikler, A., Essig, C. F., and Isbell, H. (1958): Degree of physical dependence induced by secobarbital or pentobarbital. *Journal of the American Medical Association*, 166:126–129.

Freund, G. (1969): Alcohol withdrawal syndrome in mice. *Archives of Neurology*, 21:315–320.

Freund, G. (*in press*): Alcohol, barbiturate and bromide withdrawal syndromes in mice. In: *Recent Advances in Studies of Alcohol*. Edited by N. K. Mello and J. H. Mendelson. U.S. Govt. Printing Office, Washington.

Isbell, H. (1959): Addiction to hypnotic and sedative drugs. *Association of Food and Drug Officials of the United States*. 23:35–43.

Isbell, H., Altschul, S., Kornetsky, C. H., Eisenman, A. J., and Fraser, H. F. (1950): Chronic barbiturate intoxication. An experimental study. *A.M.A. Archives of Neurology*, 64:1–28.

Isbell, H., Fraser, H. F., Wikler, A., Belleville, R. E., and Eisenman, A. J. (1955): An experimental study of the etiology of 'rum fits' and delirium tremens. *Quarterly Journal of Studies on Alcohol*, 16:1–33.

Jaffe, J. H., and Sharpless, S. K. (1965): The rapid development of physical dependence on barbiturates. *Journal of Pharmacology and Experimental Therapeutics*, 150:140–145.

Meisch, R. A. (1969): Self-administration of pentobarbital by means of schedule-induced polydipsia. *Psychonomic Science*, 16:16–17.

Seevers, M. H., and Deneau, G. A. (1963): Physiological aspects of tolerance and physical dependence. In: *Physiological Pharmacology*, Vol. 1, part A, edited by W. S. Root and F. G. Hoffman. Academic Press, New York, pp. 535–540.

Seevers, M. H., and Tatum, A. L. (1931): Chronic experimental barbital poisoning. *Journal of Pharmacology and Experimental Therapeutics*, 42:217–231.

Swinyard, E. A., Chin, L., and Fingl, E. (1957): Withdrawal hyperexcitability following chronic administration of meprobamate to mice. *Science*, 125:739–741.

Victor, M. (1968): The pathophysiology of alcoholic epilepsy. *Proceedings of the Association for Research in Nervous and Mental Diseases*, 46:431–454.

Wikler, A., and Essig, C. F. (1970): Withdrawal seizures following chronic intoxication with barbiturates and other sedative drugs. In: *Epilepsy (Modern Problems of Pharmacopsychiatry)* Vol. 4, edited by E. Niedermeyer. Karger, Basel, pp. 170–184.

Woods, J. H., and Schuster, C. R. (1970): Regulation of drug self-administration. In: *Drug Dependence*, edited by R. T. Harris, W. M. McIsaac, and C. R. Schuster. University of Texas Press, Austin, pp. 158–169.

Yanagita, T., Deneau, G. A., and Seevers, M. H. (1965): Evaluation of pharmacologic agents in the monkey by long-term intravenous self- or programmed administration. *Excerpta Medica International Congress Series*, 87:453–457.

21

Phylogenetic Correlations

Z. Servít

OUTLINE

I. BASIC IDEAS ON THE COMPARATIVE (PHYLOGENETIC) APPROACH TO THE PHYSIOPATHOLOGY OF EPILEPTIC PHENOMENA

The evolutionary theory is one of the foundations of modern biology. In the last century it influenced almost all branches of biological sciences in various ways and to different degrees.

In biological studies, the evolutionary approach may be applied in two ways. Development can be studied in order to bring insight into the laws governing evolution. On the other hand, the follow-up of phylogenetic development may be used as a method of research for a better understanding of biological structure and function under normal and pathological conditions at the highest levels of evolution—in higher mammals and in man.

In this case the basic methodology may be deduced from the following idea: a complex structure may be better understood if we follow its phylogenetic development from the simple to the complex. An analogy and, at the same time, an experimental model of a complex function may be found in a simpler form at lower stages of evolution of this structure, where it can be analyzed more easily. At the same time differences, evolutionary changes of a certain structure and/or function, may be followed and compared at different levels of phylogeny (comparative approach). From these comparative observations, conclusions may be drawn concerning the relations between structure and function of the organ under observation.

At present, the terms "evolutionary" and "comparative" are used without specification. Perhaps "evolutionary" should be applied in studies where mechanisms of evolution are the aim of the study, and "comparative" could be reserved for all other studies where the evolutionary approach is used as a method for other research aims.

In neurology, anatomy has gained most from the application of this evolutionary method. Much of the knowledge we have today of the anatomy of the human brain is based on comparative studies. Comparative neurophysiology has also developed into a separate and important branch of science. In physiopathology of the nervous system the comparative approach has been applied to a much smaller extent. This may be connected with some controversial opinions concerning the use of experimental models in physiopathology and medicine.

In medical research we often encounter the opinion that the best model of man is man himself. When we are obliged (because of ethical restrictions) to use experimental animals, the most suitable are those which can reproduce the human "original" with the highest fidelity. In my opinion, this cannot be accepted as a general rule. Man is not always the best experimental subject. It is not only for ethical reasons that we use experimental animals. One of the purposes of using an experimental model is to simplify a complex situation. The best model is the simplest one which can reproduce the function to be studied with sufficient fidelity.

There are, of course, functions, structures, or even organs that are unique in man or higher mammals. These cannot be studied in their full complexity at lower levels of phylogeny. It is one of the tasks of the comparative approach to single out these qualitative differences. The mammalian neocortex may be an example here.

Even in the case of qualitative differences, however, some structural principles and/or some components of the complex function may appear or remain unchanged at different levels of evolution. Comparative morphology and physiology should uncover such similarities. Collateral and recurrent inhibition may serve as an example of a functional principle which was developed at rather primitive stages of phylogeny of the forebrain cortex and which remained equally valid for the mammalian neocortex.

By discovering such similarities and differences, as well as by comparing the function and morphological organization at each level of evolution, a more profound insight into and a more rational explanation of a complex function may be acquired at the highest levels of phylogeny. Of course, it should be remembered that the comparative approach is the very methodical principle of comparative physiology and that man is also a link in the phylogenetic line and, perhaps, the top of our family tree.

In medical research all comparative studies must eventually lead to human physiology and physiopathology. When this is accomplished, another important contribution of comparative physiology emerges. We must realize that all animal experiments (even experiments on higher mammals) are in principle comparative studies at lower stages of phylogeny. We can interpret them correctly with regard to medical requirements only in the case when we appreciate fully the place of our experimental model on the phylogenetic scale, its similarities and differences in comparison with the human organism. The reconstructions of the important stages, pathways and crossroads of phylogeny may thus aid in rightly interpreting our experiments.

II. SOME CHARACTERISTIC FEATURES OF EXPERIMENTAL MODELS DERIVED FROM THE INFRAMAMMALIAN STAGES OF BRAIN PHYLOGENY

Because experimental models derived from higher (mammalian) stages of brain phylogeny are extensively treated in other chapters of this volume, attention in this chapter will be directed toward the reproduction of epileptic phenomena in the brains of inframammalian vertebrates. These animals (sometimes not quite adequately called "lower vertebrates") have, from the experimental point of view, some common properties which may be both advantageous and disadvantageous in experimental work.

One of the advantages is the more modest requirements for maintaining the inner homeostasis of the brain. The brains of fish, amphibia, and reptiles are much less sensitive to oxygen lack than the mammalian brain. In amphibia (frogs), body surface respiration is usually sufficient to last for several hours. We can work on curarized animals without artificial respiration. Reptiles can easily be ventilated orally. The vitality of the brain is rather high. This makes it possible to work on the brain exposed by a large trephine opening, or even using isolated heads or brains (or parts of brains) for experimentation under very simple experimental conditions. On the other hand, experiments can also be done under the same conditions as in mammals on freely moving animals with implanted electrodes.

Basic methodological information dealing with electrophysiological experimental work on brains of submammalian vertebrates can be found in the following papers.

Acute experiments

(a) Fish: Schadé and Weiler (1959); Strejčková (1969); Servít and Strejčková (1970)
(b) Frogs: Caspers and Winkel (1952); Servít et al. (1965, 1966*b*, 1968)
(c) Reptiles: Winkel and Caspers (1953); Orrego (1961); Belekhova (1963); Karamyan et al. (1966); Volanschi and Servít (1969*a,b*)

Chronic experiments with implanted electrodes

(a) Fish: Peyrethon (1968)
(b) Frogs (toads): Segura and Juan (1966); Hobson (1967)
(c) Reptiles: Peyrethon (1968); Tauber et al. (1968)

Isolated head

(a) Fish: Buser (1955)
(b) Frogs: Buser (1955); Takagi and Shibuya (1960)
(c) Turtles: Vasilescu (1970)

Isolated brain

(a) Fish: Strejčková (1969)
(b) Frogs (toads): Libet and Gérard (1939); Watanabe and Matsumoto (1968)

Inframammalian vertebrates are poikilotherms. (Birds, being on a side branch of the phylogenetic tree, are not strictly speaking "inframammalian.") This enables us to modify easily their body temperature by changing the temperature of the external environment and to study the influence of temperature on brain functions.

On the other hand, lower dependence of the brain upon oxygen supply and the dependence of body temperature upon external environment indicate rather important metabolic differences between the mammalian and inframammalian brains. Because these differences are poorly understood at present, the brains of these animals cannot be used as models for metabolic studies relevant for mammals and man. For the same reason, pharmacological studies should be interpreted with caution.

Another important advantage of using the brain of lower vertebrates lies in its simpler structural organization, which enables it to be used as a simplified model of a more complex brain. This simplicity appears not only in the inner organization, but also in the gross anatomy of the brain. For instance, in fish and frog and for a great part also in reptiles, the original anatomical sequence of individual brain levels is preserved, the telencephalon, diencephalon, mesencephalon, and rhombencephalon being situated one after another in the rostro-caudal order. Here we do not have to deal with anatomical distortions and overlappings which complicate the surgery and placement of electrodes in the mammalian brain. This (together with the great vitality of the brain) makes it possible to separate relatively easily or to eliminate individual brain structures, as well as to introduce electrodes into them under visual control without stereotactic equipment. In the frog, for instance, we may easily separate the forebrain from the thalamus and hypothalamus and work on a *télencéphale isolé* preparation (Servít et al., 1966*b*).

A disadvantage of the lower vertebrates (at least of the great majority of those generally used for experimentation) is the very small size of their brains, which usually necessitates a rather elaborate technique.

The most important structural differences between individual animal species will be discussed in the next section in connection with problems encountered when choosing representatives of different zoological classes for comparative studies.

III. CHOICE OF MODELS

The choice of an appropriate experimental model should primarily be influenced by the problems to be solved. The main aspects of epileptology which can be studied at present in comparative studies will be discussed in more detail below. These can be divided into two groups.

(A) In the first group, the influence of the external environment and of living conditions of the animal are observed in relation to seizure susceptibility and the stimuli which are able to evoke seizures. These are not phylogenetic studies in the strict sense of the word, because in this case ecology of the animal plays the major role in the choice of a suitable model. The actual stage of phylogenetic development of the brain plays only a secondary role here. The influence of nourishment on seizure susceptibility and the role of the epileptogenic stimulus in triggering seizures are the main problems in this category.

A few examples may be given here for illustration. Audiogenic epilepsy of rodents is a typical form of sensory or reflex epilepsy. Special strains of rats or mice are mainly used as experimental models, but wild rats are also sensitive. The disposition of these animals can be influenced genetically and by different metabolic factors. However, this special susceptibility may be caused in the first place by the extreme sensitivity of the acoustic apparatus of these rodents which is related to their special ecology (life in the dark). (For review, see Busnel, 1963; Servít, 1963). Another example of the special sensitivity to an epileptogenic stimulus may be photogenic epilepsy in baboons (Killam et al., 1966; see also Naquet and Meldrum, this volume).

As an example of epilepsy caused primarily by components of nourishment observed predominantly in dogs, the so-called glutene or methionine sulfoximine epilepsy may be considered. Ecological metabolic differences may probably play a role in the special sensitivity of different animal species to the toxic agent, the phylogenetic level of brain development being of secondary significance (for review, see Servít, 1963).

(B) The second group of epileptological problems concerns the relations between structure and functional organization of the brain on the one hand and disposition to the genesis of epileptic phenomena and their symptomatology on the other. In these problems the phylogenetic approach, i.e., the study of structural and functional organization of the brain in relation to the location of the experimental animal in the phylogenetic tree, should be crucial in the choice of the model. Of course, the ecology of the animal must also be considered in this case since it represents a major factor in phylogeny.

The main task of the experimenter is not to "reconstruct," more or less adequately, the phylogenetic family tree of the human brain (this being impossible, in any case, from the living representatives of vertebrates), but to choose animals whose brains represent important steps in brain evolution, i.e., significant changes in organization of the brain which could play a role in the origin, course or symptomatology of the epileptic process.

This depends in the first place on the actual level of our knowledge of comparative anatomy and physiology and may be rather difficult in special cases, since the problems of homology or analogy of brain structures at different levels of development are far from being elucidated.

In addition to the classical work of Kappers (1947), Herrick (1956), and Kuhlenberg (1967), pertinent information concerning evolutionary anatomy and physiology (especially electrophysiology) of inframammalian vertebrates may be found in the following monographs and papers.

Monographic works on brain physiology and anatomy
Guselnikov (1965); Karamyan (1970).

Special papers
(a) Arterial blood supply of the brain: Gillilan (1967)
(b) Fish — anatomy: Sheldon (1912); Ingle (1968)
    — electrophysiology: Schadé and Weiler (1959)
(c) Amphibia — anatomy: Hoffmann (1963); Lazár and Székely (1969)
    — electrophysiology: Segura and Juan (1966); Hobson (1967)
(d) Reptiles — anatomy: Bishop (1957, 1961); Kruger (1969); Hall and Ebner (1970)
    — electrophysiology: Orrego (1961); Belekhova (1963); Karamyan et al. (1966)

I have tried to summarize some data which seem of importance for comparative epileptology in Tables 1 and 2.

A simplified scheme of a part of the development of the vertebrate brain is outlined in Table 1. The scheme should not be considered as a "phylogenetic family tree," but as an attempt to outline some important features of brain development from the representatives of recent, living animals.

A direct evolutionary line leads from cyclostomes through amphibia and reptiles to mammals. It is characterized by two important features: by a progressive integration of the brain into a functionally unified organ and by the transposition of the leading integrative structures rostrally into the forebrain. Projection of afferent pathways from all receptors into a single brain structure, i.e., the neocortex, differentiation of afferent pathways into the specific and nonspecific ones, and transformation of the forebrain (especially the thalamocortical complex) into an organ processing information from different receptors play a major role here.

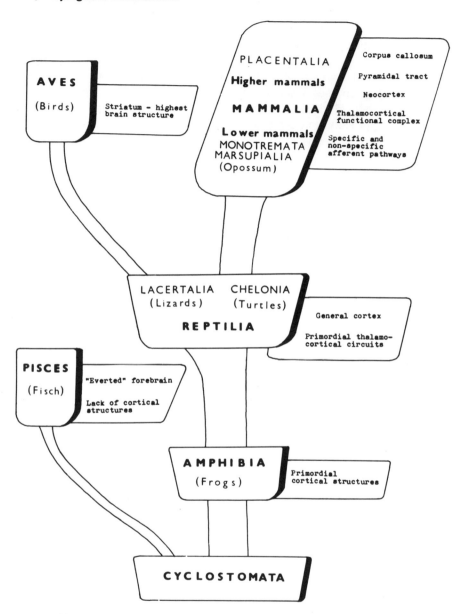

TABLE 1. Simplified outline of development of the vertebrate brain.

At lower, inframammalian stages of evolution, the brain is much less functionally integrated than in mammals. In communication with the external world, some of the sense organs usually play a leading role and determine the behavioral reactions of the animal rather independently. This has been proved in reflexological studies (Guselnikov, 1965; Sergeev, 1965).

In cyclostomes and fish, the principal brain centers are situated in the rhombencephalon and mesencephalon. The leading sense organs are chemoreceptors (in some fish they are spread over a large part of the body surface) and the receptors of the lateral line with corresponding centers in the medulla, and, in some species, the optic sense with its highest center in the midbrain (superior colliculus–tectum opticum). The communication of lower brain parts with the forebrain, which is primarily the olfactory brain, is rather poor here. The projection of optic and other afferent pathways into the forebrain does not exist or is functionally without significance.

Fish are situated on a side branch of the mammalian family tree. Their forebrain differs structurally from the brain of cyclostomes and amphibia. It was probably formed by a process of "eversion" (in comparison with the "inverted" forebrain of other vertebrates) and lacks any layered structure of the cortical type completely.

In amphibia, the leading brain part is the optic centers in the midbrain. The first steps of ascending communication from the midbrain through the diencephalon to the forebrain (primordium hippocampi) have been demonstrated using evoked potentials (see Orrego, 1961; Karamyan et al., 1966; Guselnikov, 1965). Nevertheless, the functional integration of the brain is still very poor. Amphibia (frogs) do not have any behavioral and/or electroencephalographical signs of "integrated" sleep (i.e., simultaneous suppression of activity of all structures which are decisive for the communication with the external environment; Hobson, 1967). A primitive two-layer cortical structure is formed in the dorsolateral part of the amphibian forebrain, especially in the primordial pyriform cortex. There is no white matter below it; all afferent and efferent pathways are situated in the superficial molecular layer.

Reptiles are situated on an important cross-road of evolutionary pathways. The "mammalian" line is characterized by progressive corticalization, the point of integration being transposed into the thalamocortical complex of the brain (see Hall and Ebner, 1970).

The side line of birds represents another variety of the evolutionary process in which the striatum represents the leading integrative center, the role of the thalamocortical complex being of secondary order. *La-*

certalia (lizards) may already be placed in this line, whereas *Chelonia* (turtles) are on the more direct line of phylogeny of the mammalian brain.

At the same time, reptiles represent an important step in brain phylogeny, in which the first signs of thalamocortical cooperation of the mammalian type can be seen. A new cortical structure appears in the dorsal forebrain wall – the general cortex (Crosby, 1917; Smith, 1910; Kruger and Berkowitz, 1960; Kruger 1969; Hall and Ebner, 1970). It is inserted between the primordium hippocampi medially and pyriform cortex laterally. Afferent optic, acoustic, and somatosensory pathways are terminated here, most of them probably having diencephalic (thalamic) relays. The origin, homology, and functional significance of this cortical region is still under discussion (see Bishop, 1957, 1961; Kruger, 1969; Hall and Ebner, 1970). Most probably the general cortex plays a role of an associative region, where the first steps of correlating different sensory information takes place. Direct thalamocortical connections of this region have recently been proved (Hall and Ebner, 1970).

There exist conflicting opinions about the specific and nonspecific nature of these afferent pathways (see Bishop, 1961; Guselnikov, 1965; Mazurskaya and Smirnov, 1966; Karamyan et al., 1966; Karamyan, 1970). It seems most probable that at this stage of phylogeny cortical afferent pathways are not yet differentiated into specific and nonspecific channels. They may, however, also operate as nonspecific afferent pathways of the mammalian neocortex in modulating the reactivity of forebrain structures (Karamyan et al., 1966; Karamyan, 1970).

As in the mammalian brain, thalamocortical circuits could also be demonstrated electrophysiologically in turtles. Recruiting potentials could be elicited in the general cortex by rhythmic stimulation of thalamic structures (Belekhova, 1963; Servít and Strejčková, 1972). Spontaneous electrographic spindles appear under certain conditions in this cortical region, which could be recorded simultaneously in the thalamus and triggered from thalamic structures with single stimuli (Volanschi and Servít, 1969*a,b;* Servít et al., 1971; Servít and Stréjčková, 1972).

The existence and character of sleep in reptiles still remain an open question (Tauber et al., 1968; Peyrethon, 1968). Reptiles probably do not sleep in the "mammalian" manner (do not have "integrated sleep"). Nevertheless, some electrographic correlates (e.g., electrographic spindles) indicate the presence of certain functional patterns (dealing with the activity of thalamocortical circuits) which are included in the mechanisms of sleep at higher levels of phylogeny.

Inframammalian vertebrates do not have lemniscal (specific) afferent pathways, true specific sensory (projection) areas in the forebrain cortex, the pyramidal efferent tract and corpus callosum.* All direct commissural pathways between forebrain hemispheres are homologous to the mammalian hippocampal commissures. The lowest mammals (*Marsupialia*) also lack a corpus callosum, the neopallial regions of their brains being joined only with the commissura anterior (see Putnam et al., 1968, in a study on *Didelphis virginiana*). On the other hand, both forebrain hemispheres are connected in amphibia and more extensively in turtles by multineuronal pathways leading through subcortical regions (Servít, 1970).

In this very simplified outline, some features of brain evolution have been stressed which could be significant in epileptogenesis. These are: the appearance of a laminar cortical structure (absent in fish, present in its sim-

TABLE 2. *Three classes of vertebrates convenient for comparative epileptological studies. Structural and functional characteristics of their brains.*

	Fish (Teleostean fish)	Amphibians (Frogs)	Reptiles (Turtles)
Localization of leading brain structures	Rhombencephalon Mesencephalon	Mesencephalon	Mesencephalon Diencephalon Telencephalon
Characteristic features of the forebrain	"Everted" forebrain Lack of laminar cortical structures Predominantly olfactory function of the telencephalon Poor connections with diencephalic and mesencephalic structures (mostly descendent)	Primordial cortical structures (no white matter below cortex) Predominantly olfactory function of the telencephalon, first optic and somatosensory projections to the hippocampus First signs of thalamocortical cooperation	Primordial cortical structures (formation of white matter) Origin of the general cortex with optic, somatosensory and acoustic projections (specific and non-specific afferent systems not yet differentiated) Origin of thalamocortical functional complex
General functional characteristics		Brain poorly integrated No sleep	First signs of functional integration Some electrographic signs of sleep

---

*Editor's Note: The reader is encouraged to examine a further analysis of this problem in Nauta, W. J. H., and Karten, H., in: *The Neurosciences: A Second Study Program.* Rockefeller University Press, New York, 1970, pp. 7–26.

plest form in amphibia), emergence of an associative general cortex in the forebrain, and emergence of the thalamocortical functional complex (absent in amphibia, present in turtles in a primitive form).

From this point of view, three classes of lower vertebrates seem to be especially convenient for comparative epileptological studies: fish, amphibia, and turtles. Some functional and structural characteristics of their brains are summarized in Table 2.

IV. SELECTED PROBLEMS OF PATHOPHYSIOLOGY OF EPILEPSY IN WHICH THE COMPARATIVE APPROACH MAY BE USEFUL

In this section, I review some problems which seem to be especially convenient for comparative pathophysiological studies, and deal with these together in a short review of results already achieved in this field.

The factors involved in the pathogenesis of epilepsy may be divided into three groups: epileptogenic stimulus, epileptic focus, and seizure susceptibility (Servít, 1959, 1962).

Seizure susceptibility—i.e., the tendency of brain structures to exhibit paroxysmal autorhythmic synchronized activity—may have cellular and structural components dealing with the predisposition of the neuronal membrane toward autorhythmic activity and structural prerequisites for the genesis of epileptic neuronal aggregates (Jasper, 1969; Ajmone Marsan, 1969).

Problems of the epileptogenic stimulus (i.e., the stimulus precipitating the seizure) deal more with the ecology of the animal than strictly with brain phylogeny (i.e., the development of the functional organization of the brain).

Seizure susceptibility may be defined as a general disposition of the whole brain to generalized paroxysmal reactions. Generalized seizures in experiments are usually elicited by so-called diffuse stimuli—electrical (electroshock) or pharmacological (systemic application of convulsive drugs). When these stimuli are applied, many cerebral structures are simultaneously invaded by the epileptogenic agent, while several regulatory mechanisms of the brain acting against seizure genesis and irradiation are suddenly broken down. This general seizure susceptibility can be measured by determining the paroxysmal (seizure) threshold. This method is often used in pharmacological experiments. Comparative studies have been published proving that this general seizure susceptibility to diffuse electrical and pharmacological stimuli increases in the phylogenetic scale of the vertebrate brain (Servít, 1959, 1962, 1963; Fig. 1).

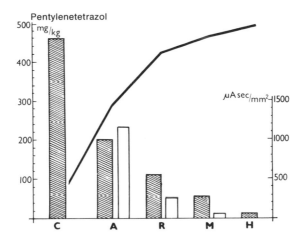

FIG. 1. Phylogenetic development of seizure susceptibility. *Shaded columns:* seizure threshold to pentylenetetrazol. *White columns:* seizure threshold to electroshock (expressed in
density of electric current per mm² of brain tissue). *C:* cyclostomata; *A:* amphibia (frogs);
R: reptiles (lizards); *M:* mammals (mice); *H:* man. (Modified from Servít, 1962.)

Symptoms of epilepsy may be classified into behavioral (motor) and
electrographic. Comparative observations dealing with behavioral symptomatology of the epileptic seizure have provided some information about
the symptoms of the generalized convulsive seizure. It develops from a
noncharacteristic composite phenomenology of tonic and clonic symptoms
to the typical sequence of tonic and clonic convulsions, well known in mammals. The first signs of this organization of convulsive symptomatology
are just discernible in amphibians (Servít, 1959, 1962, 1963).

The local disposition of different brain structures to generate epileptic
electrographic activities may have a different phylogenetic development.
It has been shown, for instance, that the disposition of forebrain structures
to generate an experimental epileptic focus (created by local penicillin application) decreases in the phylogenetic line of submammalian vertebrates.
The transition of interictal activity into electrographic seizures also becomes
less frequent (Wilder et al., 1968; Servít, 1970). In fish, this local seizure
susceptibility is very high, and, in addition, the mechanisms arresting the
self-sustained ictal activity after several tens of seconds are insufficient.
Paroxysmal activity here may last up to several tens of minutes (Strejčková,
1969; Servít, 1970; Table 3).

The main topics to be studied in comparative experiments include
problems of generation of the epileptic focus, the transition of interictal
focal activity into a self-sustained electrographic seizure, some problems

TABLE 3. *Differences in focal and seizure activity in fish, frog, and turtle*

	FISH	AMPHIBIA	REPTILES
Species (↓ = localization of the primary focus)	TENCH	FROG	TURTLE
Focus			
Genesis of the primary focus	100%	100%	100%
Onset of activity (min after penicillin application)	2–4	2–10	2–19
Firing interval (sec)	9–10	15–17	21–30
Electrographic pattern	in all species the same: spike complex, − wave, + wave		
Duration of the discharge (msec)	1500–2500	1000–2000	600–900
Genesis of the projected focus	100%	100%	100%
Genesis of an independent secondary focus	50%	rarely	never
Seizure			
Genesis of an electrographic seizure (% of experiments)	spontaneously (100%)	after pentylene-tetrazol application (35%)	very rarely (even after pentylenetetrazol)
Start	abruptly	shortening of the firing interval	prolongation of the after-discharge
Duration	several min	tens of sec	tens of sec
Termination	indefinite	abrupt	abrupt
Electrographic pattern	spike and wave, 2/sec	spike and wave, 2.5/sec	spike and wave, 2–3/sec
Pathways of propagation of the epileptic activities			
Latency of the secondary focal discharge	50ms	24ms, 130ms	30ms, 37ms

TABLE 3. Differences in focal and seizure activity in fish, frog and turtle. (Reproduced from: Z. Servít, Focal epileptic activity and its spread in the brain of lower vertebrates. A comparative electrophysiological study. *Epilepsia*, 11 (1970), 227–240, Table I, page 230.)

of seizure irradiation, the role of different mechanisms of synchronization, and selected questions of electrogenesis of epileptic electrographic phenomena. The published results in this field may be summarized as follows.

It is possible to create an epileptic focus with locally applied penicillin in the forebrain of different species of inframammalian vertebrates (Holubář et al., 1966; Wilder and Morrell, 1967a,b; Wilder et al., 1968; Servít and Strejčková, 1967, 1970; Strejčková, 1969; Servít et al., 1968, 1971; Volanschi and Servít, 1969a,b; Servít, 1970), as well as in the cortex of the lowest mammals (opossum — Wilder et al., 1968). The generation of an independent secondary focus has been observed in all these species. The tendency for primary focus introduction for the generation of an independent secondary (mirror) focus in the contralateral brain hemisphere, as well as the possibility of the transition of interictal activity into an electrographic seizure, seem to diminish at the submammalian vertebrate scale (Wilder et el., 1968; Servít, 1970).

The macroelectrographic symptomatology of interictal focal discharges does not change essentially with the brain phylogeny (Servít, 1970; Fig. 2). At present, there are very few observations concerning the activity of individual neurons in the penicillin focus (in frog — Wilder and Morrell, 1967b).

The generation of paroxysmal electrographic activities could be created by different means in all species of lower vertebrates studied until now (fish, frogs, lizards, and turtles). Spike-and-wave activity has been elicited with pentylenetetrazol in frogs (Morocutti and Vizioli, 1957), with electroshock in frogs, lizards, and turtles (Servít et al., 1965; Volanschi and Servít, 1969b), and with locally applied penicillin sometimes supplemented by subthreshold doses of pentylenetetrazol in fish and frogs (Strejčková, 1969; Servít and Strejčková, 1967, 1970; Wilder and Morrell, 1967a,b; Servít, 1970). Often this activity has a characteristic form and frequency very similar to the episodic epileptic activity well known in the human EEG. In frogs, a very regular paroxysmal 10 Hz activity was also observed (Servít et al., 1965; Krekule et al., 1966).

These paroxysmal activities arise in brains with primitive cortical structures (amphibia, reptiles), but also in the fish forebrain, which completely lacks neuronal structures with a laminar arrangement (Strejčková, 1969).

In frogs and fish, the independence of paroxysmal spike-and-wave and 10 Hz activities on diencephalic and mesencephalic structures could be proved. It is also possible to elicit them with electric stimuli in the isolated forebrain of the frog and fish (Servít et al., 1966b; Servít and Strejčková, 1970).

The similarity of the paroxysmal spike-and-wave activity in lower vertebrates with the analogous electrographic pattern in vertebrates is rather striking. The similarity of the macroelectrogram does not imply, of course, the similarity or identity of electrogenesis. The elucidation of the electrogenetic mechanisms needs further study. Only the first steps have been taken here in the frog pyriform cortex (laminar field analysis with local application of pharmacological agents — Servít et al., 1967).

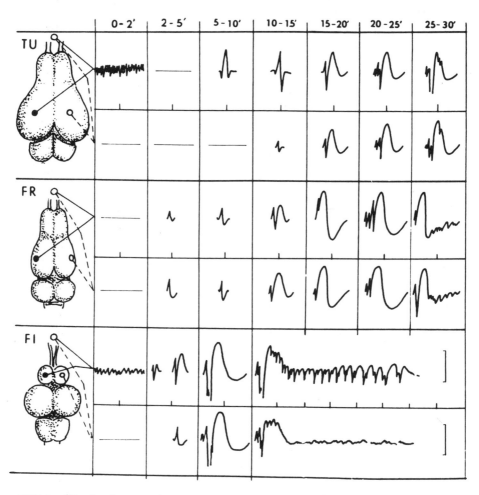

FIG. 2. The development of the pattern of discharge at the site of applied penicillin and at the contralateral projected focus in turtle (*TU*), frog (*FR*), and fish (*FI*) (semischematic drawing, monopolar recording). *Left:* primary focus; *right:* secondary focus; time after application of penicillin in min; calibration: 1 mV. (Reproduced from: Z. Servít, Focal epileptic activity and its spread in the brain of lower vertebrates. A comparative electrophysiological study. *Epilepsia,* 11 (1970), 227–240, Figure 2, page 229.)

Phylogenetic development of irradiation pathways of paroxysmal activities between both forebrain hemispheres was studied in three species of lower vertebrates: fish, frog, and turtle (Wilder and Morrell, 1967a; Servít et al., 1968; Volanschi and Servít, 1969b; Servít, 1970; Servít and Strejčková, 1970). In fish, the short forebrain commissures are the sole pathways along which epileptic activity is propagated from one hemisphere to the other. In amphibia and reptiles, ascending and descending pathways through lower brain structures may be more important both in propagation of focal activity and in the dissemination of the seizure (Table 3). As has already been mentioned, the corpus callosum is absent in all these animals. A comparison with lower mammals who also lack callosal commissural pathways (Marsupialia) may be of interest here. (For interhemispheric relations in Didelphis virginiana, see Putnam et al., 1968.)

An interesting problem of the physiopathology of epileptic phenomena is their relation to the activity of thalamocortical circuits. Turtles may serve as an important model here for comparative studies. As mentioned above, thalamocortical relations similar to those of the mammalian brain could also be shown in turtles (e.g., electrographic spindles, recruiting response). Several observations also speak in favor of the assumption that epileptic activities in the turtle forebrain are similarly correlated with the thalamocortical functional complex (Servít et al., 1971; Servít and Strejčková, 1972). The brain of turtles seems to be a very appropriate model for comparative studies of mechanisms of synchronization and some other cortico-subcortical relations of importance in epileptogenesis. Comparisons with the brains of the lowest mammals could prove to be very fruitful.

V. PERSPECTIVES OF COMPARATIVE EPILEPTOLOGICAL STUDIES

The possibilities of phylogenetic studies in epileptology should be evaluated with respect to the problems to be solved.

In the preceding section I have tried to give a survey of questions which are or may be suitable for comparative research in this field. Full advantage has not been taken of the models described here. Other models may be found, the phylogenetic transition between submammalian vertebrates and the lowest mammals being especially interesting.

Finally, I would like to mention a question which is still under discussion. It is the problem of the epileptic neuron, including the possibility of creating and studying the model of epileptic neuronal pathology in lower vertebrates and/or in invertebrates.

The question of participation of specially deteriorated epileptic neurons in the genesis of epileptic activities and of the activity of normal and/or abnormal neurons in epileptic neuronal aggregates (Ajmone Marsan, 1961) has repeatedly been the subject of research and discussion (see the symposium on *Comparative and Cellular Pathophysiology of Epilepsy* (1966), especially the papers of Grundfest and Ajmone Marsan, as well as the papers of Ajmone Marsan and Jasper in *Basic Mechanisms of the Epilepsies* (1969).

Until now only one study of the behavior of individual neurons in an epileptic focus in the frog forebrain (Wilder and Morrell, 1967*b*) and a few papers dealing with "convulsive" reactivity of neurons of invertebrate animals have been published (see, for instance, Johnson and O'Leary, 1965; Ayala et al., 1970; Washizu et al., 1961). Comparative physiopathological studies in this field could be of great interest; however, the comparative physiology of vertebrate and invertebrate neurons is unfortunately still an incompletely investigated field. The evaluation and interpretation of these experiments with respect to medical pathology and pharmacology must therefore be approached with some caution.

VI. REFERENCES

Ajmone Marsan, C. (1961): Electrographic aspects of "epileptic" neuronal aggregates. *Epilepsia*, 2:22–38.

Ajmone Marsan, C. (1966): Microstructural mechanisms of seizure susceptibility. In: *Comparative and Cellular Pathophysiology of Epilepsy*, edited by Z. Servít. Excerpta Medica Foundation, Amsterdam, pp. 47–59.

Ajmone Marsan, C. (1969): Acute effects of topical epileptogenic agents. In: *Basic Mechanisms of Epilepsy*, edited by H. H. Jasper, A. A. Ward, Jr., and A. Pope. Little, Brown and Company, Boston, pp. 299–319.

Ayala, G. F., Lin, S., and Vasconetto, C. (1970): Penicillin as epileptogenic agent: Its effect on an isolated neuron. *Science*, 167:1257–1260.

Belekhova, M. G. (1963): Electrical activity of cerebral hemispheres evoked by stimulation of diencephalic structures in Varanus. *Fiziologicheskii Zhurnal SSSR imeni I. M. Sechenova*, 49:1318–1329 (in Russian).

Bishop, G. H. (1957): The place of cortex in a reticular system. In: *Reticular Formation of the Brain*, edited by H. H. Jasper, L. D. Proctor, and R. S. Knighton. Churchill, London, pp. 413–421.

Bishop, G. H. (1961): The organization of cortex with respect to its afferent supply. *Annals of the New York Academy of Sciences*, 94:559.

Buser, P. (1955): Etude de l'activité électrique des vertébrés inférieurs. *Journal de Physiologie*, 47:737–768.

Busnel, R. G. (1963): *Psychophysiologie, Neuropharmacologie et Biochimie de la Crise Audiogène*. Colloques internationaux C.N.R.S. No. 112, Editions C.N.R.S., Paris.

Caspers, H., and Winkel K. (1952): Untersuchungen über die Bedeutung des Thalamus und Lobus opticus für die Grosshirnrhythmik beim Frosch. *Pflügers Archiv*, 255:391–416.

Crosby, E. C. (1917): The forebrain of *Alligator mississippiensis. Journal of Comparative Neurology*, 27:325–402.

Gillilan, L. A. (1967): A comparative study of the extrinsic and intrinsic arterial blood supply to brains of submammalian vertebrates. *Journal of Comparative Neurology*, 130:175–196.

Grundfest, H. (1966): Some determinants of repetitive electrogenesis and their role in the electrical activity of the central nervous system. In: *Comparative and Cellular Pathophysiology of Epilepsy*, edited by Z. Servít. Excerpta Medica Foundation, Amsterdam, pp. 19–46.

Guselnikov, V. I. (1965): *Elektrofiziologicheskoe Issledovanie Analizatornykh Sistem v Filogeneze Pozvonochnykh.* Izdatelsto Moskovskogo Universiteta, Moskva.

Hall, W. C., and Ebner, F. F. (1970): Thalamoencephalic projections in the turtle (*Pseudemys scripta*). *Journal of Comparative Neurology*, 140:101–122.

Herrick, H. (1956): *The Evolution of Human Nature.* University of Texas Press, Austin.

Hobson, A. J. (1967): Electrographic correlates of behavior in the frog with special reference to sleep. *Electroencephalography and Clinical Neurophysiology*, 22:113–121.

Hoffman, H. H. (1963): The olfactory bulb, accessory olfactory bulb and hemisphere of some anurans. *Journal of Comparative Neurology*, 120:317–368.

Holubář, J., Strejčková, A., and Servít, Z. (1966): Penicillin and mirror epileptogenic foci in the brain hemispheres of the frog. In: *Comparative and Cellular Pathophysiology of Epilepsy*, edited by Z. Servít. Excerpta Medica Foundation, Amsterdam, pp. 214–220.

Ingle, D. (1968): *The Central Nervous System and Fish Behavior.* University of Chicago Press, Chicago.

Jasper, H. H. (1969): Mechanisms of propagation: extracellular studies. In: *Basic Mechanisms of Epilepsy*, edited by H. H. Jasper, A. A. Ward, Jr., and A. Pope. Little, Brown and Company, Boston, pp. 421–440.

Johnson, W. L., and O'Leary, J. L. (1965): Assay of convulsants using single unit activity. *Archives of Neurology*, 12:113–127.

Kappers, A. (1947): *Anatomie Comparée du Système Nerveux, particulièrement du celui des Mammifères et de l'Homme.* Haarlem de Erven F. Bohn, Paris.

Karamyan, A. I. (1970): *Funktsionalnaya evolutsiya mozga pozvonochnykh (Functional Evolution of the Vertebrate Brain).* Izdatelstvo Nauka, Leningrad.

Karamyan, A. I., Vesselkin, N. P., Belekhova, M. G., and Zagorulko, T. M. (1966): Electrophysiological characteristics of tectal and thalamocortical divisions of the visual system in lower vertebrates. *Journal of Comparative Neurology*, 127:559–576.

Killam, K. F., Naquet, R., and Bert, J. (1966): Paroxysmal responses to intermittent light stimulation in a population of baboons (*Papio papio*). *Epilepsia*, 7:215–219.

Krekule, I., Weiss, T., and Servít, Z. (1966): Comparison by means of probabilistic methods of "ten per second" quasiperiodic activities recorded in man and frog. In: *Comparative and Cellular Pathophysiology of Epilepsy*, edited by Z. Servít. Excerpta Medica Foundation, Amsterdam, pp. 129–138.

Kruger, L. (1969): Experimental analyses of the reptilian nervous system. *Annals of the New York Academy of Sciences*, 167:102–117.

Kruger, L., and Berkowitz, E. C. (1960): The main afferent connections of the reptilian telencephalon as determined by degeneration and electrophysiological methods. *Journal of Comparative Neurology*, 115:125–141.

Kuhlenberg, H. (1967): *The Central Nervous System of Vertebrates.* N. Y. Karger, Basel.

Lázár, G., and Székely, G. (1969): Distribution of optic terminals in the different optic centers of the frog. *Brain Research*, 16:1–14.

Libet, B., and Gerard, R. W. (1941): Steady potential fields and neuron activity. *Journal of Neurophysiology*, 4:438–455.

Mazurskaya, P. Z., and Smirnov, G. D. (1966): Nekotorye kharakteristiki zritelnykh proektsii perednego mozga cherepakhi. *Doklady Akademii Nauk SSSR*, 167:1414–1417.

Morocutti, C., and Vizioli, R. (1957): Osservazioni sull'attivita elettrica del cervello e sulle crisi convulsive di "Bufo vulgaris." *Rivista di Neurologia*, 27:669–676.

Orrego, F. (1961): The reptilian forebrain. I. The olfactory pathways and cortical areas in the turtle. *Archives Italiennes de Biologie,* 99:425–445.

Peyrethon, J. (1968): *Sommeils et Evolution. Etude Polygraphique des Etats de Sommeil chez les Poissons et les Reptiles.* Thèse de Médecine, Lyon, France.

Putnam, S. J., Megirian, D., and Manning, J. W. (1968): Marsupial interhemispheric relation. *Journal of Comparative Neurology,* 132:227–233.

Schadé, J. P., and Weiler, I. J. (1959): EEG patterns in the goldfish (*Carassius auratus L.*). *Journal of Experimental Biology,* 36:435–452.

Segura, E. T., and Juan, A. (1966): Electroencephalographic studies in toads. *Electroencephalography and Clinical Neurophysiology,* 21:373–380.

Sergeev, B. F. (1965): Elektrofiziologicheskij analiz obrazovaniya vremennykh svyazei tipa assotsiyatsii u nizshikh pozvonochnykh. *Zhurnal vysshei nervnoi dejatelnosti,* 15:425–432.

Servít, Z. (1959): Phylogenetic development of susceptibility to and symptomatology of epileptic seizures. *Epilepsia,* 1:95–104.

Servít, Z. (1962): Phylogenesis and ontogenesis of the epileptic seizure. *World Neurology,* 3:259–274.

Servít, Z. (1963): *Epilepsie. Grundlagen einer Evolutionären Pathologie.* Akademie-Verlag, Berlin.

Servít, Z. (1970): Focal epileptic activity and its spread in the brain of lower vertebrates. A comparative electrophysiological study. *Epilepsia,* 11:227–240.

Servít, Z., Machek, J., and Fischer, J. (1965): Electrical activity of the frog brain during electrically induced seizures. A comparative study of the spike and wave complex. *Electroencephalography and Clinical Neurophysiology,* 19:162–171.

Servít, Z., Machek, J., Strejčková, A., and Fischer, J. (1966a): Laminar analysis of the electrogenesis of spike and wave activity in the frog telencephalon. In: *Comparative and Cellular Pathophysiology of Epilepsy,* edited by Z. Servít. Excerpta Medica Foundation, Amsterdam, pp. 144–150.

Servít, Z., and Strejčková, A. (1967): Epileptogenic focus in the frog telencephalon. Seizure irradiation from the focus. *Physiologia Bohemoslovaca,* 16:522–530.

Servít, Z., and Strejčková, A. (1970): An electrographic focus in the fish forebrain. Conditions and pathways of propagation of focal and paroxysmal activity. *Brain Research,* 17:103–113.

Servít, Z., and Strejčková, A. (1971): Thalamocortical relations and the genesis of epileptic electrographic phenomena in the forebrain of the turtle. *Experimental Neurology,* 35:50–60, 1972.

Servít, Z., Strejčková, A., and Fischer, J. (1966b): Paroxysmal electrical activity in the isolated forebrain of the frog (*Rana temporaria*). Comparative pathophysiology of the thalamic pacemaker of paroxysmal activity. *Physiologia Bohemoslovaca,* 15:319–326.

Servít, Z., Strejčková, A., and Fischer, J. (1967): Effect of strychnine and gamma-aminobutyric acid on spike and wave activity in the frog telencephalon. *Experimental Neurology,* 17:389–402.

Servít, Z., Strejčková, A., and Volanschi, D. (1968): An epileptogenic focus in the frog telencephalon. Pathways of propagation of focal activity. *Experimental Neurology,* 21:383–396.

Servít, Z., Strejčková, A., and Volanschi, D. (1971): Epileptic focus in the forebrain of the turtle (*Testudo graeca*). Triggering of focal discharges with different sensory stimuli. *Physiologia Bohemoslovaca,* 20:24–29.

Sheldon, R. E. (1912): The olfactory tracts in teleosts. *Journal of Comparative Neurology,* 22:177–339.

Smirnov, G. D., and Manteifel, Yu. B. (1962): Sravnitelnoe elektrofiziologicheskoe izuchenie mozga v ryadu pozvonochnykh zhivotnykh. *Uspekhi sovremennoi biologii,* 54:309–332.

Smith, E. G. (1910): *Some problems relating to the evolution of the brain.* Lancet, 1–16, 147–153, 221–227.

Strejčková, A. (1969): Epileptogenic focus in the forebrain of the fish. *Physiologia Bohemoslovaca,* 18:209–216.

Takagi, S. F., and Shibuya, T. (1960): The "on" and "off" responses observed in the lower olfactory pathway. *Japanese Journal of Physiology,* 10:99–105.

Tauber, E. S., Rojas-Ramírez, J., and Hernández, P. R. (1968): Electrophysiological and behavioral correlates of wakefulness and sleep in the lizard, *Ctenosaura pectinata.* *Electroencephalography and Clinical Neurophysiology,* 24:424–433.

Toman, J. E. P., and Sabelli, H. C. (1969): Comparative neuronal mechanisms. *Epilepsia,* 10:179–192.

Vasilescu, E. (1970): Isolated head of the tortoise (*Emys orbicularis*). *Revue Roumaine de Biologie – Zoologie,* 15:273–276.

Volanschi, D., and Servít, Z. (1969a): Epileptic focus in the forebrain of the turtle. *Experimental Neurology,* 24:137–146.

Volanschi, D., and Servít, Z. (1969b): Epileptic focus in the forebrain of the turtle. Pathways of propagation of epileptic activity. *Physiologia Bohemoslovaca,* 18:381–386.

Watanabe, S., and Matsumoto, J. (1968): Effects of potassium ferricyanide on the electroencephalogram of isolated toad brain. *American Journal of Physiology,* 214:192–196.

Wilder, B. J., and Morrell, F. (1967a): Cellular behavior in secondary epileptic lesions. *Neurology,* 17:1193–1204.

Wilder, B. J., and Morrell, F. (1967b): Secondary epileptogenesis in the frog forebrain. *Neurology,* 17:1041–1051.

Wilder, B. J., King, R. L., and Schmidt, R. P. (1968): A comparative study of secondary epileptogenesis. *Epilepsia,* 9:275–289.

Winkel, K., and Caspers, H. (1953): Untersuchungen an Reptilien über die Beeinflussung der Grosshirnrindenrhythmik durch Zwischenhirnreizungen mit besonderer Berücksichtigung des Thalamus. *Pflügers Archiv,* 258:22–37.

Washizu, Y., Bonewell, G. W., and Terzuolo, C. A. (1961): Effect of strychnine upon the electrical activity of an isolated nerve cell. *Science,* 133:333–334.

22

Ontogenetic Models in Studies of Cortical Seizure Activities

Dominick P. Purpura

OUTLINE

I. INTRODUCTION

The epidemiological fact that seizure disorders frequently have their onset prior to early adulthood has usually been ignored in the design of experimental models of epilepsy in laboratory animals. It is during the prolonged period of postnatal maturation of the human brain that the tendency to exhibit seizures as a consequence of perinatal traumatic and metabolic insults or "constitutional factors" is most pronounced. Why this is so is more a matter of speculation than established fact. Very little is known concerning the properties of immature neurons and their synaptic organizations at different neuraxial sites (Purpura, 1969, 1971a). Still less is known concerning the response of the immature brain to perturbations of its internal or external milieu which may result in structural and functional alterations in the orderly progression of maturational processes. Thus the study of normal developmental events during brain maturation is no less important than the search for appropriate models for inducing abnormalities in structure and function that are associated with convulsant activity in the immature animal.

Ontogenetic studies of epileptogenic processes can be expected to provide a wide spectrum of information depending upon the resolving power of the technical approach and the imagination and endurance of the investigator. Studies of differences in overt seizure thresholds and seizure characteristics as a function of postnatal age and of their modification by pharmacological agents provide some clues as to the influence of maturation *per se* on seizure susceptibility. In some instances such studies may also permit inferences as to the predominant site of action of the seizure-inducing or anticonvulsant agent in the immature brain. Inasmuch as the overt pattern of seizure activity produced by a convulsant agent is dependent upon the maturational status of different neuraxial organizations, it is possible to obtain information on the maturation of these organizations by analysis of such patterns. For example, Table 1 summarizes the sequence and appearance of maximal electroshock responses in the maturing rat from the data of Vernadakis and Woodbury (1969). According to these workers, the factors which influence the sequential development of different phases can be related to the myelination process and other chemical manifestations of maturation. It is also of importance to point out that, as is the case for electrically induced seizures, the pattern of convulsions induced by strychnine, pentylenetetrazol, and picrotoxin develops in phases in the maturing rat (Fig. 1, Vernadakis and Woodbury, 1969). This general approach to the study of seizure processes in the immature animal is par-

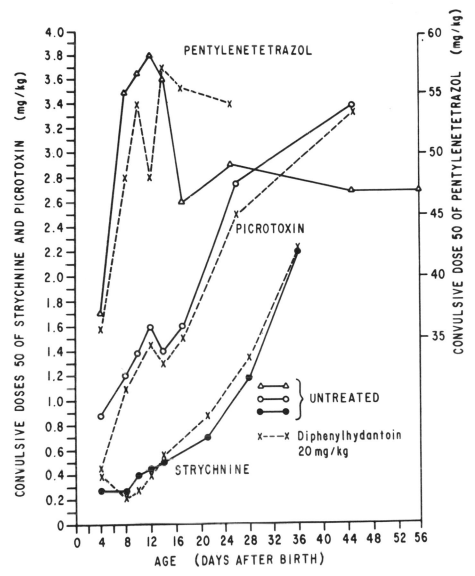

FIG. 1. Changes with age in the susceptibility of rats to seizures induced by strychnine, picrotoxin, and pentylenetetrazol. From Vernadakis and Woodbury (1969) with permission of the publisher.

ticularly valuable in identifying problems for more detailed analysis. At the other end of the spectrum of analytical approaches are those involving the use of microphysiological techniques for extracellular and intracellular studies of immature neurons whose functional activity has been altered by various means for inducing abnormal synchronized discharges.

TABLE 1. *Sequence and appearance of seizure patterns in developing rats*

Age (days after birth)	Pattern
1–8	hyperkinesia
8–9	forelimb clonus
10–12	forelimb flexion
13–15	forelimb flexion followed by forelimb extension and hindlimb flexion
16 and older	tonic hindlimb flexion and extension

From Vernadakis and Woodbury (1969), with permission of the publisher.

The advantages of the microphysiological approach are self-evident in permitting analysis of the relationship of changes in synaptic events to alterations in the type of seizure activity manifested by different neuronal organizations at different stages of their postnatal morphogenesis. When combined with appropriate light- and electron-microscopic studies of organizations investigated with electrophysiological and pharmacological techniques, conclusions may be drawn concerning the nature of seizure processes that are unique to the immature brain. These features provide necessary contrasts for sharpening the focus of studies of seizure mechanisms in the adult animal as well, since it is likely that responses of the mature brain to insult or injury have a natural history of ontogenetic development. In view of this, it is of importance to determine the extent to which pathological excitability changes observed in mature neuronal organizations reflect processes characteristic of the immature brain.

The foregoing rationale for employing ontogenetic models in studies of epileptogenic processes in laboratory animals has guided the present writer in a variety of studies, each of which has required a particular type of experimental design. The problems investigated have ranged from intracellular studies of the organization of synaptic activities in the neonatal period to consideration of the electrographic characteristics of seizure activities induced in the immature brain by dibutyryl cyclic AMP. Since the methods employed in these ontogenetic studies have been basically similar to those utilized in adult animals only those aspects which require special attention in studies of immature animals will be emphasized in this survey. The major focus of this chapter will be on the usefulness of different experimental ontogenetic models in attempts to answer specific questions concerning epileptogenic processes in the immature brain.

II. CHOICE OF LABORATORY ANIMALS IN ONTOGENETIC STUDIES

Were it possible to insure an unlimited and inexpensive supply of newborn and young monkeys for acute and chronic studies, there is no question but that this animal would be the ideal subject for ontogenetic investigations of epileptogenic processes. Unfortunately, logistics and financial considerations preclude extensive usage of newborn monkeys in the vast majority of laboratories. In those instances in which immature monkeys have been utilized in developmental studies of penicillin-induced focal discharges of motor cortex, important relationships have been disclosed between electrophysiological, behavioral, and morphological observations (Caveness, 1969).

It is to be recalled that the newborn monkey, unlike the normal human infant at birth, exhibits a relatively wide range of motor and exploratory behaviors. This is indicative of a relatively advanced state of brain maturation in the newborn monkey, when compared with the newborn of the more common laboratory mammals, such as the mouse, rat, rabbit, dog, and cat. The investigator who plans to undertake an experimental study of seizure activities in immature animals should be aware of the sequential temporal development of some overt behaviors in different species. Table 2 is a summary of the comparative development of simple and complex responses in man, dog, mouse, and cat, reproduced from the recent review by Fox (1970). Additional surveys of ontogenetic studies of the EEG, steady potentials, evoked cortical and subcortical potentials, and conditioned responses in different species are to be found in the volume edited by Himwich (1970).

The author has found the kitten to be particularly suitable for detailed ontogenetic investigations of seizure mechanisms for several reasons. Much of what is currently known concerning normal and abnormal electrocortical physiology in animals has been derived from investigations on adult cats. Thus studies of newborn and young kittens have the advantage of ready comparison with findings in mature animals. A second advantage lies in the size of the newborn kitten brain which, despite the immaturity of

TABLE 2. *Approximate age when adult-like response appears or neonatal response disappears.*

Reflex	Man (Dekeban, 1959)	Dog (Fox, 1964)	Mouse (Fox, 1965)	Cat (Fox[a])
Rooting[b]	11–12 months	24 days	9 days	20 days
Hyperkinesias (coarse tremors)[b]	2 months	21 days	10 days	–
Magnus (tonic neck and labyrinthine)	3–6 months	21 days	6–8 days	15 days
Mass movements (generalized responses, for example, to pain)[b]	3 months	21 days	9 days	–
Postural flexion (in vertical suspension)[b]	3–4 months	4 days	6 days	–
Postural extension (-do-)[b]	4–6 months	19 days	10 days	–
Righting	2–3 months	birth	birth	birth
Crossed extensor[b]	3–4 months	15 days	4 days	15 days
Mature relaxed phase	–	26 days	12–14 days	–
Primitive stepping[b]	7 months	–	–	–
Forelimb placing (visual)	5–6 months	27 days	12–14 days	21 days
Forelimb contactual placing	–	4 days	birth	birth
Subcortical and spinal responses weaken (cortical dominance)	3 months	16–21 days	8–10 days	11–14 days
Reciprocal kick reaction	4 months	15 days	5 days	–
Voluntary elimination	22–24 months	23 days	12–14 days	5–6 wks.
Emotional reactions	6–12 months	21 days	12 days	15–21 days
Eyes open	at birth	10–13 days	11–12 days	5–9 days
Visual fixation	4 months	28 days	–	17 days
Auditory startle	at birth	25 days	12–14 days	15 days
Visual orientation (following response)	at birth	26 days	–	17 days
Auditory orientation	4 months	26 days	16 days	16 days

[a] Present data.
[b] Neonatal responses.

its constituent neurons, renders it amenable to the placement of considerable stimulating and recording hardware and permits surgical intervention with preservation of important landmarks.

Finally, it should be noted that much information is available on the maturational status of cortical neurons and synaptic organizations in the kitten brain at different postnatal stages (Noback and Purpura, 1961; Scheibel and Scheibel, 1964; Voeller et al., 1963). In the immediate neonatal period, pyramidal neurons exhibit well-developed apical dendrites but the basilar dendrites of most pyramidal neurons are poorly represented (Fig. 2). The major synaptic relations at this stage are effected largely by axodendritic synapses (Voeller et al., 1963). By the second postnatal week, basilar dendrites and axon-collateral systems undergo a phase of rapid development along with the elaboration of axospinodendritic and axosomatic synapses. In the ensuing few weeks, cortical neurons acquire all the morphological characteristics typical of mature neurons, with the exception that the axons of large pyramidal elements do not possess their full complement of myelin until the end of the 4th or 5th month postnatally

(Purpura et al., 1964). This brief account of the major morphogenetic events in immature feline cerebral cortex indicates that although cortical neuronal maturation is completed within 4 to 5 weeks after birth in the kitten, distinct phases are definable for examining the effects of epileptogenic

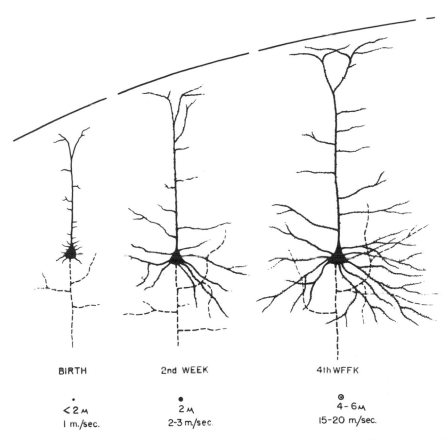

BIRTH

2nd WEEK

4th WFFK

<2 M
I m./sec.

2 M
2-3 m./sec.

4-6 M
15-20 m/sec.

FIG. 2   General characteristics of neocortical pyramidal neurons in the kitten at birth, 2 weeks, and 4 weeks postnatally. Relative diameter of axons and conduction velocities of largest fibers in medullary pyramidal tract are indicated below each cell for the different ages. Axons and axon-collaterals are shown as dashed lines. In the newborn kitten, pyramidal neurons have well-developed apical dendrites and many have rudimentary basilar dendritic systems. Axon-collaterals are poorly developed, and dendrites are devoid of typical spines. During the second postnatal week, basilar dendrites grow extensively, and apical dendrites increase in length and contain more tangential branches. Spines appear on dendrites at this stage and axon-collateral growth is prominent. In the 1-month-old kitten, neocortical pyramidal neurons have attained adult characteristics. Myelination of the largest corticospinal axons is completed by the 4th or 5th month. Modified from Purpura et al. (1964).

processes at different postnatal stages. Thus the ontogenetic approach to the study of seizure phenomena offers the possibility of effecting structure-function correlations which are frequently obscured by the overwhelming complexity of the mature brain (Purpura, 1964).

III. INTRACELLULAR STUDIES OF IMMATURE NEURONS: ADVANTAGES AND DISADVANTAGES

Satisfactory intracellular recordings have been obtained from neo-cortical and hippocampal neurons in neonatal and very young kittens (Purpura et al., 1965, 1968). However, the investigator who has not utilized the intracellular recording method in studies of cortical neurons in adult animals will be hard pressed to develop these techniques for the first time in studies of the immature brain. The young investigator may chart his progress in perfecting the manufacture of ultramicropipettes and in achieving a stable "non-pulsatile" preparation by noting the ease with which he can obtain recordings first from spinal motoneurons, then pyramidal tract neurons, hippocampal pyramidal cells, and finally thalamic neurons in adult animals. This progression from large to small neurons must be accompanied by careful attention to micropipette characteristics which are major determinants of successful penetration of small and fragile neurons. (See Appendix I.)

The chief disadvantage of the intracellular recording technique in studies of the immature brain is that very few data may be forthcoming even in the most experienced hands. In the immediate neonatal period, impalements of cortical neurons that yield 40 to 60-mV spike potentials are few and far between. Fortunately the yield of data rapidly increases with the age of the preparation so that studies utilizing 7 to 21-day-old kittens are usually much more productive.

The investigator who seeks a special challenge in developmental neurobiology will immediately recognize the enormous advantages to be gained by determined efforts to obtain intracellular data during the normal and abnormal functional operations of immature cortical neurons. Examples of the different varieties of data that have been obtained in such studies of normal immature neocortex and hippocampus are illustrated in Fig. 3. It has been shown that, despite the relative paucity of synapses on neo-cortical neurons in the immediate neonatal period, stimulation of thalamo-cortical pathways is capable of eliciting in these elements prominent and prolonged excitatory postsynaptic potentials (EPSPs) which rarely trigger

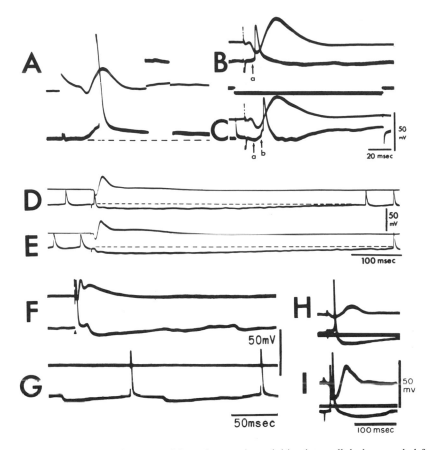

FIG. 3. Examples of spike potentials and synaptic activities intracellularly recorded from neocortical and hippocampal neurons in the neonatal and young kitten. *A:* Prolonged EPSP (80 to 100 msec) evoked by ventrolateral thalamic stimulation in a sensorimotor cortex neuron from a 6-day-old kitten. In this and other dual-channel recordings, the upper channel records indicate cortical surface activity, negativity upwards. Weak stimulation elicits an 18- to 20 msec latency EPSP with a slow rise time and prolonged declining phase. Calibration: 50 mV, 20 msec. *B* and *C:* Appearance of partial response during induced soma hyperpolarization in a neuron from a 24-day-old kitten. *B:* Ventrolateral thalamic stimulation elicits a 5-msec latency small EPSP (at arrow, A) and a cell discharge. *C:* During soma hyperpolarization (indicated by first trace), the EPSP is augmented and a second component is revealed, b, which is succeeded by a spike potential. The response revealed at b, is presumably due to a dendritic partial spike. *D* and *E:* Prolonged IPSPs recorded from a sensorimotor cortex neuron in a 24-day-old kitten. Examples are shown of two responses to single-shock stimulation of the ventrolateral thalamus. Broken horizontal lines are drawn through base lines to facilitate estimation of IPSP duration, which may attain a value of 600 msec. *F* and *G:* Spontaneous and evoked IPSPs in a hippocampal pyramidal neuron from a 3-day-old kitten. Upper trace, hippocampal surface evoked response to fimbrial stimulation. *H* and *I:* Examples of changing characteristics of spike potentials recorded in a sensorimotor cortex neuron from a 3-week-old kitten during single shock (*H*), and during 5/sec ventrolateral thalamic stimulation (*I*) which elicited cortical surface augmenting responses. In *H*, the thalamic stimulus evokes a typical spike potential which arises from an EPSP. During summation of IPSPs, thalamic stimulation elicits spikes without depolarizing prepotentials which arise from a level of increased membrane polarization. Such spikes are generated in dendrites and propagate in an all-or-none fashion into the soma. *A–E, H,* and *I,* modified from Purpura et al. (1965); *F* and *G* from Purpura et al., (1968).

more than one spike potential (Purpura et al., 1965) (Fig. 3*A*). This is in marked contrast to findings in similar types of studies carried out in adult cats (Purpura, 1972). In both neocortical and hippocampal neurons of neonatal and very young kittens, prolonged inhibitory postsynaptic potentials (IPSPs) are readily obtained (Fig. 3*D–G*). Since axodendritic synapses provide the major type of neuronal relation at this early postnatal developmental stage, it follows that such IPSPs are generated in dendrites. The fact that IPSPs elicited in immature cortical neurons have all the characteristics that are observed in adult animals suggests that there is a precocious development of inhibitory synaptic pathways in immature cerebral cortex.

The implications of this suggestion for the pathophysiology of seizures as well as other abnormalities of the maturing brain are worthy of further comment. If inhibitory neurons are relatively more mature in functional development than excitatory elements at birth, these inhibitory neurons may be selectively vulnerable to major metabolic, asphyxial, or toxic insults in the antenatal or immediate neonatal period. This vulnerability may be a consequence of the high metabolic demands of inhibitory neurons which have attained a stage of functional differentiation in the immature brain comparable to that of inhibitory neurons in the mature animal. Selective destruction of inhibitory neurons could result in loss of inhibitory activities in neuronal organizations requiring an admixture of excitatory and inhibitory events for the normal processing of input-output functions. Thus the further study of inhibitory activities in immature brain may serve to clarify the epileptogenic effects of a number of severe disturbances peculiar to the perinatal period.

Intracellular recording from a small proportion of immature neurons has also disclosed the tendency for these elements to exhibit partial dendritic responses as well as propagating spikes in dendrites (Purpura, 1967). (Fig. 3*B, C, H,* and *I*).

Findings of prolonged PSPs and low-level responsiveness of immature neurons have been recently confirmed in intracellular studies of immature neurons involved in penicillin-induced focal paroxysmal discharges (Prince and Gutnick, 1972). Additional data obtained in the latter studies indicate important differences between the functional organization of immature and mature neurons during focal epileptogenic activity.

The usefulness of the intracellular method may be greatly enhanced when combined with techniques for producing alterations in steady potential gradients in immature cortex. Such effects of steady polarizing currents on spontaneous and evoked potentials, seizure discharges, and intracellularly recorded activities have been extensively examined in the adult animal (Purpura and McMurtry, 1965). (See Appendix II.)

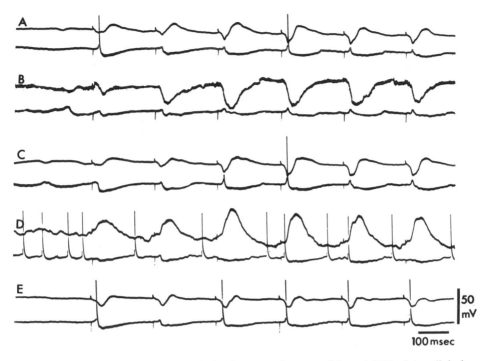

FIG. 4. Effects of transcortical polarization on spike potentials and PSPs intracellularly recorded in a sensorimotor cortex neuron from a 3-week-old kitten. *A:* Responses to 5/sec stimulation of the ventrolateral thalamus. Short-latency EPSPs occasionally trigger spike potentials. These are succeeded by prolonged IPSPs. *B:* Cortical-surface cathodal polarization results in marked enhancement of surface-positive component of evoked responses. Spike potentials are eliminated and IPSPs are somewhat attentuated. *C:* Recovery after cessation of cathodal polarization. *D:* During cortical-surface anodal polarization, spike discharge frequency is enhanced and spikes appear to arise directly from baseline indicating their dendritic origin. Evoked potentials exhibit loss of surface positivity and marked enhancement of surface-negativity. *E:* Recovery of responses after cessation of anodal polarization. Unpublished observations of Purpura and Shofer.

The feasibility of the combined methods is evident in the effects of cortical polarization on spike potentials and PSPs recorded from immature neurons (Fig. 4). In view of the different thresholds for inducing seizures by diffusely applied polarizing currents in neocortical and hippocampal neuronal organizations in the adult animal, similar studies in immature animals should provide information on the susceptibility of these two types of cortex to induced alterations in steady potentials as a function of postnatal age (Purpura, 1969).

Apart from the general difficulties of the method, intracellular studies favor observations on the largest and less fragile elements of the immature brain. Thus the vast majority of interneurons may be poorly represented in samples of neuronal populations studied with intracellular techniques. Another limitation of the method is inherent in the fact that intrasomatic registration may fail to detect synaptic and nonsynaptic processes localized to remote dendritic sites. (Purpura, 1967). (However, both criticisms are also applicable to studies of neurons in the mature brain.) Fortunately, less demanding techniques are available for studying the development of convulsant activities involving axodendritic synaptic activities in the immature cerebral cortex by judicious employ of the evoked potential method as noted in the following section.

IV. SUPERFICIAL CORTICAL RESPONSES IN IMMATURE BRAIN: COMPARATIVE DEVELOPMENT OF SYNAPTIC PATHWAYS REVEALED BY CONVULSANTS

The problem with the evoked potential technique in general is that it provides a plethora of data that are usually difficult to interpret. For this reason it is useful to examine the simplest evoked response of the immature brain, the surface-negative wave elicited by local cortical stimulation. The fact that this response is readily obtained in the near-term and neonatal kitten has been attributed to the presence of relatively well-developed superficial axodendritic synaptic pathways in the perinatal period (Purpura, 1961a).

The middle suprasylvian gyrus of the kitten is a particularly favorable site for examining the changing characteristics of the superficial cortical response (SCR) and the effects of consulvant agents during postnatal ontogenesis. A pair of 0.1-mm Teflon-coated silver wires cemented together may be employed for surface stimulation. Wick electrodes or small (0.2 mm) chlorided silver ball electrodes placed at varying distances from the stimulating electrodes are satisfactory for registering SCRs. Monopolar recording electrodes may be placed in linear array along the length of the mid-suprasylvian gyrus for distances up to 10 mm. Comparison of the SCR recorded very close to the site of stimulation and at, for example, 2, 4, or 6 mm, away permits observations of the spread of the SCR along superficial axodendritic synaptic pathways as a function of postnatal age. (Purpura et al., 1960). This is of value in providing information on the development of tangential as well as intracortical synaptic pathways to dendrites of distant cortical neurons. It can be demonstrated in this fashion that distant SCRs may exhibit synaptic facilitation at different sites from the locus of stimulation during postnatal development.

The foregoing experimental design has served as a model for examining the changing responsiveness of superficial axodendritic synaptic pathways to simple convulsant agents such as the six-carbon aliphatic ω-amino acid, ϵ-amino caproic acid. (Purpura, 1961b). This ω-amino acid, unlike the four-carbon member of the aliphatic series γ-aminobutyric acid (GABA), produces convulsant activity when topically applied to mature cat cortex. (Purpura et al., 1959). (In contrast, the inhibitory synaptic actions of GABA are now well established; see Curtis, this volume.)

Examples of the effects of ϵ-amino-caproic acid (C_6) on near and distant SCRs of immature neocortex are shown in Fig. 5. When a few drops containing a 1% Tris-buffered Ringer solution of the amino acid are placed at the recording site of the SCR evoked in the newborn kitten, the response is somewhat depressed (Fig. 5A2). Even with prolonged application of C_6,

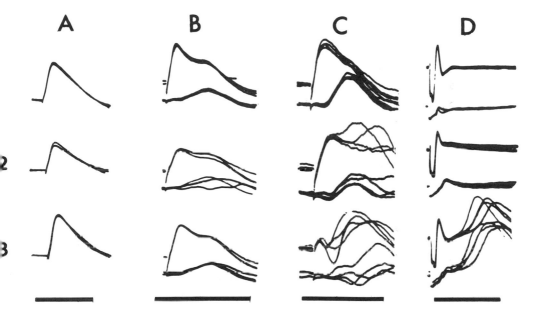

FIG. 5. A–C: Changing responsiveness of superficial neocortical axodendritic synaptic pathways to topically applied ϵ amino caproic acid (C_6). A, newborn kitten; B, 7 day old kitten; C, 15-day-old kitten. In A and upper-channel records of B and C, superficial (negative) cortical responses (SCRs) were recorded close to the site of cortical-surface stimulation. Lower-channel responses in B and C were recorded at 5 and 6 mm, respectively, from the site of stimulation. 1, control responses; 2, effect of topically applied C_6; 3, responses observed after removal of C_6. Note in C onset of seizure activity. D: Responses recorded at two sites along the ventricular surface of the exposed hippocampus in a 2-day-old kitten. Upper channel, response to fimbrial stimulation recorded at the fimbrial-hippocampal junction. Lower channel, responses several millimeters away. 1, control; 2, few seconds after C_6 application to hippocampal surface; 3, development of convulsant activity due to C_6. Time bar: 1 sec throughout. A–C, modified from Purpura, 1961b; D, unpublished observations.

there is only a minimal alteration in background activity. In the 1-week-old kitten, SCRs generally exhibit a late surface negativity in addition to the early negativity when the responses are recorded close to the site of stimulation. Distant responses consist of a long-latency slow-negativity. At this developmental stage, C_6 depresses the early SCR and induces marked variation in late components (Fig. 5B). An entirely different situation is encountered in 10- to 15-day-old kittens. At this age, C_6 application results in prompt and pronounced enhancement of late components of near-responses with depression of early components. Convulsant activity is evident in very long latency components of the overt responses (Fig. 5C). In contrast to the depressant effects of C_6 on superficial axodendritic synaptic pathways of neocortex in the neonatal and very young kitten, hippocampal surface responses elicited by fimbrial stimulation in neonatal animals are augmented and paroxymal discharges readily elicited by topical C_6 (Fig. 5D).

The most parsimonious interpretation of the data illustrated in Fig. 5 is that the convulsant action of ϵ-amino caproic acid is dependent upon the functional development of a synaptic substrate that becomes progressively more sensitive to the amino acid during the early phases of postnatal development. The fact that there is a marked difference in the C_6 sensitivity of hippocampal as opposed to neocortical synaptic pathways in the neonatal kitten may be explicable on the basis of the relatively advanced maturational status of neurons and synaptic organizations in the hippocampus at birth (Purpura and Pappas, 1968; Schwartz et al., 1968).

Whether the progressive increase in C_6 sensitivity of neocortical synaptic pathways is due to the morphogenesis of new synapses or to the increasing receptor sensitivity of synapses already present at birth is not known. For present purposes, it is sufficient to indicate the advantages of the model in the analysis of the different effects of convulsant agents on developing synaptic pathways in the immature mammalian cerebral cortex. Such studies which attempt to relate changing pharmacological effects to changes in synaptic substrate may provide a more rational approach to developmental neuropharmacology than is currently available.

V. AN ONTOGENETIC MODEL OF ENHANCED SEIZURE SUSCEPTIBILITY OF ISOLATED IMMATURE CORTEX

Weak cortical stimulation which elicits superficial cortical responses, such as illustrated in Fig. 5, never produces repetitive after-discharges or seizure activity in newborn and young kittens. In the author's experience, a single brief stimulus which elicits the SCR and only a minimal late surface positivity is always subthreshold for producing rhythmically recurring after-discharges in the intact cortex of unanesthetized adult cats. A dramatically different effect of weak cortical surface stimulation is observed following chronic subpial isolation of a slab of immature neocortex (Purpura and Housepian, 1961). Under these conditions, a single, weak cortical-surface stimulus generally elicits an SCR which is succeeded by repetitive after-discharges with rather stereotyped though complex characteristics (Fig. 6).

Isolated slabs of suprasylvian gyrus in very young kittens can be studied within 2 to 9 days after preparation of the slabs. (See Appendix

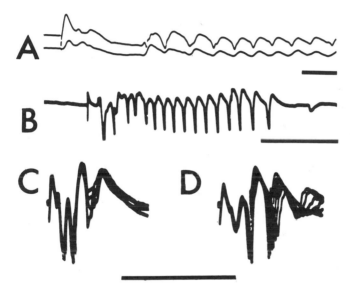

FIG. 6. Responses of chronically isolated immature neocortex to weak stimulation of the isolated slab. *A:* Superficial cortical responses and repetitive discharges recorded 1.5 mm (upper channel) and 3.5 mm (lower channel) from the site of stimulation in a region of chronically isolated neocortex in a 10-day-old kitten, 7 days after preparation of the isolated slab. The SCRs recorded at both sites exhibit multiple additional surface-negativities on the late phases. These are succeeded by very long-latency, predominantly surface-positive, 10 to 14/sec repetitive responses. *B:* SCR and repetitive burst response recorded from an isolated cortical slab in a 5-day-old kitten, 3 days after cortical isolation. Recording electrode 1 mm from site of weak local stimulation of the slab. *C* and *D:* Responses elicited during surface stimulation of an isolated slab in a 5-day-old kitten, 3 days after cortical isolation. Surface responses recorded 1.5 mm from site of stimulation. Stimulus frequency, 0.5/sec. Note extraordinary regularity of complex and stereotyped paroxymal discharges following the SCR. Time bar: 1 sec throughout. Modified from Purpura and Housepian, 1961.

III, and Halpern, this volume.) Stimulating and recording arrangements for eliciting SCRs in such preparations are identical to those utilized in unoperated kittens of the same age. The laminar distribution and pharmacological responsiveness of the repetitive discharges evoked in isolated immature cortex can be examined with extracellularly located microelectrodes (Purpura and Housepian, 1961). At the conclusion of the physiological studies, the kittens are sacrificed and the rectangular slabs of cortex removed and placed in various fixatives for cytological studies. (Detailed descriptions of currently utilized neuroanatomical techniques may be found in the volume edited by Nauta and Ebbesson, 1970).

Golgi-Cox preparations have been particularly valuable in providing morphological information on the alterations in neuronal cytoarchitecture that could contribute to the repetitive after-discharges observed in immature cerebral cortex within 2 to 9 days after subpial isolation of a cortical slab. The finding of precocious axon-collateral proliferation of immature pyramidal neurons whose mainstem axons have been interrupted during the isolation procedure has been of considerable importance in attempts to establish satisfactory morphophysiological correlations of the data.

This ontogenetic model has additional advantages in providing a preparation in which seizure phenomena are associated with alterations in synaptic pathways that may be examined in the electron microscope or studied pharmacologically with iontophoretic methods. (See Curtis, this volume.) Correlations may also be effected between morphophysiological data and biochemical alterations in the isolated immature cortex. This wide range of possible investigations addresses some of the most fundamental issues relating to the effects of trauma on the development of seizure activity in the immature brain.

VI. APPLICATION OF THE FREEZE-LESION TECHNIQUE TO ONTOGENETIC STUDIES OF FOCAL DISCHARGES

The freeze-lesion of neocortex in adult animals has served as a useful model for reliably producing focal EEG spikes and sharp waves in a circumscribed area of cortex immediately adjacent to the area contacted by the cold probe (Smith and Purpura, 1960). In adult unanesthetized-paralyzed cats, best results have been obtained by gentle application to the cortical surface of a 4- to 5-mm diameter metal rod in contact with a chamber of dry ice. Within 10 to 15 sec after application, close inspection of the area of contact will usually reveal a peripheral rim of hyperemia. The rod is allowed to remain in contact for 0.5 to 1.0 min and is then released from the cortical surface after generous application of warm Ringer's to melt the ice formed between rod and pial surface. From 0.5 to 2 hr after the freeze-lesion, initially negative focal spikes rhythmically recurring at a frequency of 0.5 to 1.5/sec can be detected in the lesion area with monopolar surface electrodes. In most instances, a single spike focus characterizes the lesion; occasionally, however, two independent foci are observed. The cold rod may be reapplied to the same or closely adjacent site if spiking fails to occur after 2 hr. Failures to produce epileptogenic lesions are generally referable to cortical depression secondary to respiratory or hemodynamic disturbances. Successful lesions may be produced in 80% of *encéphale isolé* preparations.

Placement of the freeze-lesion in somatosensory or association cortex permits analyses of the effects of different varieties of evoked cortical responses on focal discharges. Additionally, information may be obtained on the manner in which focal epileptogenic discharges interact with evoked responses and are in turn modified by repetitive stimulation of intracortical and corticipetal pathways (Smith and Purpura, 1960). Since focal epileptogenic discharges generally begin from 0.5 to 2 hr after production of the freeze-lesion, it has been possible to utilize the model in adult animals to follow the temporal course of alterations in amino acids and their compartmentation at the lesion site prior to and after the onset of seizure activity. These values may be compared with observations from normal cortex in the same preparation (Berl et al., 1959, 1960).

If the foregoing technique for producing freeze-lesions in adult animals is applied to the immature cortex, largely negative results are obtained in newborn and very young kittens (Goldensohn et al., 1963). Inasmuch as the freeze-lesion can be expected to produce the same traumatic effect on cortical elements in immature and mature brain, the failure of such trauma to initiate focal discharges in the young kitten is a *negative* finding of considerable importance. This is an instance in which attempts to disclose the *basis* for the negative epileptogenic effect of a traumatic insult to the immature brain may provide information on factors responsible for the low-level excitability of immature cortex. Whatever factors underlie the failure of freeze-lesions to induce rhythmically recurring focal discharges in immature brain, it is evident that these have little to do *per se* with the morphological maturation of cortical neurons and their synaptic relations. This follows from the fact that focal discharges with characteristics similar to those encountered in adult animals are rarely observed before the 2nd postnatal month in the kitten. At this time cortical neurons and synaptic pathways have completed their maturational sequences. Other data indicate that the *capacity* for focal epileptogenesis secondary to the freeze-lesion is present at a much earlier postnatal age but this is not expressed, for reasons which remain obscure. Indeed, factors which suppress the normal operations of cortical neuronal organizations in young kittens may unmask or activate focal epileptogenic discharges in a freeze-lesion of immature cortex.

The investigator interested in the ontogeny of post-traumatic epileptogenic lesions such as exemplified by the freeze-lesion of cortex should be aware of the possible role of non-neural developmental events in the late appearance of seizure susceptibility. The fact that the elaboration of glial elements, which is reflected in part in myelination of cortical efferent and afferent pathways, occurs relatively late in respect to neuronal maturation may be a significant clue worth pursuing (Purpura, 1964). Studies of the development of "silent cell," presumably glial, membrane potentials and their alterations by extracellular and intracellular potassium ion concentrations as a function of postnatal age can be carried out with the intracellular techniques described above. This again emphasizes the importance of applying the information obtained in studies of neural and non-neural elements in the adult cat to problems of the stability and seizure susceptibility of the immature brain.

VII. USEFULNESS OF ONTOGENETIC MODELS IN BIOCHEMICAL STUDIES OF SEIZURE ACTIVITIES

No attempt will be made here to indicate the importance of the new wave of biochemical studies that has appeared in recent years in the area of developmental neurobiology (Himwich, 1970). Clearly, the normative data obtained in these investigations will be fundamental to an adequate understanding of the disturbances in biochemical processes underlying seizure disorders in the immature brain.

Collaborative morphophysiological and biochemical approaches are of course the most productive avenues of attack upon this problem. However, if any success is to be expected in these collaborative investigations, it is required that data obtained from one discipline be "translatable" into the special languages of the other disciplines. This point may be illustrated with reference to the relationship of the adenyl cyclase–cyclic AMP–phosphodiesterase system to the morphological features and synaptic events of immature cerebral cortex. In view of the critical importance of this system in a variety of hormonal and transmitter-mediated processes (Greengard and Costa, 1970), it is reasonable for the neurophysiologist to pose the following questions. What is the role of the cyclic AMP system in synaptic processes in the immature brain? What effects are produced by cyclic AMP on immature cortex? How do traumatic or metabolic insults to the immature cortex or pharmacological agents influence the cyclic AMP system? The biochemist may inquire into the tissue levels of adenyl cyclase, cyclic AMP, phosphodesterase, and protein kinases in immature cerebral cortex as a function of postnatal age. These parameters might also be examined in focal epileptogenic areas or isolated cortical slabs. The neuromorphologist may be concerned with the subcellular localization of elements of the system as well as the type of synaptic substrate involved in physiological events triggered by cyclic AMP.

The potential usefulness of the foregoing experimental design is evident in results obtained in recent studies which have dealt with various aspects of these problems (Purpura and Shofer, 1972). It has been established that in very young kittens (< 1 week old) cortical-surface application of dibutyryl cyclic AMP (0.2 mM) produces within 10 min enhancement of transcallosally evoked responses (TCRs) elicited as shown in Fig. 7. In these studies, TCRs were recorded from three, closely spaced monopolar electrodes located on the anterior middle suprasylvian gyrus. Under these conditions, spread of TCRs from nonhomotopic sites is minimal but becomes greatly facilitated after dibutyryl cyclic AMP. Several minutes after the appearance of enhanced TCRs, paroxysmal activity and repetitive after-discharges are observed. Typically, at a later stage convulsant activity appears independently at the three recording sites (Fig. 8). The fact that convulsant discharges recorded from closely spaced monopolar electrodes may be completely independent at the different sites indicates little or no "functional coupling" between small areas of cortex in the immature brain. The morphological basis for this weak "functional coupling" between closely spaced regions of cortex may be sought in the relative immaturity of tangentially organized intracortical synaptic pathways in the early postnatal period. The physiological observations are reminiscent of the data obtained on the tangential spread of the SCR (Fig. 5). The ability of dibutyryl cyclic AMP to produce prominent convulsant activity in the cortex of the very young kitten (although ε-amino-caproic acid and freeze-lesions are ineffective) again emphasizes the fact that appropriate manipulations of immature brain are required to reveal its seizure susceptibility.

It is beyond the scope of this brief survey to pursue the implications and interpretations of the data illustrated in Figs. 7 and 8. Suffice it to say that ontogenetic studies have provided a useful model for a major collaborative program on the role of the cyclic AMP system in the control of

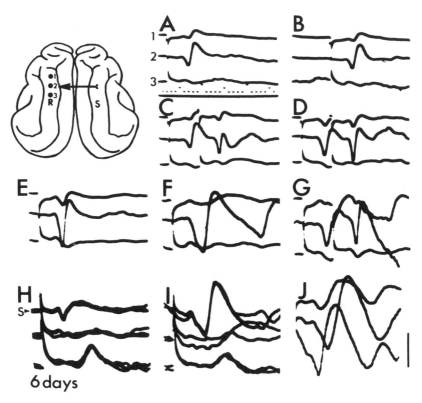

FIG. 7. Effects of topically applied dibutyryl cyclic AMP on transcallosal evoked responses (TRC) and spontaneous activity of immature feline cerebral cortex (6-day-old kitten). *Inset* shows arrangement of three monopolar recording electrodes on left suprasylvian gyrus (indifferent electrode on temporal muscle). Separation of 2 mm between adjacent pairs of recording electrodes. The homotopic site opposite the R_2 recording electrode was stimulated to evoke the responses shown in A–G. A and B: conditioning and testing responses, respectively (negativity upwards). C: Paired responses. D: 10 min following application of 0.2 mM dibutyryl cyclic AMP. E: 5 min. after D. F and G: 10 min after additional dibutyryl cyclic AMP. Convulsant activity is evident. In H and I, stimulation was homotopic to R_1. Note the appearance of a prominent surface negative response at R_3. J: Seizure activity recorded with different temporal and electrographic characteristics at the three recording sites. Time bar: 10-msec intervals. Amplitude, 0.2 mV. From Purpura and Shofer (1972) with permission of the publisher.

neuronal excitability in the immature brain. The investigator who seeks a similar advantage in effecting other types of morphophysiological and biochemical correlative studies of seizure phenomena is encouraged to explore the value of ontogenetic models.

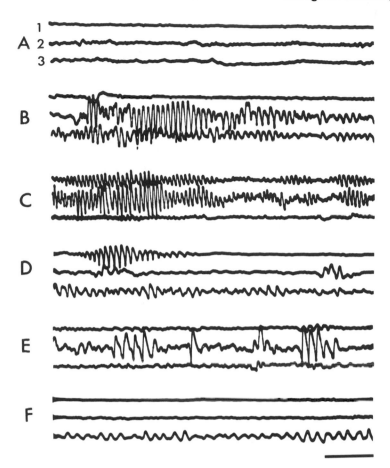

FIG. 8. Convulsant action of topically applied dibutyryl cyclic AMP in a 6-day-old kitten. 1,2,3: Activity recorded monopolarly from a linear array of electrodes located on the middle suprasylvian gyrus, each electrode separated by 2 mm. A: Interictal activity. B–F: various stages during the action of the dibutyryl cyclic AMP. Note that convulsant activity may be limited to sites 2 and 3 (B), 1 and 2 (C), 2 (E), or 3 (F). This independence of convulsant activity is indicative of loose synaptic coupling between areas of registration. Unpublished observations of Purpura and Shofer.

VIII. SUMMARY

Ontogenetic studies provide the investigator with suitable models for examining the role of developmental events in seizure disorders and permit identification of morphophysiological and biochemical factors in epileptogenesis as a function of postnatal age. Intracellular and extracellular recording techniques greatly enhance the power of ontogenetic investigations especially when these are considered in relation to morphological data on postnatal synaptogenesis. Ontogenetic models of the effects of convulsant agents on definable axodendritic synaptic pathways and of traumatic lesions associated with epileptogenesis in immature cortex are also described. These emphasize the value of judicious employ of evoked potential and extracellular recording techniques in combination with morphological investigations on the immature brain. An experimental design for correlating morphophysiological and biochemical studies in immature cerebral cortex is illustrated in relation to the problems of the role of the cyclic AMP system in seizure activities. These and other models are described with the intent to encourage a wider utilization of the ontogenetic approach in experimental studies of epileptogenic processes in the mammalian brain.

IX. APPENDIX I

Glass is a complex mixture of silicates and other substances. It varies considerably in "hardness" from batch to batch obtained from the same manufacturer despite the fact that the investigator may specify a uniform internal and external diameter of "Pyrex" capillary tubing. Such variations in properties will determine the slow and rapid pull-phases of micropipette-pullers and thus the shape and resistance of the micropipette. Best results in the author's laboratory have been obtained with saturated (1.5 to 2.0 M) potassium citrate-filled micropipettes pulled with relatively long tapers and exhibiting resistances of 20 to 40 MΩ. Not infrequently, optically satisfactory micropipettes within this range of resistances produce disappointingly negative results in the immature cerebral cortex. Failure to observe DC shifts and spike potentials of appreciable magnitude (>10 to 20 mV) in penetration after penetration of immature cortex with electrodes exhibiting "ideal" characteristics is more the rule than the exception. This is usually due to a combination of factors: plugging of micropipette tips, poor cerebral circulation, reduced cortical oxygenation, vascular pulsations, and hypothermia. Passing current through the electrode via a bridge circuit (Araki and Otani, 1955) is occasionally effective in unplugging tips. Discarding the micropipette is equally effective. Meticulous attention to blood loss during surgical procedures on neonatal and young kittens is essential. A single 2 × 2-inch surgical sponge that becomes homogeneously pink with absorbed blood means excessive blood loss in operations on young kittens. An adequate airway can be achieved by intratracheal installation of the best-fit uretheral catheter with side holes to reduce dead space and resistance to expiratory air flow. Body and brain temperature must be maintained at 37 to 39°C since newborn and young kittens are exquisitely sensitive to heat loss. An effective maneuver is to wrap the hindlegs, abdomen, and thorax in biochemical heating tapes operated from a DC source. Oxygen may be employed during artificial ventilation with attention to the CO_2 content of expired air. The tendency to hyperventilate paralyzed, artificially ventilated kittens in which bilateral pneumothorax has been established must be guarded against. Experience dictates that this may be a major contributor to brain pulsations. The latter are difficult to eliminate in the very young kitten by means of agar–Ringer-filled chambers secured over the site of recording. If cisternal drainage is performed, care taken in control of respiration, and the kitten suspended from vertebral processes, so that its heart is approximately at the level of its head, pulsations may be diminished, but rarely abolished. It is a remarkable fact that although no evidence of cortical pulsation may be detected with the unaided eye or with a dissecting microscope, maddening pulsations may often be detected with a probing high-resistance micropipette, especially when the tip becomes partially plugged with cellular debris. Such preparations are best discarded early in the day rather than in the wee hours of the morning after a frustratingly negative 8 to 10 hrs, assuming the kitten survives the ordeal.

X. APPENDIX II

Studies of the effects of cortical-surface polarizing currents on intracellular activities of immature neurons require preparation of non-polarizable electrodes for delivering low-level polarizing currents. Ag-AgCl electrodes in Ringer-filled glass tubes fitted with cotton wicks have been successfully employed in the author's laboratory for this purpose. The electrodes are incorporated in a 1.5-V battery-operated circuit in which current intensity is regulated by a potentiometer and measured with a milliameter in series with the preparation. For polarizing small areas of immature cortex, the cotton wick of one electrode may contact a cortical surface area of approximately 4 mm^2. The other electrode of the pair may be placed at various non-cortical sites (e.g., roof of the orbit, frontal sinus, temporal muscle). Micropipettes for intracellular recording should be placed for cortical penetration as close as possible to the wick electrode and to the recording surface electrode. In the intracellular studies involving cortical polarization, intracellular potentials were led into a neutralized input-capacity amplifier and displayed on an oscilloscope operated on AC mode because of the large and occasionally erratic potential fields established by the polarizing currents. Under such conditions depolarizing and hyperpolarizing effects of cortical-surface polarization may be inferred from changes in intracellular spike characteristics and alterations in spontaneous and evoked PSPs. Estimates of transcortical voltage gradients produced by polarizing currents have been obtained by oscilloscopic registration of the potential differences between two microelectrodes connected to neutralization amplifiers. One microelectrode is placed on the cortical surface close to the polarizing electrode while the other is employed for intracellular recording (Purpura and McMurtry, 1965).

XI. APPENDIX III

The method employed for producing such hyperexcitable slabs of immature cortex is essentially that described by Echlin (1959) in adult animals. (See also Halpern, this volume.) Young kittens are anesthetized with ether and the membranous bone overlying the dorsolateral connexity is cut with sharp scissors in order to turn a small bone flap. With dura intact, a rectangular area 15 to 20 mm by 8 to 10 mm is outlined which includes mid- and posterior suprasylvian gyrus. A #22 hypodermic needle is inserted to a depth of 8 to 10 mm at one corner of the rectangular area. The needle is then rotated upwards until its shaft is flush with the dura. Gentle pressure is applied with a finger so as to compress cautiously the needle shaft against the meninges. The needle is again rotated to the perpendicular position and the same procedure is followed along the adjacent side of the rectangular area. When this is completed, the needle is swept in a 90° arc at a depth of 8 to 10 mm to sever underlying white matter. The entire procedure is repeated after inserting the needle into the diagonally opposite corner of the rectangular area. The method effectively interrupts intracortical and subcortical connections of the rectangular slab of cortex without compromising the pial circulation. The bone flap is replaced and skin closure secured with clips or sutures. It is advisable that kittens not be returned to their mothers until they have recovered from anesthesia. Some mother cats become agitated when kittens are returned with excessive ether vapors or bloody wound margins evident. Such cats may refuse to nurse, or may tear open wounds or destroy the operated kittens. An effective maneuver is to "habituate" the environment by spraying the home cage with a few drops of ether for several days prior to the surgery. More important is to utilize cats familiar with the laboratory setting or with a past history of being "good" mothers. (Caution: Pregnant stock cats recently confined to small cages and poorly handled may make poor mothers with infanticide tendencies!)

XII. ACKNOWLEDGMENTS

This investigation was supported in part by the Alfred P. Sloan Foundation and by U.S. Public Health Service grant NS–07512 from the National Institute of Neurological Diseases and Stroke.

XIII. REFERENCES

Araki, T., and Otani, T. (1955): Response of single motoneurons to direct stimulation in toad's spinal cord. *Journal of Neurophysiology*, 18:472–485.

Berl, S., Purpura, D. P., Girado, M., and Waelsch, H. (1959): Amino acid metabolism in epileptogenic and non-epileptogenic lesions of the neocortex (cat). *Journal of Neurochemistry*, 4:311–317.

Berl, S., Purpura, D. P., Gonzalez-Monteagudo, O., and Waelsch, H. (1960): Effects of injected amino acids on metabolic changes occurring in epileptogenic and non-epileptogenic lesions of the cerebral cortex. In: *Inhibition in the Nervous System and Gamma-Aminobutyric Acid*, edited by E. Roberts. Pergamon Press, New York, pp. 445–453.

Caveness, W. F. (1969): Ontogeny of focal seizures. In: *Basic Mechanisms of the Epilepsies*, edited by H. H. Jasper, A. A. Ward, and A. Pope. Little, Brown and Co., Boston, pp. 517–534.

Dekeban, A. (1959): *Neurology of Infancy*. Williams and Wilkens, Baltimore.

Echlin, F. A. (1959): The supersensitivity of chronically "isolated" cerebral cortex as a mechanism in focal epilepsy. *Electroencephalography and Clinical Neurophysiology*, 11:697–722.

Fox, M. W. (1970): Reflex development and behavioral organization. In: *Developmental Neurobiology*, edited by W. A. Himwich. Charles C Thomas, Springfield, Ill., pp. 553–580.

Goldensohn, E. S., Shofer, R. J., and Purpura, D. P. (1963): Ontogenesis of focal discharges in epileptogenic lesions of cat neocortex. *Electroencephalography and Clinical Neurophysiology*, 15:163–164.

Greengard, P., and Costa, E., editors (1970): *Role of Cyclic AMP in Cell Function*. Raven Press, New York.

Himwich, W. A. (1970): *Developmental Neurobiology*. Charles C Thomas, Springfield, Ill.

Nauta, W. J. H., and Ebbesson, S. O. E. (1970): *Contemporary Research Methods in Neuroanatomy*. Springer-Verlag, New York.

Noback, C. R., and Purpura, D. P. (1961): Postnatal ontogenesis of neurons in cat neocortex. *Journal of Comparative Neurology*, 117:291–308.

Prince, D. A., and Gutnick, M. J. (1972): Neuronal activities in epileptogenic foci of immature cortex. *Brain Research (in press)*.

Purpura, D. P. (1961a): Analysis of axodendritic synaptic organizations in immature cerebral cortex. *Annals of the New York Academy of Sciences*, 94:604–654.

Purpura, D. P. (1961b): Ontogenetic analysis of some evoked synaptic activities in superficial neocortical neuropil. In: *Nervous Inhibition*, edited by E. Florey. Pergamon Press, New York, pp. 495–514.

Purpura, D. P. (1964): Relationship of seizure susceptibility to morphologic and physiologic properties of normal and abnormal immature cortex. In: *Neurological and Electroencephalographic Correlative Studies in Infancy*, edited by P. Kellaway and I. Petersen. Grune and Stratton, New York, pp. 117–154.

Purpura, D. P. (1967): Comparative physiology of dendrites. In: *The Neurosciences: A Study Program*, edited by G. C. Quarton, T. Melnechuck, and F. O. Schmitt. Rockefeller University Press, New York, pp. 372–393.

Purpura, D. P. (1969): Stability and seizure susceptibility of immature brain. In: *Basic Mechanisms of the Epilepsies*, edited by H. H. Jasper, A. A. Ward, and A. Pope. Little, Brown and Co., Boston, pp. 481–505.

Purpura, D. P. (1971a): Synaptogenesis in mammalian cortex: Problems and perspectives. In: *Brain Development and Behavior*, edited by M. B. Sterman, D. J. McGinty, and A. M. Adinolfi. Academic Press, New York, pp. 23–41.

Purpura, D. P. (1972): Intracellular studies of synaptic organizations in the mammalian brain. In: *Structure and Function of Synapses*, edited by G. D. Pappas and D. P. Purpura. Raven Press, New York, pp. 257–302.

Purpura, D. P., Carmichael, M. W., and Housepian, E. M. (1960): Physiological and anatomical studies of development of superficial axodendritic synaptic pathways in neocortex. *Experimental Neurology*, 2:324–347.

Purpura, D. P., Girado, M., Smith, T. G., Callan, D., and Grundfest, H. (1959): Structure-activity determinants of pharmacological effects of amino acids and related compounds on central synapses. *Journal of Neurochemistry*, 3:238–268.

Purpura, D. P., and Housepian, E. M. (1961): Morphological and physiological properties of chronically isolated immature neocortex. *Experimental Neurology,* 4:377–401.

Purpura, D. P., and McMurtry, J. G. (1965): Intracellular activities and evoked potential changes during polarization of motor cortex. *Journal of Neurophysiology,* 28:166–185.

Purpura, D. P., and Pappas, G. D. (1968): Structural characteristics of neurons in the feline hippocampus during postnatal ontogenesis. *Experimental Neurology,* 22:379–393.

Purpura, D. P., Prelevic, S., and Santini, M. (1968): Postsynaptic potentials and spike variations in the feline hippocampus during postnatal ontogenesis. *Experimental Neurology,* 22:408–422.

Purpura, D. P., and Shofer, R. J. (1972): Excitatory action of dibutyryl cyclic adenosine monophosphate on immature cerebral cortex. *Brain Research,* 38:179–181.

Purpura, D. P., Shofer, R. J., Housepian, E. M., and Noback, C. R. (1964): Comparative ontogenesis of structure-function relations in cerebral and cerebellar cortex. In: *Progress in Brain Research, Vol. IV. Growth and Maturation of the Brain,* edited by D. P. Purpura and J. P. Schade. Elsevier, Amsterdam, pp. 187–221.

Purpura, D. P., Shofer, R. J., and Scarff, T. (1965): Properties of synaptic activities and spike potentials of neurons in immature neocortex. *Journal of Neurophysiology,* 28:925–942.

Scheibel, M., and Scheibel, A. (1964): Some structural and functional substrates of development in young cats. In: *Progress in Brain Research, Vol. IX. The Developing Brain,* edited by W. A. Himwich and H. E. Himwich. Elsevier, Amsterdam.

Schwartz, I. R., Pappas, G. D., and Purpura, D. P. (1968): Fine structure of neurons and synapses in the feline hippocampus during postnatal ontogenesis. *Experimental Neurology,* 22:394–407.

Smith, T. G., Jr., and Purpura, D. P. (1960): Electrophysiological studies on epileptogenic lesions of cat cortex. *Electroencephalography and Clinical Neurophysiology,* 12:59–82.

Vernadakis, A., and Woodbury, D. M. (1969): The Developing Animal as a Model. *Epilepsia,* 10:163–178.

Voeller, K., Pappas, G. D., and Purpura, D. P. (1963): Electron microscope study of development of cat superficial neocortex. *Experimental Neurology,* 7:107–130.

23

Applications to Drug Evaluations

Dixon M. Woodbury

OUTLINE

I. INTRODUCTION

The potential hazards of testing new therapeutic agents in humans necessitates the use of experimental models for preliminary screening and evaluation. The relevance of such screening procedures is clearly related to the degree to which the experimental models approximate the disease in humans. The ideal model for testing the effects of potential antiepileptic drugs would be one that closely approximates human epilepsy, is simple and inexpensive, and from which rapid results could be obtained. No model at present meets all these criteria, but all models are potentially useful for evaluation of anticonvulsant drugs. The models presently used, therefore, represent compromises; those which are simple and rapid may not be closely related to epilepsy in humans, whereas those which are probably closely related to the human disease are more expensive and provide less rapid answers.

Which of these models to use, therefore, depends on the stage of development of the antiepileptic drugs being evaluated. Thus, for initial screening of a large number of drugs for anticonvulsant activity, the simple and rapid models are generally used, whereas for determination of the selectivity of a drug and for in-depth studies of the neurophysiological and biochemical effects of the drug and of its mechanisms of action, the more sophisticated, possibly slower and more expensive human-related models should be used. However, in the use of the simple methods for initial and preliminary screening, the models to be used hopefully should not exclude potentially useful drugs. In order to avoid this possibility, a battery of simple and rapid experimental models have been advocated, and the overall spectrum of the results evaluated rather than the results of a single test (Swinyard, 1969). It has been demonstrated that the accuracy of predicting is enhanced by this means.

It is obvious, of course, that the best approach to the development of new antiepileptic drugs is to elucidate the mechanism of action of the present drugs used in the different types of the disease. Once the mechanism by which the drug prevents seizures is known (which also implies that the mechanism of seizure production is also understood), a model can be set up to test new drugs that may exert the same effect. New antiepileptic drugs can be tailor-made by this approach, as has been the case for the development for the treatment of gout of allopurinol to influence uric acid metabolism.

It is obvious from the foregoing that the objective of this chapter is to discuss the application of experimental models of epilepsy to evaluation of anticonvulsant drugs. As mentioned, this must be done in animals because humans cannot be used in the initial phase of drug testing. To accomplish this objective, an attempt will be made to answer the following questions that seem pertinent to the evaluation of anticonvulsants in experimental models. (1) Can anticonvulsant activity in man be predicted from present experimental models? (2) As a corollary to (1), can anticonvulsant activity for a specific type of epilepsy (e.g., grand mal, absence) be predicted from present experimental models? (3) What is to be accomplished by the testing of anticonvulsants in experimental models? (4) What aspects of anticonvulsant activity are tested by the presently available experimental models?

To answer these questions, it is first necessary to discuss some general principles of anticonvulsant evaluation in experimental animals and then to consider each model with respect to its usefulness for anticonvulsant drug evaluation and determination of the mechanism of action of these drugs.

II. GENERAL PRINCIPLES OF EVALUATION AND ACTIONS OF ANTICONVULSANT DRUGS

Epilepsy in man is characterized by chronically recurring, spontaneous clinical seizures. It is clear, therefore, that a model in experimental animals should also exhibit these fundamental properties. If such a model could be obtained, it would be ideal for the evaluation of anticonvulsant drugs. However, this model has not yet been developed although certain ones to be discussed approach the ideal. The question that arises is whether the basic properties of seizures, regardless of the etiology, are similar. If this is the case, then any model that measures all or a part of these properties should be useful for drug evaluation. The major difficulty is that only a very few models have been evaluated as predictors of useful anticonvulsants in man. In fact, for some of the models to be discussed, presently used antiepileptic drugs have not been tested to see if they are effective. One of the greatest needs is to evaluate antiepileptics in all of these models. As pointed out by Ajmone-Marsan (1969),

> "the gap between . . . an experimental situation and the focal form of human epilepsy—a clinical entity characterized by exquisitely chronic features—is only apparent. In an investigation of the *development of pathological changes and related electrical phenomena* in the epilepto-genic lesion (and its concomitant motor manifestations), other experimental approaches should be designed, and for instance, the use of alumina cream or metal-pellets implantation would be more appropriate. Once an epileptic process has become established, its sporadic electrical manifestations, at least in their main qualitative aspects, appear to be rather stereotyped, and *there is no convincing evidence for the existence of important differences in their underlying basic mechanisms that might be related to its type of development.* Thus it should be obvious that use of local epileptogenic agents and analysis of their acute effects offer the great advantage of convenience of a relatively simple experimental design" (italics by the author).

Similarly, the analysis of potential anticonvulsant drugs in experimental models should yield information on their effectiveness regardless of the manner in which the seizures were produced. However, because of the variety of clinical types of epilepsy and their differences in response to drugs, a complete analysis of the spectrum of drugs and their potential usefulness in epilepsy obviously requires more detailed study in various types of models after not only acute but also chronic administration. This is essential since each model is different and possesses only one or a few but not all of the properties of human epilepsy; potential anticonvulsants should, therefore, be evaluated in a battery of tests that approximate as closely as possible the human disease. Information provided through such tests, in addition to providing data on the clinically useful properties of the drugs, also contributes to the understanding of the mechanism of action of the drugs employed in the tests.

Briefly, the *pathophysiological events in epilepsy* can be considered in three steps: (1) the abnormalities which generate the discharge of an epileptogenic focus; (2) the local spread and the changes which precipitate the interictal activity into a seizure; and (3) the propagation of discharge during a major seizure (see Halpern et al., 1969; Ward, 1969; Toman, 1970). An abnormal feature of the neuron engaged in seizure activity is the paroxysmal depolarizing shift (PDS), often associated with high-frequency action-potential bursts, loss of inhibitory postsynaptic potentials, and synchronous discharge of other cells of the same group. Neurons in a chronic seizure focus exhibit a phenomenon close to denervation sensitivity (probably of the dendrites) with regard to excitatory stimuli, and may also be relatively lacking in inhibitory input. Such hyperactive cells appear to differ in pharmacological properties from those of more normal neighboring neurons. The high-frequency firing in the seizure focus is probably a result of local biochemical changes, ischemia, and loss of vulnerable small-cell inhibitory systems. The focus may remain quiescent over long periods of time, discharging only intermittently as revealed from EEG studies, and may cause no signs and symptoms. The spread of convulsive activity to neighboring normal cells appears to be restrained by normally present inhibitory processes. However, many factors that by themselves do not precipitate seizures may trigger the focus or facilitate seizure spread to normal tissue. These include changes in blood-sugar level, blood-gas tensions, pH, total osmotic pressure and electrolyte composition of extracellular fluid, and endocrine function; fatigue, emotional stress, and nutritional deficiencies also may play a role. In addition, these factors are important in assessing anticonvulsant drug effects on animals or humans with such foci.

If suitable precipitating factors are present, the abnormal activity in the focus may spread to normal brain tissue. If this spread is sufficiently extensive, the entire brain is activated and a tonic-clonic seizure with unconsciousness ensues. If the spread is localized, the seizure is characteristic only of the anatomical focus. Once a seizure has begun, it maintains itself by recirculation of excitatory impulses in a closed feedback pathway that may or may not necessarily include the original seizure focus. Self-maintenance and spread appear to involve the phenomenon of post-tetanic potentiation (PTP), a progressive enhancement of synaptic transmission during rapid, repetitive stimulation. The seizure usually is terminated by the elevated threshold and prolonged refractoriness that result from hyperactivity, and also by inhibition from pathways external to the discharging seizure focus.

It is obvious from the above discussion of seizure mechanisms that drugs might act in many ways to abolish or attenuate seizures (see, for example, Toman, 1970; Toman and Goodman, 1948). General mechanisms include: (1) effects on non-neural lesions, such as normalization of the ischemic blood supply of cortical seizure foci; (2) effects confined to the pathologically altered neurons of the seizure focus to prevent their excessive discharge; and (3) effects also on normal neurons to prevent their detonation by the seizure focus. Most anticonvulsant drugs probably act by the latter mechanism since they all produce side-effects related to effects on normal tissue. The effects on normal tissue include such processes as elevation of the threshold for excitatory synaptic transmission, enhancement of inhibitory processes, prolongation of the refractory period, or prevention of seizure spread by reduction of PTP.

A. Basic actions of anticonvulsant drugs on neuronal processes

At least three distinct actions of anticonvulsant drugs on neuronal processes (see review by Woodbury, 1969) can be cited as underlying the effects of anticonvulsants in experimental seizures, no matter how induced: stabilization of the neuronal membrane, decrease in tendency to repetitive discharge, and reduction in spread of seizure discharge (Woodbury and Esplin, 1959). All three actions may underlie alteration of the tonic-clonic maximal seizure pattern, whereas only the first two would appear to be concerned in altering the threshold for discharge of the focus.

An evaluation of anticonvulsants in various experimental models of epilepsy, together with studies of their effects on synaptic transmission, have revealed that certain agents possess one or another of the actions mentioned in rather pure form. Among such agents appear to be diphenylhydantoin (DPH) and trimethadione (TMO). In Table 1 are given the spectra of anticonvulsant properties exhibited by these two drugs when they are administered in fully effective doses. Central nervous system depression is not a prominent feature of either agent. Of the two drugs shown, only TMO has a marked ability to elevate seizure threshold; there is moderate elevation of electrical threshold and striking elevation of pentylenetetrazol threshold. In contrast, DPH is effective in abolishing the tonic phase of the maximal seizure induced by electroshock stimulation. Also shown in this table are the effects of these two drugs on various aspects of spinal cord synaptic transmission in cats in anticonvulsant-nontoxic doses. Both show some evidence of a direct depressant action as indicated by reduction in either monosynaptic or polysynaptic discharge. It is significant that TMO, which is the more effective of the two agents in elevating electrical and chemical seizure thresholds, is the one which markedly decreases spinal cord transmission during repetitive stimulation. Of the three general ac-

TABLE 1. *General characteristics of diphenylhydantoin and trimethadione as revealed by conventional laboratory tests and their effects on spinal cord synaptic transmission*

	Diphenylhydantoin	Trimethadione
Tests		
CNS depression	0	+
Elevation of EST	+	+++
Elevation of pentylenetetrazol threshold	0	++++
Abolition of tonic phase of MES	++++	+
Effects		
Depression of mono-synaptic spike			0
Depression of poly-synaptic response	++	++
Decrease in response to repetitive stimulation	+	++++
Antagonism of anticon-vulsant effects of pentylenetetrazol	0	++++
Depression of posttetanic potentiation	++++	0

Data obtained from Woodbury and Esplin, 1959.

tions of anticonvulsants proposed above to underlie modification of maximal electroshock pattern, it is suggested that DPH abolishes the tonic phase of the convulsion primarily by *reducing spread of seizure discharge,* through an effect on PTP. Thus the effects of these two agents on experimental seizures illustrate two principle effects of anticonvulsants that are seen in all models of epilepsy, namely, *elevation of threshold for seizure discharge* and *reduction of spread of seizure discharge.* The fine details of the mechanisms by which these effects are accomplished must be studied in more precise models with more elegant techniques than are generally used for the simple models. Examples of these techniques are presented in earlier chapters in this book and are illustrated herein by the studies in the spinal cord carried out by Esplin and colleagues (Esplin, 1957; Esplin and Curto, 1957).

The example illustrated here of effects of anticonvulsants on spinal cord synaptic transmission which are in general harmony with their antiepileptic properties lends support to the assumption that these agents do not exert their effects at specific supraspinal loci but that they influence neuronal processes which underlie transmission at various sites. Thus,

DPH and TMO exert effects on the stellate ganglion and the neuromuscular junction qualitatively identical to those observed in spinal cord experiments. Experiments on cortical and subcortical areas of the brain also suggest that these two drugs exert the same effects as on the spinal cord. The other clinically effective antiepileptics that have been studied (bromide, phenobarbital, and phenacemide) do not provide such clear-cut correlations between anticonvulsant properties and effects on spinal cord transmission. However, it is probable that the three mechanisms discussed above also underlie the action of these and other antiepileptics, although each of these drugs appears to act by more than a single mechanism.

B. Effects of anticonvulsant drugs on excitatory and inhibitory processes

It is essential for a complete understanding of the actions of anticonvulsants and for their rational therapeutic use that they be evaluated in experimental models with respect to actions on inhibitory and excitatory processes in the brain. This is necessary because the normal functioning of the central nervous system is dependent on a balance between these two processes. A reduction of inhibition (as, for example, is induced by strychnine) or enhancement of excitation (as induced by pentylenetetrazol) will tip this delicate balance toward seizure activity. This balance is upset in human epilepsy. Thus anticonvulsant drugs can act by increasing the degree of inhibition or by blocking excitation in the brain, a process that involves an action at synapses. An example of the use of experimental models for elucidating the effects of antiepileptics on excitatory and inhibitory processes is the effects of DPH on the development of seizures in the maturing rat (Vernadakis and Woodbury, 1969*a,b*). The sequence of development of seizures in response to various seizure-inducing procedures and agents in neonatal rats has been described previously and will be only briefly presented here. The sequence begins with hyperkinetic movements in neonatal rats and progresses to clonus, tonic flexion, and then tonic extension in 17- to 21-day-old animals. These changes indicate progressive maturation of different areas of the neuroaxis with age and also maturation of inhibitory systems. DPH, in rats less than 12 days of age, has only excitatory effects as measured by increased susceptibility to electroshock, pentylenetetrazol, strychnine, and picrotoxin. After this period, DPH abolishes the tonic flexor phase of the maximal electroshock seizure pattern and decreases susceptibility to electroshock and chemically induced seizures. It is evident that DPH has a biphasic effect on the brain of maturing rats: excitatory effects early in life and inhibitory effects later when these systems have developed to a fuller extent. These data suggest that one of the basic effects of DPH is excitation and that part of its characteristic antispreading effects is a result of stimulation of inhibitory processes that predominate in the adult brain, but which are reduced during epileptic seizures. These data in experimental animals correlate with the known effects of this drug in man. DPH is ineffective in the treatment of seizure in infants and young children induced by fever, or by other etiologies (Melchior et al., 1971). In addition, there is evidence of excitatory effects of DPH in high doses in adults. It is evident from this example that the developing animal is a useful model for testing anticonvulsants that are to be used in children and also for elucidating effects of inhibitory and excitatory systems.

C. Acute versus chronic evaluation of anticonvulsant drugs in experimental models

Since antiepileptic drugs in man are given for extended periods of time, it is essential that they be evaluated in experimental models during long-term treatment. It is important, therefore, to choose a suitable model for such chronic studies of drug action. Certain species such as the cat are particularly sensitive to chronic administration of antiepileptics and hence are not suitable for such studies, although they are excellent animals for the study of the acute neurophysiological effects of these drugs. Many examples are presented in previous chapters of this volume on the usefulness of the cat for detailed studies of anticonvulsant drug action. The most useful models for chronic study of drug effects are those in which focal lesions of the brain have been induced by the heavy metals. This induces in some species chronic, paroxysmal, and recurrent seizures resembling human epilepsy. The most suitable animal for these studies is the monkey. A description of this technique is presented in Chapter 1 by Ward.

D. Role of species differences in the evaluation of anticonvulsant drugs

The most useful species to study in the evaluation of antiepileptic drugs depends on the models to be used and whether acute or chronic treatment is to be given (see above). However, many models can be duplicated in various species and it is desirable to test drugs in these models in a variety of species. This is the case because such factors as the absorption, distribution, biotransformation, and excretion of the drugs may vary vastly from species to species and even from man to man. It is also useful, since methods are now available, to determine plasma levels of the drug in the various species because in most instances the pharmacological responses to the drugs are similar in all species including man for equal plasma levels of drug (Brodie and Reid, 1969).

Some species are better for some models than are others. For example, the mouse is the most useful animal for the maximal electroshock seizure test (MES), for the EST tests, for studies with intravenous pentylenetetrazol, and for the audiogenic seizure model, whereas the rat and monkey are useful for models involving chronic studies with irritant metal induced foci, and the baboon (*Papio papio*) for studies of photomyoclonic seizures. Acute neurophysiological studies are best done in cats.

E. Age factors in the evaluation of anticonvulsant drugs

The different responses of maturing rats to anticonvulsant drugs are discussed in a previous section. It is important to realize that sensitivity to seizures varies with age, and, consequently, susceptibility to antiepileptic drugs also varies with age. There are not only quantitative changes in seizure susceptibility with age but often qualitative changes as well, as already described. For example, the threshold for electrically induced seizures in rats decreases after the 12th postnatal day until 28 days after birth and then increases thereafter. Thus, the 28-day-old rat is the most susceptible to seizures. Also, as demonstrated by Petty and Karler (1965), the ED_{50} of phenobarbital, acetazolamide, and CO_2 to abolish the tonic extension component of the MES pattern decreases with age in rats, but that for CO_2 and acetazolamide increases with age in mice. It is obvious that care must be taken to know the age of the animals when evaluating antiepileptic drugs in experimental models.

F. Role of genetic factors in the evaluation of anticonvulsant drugs

Genetic factors play a role in evaluation of antiepileptic drugs mainly from two aspects. Inbred strains of animals are more uniform in their response to the evoking stimulus and to anticonvulsant drugs; hence, they give more reliable statistical information. Rats and mice, therefore, are better in this respect. The other aspect is in terms of the use of genetic models of epilepsy for evaluation of anticonvulsant drugs. Audiogenic seizures in mice and photomyoclonic seizures in baboons are examples of models that are genetically determined. Some strains of beagle dogs also appear to have spontaneous seizures.

III. EVALUATION OF EXPERIMENTAL MODELS FOR
ANTICONVULSANT DRUG TESTING

In order for an experimental model to be classified as an epileptic-like model and to be useful as a method for evaluation of anticonvulsant drugs, it must be evaluated from two criteria: (1) electrographic studies must show the presence of epileptic-like activity in the EEG, e.g., spikes and waves, and (2) clinical seizure-like activity must be manifested, e.g., motor movements such as clonus and tonus and behavioral changes such as originate in the temporal lobe. Once these criteria have been established, a particular procedure is a potentially useful model of epilepsy. It is pertinent to summarize here the methods described in previous chapters in this book with respect to whether they meet these criteria and whether they are useful for assay of anticonvulsant drugs. In the next section will be discussed the value of these models for predicting antiepileptic drug activity in man especially with respect to those that can be used to detect drugs of potential value in the different types of epilepsy in man (e.g., grand mal, petit mal, temporal lobe seizures).

A. Models for inducing local epileptogenic activity

1. Epileptic-like models. In the case of epileptic-like models, both electrographic and clinical evidence of seizures has been established. They include the topical convulsant metals (see Chapter 1), topical freezing (Chapter 2), and topical convulsant drugs and metabolic antagonists (Chapter 3). These models of epilepsy have been studied in both acute and chronic situations. Acute studies have shown that of the limited number of conventional antiepileptic drugs tested in these models all have been active both in preventing the spontaneous seizures and in modifying the electrographic manifestation of the seizures. In these models, the clinical manifestations and the response to anticonvulsant drugs depend on the location of the lesion and the type of clinical seizure that results. If the evoking agent is applied to the cerebral cortex, generally clonic-type seizures are produced; occasionally tonic-clonic seizures occur. Therefore, drugs such as phenobarbital and primidone, but not DPH, are effective in preventing the focal discharge that results in clonic activity induced by the evoking agents or procedure. The spread of the impulse to involve the whole cortex which results in tonic-clonic seizures can be blocked by DPH, as would be predicted from its known action to prevent seizure spread or propagation.

TABLE 2A. *Summary of effects of selected clinically useful drugs on various experimental models that induce local epileptogenic activity*

Experimental model	Response measured	Species	Clinically useful drugs						
			DPH	Phenobarbital	Primidone	Phenacemide	TMO	Ethosuximide	Diazepam
Topical metals									
Tungstic acid	Interictal spike	cat		++			+++		
	Spike after-discharge			++++			++++		
	Clonic seizure			++++			++++		
Alumina cream									
Acute	EEG	rat, cat, monkey							
Chronic	Clonus	monkey	+	+++					
Freezing	Spike frequency (primary focus)	rabbit	0	+			+		
	Spread of activity								
	Basal	cat	0	++			++		
	Cortical	monkey	++	+			0		
Topical chemicals									
Penicillin	EEG	rat, cat, monkey	+						++
	Clonus								+++
	Tonus-clonus		++++						
Focal electrical stimulation	Motor threshold[a]	cat,	++++	+++			++		+
	Threshold for convulsions[b]	monkey	++++	++			+		
	Threshold for EAD[c]		+++	+++			++		+++
Isolated cortex	Threshold for EAD[c]	cat	+++	++++			±	0	
Stimulated brain slices	Electrical activity	guinea pig, rat		depresses postsynaptic response but not conducted response					
	Metabolic activity								
Single cells	Action potential								
	Membrane potential								
Spinal cord	PTP	cat	++++	±			0		
	Repetitive stimulation	cat	±	+			++++		
	Clonus	rat, cat	0	+			++		
	Tonus-clonus	rat, cat	++	++			±		
Mirror focus	Electrical activity in focus	cat							

[a]Threshold for minimal motor response.
[b]Threshold for local motor (clonic) convulsive effects.
[c]Threshold for electrical after-discharge.

Since the lesions persist for a long period of time, these models, especially when the monkey is the experimental animal, are particularly suited for chronic evaluation of anticonvulsant drugs and should be used for final testing before evaluating the drug in man. A summary of the few drugs that have been evaluated by these procedures is shown in Table 2A (see also Elazar and Blum, 1971). One disadvantage of these models is the high cost of maintaining monkeys with chronic brain lesions and of recording electrographic and seizure manifestations. Also, the lesions are not always reproducible (see Chapter 1).

    2. Models for inducing localized electrical discharge (spiking). In these models, electrical after-discharge (EAD) is elicited by localized stimulation of various areas of the brain. They include *focal electrical stimulation* models (Chapter 6) in which electrodes are implanted in various areas of the brain and the results of stimulation recorded. The responses measured are the threshold for EAD, or the threshold for local motor convulsive (clonic) activity (CT). This model is the best example of the acute induction of seizures by local effects. Both DPH and phenobarbital increase the threshold for EAD and CT. TMO is less effective (see, for example, Delgado and Mihailović, 1956, and Table 2A).

    Another model of this type involves the use of the *isolated cortical slab* (Chapter 8) where spiking activity is elicited by electrical stimulation but spontaneous seizures do not occur. The EAD threshold or the duration of after-discharge is used to measure responses to drugs. Phenobarbital blocks the focal spiking or discharge but DPH does not, although DPH does block the spread of activity as indicated by an increase in EAD threshold and a decrease in the duration of after-discharge (see Halpern et al., 1969). Thus, these tests can determine the differential effects of drugs to increase the threshold for local motor seizures or for EAD in different areas of the brain. In the *mirror focus* models (Chapter 4), electrographic changes are recorded and also the ability of the impulse to spread from the primary focus to the secondary or mirror focus. Again, phenobarbital raises the threshold for firing of the focal discharge whereas DPH does not affect the focal discharge; however, DPH does inhibit the projection of the discharge to the mirror focus.

    The *spinal cord models,* particularly those studied by Esplin (see Chapter 9), are also examples of this approach (see Table 2A). These models are discussed elsewhere.

    All these models are useful for localizing the sites of drug action in different areas of the brain and for obtaining finer details of the mechanism of action of anticonvulsant drugs. They serve to separate drugs that raise threshold for focal discharge (e.g., phenobarbital) from those that prevent the propagation or spread of the discharge to involve the whole brain and cause tonic-clonic seizures (e.g., DPH), as well as those that have effects on the cortex and those on subcortical areas. By use of the EAD, the focal electrical stimulation models are excellent for studying factors affecting seizure discharge. This model can also be used for chronic experiments since the focal electrodes can be kept in place for long periods of time. The isolated cortical slab model is useful for drug assay mainly in acute experiments since a fatigue effect occurs in chronic trials of anticonvulsant drugs. However, the model is useful for studying the role of deafferentation and supersensitivity in seizure mechanisms and drug effects.

The *electrical stimulation of tissue slices* (Chapter 11) and *tissue culture models* (Chapter 12) are potentially useful for studies on mechanisms of action of drugs from both a neurophysiological and biochemical standpoint, but a sufficient number of drugs have not been tested in these models to evaluate their usefulness in anticonvulsant testing. However, the McIlwain model has been shown to differentiate DPH and phenobarbital from other drugs. Further work is certainly warranted. The exciting tissue culture models of Crain, however, have properties that suggest they will prove of value for anticonvulsant drug testing, but the preparations have not been sufficiently standardized to make extensive drug evaluation possible at present.

The *microiontophoresis and single-cell models* discussed by Curtis (Chapter 10) also appear to be useful for anticonvulsant drug testing but extensive analysis has not been done. They are of particular value for studying effects of drugs on synaptic transmission and transmitter action, ionic fluxes, mechanisms of initiation of a focus, and mechanism of propagation of seizures.

B. Models for inducing generalized epileptogenic activity

1. Sensory-precipitated generalized seizure models. The *audiogenic seizure* (Chapter 14) and *photogenic seizure* (Chapter 15) models are both useful for testing of anticonvulsant drugs. Although the clinical manifestations of audiogenic seizures—running movements, flexion, extension, and clonus—have been clearly documented, the electrographic evidence for such seizures has not been adequately established. Nevertheless, as seen in Table 2B, drugs such as DPH, phenobarbital, phenacemide, and TMO have been shown to abolish the tonic extensor component of these seizures in the same relative doses as they block tonic extensor seizures induced either by maximal electrical stimulation of the brain or by pentylenetetrazol. The running movements are blocked by drugs such as phenobarbital and

TABLE 2B. *Summary of effects of selected clinically useful drugs on various experimental models that induce generalized epileptogenic activity*

Experimental model	Response measured	Species	Clinically useful drugs						
			DPH	Phenobarbital	Primidone	Phenacemide	TMO	Ethosuximide	Diazepam
Audiogenic	Running movements	mouse	±	+++		++	+		
	Tonus-clonus	rat (rare)	++++	+++		++	+		
Photomyoclonic	EEG, myoclonus	baboon	0 (acute) + (chronic)	++++					++++
Derangements of brain extracellular fluid									
High K⁺	Implanted electrode in hippocampus-EEG spike discharge	cat							
Systemic chemicals									
Pentylenetetrazol	EEG, clonus	mouse rat rabbit	−	+++	++	++	++	+++	++++
	Tonus-clonus	mouse rat, man rabbit monkey	++	+++	++	++	++	+++	+++
Flurothyl (Hexafluorodiethyl ether)	Myoclonus	rat		+++	++				
	Tonus-clonus	rat		+++	++				
Electrically induced									
6 Hz-EST	Clonus	mouse	++	++++	+++	++++	++		
60 Hz-EST	Clonus	mouse	++	++++	++	+++	++		++
Extensor EST	Threshold for extension	mouse rat	+++	++++	++++	++	+		
MES	Tonus-clonus	mouse rat cat	++−−	+++	+++	+++	+		+++
Oxygen at high pressure	Tonus-clonus EEG	mouse rat cat dog, man		Protects					
CO₂ seizures	Clonus, EEG	rat	−	+++			++		
CO₂ withdrawal	Clonus, EEG	rat dog	−	+++			++		
Barbiturate withdrawal	Clonus, EEG	rat dog	0	++++					
Spreading depression	Electrical	man							

TMO that raise the threshold for localized discharge, but not by DPH which limits propagation (spread) of the nerve impulse but has little effect on focal discharge. Thus this model is useful for screening of anticonvulsant drugs.

Photogenic myoclonic seizures in baboons (*Papio papio*) have been validated as a seizure model by the fact that photic stimulation has been demonstrated to cause seizures identified both clinically and electrographically as myoclonus. This model has also been shown to be useful in the testing of anticonvulsant drugs (see Table 2B and Stark et al., 1970). It seems particularly suitable for evaluation of drugs after chronic administration. Drugs effective in elevating the threshold for epileptic discharge seem to be of particular value in this model.

2. *Electrically or chemically induced generalized seizure models* (Table 2B). In the category of electrically or chemically induced seizure models are included the most commonly used of all models for assay of anticonvulsant drugs. These models have been validated both clinically and electrographically. The *electroshock* tests (Chapter 17) have been used most extensively for evaluation of anticonvulsants and are the ones used in the drug industry for screening of drugs for anticonvulsant activity. The electrical threshold tests (e.g., 6 Hz-EST, 60 Hz-EST) are useful for drugs such as phenobarbital and TMO whereas the MES pattern tests are useful for drugs such as DPH and acetazolamide (Diamox ®).

The most commonly used and valuable *chemical convulsant* model is the *pentylenetetrazol* test (Chapter 16) which, as discussed later, appears best suited for evaluation of drugs useful in petit mal epilepsy. Other convulsant agents such as strychnine and picrotoxin are of value only in elucidating the mechanism of action of drugs that block these seizures on transmitter function. This is the case since strychnine appears to act by competing with the inhibitory transmitter (probably glycine) affecting spinal motoneurons, and picrotoxin may compete, as one of its effects at least, with the transmitter involved in presynaptic inhibition. Seizures induced by methionine sulfoximine (which inhibits glutamine synthetase) and by fluoroacetate (which inhibits oxidative metabolism of acetate) are potentially useful screening models but have not been tried adequately against the various clinically useful drugs. They, therefore, should be evaluated by testing with a variety of anticonvulsant drugs. The EEG patterns induced by both these convulsants are similar to those occurring in patients with petit mal seizures.

Myoclonic jerks and tonic-clonic seizures induced by inhalation of *flurothyl* (hexafluorodiethyl ether) (see Table 2B) would appear to provide a good model for testing of anticonvulsants. Primidone and phenobarbital protect against both these types of seizures but other drugs have not been evaluated (Gallagher et al., 1970). Whether the test is selective for sorting out drugs effective in a specific type of epilepsy cannot be determined from the limited number of drugs tested, but it is probably no better than the MES test. However, the test is readily set up and reliable and provides a simple model for testing drugs and factors affecting seizure activity.

Tonic-clonic seizures induced in animals by *oxygen at high pressure* (Chapter 18) have been identified electrographically and have been shown to occur in man. No systematic study of the effects of anticonvulsants on these seizures has been made. One would expect, however, that the tonic-clonic seizures would be blocked by drugs such as DPH and phenobarbital that are useful in grand mal. Nevertheless, these seizures are of value in studying the role of gamma-aminobutyric acid (GABA) in seizure processes and how anticonvulsants effect GABA metabolism.

3. Withdrawal seizure models. Seizures induced by withdrawal from high concentrations of *carbon dioxide* (Chapter 19) have been shown to be clonic in nature, and the EEG pattern demonstrates that seizure activity is present. TMO, phenobarbital, and acetazolamide prevent these seizures whereas DPH exacerbates them. The effects of the succinimides and benzodiazepines should also be tried to assess whether this model is useful for predicting drugs effective in petit mal epilepsy.

Barbiturate withdrawal seizures in animals (Chapter 20) have also been validated as a potentially useful model of epilepsy by both clinical and EEG criteria. Phenobarbital protects against such seizures whereas DPH exerts no such effect. The effects of other anticonvulsants have not been assessed. However, it is a good model of drug-induced withdrawal seizures and as such can be used to determine the mechanism of seizures induced by abrupt withdrawal from sedative-hypnotic drugs.

4. Spreading depression (Chapter 7). Little is known about the usefulness of the phenomenon of spreading depression for assay of anticonvulsant drugs since the ability of these substances to prevent the spread has not been tested. The results of studies on spreading depression would be of great interest not only from the practical point of developing a model for evaluation of drugs but also for their heuristic value of showing more about spreading depression and how drugs effect it.

IV. APPLICATION OF MODELS TO THE DEVELOPMENT OF DRUGS USEFUL AS ANTIEPILEPTICS IN MAN

In Table 3 is presented a summary of the experimental models of epilepsy that have proved of value or potentially are valuable in predicting antiepileptic activity in various types of epilepsy in man. These tests are presented in outline form and separated into tests useful for preliminary screening of drugs for anticonvulsant activity, and into tests useful for predicting drugs effective in grand mal, petit mal and temporal lobe epilepsy. The following discussion elaborates some of the features of these models listed in Table 3.

TABLE 3. *Summary of experimental animal models of epilepsy of demonstrated value or potential usefulness that can predict antiepileptic activity in different types of epilepsy in man*

A. Gross Screening Models in Animals That Are Used to Predict Drugs That Have Antiepileptic Activity in Man
   These tests are used for preliminary screening of any drug for anticonvulsant activity.
   1. *Maximal electroshock seizure test (MES) in mice*
      Measure ability of drugs to abolish tonic extension component of the seizure.
   2. *Pentylenetetrazol (Metrazol®)-induced seizures in mice*
      Measure ability of drugs to block seizures induced by pentylenetetrazol.
B. Experimental Models That Predict Drugs Effective in Generalized Seizures of the *Grand Mal* Type (Tests in Which Diphenylhydantoin, Phenobarbital, and Primidone Are Effective)
   1. *Maximal seizure pattern tests*
      a. Maximal electroshock seizures (MES)
      b. Maximal pentylenetetrazol (Metrazol®) (MMS)
      c. Maximal audiogenic seizures (MAS)
      d. Flurothyl-induced maximal tonic-clonic seizure
   2. *Post-tetanic potentiation in spinal cord of cats*
      Measure ability of drugs to abolish PTP.
   3. *Local lesions of cerebral cortex*
      Measure ability of drugs to prevent propagation of seizure activity to opposite cortex.
      a. Chronic alumina cream lesions
      b. Freezing lesions
   4. *Topical cortical convulsant drugs such as penicillin*
      Measure ability of drugs to prevent clinical manifestations and EEG alterations.
   5. *Focal electrical stimulation with implanted cortical electrodes*
      Measure ability of drugs to elevate the threshold for local motor convulsive activity in cortex and threshold for electrical after-discharge (EAD) in cortex.
C. Experimental Models That Predict Drugs Effective in Generalized Seizures of the *Petit Mal (Absence)* Type (Tests in Which Trimethadione, Succinimides, and Benzodiazepines Are Effective, and in Which Diphenylhydantoin Is Ineffective or Produces an Excitatory Response)
   1. *Pentylentetrazol (Metrazol®)-induced seizures in mice*
   2. *Photomyoclonus in* Papio papio
      Measure ability of drug to prevent EEG and clinical seizure manifestations.
   3. *CO_2-withdrawal seizures in rats*
      Measure ability of drugs to prevent the clinical seizure on withdrawal of animals from high concentrations of CO_2.
   4. *Response to repetitive stimulation in spinal cord of cats*
   5. *Focal lesions of subcortical areas or of cortex*

TABLE 3 (continued)

Measure ability of drugs to prevent typical spike-wave EEG activity and clinical seizure manifestations or to prevent spread of activity from cortex to subcortical areas or vice versa.
  a. Freezing lesions
  b. Alumina cream lesions
  6. *Topical convulsants applied to subcortical areas*
  7. *Focal electrical stimulation with subcortically implanted electrodes*
  8. *Fluoroacetate-induced seizures*
    Of only theoretical value at the present time. May be useful because this convulsant induces clonic-like seizures and an EEG with typical spike-wave seizure activity.
D. Experimental Models That Predict Drugs Effective in Focal Seizures of the *Complex Temporal Lobe Type* (Includes Psychomotor Seizures) (Tests in Which Phenacemide Is Effective)
    There is insufficient work in this area to define a test as being of predictive value in temporal lobe epilepsy.
  1. *6 Hz-EST in mice*
    Measure ability of drugs to raise threshold for 6 cycles/sec stimulation of brain.
  2. *Potentially useful models*
    a. Focal lesions in temporal lobe area or amygdala and hippocampus
      Measure ability of drug to prevent electrographic changes and inhibit behavioral responses.
      (1) Alumina cream lesions in monkeys
    b. Focal electrical stimulation with implanted temporal lobe electrodes
      Measure ability of drugs to raise the threshold for electrical after-discharge. Monkeys are probably the most suitable animals.
    c. Potassium perfusion experiments with electrodes implanted in hippocampus
      Measure ability of drugs to prevent EEG changes and convulsive manifestations resulting from infusion in CSF of high K+ solution.
E. Untried But Promising Models
  1. *Ontogenetic models* (see Chapters 15 and 21)
    Same procedures as in adults but used to evaluate drugs potentially useful in children with epilepsy. The best experimental animals for ontogenetic studies are mice, rats, cats and monkeys.
  2. *Surgically isolated or partially isolated cortical slabs* (see Chapter 5)
    Measure electrical after-discharge and other parameters.
  3. *Short-circuit current and ionic flux measurements in toad urinary bladder*
    Measure effect of drugs on short-circuit current, and Na+, Cl-, and K+ fluxes in toad urinary bladder.
F. Specialized Models
    Mostly untried but may be useful in predicting drugs of value in the therapy of epilepsies caused by metabolic or genetic deficiencies in man. Measure ability of drugs to prevent seizures caused by metabolic or genetic defects.
  1. *Seizures induced by oxygen at high pressure* (see Chapter 16)
    Seizures are probably due to a deficit in GABA metabolism hence should measure ability of drugs to prevent these seizures by increasing GABA levels in body.
  2. *Methionine sulfoximine seizures* (see Chapter 14)
    Measure ability of drugs to effect glutamine synthetase activity and thereby prevent seizures.
  3. *Vitamin B6 deficiency* (see Chapter 14)
    Seizures result from a deficiency of this vitamin. Probably also related to GABA metabolism. Measure ability of drugs to prevent seizures induced by B6 deficiency.

A. Gross screening models in animals that are used to predict drugs that have antiepileptic activity in man

1. Maximal electroshock seizure (MES) pattern test in mice. The MES pattern test is probably the single most useful test for rapid determination of potential anticonvulsant activity of a drug. MES have been induced in psychiatric patients, and antiepileptic drugs useful in grand mal have been shown to abolish the tonic extension phase as they do in mice and other experimental animals (Toman et al., 1947). Electrographic recordings have been made in such cases and the EEG's were found to be like those in patients with grand mal epilepsy. Thus this is one of the few models completely validated in man. (See next section for further discussion of this model and Chapter 17 for discussion of the methods for carrying out the test.)

2. Pentylenetetrazol-induced seizures in mice. This is also a rapid screening method for assessing an anticonvulsant drug potentially useful in epilepsy. The ability of drugs to inhibit seizures induced by pentylenetetrazol is measured in this test. Many variations of the methods of carrying out this test have been reported and are described in Chapter 16 and in earlier articles by Swinyard (1969) and by Ahmad and Dhawan (1969). Pentylenetetrazol seizures have been induced in man and the EEG recorded. Both the seizures and EEG's are similar to those seen in patients with petit mal. Thus, this test has also been validated in man. Drugs useful in petit mal epilepsy are particularly effective in blocking pentylenetetrazol seizures. See below for further discussion of this test.

B. Experimental models that predict drugs effective in generalized seizures of the grand mal type (tests in which diphenylhydantoin, phenobarbital, and primidone are effective)

1. Maximal seizure pattern models. a. The maximal electroshock seizure (MES) pattern test (see Chapter 14) involves measurement of the dose of a drug that abolishes the tonic extensor component of the seizure induced by supramaximal stimulation of the brain in 50% of animals. Mice are the best experimental animals for this method. This model is probably the best validated of all tests for evaluating anticonvulsant drugs. All drugs clinically useful in the therapy of grand mal epilepsy are effective by this test when given either to experimental animals or to man. Thus, it is one of the few models which have been validated in both animals and man from both clinical and EEG data. If the drug is present in the plasma, as far as can be ascertained, all drugs that are effective by the MES technique in animals have anti-grand mal activity in man. Whether a drug effective in this test in animals will become a clinically useful antiepileptic agent in man cannot be predicted from the results, only that it will have anticonvulsant activity in man. Other factors, such as toxicity and the absorption, distribution, biotransformation, and excretion of the drug in man, determine its ultimate value. The test determines the ability of the drug to prevent propagation (spread) of the epileptic discharge as described earlier.

    b. Other maximal seizure pattern models. The maximal pentylene-tetrazol (Metrazol®) seizure (MMS) (Chapter 16), the maximal audiogenic seizure (MAS) (Chapter 14), and the maximal fluorothyl seizure tests measure the same phenomena as does the MES test. Anti-grand mal drugs abolish the tonic extensor component of these seizures and it is likely that drugs which abolish this component will be effective in grand mal, but this has not been validated as yet.

    2. Post-tetanic potentiation (PTP) in the spinal cord (Chapter 9). The clinically useful drugs that inhibit PTP in the spinal cord (DPH and, to a much smaller extent, phenobarbital) have anti-grand mal activity in man. However, the effects of these drugs on PTP in the spinal cord of man have not been assessed. Also, it has not been ascertained as yet if all drugs that block PTP will have antiepileptic activity in man. This is potentially a useful model for selecting out drugs, particularly, of the DPH type that act to prevent propagation of the epileptic discharge by preventing PTP, an effect that the DPH studies suggest may be one important mechanism by which anticonvulsant drugs act.

    Certainly this test is important for elucidating the finer mechanisms of anticonvulsant drug action.

    3. Local lesions of the cerebral cortex. a. Alumina cream lesions of the cerebral cortex in monkeys (Chapter 1). The types of seizures resulting from this procedure are usually clonic but occasionally tonic-clonic. However, the tonic-clonic seizure is not reproducible in chronic animals. DPH is slightly protective, and then only on chronic administration, in preventing the clonic seizures in such animals; phenobarbital and probably primidone are very effective. Electrographic data indicate the similarity of this type of seizure to that in man. The test is most useful for chronic testing of drugs of the phenobarbital type in all animal species phylogenetically close to man. If possible, this test should be the final stage in evaluation of a potentially useful antiepileptic agent before using it in man. How useful the test is for evaluation of new agents with characteristics like those of DPH cannot be predicted from the available evidence. This model is also excellent for prediction of drugs useful in therapy of epilepsy characterized only by clonic activity or myoclonus.

b. Freezing lesions of the cerebral cortex (Chapter 2). If the drugs are tested for ability to prevent propagation of the epileptic discharge induced by the freezing lesion, drugs of the DPH type can be readily discovered. If tested for ability to reduce the frequency of the focal discharge, then drugs of the phenobarbital type can be found. Thus, this procedure can be used for assaying acutely anti-grand mal drugs of both types. An example of the use of this model for testing anticonvulsants is found in the paper of Morrell et al. (1959); the results of such tests are shown in Table 2A. Also, Musgrave and Purpura (1963) demonstrated that DPH did not prevent focal spiking induced by a freezing lesion on the cat cortex, but did reduce discharge frequency and spread from secondary foci.

4. Topical convulsant drugs such as penicillin (Chapter 3). This model is similar to that of the freezing lesion model just described, and can be used to assay anti-grand mal drugs of the DPH and phenobarbital types. For example, Louis et al. (1968) have used this model in cats for testing the effects of DPH to modify the seizures and electrographic alterations induced by topical application of penicillin.

5. Focal electrical stimulation with implanted cortical electrodes (Chapter 6). This model has been discussed in Section III in relation to its usefulness for evaluation of anticonvulsant drugs in general. Its specific use for predicting drugs useful in grand mal stems from the fact that drugs such as DPH and phenobarbital (see Table 2A) are effective in raising the electrical threshold for local motor convulsions and for EAD induced in the various areas of the brain by stimulation through electrodes implanted in these areas (see, for example, Delgado and Mihailović, 1956). TMO was much less effective. Other drugs have not yet been evaluated, but this is a very promising technique for evaluating anti-grand mal drugs.

C. Experimental models that predict drugs effective in generalized seizures of the petit mal (absence) type (tests in which trimethadione, succinimides, and benzodiazepines are effective, and in which DPH is ineffective or produces an excitatory response)

No well-established model of petit mal epilepsy is available but some potentially excellent models have been developed and require only extensive drug testing to validate them. The following represent the most promising of these models.

1. Pentylenetetrazol-induced seizures in mice. This test has already been discussed. It has been validated in man, and all drugs that are effective anti-petit mal agents in man protect against pentylenetetrazol seizures in animals. Also, probably all drugs effective against seizures induced by this drug have anti-petit mal activity in man, but all are not clinically useful for this type seizure because of the limitations imposed by their toxicity, or by absorption, distribution, biotransformation, and excretion factors that prevent their access to the receptors. This is probably the best available model of petit mal since this type of epilepsy is generalized and not focal. Pentylenetetrazol appears to simulate the disease more than the focal models discussed below.

2. *Photomyoclonus in baboons (Papio papio)*. Phenobarbital, TMO, and diazepam prevent the seizures in these animals induced by photic stimulation in doses not producing CNS toxicity on either acute or chronic administration. However, this model has not been evaluated in sufficient detail to ascertain how specific it is for other anti-petit mal drugs. This is particularly true since DPH to a slight extent, but generally in toxic doses, protects against these light-induced seizures, especially on chronic administration. It does, however, appear to be a very promising model since the seizure is generalized as is the case with pentylenetetrazol.

3. CO_2-*withdrawal seizures in rats* (Chapter 19). This is a relatively good model for predicting drugs effective in petit mal-type seizures (see Table 2B for summary of drug effects). TMO, phenobarbital, and acetazolamide protect against such seizures and DPH enhances them, as it does petit mal epilepsy in man. The succinimides and benzodiazepines have not yet been evaluated in this test, and this should be done before the model is demonstrated to be a useful test for petit mal drugs. CO_2-withdrawal seizures have, however, been reported in man and thus it is validated as a model of epilepsy (Gibbs et al., 1938).

4. *Response to repetitive stimulation in spinal cord of cats* (Chapter 9). TMO is markedly effective in decreasing spinal cord transmission during repetitive stimulation (see Tables 1 and 2A). Phenobarbital has a slight effect and DPH is only marginally active. Other anti-petit mal drugs have not been assessed in this test; hence this procedure remains as a potentially useful model until further work is accomplished.

5. *Focal lesions of subcortical areas or of cortex* (Chapters 1 and 2). These are only potentially useful models until all clinically valuable anti-petit mal drugs are tested. Petit mal-type drugs, however, do appear to be effective in preventing the electrographic and clinical seizure manifestations of these models or to prevent the spread of activity from the cortical to subcortical areas or vice versa.

6. *Topical convulsants applied to subcortical areas* (Chapter 3). Again, insufficient drug data are available to evaluate these models. Anti-petit mal drugs probably prevent seizures induced by focal implantation of convulsants (e.g., penicillin) in subcortical areas.

7. Focal electrical stimulation with subcortically implanted electrodes (Chapter 6). As with the models described in Chapters 11 and 12, insufficient data are available for evaluation of this model as a predictor of anti-petit mal drugs. However, when electrodes are in the thalamic area, TMO does raise the CT and EAD thresholds. It is thus a potentially useful model.

All of the focal methods are probably not adequate models of petit mal since, as noted previously, petit mal is a generalized seizure and not a focal one. The systemic convulsants are, therefore, probably better models.

8. Fluoroacetate-induced seizures. These are included since seizures induced by this drug, which inhibits metabolism of acetate, are clonic in nature and the electrographic recordings show typical spike-wave seizure activity in rats, dogs, and cats. Fluoroacetate-induced seizures in man have been reported from accidental poisoning. The convulsive manifestations are prevented by treatment with barbiturates, CO_2, and TMO. These data suggest that this is a potentially useful model for assessing drugs of value in petit mal epilepsy and that further work should be done to validate this possibility. (See Toman and Davis, 1949, for summary of this drug.)

D. Experimental models that predict drugs effective in focal seizures of the complex temporal lobe types (includes psychomotor seizures) (tests in which phenacemide is effective)

Experimental models that simulate temporal lobe epilepsy are available, but none of them has been used to evaluate their ability to predict drugs useful in the therapy of this type of seizure, although phenacemide has been used in some of them.

1. 6 Hz-EST in mice. Of the available models, the only one that has been used extensively is the *6 Hz-EST* test in which the ability of drugs to raise the threshold for 6 cycles/sec electrical stimulation of the brain is measured. However, this test is not selective for phenacemide, since phenobarbital, DPH, primidone, and TMO all elevate the threshold for these low-frequency-induced seizures. Phenacemide is relatively more effective in this test than in others. It is obvious that better models are urgently needed.

2. Potentially useful tests. Of the potentially useful models for evaluation of drugs useful in temporal lobe epilepsy, the ones involving production of *focal lesions* in the temporal lobe area or in the amygdala and hippocampus or *implanted electrodes* in these same areas are most promising. Such procedures produce behavioral modifications, seizure activity, and electrographic charges, particularly in monkeys, similar to those present in temporal lobe epilepsy. Since anticonvulsant drugs have not been tested in such models, however, evaluation of their use as predictors of drugs for temporal lobe epilepsy cannot be made at the present time.

Another model that appears of great promise is the one described in Chapter 13 by Glaser involving activation of the hippocampus, as measured by implanted electrodes, by perfusion of high-potassium solutions in the CSF in either control cats or cats with chronic alumina cream or cobalt lesions in the hippocampus (see Zuckermann and Glaser, 1970). Activation by potassium causes both clinical and electrographic seizures like those seen in temporal lobe epilepsy. Drug evaluations have not been done, so its value in predicting drugs useful in this type of epilepsy cannot yet be assessed.

E. Untried but promising models

1. Ontogenetic models (see Chapters 17 and 22). These are summarized in Table 3.

2. Surgically isolated or partially isolated cortical slabs (see Chapter 8). This model is discussed in a previous section and is presented here since it represents a model with potential that is as yet untested and the type of seizure for which it would be useful undefined. However, Krip and Vazquez (1971) suggest that this preparation is a potentially excellent model for evaluation of drugs effective in grand mal. This was based on the fact that in chronically isolated slabs of cerebral cortex in cats DPH decreased the duration of EADs whereas trimethadione and ethosuximide had no effect (see Table 2A).

3. Short-circuit current and ionic flux measurements in toad urinary bladder and in frog skin. An example of this approach is the use of the epithelial cells of toad bladder or frog skin to test the effects of convulsant and anticonvulsant drugs on electrolyte transport processes. Gross and Woodbury (*unpublished observations*), for example, have shown that pentylenetetrazol and various other tetrazole derivatives increase short-circuit current across toad bladder by increasing selectively the permeability of the cell membrane on the serosal side of the cell to the K ion. The ratios of the effect of the various tetrazole derivatives on K^+ permeability was the same as their ratios of effect for producing seizures in mice. TMO blocked the increase in permeability to K^+ induced by pentylenetetrazol in the toad bladder in the same ratio of doses as it blocks the seizures in mice induced by this convulsant. It might be possible, therefore, to discover new anticonvulsants that act in a manner similar to that of TMO by evaluating their ability to inhibit the increase in K^+ permeability induced by pentylenetetrazol in toad bladder. Similarly, DPH also increases short-circuit current across frog skin and toad bladder epithelial cells, but in this case the increase is a result of enhanced movement of Na ions across the cells (Watson and Woodbury, 1972). Thus, DPH acts by a different mechanism than TMO on ion transport across epithelial cells. Drugs similar in action to that of DPH might, therefore, be discovered by testing their effects on Na^+ movement across these epithelial membranes. These are just examples where detailed studies of the mechanism of action of antiepileptic drugs might lead to new methods of evaluating antiepileptics and result in the development of new drugs.

F. Specialized models

These are summarized in Table 3.

V. ACKNOWLEDGMENTS

This investigation was supported by a U.S. Public Health Service Program-Project Grant (5–PO1–NS–04553) from the National Institute of Neurological Diseases and Stroke. The author is a recipient of a Research Career Program Award (5–K6–NS–13,838) from the National Institute of Neurological Diseases and Stroke.

VI. REFERENCES

Ahmad, A., and Dhawan, B. N. (1969): Metrazol® test for rapid screening of anticonvulsants. *Japanese Journal of Pharmacology,* 19:472–474.

Ajmone Marsan, C. (1969): Acute effects of topical epileptogenic agents. In: *Basic Mechanisms of the Epilepsies,* edited by H. H. Jasper, A. A. Ward, Jr., and A. Pope. Little, Brown & Co., Boston, pp. 299–319.

Brodie, B. B., and Reid, W. E. (1969): Is man a unique animal in response to drugs? *American Journal of Pharmacy,* 141:21–27.

Delgado, J. M. R., and Mihailović, L. (1956): Use of intracerebral electrodes to evaluate drugs that act on the central nervous system. *Annals of the New York Academy of Sciences,* 64:644–666.

Elazar, Z., and Blum, B. (1971): Effect of drugs on interictal spikes and after-discharges in experimental epilepsy. *Archives Internationales de Pharmacodynamie et de Therapie,* 189:310–318.

Esplin, D. W. (1957): Effects of diphenylhydantoin on synaptic transmission in cat spinal cord and stellate ganglion. *Journal of Pharmacology and Experimental Therapeutics,* 120:301–323.

Esplin, D. W., and Curto, E. M. (1957): Effects of trimethadione on synaptic transmission in the spinal cord; antagonism between trimethadione and pentylenetetrazol. *Journal of Pharmacology and Experimental Therapeutics,* 121:457–467.

Gallagher, B. B., Smith, D. B., and Mattson, R. H. (1970): The relationship of the anticonvulsant properties of primidone to phenobarbital. *Epilepsia*, 11:293–301.

Gibbs, F. A., Gibbs, E. L., and Lennox, W. G. (1938): Cerebral dysrhythmias of epilepsy. Measures for their control. *Archives of Neurology and Psychiatry*, 39:298–314.

Halpern, L. M., Ward, A. A., Jr., Black, R. G., and Lockhard, J. W. (1969): The hyperexcitable neuron as a model for the laboratory analysis of anticonvulsant drugs. *Epilepsia*, 10:281–314.

Krip, G., and Vazquez, A. J. (1971): Effects of diphenylhydantoin and cholinergic agents on the neuronally isolated cerebral cortex. *Electroencephalography and Clinical Neurophysiology*, 30:391–398.

Louis, S., Kutt, H., and McDowell, F. (1968): Intravenous diphenylhydantoin in experimental seizures II. Effect on penicillin-induced seizures in the cat. *Archives of Neurology*, 18:472–477.

Melchior, J. C., Buchthal, F., and Lennox-Buchthal, M. (1971): The ineffectiveness of diphenylhydantoin in preventing febrile convulsions in the age of greatest risk, under three years. *Epilepsia*, 12:55–62.

Morrell, F., Bradley, W., and Ptashne, M. (1959): Effect of drugs on discharge characteristics of chronic epileptogenic lesions. *Neurology*, 9:492–498.

Musgrave, F. S., and Purpura, D. P. (1963): Effects of Dilantin® on focal epileptogenic activity of cat neocortex. *Electroencephalography and Clinical Neurophysiology*, 15:923.

Petty, W. C., and Karler, R. (1965): The influence of aging on the activity of anticonvulsant drugs. *Journal of Pharmacology and Experimental Therapeutics*, 150:443–448.

Stark, L. G., Killam, K. F., and Killam, E. K. (1970): The anticonvulsant effects of phenobarbital, diphenylhydantoin and two benzodiazepines in the baboon, *Papio papio*. *Journal of Pharmacology and Experimental Therapeutics*, 173:125–132.

Swinyard, E. A. (1969): Laboratory evaluation of antiepileptic drugs. Review of laboratory methods. *Epilepsia*, 10:107–119.

Toman, J. E. P. (1970): Drugs effective in convulsive disorders. In: *The Pharmacological Basis of Therapeutics*, 4th Ed., edited by L. S. Goodman and A. Gilman. Macmillan, New York, pp. 204–225.

Toman, J. E. P., and Davis, J. P. (1949): The effects of drugs upon the electrical activity of the brain. *Journal of Pharmacology and Experimental Therapeutics, Part 2*, 97:425–492.

Toman, J. E. P., and Goodman, L. S. (1948): Anticonvulsants. *Physiological Reviews*, 28:409–432.

Toman, J. E. P., Loewe, S., and Goodman, L. S. (1947): Physiology and therapy of convulsive disorders 1. Effect of anticonvulsant drugs on electroshock seizures in man. *Archives of Neurology and Psychiatry* (Chicago), 58:312–324.

Vernadakis, A., and Woodbury, D. M. (1969a): The developing animal as a model. *Epilepsia*, 10.163–178.

Vernadakis, A., and Woodbury, D. M. (1969b): Discussion. Maturational factors in development of seizures. In: *Basic Mechanisms of the Epilepsies*, edited by H. H. Jasper, A. A. Ward, Jr., and A. Pope. Little, Brown and Co., Boston, pp. 535–541.

Ward, A. A., Jr. (1969): The epileptic neuron: chronic foci in animals and man. In: *Basic Mechanisms of the Epilepsies*, edited by H. H. Jasper, A. A. Ward, Jr., and A. Pope. Little, Brown and Co., Boston, pp. 263–288.

Watson, E. L., and Woodbury, D. M. (1972): Effects of diphenylhydantoin on active sodium transport in frog skin. *Journal of Pharmacology and Experimental Therapeutics*, 180:767–776.

Woodbury, D. M. (1969): Mechanisms of action of anticonvulsants. In: *Basic Mechanisms of the Epilepsies*, edited by H. H. Jasper, A. A. Ward, Jr., and A. Pope. Little, Brown and Co., Boston, pp. 647–681.

Woodbury, D. M., and Esplin, D. W. (1959): Neuropharmacology and neurochemistry of anticonvulsant drugs. *Proceedings of the Association for Research in Nervous and Mental Disease*, 37:24–56.

Zuckermann, E. C., and Glaser, G. H. (1970): Activation of experimental epileptogenic foci. Action of increased K^+ in extracellular spaces of brain. *Archives of Neurology*, 23:358–364.

24

Application of Experimental Models to Human Epilepsy

Herbert H. Jasper

OUTLINE

I. INTRODUCTION

By definition, human epilepsy, or the epilepsies, are recurrent self-sustained paroxysmal disorders of brain function characterized by excessive discharge of cerebral neurons. There may be excessive inhibition as well as excessive excitation, the one predominating over the other in different types of seizures as well as at different times in the course of a single seizure.

There is a wide variety of clinical and electrical manifestations of seizures in man (Jasper and Kershman, 1941; Penfield and Jasper, 1954; Lennox, 1960; Gastaut, 1970). This is due (1) to the functional characteristics of the neuronal circuits primarily involved and their pattern of spread in the brain, and (2) to the nature of the epileptic disorder itself, e.g., whether it be predominantly excitatory or inhibitory, whether of short or long duration, whether of low or high intensity in individual neurons, and the degree of synchronization and quantity of neurons involved. There may be, however, common factors involved in the basic mechanisms of all seizures, in spite of the bewildering variety of their clinical and electrical manifestations and the many mechanisms for their induction or precipitation.

Neuropathological causes appear to be as varied as are the clinical manifestations in human epileptiform seizures. It is for this reason that epilepsy is often called a symptom of many diseases rather than a single disease entity. In at least one-half of the cases of human epilepsy, the true cause remains unknown, and in many others the cause or causes are only presumed. Hereditary predisposition seems clearly established in some cases, but it is probably not more important than in many other diseases (cardiovascular diseases, for example) and less clearly established than for some other diseases of the nervous system, such as Friedreich's ataxia or Huntington's chorea (Lennox et al., 1940; Lennox, 1960; Metrakos and Metrakos, 1969; Gastaut et al., 1969a). Precipitating causes (trauma or disease) often play a critical role even in cases with a strong hereditary predisposition.

It should be pointed out also that there are many human "models" of epileptiform seizures which are not considered to be true epilepsy as strictly defined (Gastaut et al., 1969b). Many seizures occur on the medical or surgical wards of a general hospital during the course of other diseases or incidental to their treatment. Hypoglycemia is known to cause seizures in some patients (Poiré, 1969). An overdose of insulin, for example, may result in a seizure. Seizures may be the presenting sign in pancreatic adenoma. Seizures may accompany toxemia of pregnancy or renal insufficiency (Prill et al., 1969). Antibiotic therapy with penicillin or other convulsant antibiotics may cause seizures, especially with intrathecal administration, but occasionally when large doses are administered systemically in susceptible patients. Alcohol excess is also known to precipitate seizures ("rum fits") in susceptible individuals. Seizures such as these are not called epilepsy because they are not "spontaneously" recurrent and they cease when the known cause is removed.

Seizures accompany many genetic diseases of the nervous system (see the review by Radermecker and Dumon, 1969) and may be "spontaneously" recurrent, but in these cases they are considered only symptomatic.

These human "models" serve to emphasize the point that seizures may arise from a wide variety of alterations in structure or metabolism of brain cells, or from an alteration in their external environment. Similarly, the human epilepsies may be symptoms of a variety of diseases of the brain rather than a disease in itself, providing that the "causes" can be discovered.

II. CRITERIA OF VALIDITY

How are we to judge the validity of a given experimental model for the study of human epilepsy? In the first place, it is necessary to make sure that both the electrical and the behavioral manifestations of the model are truly similar to those known to characterize human epilepsy. This presents little difficulty with major convulsive seizures associated with high-voltage repetitive discharge in the EEG. There are, however, other forms of seizure, some without convulsive movements, which are associated with disturbances in the EEG that may be called epileptiform.

To illustrate the possible dissociation which may occur between epileptiform discharge in the EEG and convulsive movements, I would like to describe some experiments recently conducted in our laboratories by Dr. Annie Courtois (1972). Focal cortical discharging lesions were produced in the precruciate gyrus of the cat by cobalt powder. Clonic convulsive movements of the contralateral forepaw, occasionally spreading to face and leg, were observed for a period of 2 to 3 days. Chronic implanted electrodes were used to record cortical electrical discharges, eye movements, and the electrical activity of neck muscles in order to have an index of muscle tone during different stages of sleep. In some experiments, electrodes were also implanted in the pyramidal tract in order to monitor impulse volleys associated with epileptiform spikes in motor cortex. During waking there was a good correlation between clonic movements of the contralateral extremities and epileptiform spikes recorded from motor cortex. During slow-wave sleep, there was a reduction in clonic movements associated with cortical discharge. During fast-wave or paradoxical sleep, convulsive movements were completely absent, in spite of an increase in cortical epileptiform discharge and a persistence of the conduction of this discharge in the pyramidal tract. Convulsive movements were apparently "uncoupled" from cortical control at the spinal level by the generalized inhibition of paradoxical or rapid-eye-movement (REM) sleep even though cortical epileptiform discharges were enhanced. Under such conditions, cortical electrical activity becomes the most reliable index of a seizure.

Recording with implanted electrodes deep in cerebral structures in human epileptic patients has revealed much electrical seizure activity not accompanied by convulsive movements and often not even apparent in the EEG from scalp surface electrodes. Sporadic spikes from focal cortical areas are characteristically without convulsive or other signs of clinical seizure during the so-called interictal periods in epileptic patients. One must depend, therefore, more upon electrical manifestations than upon clinical or behavioral manifestations of epilepsy in judging the validity of a given model of epilepsy. Electrical seizures are not, however, equivalent to behavioral seizures, especially from the clinical point of view. Mechanisms responsible for generating limited focal epileptic discharge may be different from those responsible for its spread into a full-blown clinical seizure even though both the focal disturbance and the generalized manifestation may be valid models of seizure mechanisms. In addition, we need reliable models of generalized seizure states which occur apparently independently of a focal onset, or in which the apparent focus is secondary to the more generalized affection of the brain as a whole.[1]

III. MODELS OF FOCAL EPILEPSY

Among the many models for producing a local epileptiform disturbance in experimental animals, there is only one which fulfills the criterion of prolonged "spontaneous" recurrence, and that is the topical or intracerebral application of alumina gel (see Ward, Chapter 1). Other topical metals, such as cobalt, reproduce a more active local discharging lesion for periods of several days, but they fail to produce a long-lasting chronic epileptogenic lesion. In spite of certain experimental inconveniences (delayed onset, useful mainly in primates), the alumina gel technique is nevertheless the method of choice for the reproduction of a chronic local epileptogenic lesion resembling very closely that seen in man.

---

[1] It may be of interest to note that Clementi (1929*a,b*) concluded from his pioneer studies of "reflex epilepsy" by means of topical application of strychnine to visual and auditory cortex in the dog, followed by seizure precipitation with visual or auditory stimuli, that susceptibility of some animals and not others must be due to some form of genetic predisposition.

The alumina gel technique has the disadvantage of being most useful in primates; also, it is particularly effective for the motor cortex. Spontaneous seizures are rather unpredictable also, although they can be precipitated by emotional stimuli and subconvulsant doses of pentylenetetrazol. Elaborate methods of observation with automatic videotape recording as developed by Lockard and Barensten (1967) may be necessary to make maximum use of the chronic alumina cream preparation for the study of "spontaneous" focal seizures. Patterns of focal seizures of origin in areas of cortex other than the motor region, or in subcortical structures, are not readily reproduced with the chronic alumina gel preparation even in primates since spontaneous seizures are too rare unless precipitated by subconvulsant doses of pentylenetetrazol or by other means, thus complicating the pattern of attack.

Application of more acutely acting epileptogenic agents which do not diffuse rapidly from the site are more useful for studies of the variations in pattern of behavioral attack arising from different brain areas, cortical and subcortical, if one is not interested in a chronic preparation. Local freezing, cobalt, or penicillin are probably the agents of choice for inducing seizures of focal origin in different vertebrate species and from almost any part of the cerebral gray matter, although not with equal facility.

Local electrical stimulation with implanted electrodes in either cortical or subcortical sites (see Ajmone Marsan, Chapter 6), combined with electrical recording from the area stimulated as well as from other areas to study spread or generalization of the seizure, is the most precise method for the study of relations between anatomical and behavioral patterns of seizure manifestation. This technique provides the additional advantage of being able to measure after-discharge thresholds and control of the onset and course of the epileptiform discharge in relation to behavior; it has the disadvantage of requiring a large number of implanted electrodes for adequate mapping of conduction or spread of the seizure, thereby making it possible to miss important structures which may be involved but not detected because of inadequate electrode placement. Experience with local electrical stimulation and recording in human epilepsy during craniotomy or with implanted electrodes has shown that typical clinical seizures can be reproduced in this manner comparable to those seen in experimental animals.

It should be pointed out that convulsive movements may not be observed regularly during locally induced seizures by any of the methods described above, including electrical stimulation, unless the discharge spreads to involve cortical or subcortical motor systems of the brain. The effect of the local seizure may, therefore, be hard to detect unless special methods of observation are employed, such as interruption of ongoing behavior, induction of irrelevant or irrational behavior, or interference with perception, attention, memory, or learning processes. Such seizures are common in human epilepsy, for example, in the varieties of so-called "psychomotor" attack, and in the variants of "petit mal" or "absence" attacks. Studies of the effects upon behavior of epileptic disturbances in brain areas concerned with more complex sensory, perceptual, motivational, and intellectual functions have been carried out to a limited extent in experimental animals. They deserve more attention in our attempt to understand the wide spectrum of behavioral disturbances in man which are associated with epilepsy, not all of which, however, may be considered of strictly focal onset.

IV. MODELS OF GENERALIZED SEIZURES

It is possible to induce apparently generalized seizures in experimental animals by means of focal epileptogenic lesions placed deeply in certain parts of the brain. Petit mal-like seizures have been induced in monkeys, for example, by local injection of penicillin in the mesial-orbital frontal cortex (Walker and Morello, 1967) or by injection of alumina gel in the rostral mesencephalic tegmental area (Hubel and Nauta, 1960). Petit mal-like seizures in kittens, but not in adult cats, have been produced by alumina gel injections in mesial thalamus and brainstem (Guerrero-Figueroa et al., 1963). These models may have some value for human epilepsy by showing possible complex varieties of focal seizures with generalized behavioral manifestation. However, most patients with true petit mal seizures, often combined with generalized major convulsive attacks, have not been shown to have local lesions in the brainstem or in mesio-orbital frontal cortex.

Experimental models for major or minor seizures which appear to be generalized from the onset are best obtained by procedures which modify cellular and synaptic excitability of the brain as a whole, either directly or indirectly. The best example in some respects is naturally occurring seizure-susceptible animals, such as the baboon (*Papio papio*) (see Naquet and Meldrum, Chapter 15). Sensitivity to intermittent photic stimulation for precipitation of seizures makes this a particularly valuable model for a similar variety of human epilepsy. Electrophysiological studies have shown that initial epileptiform activation with photic stimulation in *Papio papio* occurs in frontal cortex, before generalization to the major convulsive seizure, showing a degree of preferential seizure susceptibility even though behavioral manifestations appear generalized. Also, many brain structures do not seem to be involved and even the hippocampus does not participate in these seizures as it does in many forms of human epilepsy.

The production of generalized seizure states by systemic administration of convulsant drugs, such as pentylenetetrazol, is still a useful model for certain forms of human epilepsy as proved by its value in the screening of anticonvulsant drugs effective in man. Of greater interest, however, are models which produce known changes in metabolism of nerve cells and synapses or in neurotransmitter functions.

It is beyond the scope of this chapter to review the many important metabolic models of generalized seizure states of potential importance for the understanding of human epilepsy (Tower, 1969; Schneider, 1969; De Robertis et al., 1969). Methionine sulfoximine seizures (Wolfe and Elliott, 1962) have been studied extensively and shown to be associated with important changes in cortical amino acid metabolism, without changes in metabolism of acetylcholine. Likewise, thiosemicarbazide and allylglycine convulsions are related to important changes in amino acid metabolism, particularly by producing an imbalance of glutamic acid and gamma-aminobutyric acid (GABA) largely due to inhibition of glutamic acid decarboxylase (GAD), although other changes may also be of importance.

More recently, the action of the powerful convulsant drug bicuculline has been found to be most probably due to specific blockage of GABA synapses as described by Curtis in Chapter 10. It has been suggested by Wood in Chapter 18 that GAD is most sensitive to the toxic action of increased tissue O_2 tension and that decreased tissue GABA may be the cause of hyperbaric seizures, but many other enzymes may also be involved. All of these methods produce generalized seizure states by metabolic alterations involving amino acids of importance in normal metabolism and synaptic transmission in the brain, which are therefore of particular importance to human epilepsy. Many other examples could be cited, not all related to amino acid metabolism, but the principle of using metabolic models most closely related to possible disturbances which may eventually be found in human epilepsy is important.

V. ELECTROPHYSIOLOGICAL MODELS

Reproduction of valid electrophysiological manifestations of epileptiform discharge is of equal if not greater importance than behavioral manifestations. Without electrophysiological evidence, one cannot always be sure that behavioral "fits" are truly of an epileptic character, especially in more complex forms of attack (such as, for example, the "running" stage of audiogenic seizures in mice; see Chapter 14). The EEG, especially when complemented by records from deep-lying brain structures with implanted electrodes, has provided necessary evidence for the evaluation of any experimental model. The availability of comparable EEG records from all forms of human epilepsy provides an immediate and objective link between experimental models and the various forms of human epilepsy.

The use of microelectrodes, both extracellular and intracellular, in experimental seizure models of various types has provided direct evidence for unit cellular and synaptic dysfunction which characterizes both interictal and ictal seizures, as summarized in this volume and in *Basic Mechanisms of the Epilepsies* (Jasper et al., 1969). The use of microelectrode techniques has been relatively limited in man, and confined largely to studies of interictal discharges from local cortical epileptogenic lesions (Ward, 1969). As pointed out by Prince in Chapter 3, the topographical applications of convulsant drugs or metals do not all produce the same effect upon unit discharge even though surface field potentials seen in the EEG may be similar. Also, even when similar effects are observed upon unit discharge patterns, the mechanism of action may be quite different depending upon the convulsant agent used. The paroxysmal depolarization shift (PDS) with bursts of high-frequency discharge is the most striking feature of some "epileptic neurons." The high-frequency bursts have been found in human epileptogenic lesions by Ward and co-workers (1969), but periods of prolonged inhibition (Spencer and Kandel, 1969) (paroxysmal hyperpolarization) are also characteristic of some cells, even in areas which lack cells showing PDS or bursts of rapid discharge (Goldensohn and Purpura, 1963; Purpura et al., 1963; Matsumoto and Ajmone Marsan, 1964 a,b; Matsumoto, 1964; Ajmone Marsan, 1965; Goldensohn et al., 1965; Prince and Wilder, 1967; Sypert and Ward, 1967).

Important changes in pre- and postsynaptic function with changes in the excitable properties of dendrites at a distance from cell bodies may not be apparent from microelectrode studies. Also, the electrical activity of interneurons is not usually seen in microelectrode records, and yet may be most important in sustained epileptic discharge. The problem of mass synchronization of unit discharge in large populations of neurons may be recorded but not explained by studying the properties of individual neurons alone. The mass DC field potential recorded across large neuronal aggregates during epileptic paroxysm deserves further study in animals and man (Gumnit and Takahashi, 1965; Caspers and Speckmann, 1969; Mahnke and Ward, 1970; Ferguson and Jasper, 1971).

The lack of unit discharge found in acutely isolated cortex, as described by Halpern in Chapter 8, even during surface paroxysmal EEG disturbance (also reported by Ferguson and Jasper, 1971), raises many problems regarding the limitations of microelectrodes for the complete characterization of all forms of epileptic discharge. More microelectrode studies need to be carried out in different forms of human epilepsy before we can judge the applicability of experimental microelectrode models to human epilepsy in general.

The combination of microelectrode recording with microiontophoresis, as described by Curtis in Chapter 10, has provided a wealth of precise information concerning the excitatory and inhibitory action of naturally occurring transmitter substances, as well as many other pharmacological agents of potential importance to an understanding of human epilepsy. This is a highly sophisticated technique, however, and results must often be interpreted with caution. The demonstration that the convulsant action of strychnine, picrotoxin, and bicuculline may be due to their specific blockade of inhibitory controls on neuronal discharge mediated normally by glycine or GABA emphasizes the importance of further studies of amino acid metabolism in epileptic patients.

Microiontophoretic studies of cerebral cortical neurons in epileptic patients during craniotomy should soon be possible. Such studies have been carried out largely by producing small local changes in the extracellular environment of *normal* nerve cell bodies. Little is known of the nature of altered responsiveness that might be found in abnormal (epileptic) neurons. It may be, however, that most "epileptic" neurons are essentially normal, but become epileptic only when subjected to an abnormal extracellular environment, or to excessive synaptic bombardment in large neuronal aggregates. These are some of the questions which microelectrode techniques may help to answer when they are applied both to a variety of experimental models and to a variety of epileptic disorders in man.

VI. BIOCHEMICAL MODELS

Biochemical models capable of being tested in human epilepsy seem most likely to lead to an understanding of the underlying causes of certain forms of seizures in man, and to their eventual rational treatment. Of particular interest in this context are the *in vitro* models of excised tissue described by McIlwain (Chapter 11) and the tissue culture model described by Crain (Chapter 12) in this volume. When combined with electrical stimulation and recording techniques, these models make possible complete control of extracellular environment, ionic and metabolic, as well as precise studies of substances liberated at synaptic junctions. When directed toward studies of derangements of metabolism leading to epileptic discharge, these models should provide much information of potential value to the understanding of human epilepsy.

Of considerable interest also is the technique described by Glaser in Chapter 13 for the study of epileptic activation due to changes in extracellular concentration of potassium induced by perfusion of the lateral ventricle. When combined with studies of potassium liberation during seizures, some insight into possible mechanisms involved in the spread of seizures to involve larger and larger populations of neurons which would otherwise be considered "normal." In this context, the studies of spreading depression as described by Leão in Chapter 7 may also be relevant since in extracellular space both increase potassium (Fertziger and Ranck, 1970) and glutamate (Van Harreveld and Fifková, 1970) accompany the spreading wave of excitation which precedes the period of depression.

The variety and specificity of different mechanisms which may cause paroxysmal epileptiform discharge in cerebral cortex may be illustrated by the example of cholinergic seizures. Topical application of acetylcholine to cerebral cortex after pretreatment with neostigmine leads to local, sustained spontaneous paroxysmal discharge. Neostigmine alone will induce local seizures in intact, alert aroused animals, apparently due to natural liberation of acetylcholine in the presence of an anticholinesterase (Celesia and Jasper, 1966; Ferguson and Jasper, 1971). Such seizures are readily arrested by the local or systemic administration of atropine or scopolamine. However, sustained rhythmic paroxysmal discharge, resembling superficially the acetylcholine-induced paroxysm, can still be brought on by electrical stimulation in the same area of cortex with little change in threshold as compared to untreated cortex. The cholinergic seizure discharge was blocked by specific blocking agents without affecting appreciably the sensitivity of the same cortical tissue to electrically induced after-discharge.

Considering the variety of conditions leading to seizures in man, it is unlikely that any single biochemical defect will be found responsible for all forms of epilepsy, and some defects may be morphological rather than biochemical as such. Consequently, a variety of biochemical approaches need to be tried in experimental models and then tested on a variety of forms of epilepsy. For example, pyridoxine deficiency will produce a convulsive disorder presumably due in part to critical disturbances in amino acid metabolism so that the normal balance of excitatory and inhibitory amino acids is altered, permitting excessive excitation and spontaneous discharge. This is known to occur in certain pyridoxine-dependent children; such cases are rare, however, and there is no evidence that such a defect exists in the majority of patients with generalized seizures, and certainly not in focal epileptogenic lesions. However, there is evidence that significant disturbances in amino acid metabolism do occur in focal epileptogenic lesions both in experimental models and in naturally occurring lesions in man, as illustrated by the following experiments.

By way of example of parallel studies of animal models and human epileptogenic brain tissue, I would like to cite some work that has recently been carried out in our laboratories by Drs. N. M. van Gelder and Ikuko Koyama in collaboration with Drs. Theodore Rasmussen and Allan Sherwin of the Montreal Neurological Institute. Dr. van Gelder was able to obtain freshly excised cortical tissue from focal epileptogenic lesions in man during craniotomy. These were carefully selected by Dr. Rasmussen on the basis of electrocortigraphic evidence for the most actively discharging focus with comparison with a distant area which seemed to be much less involved. Controls were also obtained from normal primate cortical tissue. It was found by Dr. van Gelder (van Gelder et al., 1972) that there were significant alterations in the tissue content of certain amino acids. There was a particularly marked drop in glutamic acid and in GABA with a consistent increase in glycine confined to the area of the active focus. In parallel studies by Dr. Koyama (1972) on cobalt focal epileptogenic lesions in the cat, there was found also a significant decrease in both glutamic acid and GABA in the actively discharging focus. Curiously enough, she also found an increase in glycine, as had been found for the human tissue. In the animal model, however, Dr. Koyama was able to study the development of the lesion from the beginning and to show that the first changes were a decrease in tissue glutamic acid before changes in GABA occurred. The decrease in GABA was a later development and occurred at a time when the focal discharge was becoming more active and spreading to other cortical areas with clinical seizures. Furthermore, Dr. Koyama was able to show that the decrease in tissue glutamic acid was associated with an increase in liberation of free glutamic acid as obtained from perfusion of the cortical surface prior to excision of the tissue for analysis. Other changes were of interest and will be found in the original reports.

The important point I wish to make here is that it is possible to demonstrate parallel changes in both human and animal material with certain models of focal epilepsy. It is also important that both show similar metabolic changes with apparent increased liberation of glutamic acid early in the development of a focal discharging lesion which might be related to the development of a pool of hyperactive neurons. The later decrease in GABA (presumably due to lack of the precursor, glutamic acid) might well be related to diminished inhibitory controls which may contribute to the spread of epileptic discharge.

This serves to illustrate the value of parallel studies in man and in experimental animals for obtaining a more direct evaluation of a model with respect to human epilepsy. Similar parallel studies should be extended to other aspects of brain metabolism, as well as more detailed microphysiological studies. There are many forms of biochemical and histochemical methods now available for studies on both man and experimental animals which have yet to be applied to the problem of epilepsy.

The heterogeneity of procedures and mechanisms used to induce seizure discharge in experimental animals reviewed in this volume could probably be matched by the heterogeneity of predisposing and precipitating causes for seizures in the human epilepsies. One might assume that naturally occurring seizures in experimental animals would provide the best model for human epilepsy, such as, for example, the Sengalese baboon with seizures induced by intermittent photic stimulation. However, these animals rarely have spontaneous attacks without photic stimulation. They are, therefore, a model only for a relatively rare form of human epilepsy; about 2 to 4% of epileptic patients studied at the Mayo Clinic, as reported by Bickford and Klass (1969), exhibited this type of seizure. In the majority of patients, seizures occur "spontaneously," independent of known or deliberate sensory precipitation. There are, no doubt, precipitating factors to account for the periodicity of attacks, but these seem more frequently related to critical changes in the internal environment of the organism which cause a "susceptibility" to reach the seizure threshold. This is likely a multivariant problem as described by Bickford and Klass in their chapter in *Basic Mechanisms of the Epilepsies* (Jasper et al., 1969).

VII. ONTOGENETIC MODELS

The importance of brain maturation on the development of seizures has long been well established by clinical observations. Ontogenetic studies such as described by Purpura in Chapter 22 are obviously, therefore, of great importance to our understanding of human epilepsy.

Furthermore, detailed studies of the functional properties of brain cells and their mechanisms of control and synaptic function at different stages of maturation of the brain provide much insight into the relation between stages of maturation and certain forms and patterns of epileptic discharge in human patients. By coupling these investigations with detailed studies of morphological maturation of dendritic and synaptic structures as well as of maturation of enzyme systems in the brain, it should be possible to find important correlations between structure and function in relation to tendencies for epileptic discharge. These questions are elaborated on in Chapter 22 and need no further comment here.

In addition to studying the importance of normal stages of maturation for the development of different forms of human epilepsy, it is perhaps more important to carry out studies of developmental pathology in relation to the development of epileptic seizures. Many cases of human epilepsy have presumed or proven causes dating from birth or early infancy, or are considered "congenital" (Penfield and Keith, 1940; Penfield, 1954). With increasing knowledge, the importance of critical stages of brain growth and development for the determination of permanent defects in later life, experimental developmental pathology in relation to seizures would seem to be an important model for more extensive study in the future.

VIII. MORPHOLOGICAL MODELS

There have been many pathological studies of epileptogenic lesions of various types with or without glial proliferation and with or without important changes in neuronal structure. These pathological studies from human material have always been open to some question because it has not always been certain that they are critical to the development of a discharging lesion, as compared to a silent lesion of similar pathology (Jasper, 1970).

In the classical epileptic scar or local cerebral atrophy following a vascular accident or some other cause of local gliosis, a marked proliferation of glial tissue is found with a diminution in nerve cells and an impairment in local cerebral circulation (Foerster and Penfield, 1930; Penfield, 1954; Pope, 1969). Comparison between local epileptogenic lesions produced by alumina gel and those found in human focal scars has been made by Westrum and co-workers (1964). They were particularly impressed not only by the glial proliferation but also by marked abnormalities in dendritic structure as seen in Golgi preparations. Dendritic trees appeared deformed and denuded of spines as compared to normal tissue both in the alumina gel lesions and in examples of human focal cortical epileptogenic lesions. Such changes, when coupled with changes in ultrastructure as seen in the electron microscope, may well be of significance in the structural neuropathology of an epileptogenic process. The changes in the dendritic tree might well reflect a denervation type of sensitization, as Ward believes, especially if abnormal renervation also occurs. Changes in glial structure surrounding neurons has also been suggested as a possible structural defect in epileptogenic lesions producing an impaired glial buffer system for extracellular fluid spaces (Glaser, Chapter 13; Pollen and Trachtenberg, 1970). These suggestive findings and their interpretation need to be confirmed and extended in many other types of epileptogenic process. More comparative morphological changes with a variety of techniques including histochemical studies need to be made both in human epilepsy and in experimental models before the importance of some of these changes can be properly assessed (see Pope, 1969).

IX. CONCLUSION

Is it possible to follow a common path through this maze of multiple mechanisms and manifestations of seizures in human epilepsy as well as in experimental models? Common to all the epilepsies, it seems, is defective control of neuronal discharge. This may be at the level of single neurons or in synaptic networks controlling mass synchronization of neuronal aggregates. The defect may lie in the metabolism and membrane structure of single nerve cells, or perhaps a class of nerve cells, or it may lie in defective synaptic function controlling the interrelationship between cells. Both of these defects may be due to abnormalities in extracellular environment rather than to primary defects in the cells and synapses themselves. Furthermore, excessive discharge may be caused by an excessive excitatory process which overwhelms the capacity of normal control systems, or it may be due to deficiencies in control systems permitting excessive response to normal excitatory drive.

The various experimental models described in this volume make possible controlled studies of the relative importance of a variety of mechanisms which may play a role in the cause of seizures in human epilepsy. In the last analysis, verification in different forms of human epilepsy, and in human seizure models, should lead to a better understanding and to more rational therapy of the different varieties of human epilepsy, as well as to a better understanding of normal brain function.

X. REFERENCES

Ajmone Marsan, C. (1965): Micro-structural mechanisms of seizure susceptibility. *Excerpta Medica International Congress Series No. 124*, 47–59.

Bickford, R. G., and Klass, D. W. (1969): Sensory precipitation and reflex mechanisms. In: *Basic Mechanisms of the Epilepsies,* edited by H. H. Jasper, A. A. Ward, Jr., and A. Pope. Little, Brown and Co., Boston, pp. 543–564.

Caspers, H., and Speckmann, E.-J. (1969): DC potential shifts in paroxysmal states. In: *Basic Mechanisms of the Epilepsies,* edited by H. H. Jasper, A. A. Ward, Jr., and A. Pope. Little, Brown and Co., Boston, pp. 375–388.

Celesia, G. G., and Jasper, H. H. (1966): Acetylcholine released from cerebral cortex in relation to state of activation. *Neurology,* 16:1053–1064.

Clementi, A. (1929a): Stricninizzazione della sfera corticale visiva ed epilessia sperimentale da stimoli luminosi. *Archivio de Fisiologia,* 27:356–387.

Clementi, A. (1929b): Stricninizzazione della sfera corticale uditiva ed epilessia sperimentale da stimoli acustici. *Archivio de Fisiologia,* 27:388–414.

Courtois, A. (1972): Motor phenomenology of cobalt experimental epileptic focus in the motor cortex of the cat during various stages of vigilance. *Electroencephalography and Clinical Neurophysiology,* 32:259–267.

De Robertis, E., Rodriguez de Lores Arnaiz, G., and Alberici, M. (1969): Ultrastructural neurochemistry. In: *Basic Mechanisms of the Epilepsies,* edited by H. H. Jasper, A. A. Ward, Jr., and A. Pope. Little, Brown and Co., Boston, pp. 137–158.

Ferguson, J. H., and Jasper, H. H. (1971): Laminar DC studies of acetylcholine-activated epileptiform discharge in cerebral cortex. *Electroencephalography and Clinical Neurophysiology,* 30:377–390.

Fertziger, A. P., and Ranck, J. B., Jr. (1970): Potassium accumulation in interstitial space during epileptiform seizures. *Experimental Neurology,* 26:571–585.

Foerster, O., and Penfield, W. (1930): The structural basis of traumatic epilepsy and results of radical operation. *Brain,* 53:99–120.

Gastaut, H. (1969): Introduction to the study of organic generalized epilepsies. In: *The Physiopathogenesis of the Epilepsies,* edited by H. Gastaut, H. Jasper, J. Bancaud, and A. Waltregny. Charles C Thomas, Springfield, Ill., pp. 147–157.

Gastaut, H. (1970): Clinical and electroencephalographical classification of epileptic seizures. *Epilepsia,* 11:102–113.

Gastaut, H., Jasper, H., Bancaud, J., and Waltregny, A. (editors) (1969a): *The Physiopathogenesis of the Epilepsies.* Charles C Thomas, Springfield, Ill.

Gastaut, H., Rohmer, F., Cossette, A., and Kurtz, D. (1969b): Introduction to the study of functional generalized epilepsies. In: *The Physiopathogenesis of the Epilepsies,* edited by H. Gastaut, H. Jasper, J. Bancaud, and A. Waltregny. Charles C Thomas, Springfield, Ill., pp. 5–25.

Goldensohn, E. S. (1969): Experimental seizure mechanisms. In: *Basic Mechanisms of the Epilepsies,* edited by H. H. Jasper, A. A. Ward, Jr., and A. Pope. Little, Brown and Co., Boston, pp. 289–298.

Goldensohn, E. S., Perez, M., and Feierman, J. (1965): Intracellular potentials and unit discharge patterns in primary and mirror epileptogenic foci. *Electroencephalography and Clinical Neurophysiology,* 18:513.

Goldensohn, E. S., and Purpura, D. P. (1963): Intracellular potentials of cortical neurons during focal epileptogenic discharges. *Science,* 139:840.

Guerrero-Figueroa, R., Barros, A., Debalbian Verster, F., and Heath, R. G. (1963): Experimental "petit mal" in kittens. *Archives of Neurology,* 9:297–306.

Gumnit, R. J., and Takahashi, T. (1965): Changes in direct current activity during experimental focal seizures. *Electroencephalography and Clinical Neurophysiology,* 19:63–74.

Hubel, D., and Nauta, W. J. H. (1960): Electrocorticograms of cats with chronic lesions of rostral mesencephalic tegmentum. *Federation Proceedings,* 19:287.

Jasper, H. H. (1970): Physiopathological mechanisms of post-traumatic epilepsy. *Epilepsia,* 11:73–80.

Jasper, H. H., and Kershman, J. (1941): Electroencephalographic classification of the epilepsies. *Archives of Neurology and Psychiatry,* 45:903–943.

Jasper, H. H., Ward, A. A., Jr., and Pope, A. (editors) (1969): *Basic Mechanisms of the Epilepsies,* Little, Brown and Co., Boston.

Koyama, I. (1972): Amino acids in the cobalt induced epileptogenic and non epileptogenic cat's cortex. *Canadian Journal of Physiology and Pharmacology (in press).*

Lennox, W. G. (1960): *Epilepsy and Related Disorders,* 2 vols. Little, Brown and Co., Boston.

Lennox, W. G., Gibbs, E. L., and Gibbs, F. A. (1940): Inheritance of cerebral dysrhythmia and epilepsy. *Archives of Neurology and Psychiatry,* 44:1155-1183.

Lockard, J. S., and Barensten, R. I. (1967): Behavioral experimental epilepsy in monkeys. I. Clinical seizure recording apparatus and initial data. *Electroencephalography and Clinical Neurophysiology,* 22:482.

Mahnke, J. H., and Ward, A. A., Jr. (1970): Photic-induced seizures with DC baseline shifts. *Experimental Neurology,* 28:1-10.

Matsumoto, H. (1964): Intracellular events during the activation of cortical epileptiform discharges. *Electroencephalography and Clinical Neurophysiology,* 17:294.

Matsumoto, H., and Ajmone Marsan, C. (1964a): Cortical cellular phenomena in experimental epilepsy: "Inter-ictal" manifestation. *Experimental Neurology,* 9:286.

Matsumoto, H., and Ajmone Marsan, C. (1964b): Cortical cellular phenomena in experimental epilepsy: Ictal manifestations. *Experimental Neurology,* 9:305-326.

Metrakos, J. D., and Metrakos, K. (1969): Genetic studies in clinical epilepsy. In: *Basic Mechanisms of the Epilepsies,* edited by H. H. Jasper, A. A. Ward, Jr., and A. Pope. Little, Brown and Co., Boston, pp. 700-708.

Penfield, W. (1954): Epileptogenic lesions. In: *Epilepsy and the Functional Anatomy of the Human Brain,* edited by W. Penfield and H. Jasper. Little, Brown and Co., Boston, pp. 281-349.

Penfield, W., and Humphreys, S. (1940): Epileptogenic lesions of the brain. *Archives of Neurology and Psychiatry,* 43:240-261.

Penfield, W., and Jasper, H. (editors) (1954): *Epilepsy and the Functional Anatomy of the Human Brain.* Little, Brown and Co., Boston.

Penfield, W., and Keith, H. (1940): Focal epileptogenic lesions of birth and infancy. *Archives of Neurology and Psychiatry,* 59:718-738.

Poiré, R. (1969): Hypoglycemic epilepsy: Clinical, electrographic and biological study during induced hypoglycemia in man. In: *The Physiopathogenesis of the Epilepsies,* edited by H. Gastaut, H. Jasper, J. Bancaud, and A. Waltregny. Charles C Thomas, Springfield, Ill., pp. 75-110.

Pollen, D. A., and Trachtenberg, M. C. (1970): Neuroglia: Gliosis and focal epilepsy. *Science,* 167:1252-1253.

Pope, A., (1969): Perspectives in neuropathology. In: *Basic Mechanisms of the Epilepsies,* edited by H. H. Jasper, A. A. Ward, Jr., and A. Pope. Little, Brown and Co., Boston, pp. 773-781.

Prill, A., Quellhorst, E., and Scheler, F., (1969): Epilepsy: Clinical and electroencephalographical findings in patients with renal insufficiency. In: *The Physiopathogenesis of the Epilepsies,* edited by H. Gastaut, H. Jasper, J. Bancaud, and A. Waltregny. Charles C Thomas, Springfield, Ill., pp. 60-68.

Prince, D. A., and Wilder, B. J. (1967): Control mechanisms in cortical epileptogenic foci. "Surround" inhibition. *Archives of Neurology,* 16:194-202.

Purpura, D. P., Goldensohn, E. S., and Musgrave, F. S. (1963): Synaptic and non-synaptic processes in focal epileptogenic activity. *Electroencephalography and Clinical Neurophysiology,* 15:1050.

Radermecker, J., and Dumon, J. (1969): Genetic epilepsies. In: *The Physiopathogenesis of the Epilepsies,* edited by H. Gastaut, H. Jasper, J. Bancaud, and A. Waltregny. Charles C Thomas, Springfield, Ill., pp. 31-35.

Schneider, J. (1969): Neurophysiological and metabolic mechanisms of so-called functional epilepsies—General aspects. In: *The Physiopathogenesis of the Epilepsies,* edited by H.

Gastaut, H. Jasper, J. Bancaud, and A. Waltregny. Charles C Thomas, Springfield, Ill., pp. 36–49.

Spencer, W. A., and Kandel, E. R. (1969): Synaptic inhibition in seizures. In: *Basic Mechanisms of the Epilepsies*, edited by H. H. Jasper, A. A. Ward, Jr., and A. Pope. Little, Brown and Co., Boston, pp. 575–603.

Sypert, G. W., and Ward, A. A., Jr. (1967): The hyperexcitable neuron: Microelectrode studies of the chronic epileptic focus in the intact awake monkey. *Experimental Neurology,* 19:104.

Tower, D. B. (1969): Neurochemical mechanisms. In: *Basic Mechanisms of the Epilepsies,* edited by H. H. Jasper, A. A. Ward, Jr., and A. Pope. Little, Brown and Co., Boston, pp. 611–638.

van Gelder, N. M., Sherwin, A. L., and Rasmussen, T. (1972): Amino acid content of epileptogenic human brain: Focal versus surrounding regions. *Brain Research,* 40:385–393.

Van Harreveld, A., and Fifkova, E. (1970): Glutamate release from the retina during spreading depression. *Journal of Neurobiology,* 2:13–29.

Walker, A. E., and Morello, G. (1967): Experimental petit-mal. *Transactions of the American Neurological Association,* 92:57–61.

Ward, A. A., Jr. (1969): The epileptic neuron: Chronic foci in animals and man. In: *Basic Mechanisms of the Epilepsies,* edited by H. H. Jasper, A. A. Ward, Jr., and A. Pope. Little, Brown and Co., Boston, pp. 263–288.

Westrum, L. E., White, L. E., and Ward, A. A., Jr. (1964): Morphology of the experimental epileptic focus. *Journal of Neurosurgery,* 21:1033.

Wolfe, L. S., and Elliott, K. A. C. (1962): Chemical studies in relation to convulsive conditions. In: *Neurochemistry* (2nd ed.), edited by K. A. C. Elliott, I. H. Page, and J. H. Quastel. Charles C Thomas, Springfield, Ill., 694–727.

Guide to Experimental Materials and Methods

The following index is intended to serve as a "where to find it" guide to the preceding chapters. Only major subjects are included in the hope that the investigator's task of isolating particular aspects of experimental methods or materials will be lightened.

Anesthetics and modes of anesthetization

secondary focus studies, 91
petit mal models, 119, 128
nonbarbiturate anesthesia, 130
spreading depression, 178
preparation of isolated cortical slabs, 202
spinal cord preparations, 230
general problems of anesthesia, 412
studies of CO_2 derangement seizures, 482

Animal preparations

acute experiments, 63, 91, 178, 204, 423, 435
chronic preparations, 19, 100, 504
choice of animals, 18, 40, 100, 119, 163, 201, 229, 348, 435, 443, 483, 513, 535
animals for audiogenic seizures, 367, 368
baboons for photogenic seizure studies, 377
animal maintenance during experiments, 64, 121, 423
surgical procedures, 63, 119, 128, 202, 230, 394, 412, 423
pulsation control, intracellular studies, 65, 553
brain tissue isolation procedures, 138–140, 192, 208, 394, 554

Data analysis

Drug administration

Electrical stimulation

Electrodes and electrode fabrication

Index

Date Due